W9-CFA-743

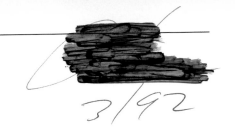

3/92

Instructional Course Lectures

Volume XLI 1992

Edited by
Robert E. Eilert, MD
Chairman, Department of Orthopaedic Surgery
The Childrens Hospital
Denver, Colorado

With 393 illustrations

American Academy
of Orthopaedic Surgeons

American Academy of Orthopaedic Surgeons

Instructional Course Lectures
Volume XLI

Director of Communications and Publications: Mark W. Wieting
Assistant Director, Publications: Marilyn L. Fox, PhD
Senior Editor: Bruce Davis
Production Manager: Loraine Edwalds
Production Editor: Monica M. Trocker
Associate Senior Editor: Joan Abern
Publications Secretary: Geraldine Dubberke
Publications Secretary: Em Lee Lambos

BOARD OF DIRECTORS 1991

President
Augusto Sarmiento, MD
Los Angeles, California

First Vice-President
Robert N. Hensinger, MD
Ann Arbor, Michigan

Second Vice-President
Bernard A. Rineberg, MD
New Brunswick, New Jersey

Secretary
Robert E. Eilert, MD
Denver, Colorado

Treasurer
Howard P. Hogshead, MD
Jacksonville, Florida

Past Presidents
Thomas B. Dameron, Jr., MD
Raleigh, North Carolina

Newton C. McCollough III, MD
Tampa, Florida

John B. McGinty, MD
Charleston, South Carolina

Members-at-Large
James W. Strickland, MD
Indianapolis, Indiana

William E. Garrett, Jr., MD, PhD
Durham, North Carolina

Lawrence B. Bone, MD
Buffalo, New York

Chairman
Board of Councilors
William W. Tipton, Jr., MD
Sacramento, California

Chairman-Elect
Board of Councilors
D. Eugene Thompson, MD
Birmingham, Michigan

Secretary
Board of Councilors
James G. Buchholz, MD
Ft. Wayne, Indiana

Chairman
Council of Musculoskeletal Specialty Societies
David F. Apple, Jr., MD
Atlanta, Georgia

Chairman-Elect
Council of Musculoskeletal Specialty Societies
Eugene R. Mindell, MD
Buffalo, New York

Executive Director
(Ex-Officio)
Thomas C. Nelson

Design: James Buddenbaum Design, Wilmette, Illinois
Typesetting: Impressions, Inc., Madison, Wisconsin
Printing: Port City Press, Inc., Baltimore, Maryland
Binding: Short Run Bindery, Medford, New Jersey
Stock: Acid-free Sterling Litho Gloss

The material presented in this volume has been made available by the American Academy of Orthopaedic Surgeons for educational purposes only. This material is not intended to represent the only, or necessarily best, methods or procedures for the medical situations discussed, but rather is intended to present an approach, view, statement, or opinion of the author(s) or producer(s), which may be helpful to others who face similar situations. Furthermore, any statements about commercial products are solely the opinion(s) of the author(s) and do not represent an Academy endorsement or evaluation of these products. These statements may not be used in advertising or for any commercial purpose.

Copyright © 1992 American Academy of Orthopaedic Surgeons

All rights reserved. No part of this publication may be reproduced, stored in a retrieval system, or transmitted, in any form or by any means, electronic, mechanical, photocopying, recording, or otherwise, without prior written permission from the publisher.

Previous volume copyrighted 1991 by the American Academy of Orthopaedic Surgeons, 222 South Prospect Avenue, Park Ridge, Illinois 60068

International Standard Book Number 0–89203–057–7

Library of Congress Catalog Card Number 91–059035

Preface

Of the making of many books there is no end.

King Solomon

The 41st volume of the *Instructional Course Lectures* is a book that represents a collection of highly regarded current opinions on a wide variety of orthopaedic topics. As such, many believe that these lectures represent the "cutting edge" of current clinical knowledge. The lecturers are chosen for their expertise, and they hold a position of respect in the orthopaedic community for their ability to educate.

Working with these authors has been a pleasure from the initial recruitment through the process of presentation orally and now in written form. The volunteer authors have been enthusiastic and energetic, devoting many hours of thoughtful deliberation to produce the fine papers in this volume.

The responsiveness of these authors and their timely production of a written exposition has made the prompt publication of these lectures possible.

The published volume is the documentation of a highly coordinated effort by many people to produce a top quality educational offering. A sampling from the 120 courses presented was used to generate the book, which includes new topics not previously presented and updates of topics not recently covered.

The papers in volume 41 were drawn from the Instructional Courses presented in Anaheim at the Annual Meeting in March 1991. The instructional course committee reviewed the applications submitted, solicited new courses, and worked hard in coordinating the course offerings as well as maintaining a consistent philosophic approach based on presenting a multifaceted view of established clinical and basic science knowledge important to the membership of the Academy. I especially appreciate their efforts and support during my tenure as chairman of the committee and as editor of this volume.

Any orthopaedist scanning the table of contents will find something which relates to his or her practice or areas of interest.

Staff support for this volume has come from Bruce Davis, senior medical editor, Monica M. Trocker, project coordinator, and Loraine Edwalds, production manager. Mark W. Wieting and Marilyn L. Fox, PhD, provided oversight and help with special problems.

Robert E. Eilert, MD
Denver, Colorado
Chairman
Committee on Instructional Courses

Walter B. Greene, MD
Chapel Hill, North Carolina

James D. Heckman, MD
San Antonio, Texas

Michael F. Schafer, MD
Chicago, Illinois

Hugh S. Tullos, MD
Houston, Texas

Contributors

Peter F. Armstrong, MD, FRCSC, FACS, Chief of Staff, Shriners Hospitals for Crippled Children, Intermountain Unit, Salt Lake City, Utah

Donald L. Bartel, PhD, Senior Scientist, Department of Biomechanics, The Hospital for Special Surgery, New York, New York

James H. Beaty, MD, Associate Professor, Orthopaedic Surgery, The Campbell Clinic, Memphis, Tennessee

Trevor N. Best, FRACS, FRCS, Orthopaedic Surgeon in Private Practice, Newcastle, Australia

John G. Birch, MD, FRCSC, Staff Orthopedist, Texas Scottish Rite Hospital, Dallas, Texas

Mark D. Brown, MD, PhD, Professor and Chairman, Department of Orthopaedics and Rehabilitation, University of Miami School of Medicine, Miami, Florida

Robert J. Brumback, MD, Associate Professor of Orthopaedic Surgery, The Shock Trauma Unit of the University of Maryland, Baltimore, Maryland

Matthew J. Bueche, MD, Clinical Instructor, Department of Orthopaedics, Loyola University Medical Center, Maywood, Illinois

Maurizio A. Catagni, MD, Associate Professor, Orthopaedic Surgeon, Lecco General Hospital, Lecco, Italy

William P. Cooney III, MD, Consultant in Orthopedic Surgery, Chief, Section of Hand Surgery, Mayo Clinic, Rochester, Minnesota

Howard B. Cotler, MD, Medical Director, Texas Back Institute–Houston, Houston, Texas

Jay S. Cox, MD, Professor of Surgery, Division of Orthopaedic Surgery, College of Medicine, Milton S. Hershey Medical Center, The Pennsylvania State University, Hershey, Pennsylvania

Charles B. Darling, BA, President, Better Business Solutions, Inc., Clearwater, Florida

Ronald L. DeWald, MD, Professor of Orthopedic Surgery, Director, Section of Spinal Surgery, Rush Medical College, Chicago, Illinois

James H. Dobyns, MD, Professor Emeritus, Department of Orthopedic Surgery, Mayo Clinic, Rochester, Minnesota

Bradley C. Edgerton, MD, Orthopaedic Surgeon, Durango Orthopedic Associates, Durango, Colorado

James A. Farmer, Jr., EdD, Associate Professor of Continuing Education, College of Education, University of Illinois at Urbana-Champaign, Champaign, Illinois

Frank J. Frassica, MD, Special Project Associate, Department of Orthopedics, Mayo Clinic and Mayo Foundation, Rochester, Minnesota

Richard J. Friedman, MD, FRCSC, Associate Professor of Orthopaedic Surgery, Medical University of South Carolina, Charleston, South Carolina

John W. Frymoyer, MD, Interim Dean, Professor of Orthopaedics, Director, McClure Musculoskeletal Research Center, University of Vermont College of Medicine, Burlington, Vermont

John P. Fulkerson, MD, Professor of Orthopaedic Surgery, University of Connecticut, School of Medicine, Farmington, Connecticut

Jorge O. Galante, MD, DMSc, Professor and Chairman, Department of Orthopedic Surgery, Rush Medical College, Chicago, Illinois

Steven R. Garfin, MD, Professor, Department of Orthopedics, University of California–San Diego Medical Center, San Diego, California

Steven Gitelis, MD, Associate Professor of Orthopedic Surgery, Director, Section of Orthopedic Oncology, Rush Medical College, Chicago, Illinois

John Golding, FRCS(Eng), Professor Emeritus, Department of Orthopaedic Surgery, University of the West Indies, Kingston, Jamaica

Robert H. Haralson, MD, Associate Clinical Professor, University of Tennessee Center for the Health Sciences, Knoxville, Tennessee

John H. Harris, Jr., MD, Professor and John S. Dunn Chair in Radiology, University of Texas Medical School, Houston, Texas

Douglas T. Harryman II, MD, Assistant Professor–Orthopaedics, Shoulder and Elbow Surgery, University of Washington, Seattle, Washington

Edward D. Henderson, MD, Emeritus Professor of Orthopedics, Mayo Medical School, Rochester, Minnesota

Harry N. Herkowitz, MD, Chairman, Department of Orthopaedic Surgery, Director, Section of Spine Surgery, William Beaumont Hospital, Royal Oak, Michigan

John A. Herring, MD, Chief of Staff, Texas Scottish Rite Hospital for Children, Dallas, Texas

Richard J. Herzog, MD, Medical Director, San Francisco Neuro Skeletal Imaging, Daly City, California

Ronald L. Huckstep, MD, FRCS, Professor and Head, Department of Traumatic and Orthopaedic Surgery, The University of New South Wales, Kensington, Sydney, Australia

Joshua J. Jacobs, MD, Assistant Professor of Orthopaedic Surgery, Rush Medical College, Chicago, Illinois

Roland P. Jakob, MD, Assistant Chief, Orthopaedic Department, Inselspitaled, University of Berne, Berne, Switzerland

Charles E. Johnston II, MD, Staff Orthopedist, Texas Scottish Rite Hospital, Dallas, Texas

Jesse B. Jupiter, MD, Associate Professor of Orthopaedic Surgery, Harvard Medical School, Boston, Massachusetts

Neil Kahanovitz, MD, Director, National Spine Center at the Anderson Clinic, Arlington, Virginia

Alexander Kalenak, MD, Professor, Department of Orthopaedic Surgery, The College of Medicine, Milton S. Hershey Medical Center, Hershey, Pennsylvania

James R. Kasser, MD, Associate Chief Orthopaedic Surgery, Children's Hospital, Boston, Massachusetts

Kurt J. Kitziger, MD, Clinical Assistant Professor of Orthopaedics, Tulane University, New Orleans, Louisiana

Martin H. Krag, MD, Associate Professor, Department of Orthopaedics and Rehabilitation, University of Vermont, Burlington, Vermont

Larry A. Kramer, MD, Director, Clinical Magnetic Resonance Imaging, The University of Texas Health Science Center at Houston, Medical School–Department of Radiology, Houston, Texas

Ronald L. Linscheid, MD, Professor of Orthopedic Surgery, Mayo Medical School, Consultant in Orthopedic Surgery and Surgery of the Hand, Mayo Clinic, Rochester, Minnesota

Frederick G. Lippert III, MD, Associate Professor of Orthopaedics, University of Washington, Seattle, Washington

Stephen J. Lipson, MD, Clinical Associate Professor of Orthopaedic Surgery, Harvard Medical School, Brigham and Women's Hospital, Boston, Massachusetts

Paul A. Lotke, MD, Professor of Orthopaedic Surgery and, Chief of the Implant Service, Hospital of the University of Pennsylvania, Philadelphia, Pennsylvania

Thomas A. Martinelli, MD, LCDR, Staff Orthopedic Surgeon, United States Naval Hospital, Naples, Italy

Michael B. Millis, MD, Associate in Orthopaedic Surgery, The Children's Hospital, Boston, Massachusetts

Srdjan Mirkovic, MD, Assistant Professor of Orthopaedic Surgery, Reconstructive Spine Surgery, Department of Orthopaedic Surgery, Northwestern University Medical School, Chicago, Illinois

Bernard F. Morrey, MD, Professor and Chairman, Department of Orthopedic Surgery, Mayo Clinic, Rochester, Minnesota

Colin F. Moseley, MD, Chief of Staff, Shriners Hospital for Crippled Children, Los Angeles, California

Stephen B. Murphy, MD, Chief, Joint Replacement Division, Department of Orthopaedic Surgery, Beth Israel Hospital, Boston, Massachusetts

James W. Ogilvie, MD, Associate Professor of Orthopaedic Surgery, University of Minnesota, Minneapolis, Minnesota

Leonard F. Peltier, MD, PhD, Professor Emeritus, Department of Surgery, University of Arizona College of Medicine, Tucson, Arizona

Daniel S. Pflaster, MS, Department of Orthopedics and Rehabilitation, University of Vermont, Burlington, Vermont

Malcolm H. Pope, DMSc, PhD, Department of Orthopaedics and Rehabilitation, University of Vermont, Burlington, Vermont

Robert Poss, MD, Professor of Orthopaedic Surgery, Harvard Medical School, Brigham and Womens Hospital, Boston, Massachusetts

Mercer Rang, MB, FRCSC, Professor of Orthopaedics, University of Toronto, Toronto, Canada

Michael G. Rock, MD, Consultant, Department of Orthopedics, Mayo Clinic and Mayo Foundation, Rochester, Minnesota

Thomas D. Rosenberg, MD, The Orthopedic Specialty Hospital, Salt Lake City, Utah

Raymond Roy-Camille, MD, Professeur de Chirurgie Orthopedique et Traumatologique, Chirurgien de l'Hopital Pitie-Salpetriere, Paris, France

Leonard K. Ruby, MD, Professor, Orthopedic Surgery, Tufts University School of Medicine, Boston, Massachusetts

Bjorn Rydevik, MD, PhD, Associate Professor, Department of Orthopaedics, University of Gothenburg, Sahlgren Hospital, Gothenburg, Sweden

Robert B. Salter, OC, MD, FRCSC, Professor of Orthopaedic Surgery, University of Toronto, Toronto, Canada

Michael F. Schafer, MD, Ryerson Professor and Chairman, Northwestern University Medical School, Chicago, Illinois

Franklin H. Sim, MD, Consultant, Department of Orthopedics, Mayo Clinic and Mayo Foundation, Rochester, Minnesota

Harry B. Skinner, MD, PhD, Professor of Orthopedic Surgery, University of California, San Francisco, California

Dale R. Sumner, PhD, Assistant Professor, Department of Orthopedic Surgery, Rush-Presbyterian-St. Luke's Medical Center, Chicago, Illinois

Hugh G. Watts, MD, Shriners Hospital for Crippled Children, Los Angeles, California

James N. Weinstein, DO, Professor, Department of Orthopaedic Surgery, Director, Spine Diagnostic and Treatment Center, University of Iowa Hospitals and Clinics, Iowa City, Iowa

Sam W. Wiesel, MD, Professor and Chairman, Department of Orthopaedic Surgery, Georgetown University, Washington, DC

Bryan Williamson, MD, Orthopaedic Resident, The University of Texas, Southwestern Medical Center, Dallas, Texas

Joel W. Yeakley, MD, Associate Professor, Chief of Neuroradiology, Department of Radiology, The University of Texas Health Science Center, Houston, Texas

Contents

Upper Extremity

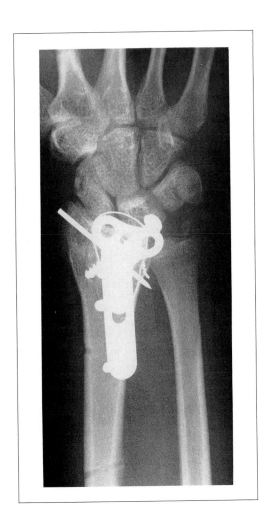

Common Surgical Approaches to the Shoulder

Douglas T. Harryman II, MD

Introduction

The purpose of this chapter is to describe the common surgical approaches used routinely by the Shoulder Team at the University of Washington. The significant anatomic structures encountered and those at risk for injury will be identified. In addition, our methods of operating room setup, patient positioning and draping, and the basic special surgical instruments necessary to develop the approach will be shown.

Principles

The principles of choosing the most appropriate surgical approach to the shoulder include: (1) preservation of normal structural anatomy without altering or endangering the surrounding anatomic structures; (2) respect for neurovascular structures; (3) use of internervous and fascial planes whenever possible; (4) provision of uncompromised access to the structures of interest; and (5) optimization of the functional recovery leading to a successful result.

To accomplish these goals, the optimal incision should be adequate in length to permit the intended procedure and be extensile. It should also avoid denervation of superficial and deep structures.

Whenever possible, cosmetically unacceptable scars are avoided by placing incisions about the shoulder parallel to Langer's lines, which follow natural skin creases. Skin incisions made in these lines generally leave only fine, hairlike scars. All shoulder incisions described, except the deltopectoral, adhere to this principle.

The deltoid muscle, which is encountered in all common surgical approaches to the shoulder, must be split, retracted, or detached. Throughout this course we will emphasize the importance of maintaining the integrity of the deltoid muscle, its osseous attachments, and its innervation.

Description of Instrumentation

Shoulder surgery requires a major orthopaedic instrument set, including standard basic instruments and retractors. The workhorse instrument for anterior or posterior shoulder procedures is the "baby" Balfour retractor, which has been modified by shortening the slide bar (Fig. 1, *top left*). We use the Fukuda humeral

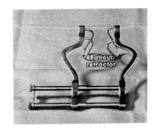
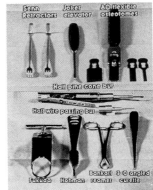
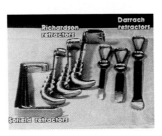

Fig. 1 Top left, The Balfour self-retaining retractor can be used during the axillary, deltopectoral and posterior approaches to the shoulder. **Right,** These instruments are used to expose and complete "Bankart" instability repairs. Joint exposure is facilitated by the Fukuda humeral head and the spiked Hohman retractors. The 3–0 angled curette, wire passing and pine cone burs, and the Bankart reamer are used to prepare the rim of the glenoid for capsular ligament fixation. The axillary, deltopectoral, and superior approach to the shoulder are facilitated by the use of the Joker elevator. Senn retractors are used to expose the subacromial space, and the AO osteotome and the pine cone bur are used for the acromioplasty. **Bottom left,** The deltoid, subscapularis, and capsule can be retracted using Richardson and Sofield retractors. Darrach retractors are especially useful around the humeral head and cuff when performing an acromioplasty and rotator cuff repair.

head retractor in concert with a spiked Hohman to expose the glenoid for instability repairs (Fig. 1, *right*). For surgery in the subacromial space we rely on Senn retractors, a Joker elevator, and a flexible AO osteotome with interchangeable blades (Fig. 1, *right*). Practically all shoulder procedures are facilitated by one of three sizes of Darrach retractors (Fig. 1, *bottom left*). Many shoulder procedures also require special equipment, such as the Hall handpiece with a wirepassing drill bit and a pine cone bur.

Draping for Anterior and Superior Surgical Approaches

In preparation for an anterior or superior surgical approach to the shoulder, the patient is placed supine in the beach chair position. We use a Roger Anderson

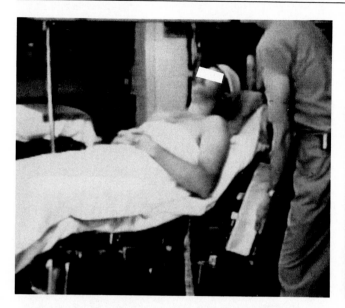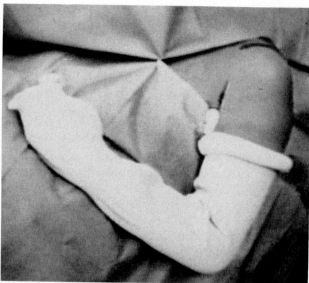

Fig. 2   Left, The patient is placed in the "beach chair" position on the Roger Anderson operating table. This table facilitates positioning and exposure for anterior, superior, and some posterior shoulder surgery. It has a removable pallet that allows the entire shoulder and scapula to be draped free and mobile. It is particularly helpful when performing shoulder arthroscopy in the seated position. (Reproduced with permission from Collins DN, Harryman DT, Lippitt SB, et al: The technique of glenohumeral arthroplasty. *Techniques Orthop* 1991; 6:50. **Right,** When sealing the triangulated drapes around the shoulder, it is important to avoid compromising the exposure when applying the adhesive incisional drape by not only retracting the barrier drapes, but also by initially placing the arm in adduction for anterosuperior application and in abduction to seal posteroaxillary.

table with a removable shoulder pallet, to allow greater access to the forequarter and extremity (Fig. 2, *left*).

The draping steps for the shoulder are as follows: A Bose bar is connected obliquely above the patient for drape attachment. The forequarter and shoulder is prepped after placement of a barrier drape across the base of the neck and posterior to the shoulder. The forequarter is triangulated with the drapes without compromising the exposure. The incision and surgical anatomy are outlined on the skin. A sterile sponge is placed in the axillary fossa, (Fig. 2, *right*), and a surgical incision drape is sealed to the patient and drapes. Finally, a lap drape is placed over the extremity and positioned about the forequarter. This draping technique allows the shoulder to be moved through a full range of motion and provides access to the anterior, superior, and posterior aspects of the shoulder.

Axillary Incision

The axillary incision is especially useful for (1) instability repairs, (eg, Bankart or a capsular shift procedure); (2) capsular release; (3) tendon lengthening (eg, subscapularis Z-lengthening or repair); (4) joint debridement; and (5) biceps tenodesis. This approach is not appropriate for subacromial operations, such as rotator cuff repair.

To achieve the best cosmetic result, the axillary skin incision is placed in the major anterior axillary skin fold (Fig. 3, *top left*). The longest and deepest skin fold and the tip of the coracoid should be marked just prior to the surgical procedure. When the arm is adducted against the side, this skin fold usually obscures the incision. We try to keep all axillary incisions low, as in the original description of Leslie and Ryan,[1] so the scar will be visible only when the arm is elevated.

The incision begins in the axilla and is centered over the pectoralis major tendon. It is usually no longer than 6 cm. If additional exposure is necessary, the incision can be extended in Langer's lines, superiorly toward the coracoid.

Once the deltopectoral fascia is encountered, the skin is undermined in all directions to allow mobilization. The identification of the deltopectoral interval proceeds after cephalad retraction of the skin. The cephalic vein marks the location of the deltopectoral interval. Often, if the cephalic vein is not readily apparent, it can be identified by palpating the tip of the coracoid and separating a small portion of the fascia immediately inferior to this bony landmark. Frequently, the cephalic vein is hidden by a thin yellow streak of subcutaneous tissue. The split in the deltopectoral interval proceeds along the medial aspect of the cephalic vein down to the clavipectoral fascia. The cephalic vein courses superiorly over the coracoid, after which it dives deep to the pectoralis musculature and drains directly into the subclavian vein.

Once the deltopectoral interval has been split, the deep surface of the deltoid is elevated bluntly by beginning dissection next to the coracoid and continuing laterally into the subacromial and subdeltoid bursa. Abducting and flexing the arm will relieve tension on the deltoid so that it can be elevated more easily.

The tip of the coracoid and lateral border of the conjoined tendon are identified. Always keep in mind that dissection medial to the coracoid musculature can be hazardous. Adhesions and bursa are released bluntly from the humeral head with rotation. The incision in the clavipectoral fascia is made along the lateral border of the conjoined tendon. Occasionally this fascia is adherent, thickened, and scarred. The surgeon can determine if this fascia has been removed completely by performing what Frederick A. Matsen III, MD, has termed a "roll-no-roll" test (Frederick A. Matsen III, MD, personal communication). The clavipectoral fascia is differentiated easily from the deeper tissues, because it will not move with internal and external rotation. Once the movement interface is defined, this fascia can be excised completely up to the coracoacromial ligament and the acromion.

Next, the "baby" Balfour retractor is inserted to retract the deltoid and coracoid muscles. To facilitate placement of the Balfour, the arm is positioned in adduction and slight forward flexion. The blades of the Balfour are placed deep to the deltoid and conjoined tendon by keeping the retractor slightly internally rotated. The inner limb of the Balfour should be just caudal to the coracoid tip. The Balfour, by maintaining exposure, is especially useful during the axillary approach. Over the past 15 years, no neurovascular injury has occurred with proper placement of the Balfour retractor. A retractor positioned in the superior aspect of the wound to retract the superior deltoid will improve exposure of the superior humeral head, rotator interval, and coracoacromial ligament.

Surgeons can appreciate that tenodesis of the biceps long head can be accomplished easily without additional exposure. The lesser tuberosity and bicipital groove are identified by palpating the humeral head while rotating the arm. Internal rotation of 15 to 20 degrees brings the bicipital groove directly anterior. The upper border of the subscapularis and the rotator interval can be palpated by passing a digit superomedially up under the coracoacromial ligament. The coracohumeral ligament is a capsular ligamentous band that originates at the base of the coracoid and crosses laterally to insert into the tuberosities. It is best palpated and released with the arm in external rotation at the side.

To enter the glenohumeral joint, a Joker elevator is placed over the superior border of the subscapularis, through the rotator interval and deep to the articular capsule and subscapularis tendon. The insertion of the Joker should be 1.5 to 2 cm lateral to the bicipital groove. The elevator is then passed deep to the capsule

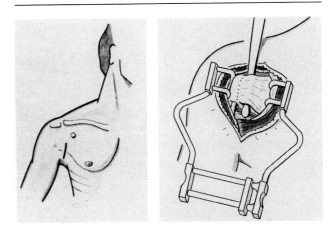

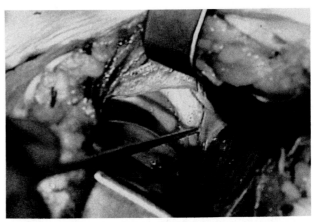

Fig. 3 **Top left,** The axillary incision is placed in the axillary skin crease following Langer's lines. **Top right,** The Joker elevator passes through the rotator interval deep to the anterior capsule and 1 cm medial to the insertion of the subscapularis tendon into the lesser tuberosity. The tip of the Joker exits superior to the anterior humeral circumflex vessels, the "three sister" vessels, and protects them during incision of the subscapularis. **Bottom,** The Fukuda humeral head retractor is locked behind the posterior lip of the glenoid, and the Sofield retractor is used to expose the articular side of the anterior capsule for placement of a spiked Hohman into the capsular defect on the anterior glenoid neck.

in an oblique anteroinferior direction parallel to the anterior anatomic neck capsular insertion (Fig. 3, *top right*). We cause the Joker elevator to exit through the anteroinferior capsule and subscapularis muscle fibers just superior to the anterior humeral circumflex vessels (often referred to as the "three sisters"). The subscapularis tendon is then tagged with a suture in the midsubstance of the tendon.

A digit passed along the anterior surface of the subscapularis muscle will encounter the axillary nerve, which feels like a firm cord-like structure. The axillary nerve, a terminal branch of the posterior cord of the brachial plexus, courses obliquely to the lower margin of the subscapularis and passes inferior to the articular capsule on its way to the quadrangular space. The nerve is joined by the posterior humeral circumflex vessels. Before an incision is made in the subscapularis, the arm

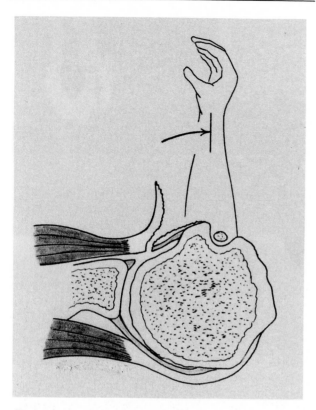

Fig. 4 The subscapularis tendon is elevated sharply from the lesser tuberosity and lengthened by completing a 2 cm coronal Z-plasty. When repairing the subscapularis, the lateral border of the tendon is sutured to the capsule attached to the lesser tuberosity. The tendon must be released from adhesions on all sides to afford a good muscular bounce.

should be externally rotated to avoid damage to the axillary nerve and circumflex vessels. It is always imperative to locate and protect this nerve during shoulder surgery.

An oblique vertical incision through the tendon and capsule follows the Joker elevator, which is aligned parallel to the articular margin. For suture repair at closure, 1 cm of capsule and tendon should remain attached to the lesser tuberosity. The inferior margin of the muscle is left intact, as are the anterior humeral circumflex vessels (the "sister" vessels). The anteroinferior capsule is incised adjacent to the articular margin for complete exposure of the humeral head. The suture tag in the subscapularis tendon is placed behind the Balfour retractor. Placement of a Joker elevator or narrow Darrach retractor outside the inferior capsule of the glenohumeral joint allows safe capsular incision from the anatomic neck. When performing an inferior capsular shift, capsular release is continued inferiorly and posteriorly along the neck of the humerus.

To expose the glenoid for a Bankart repair, the Balfour retractor must be removed and the arm internally rotated to insert the Fukuda humeral head retractor behind the posterior lip of the glenoid. A Sofield re-

tractor is used to elevate the subscapularis tendon for examination of the anterior capsule subjacent to the subscapularis tendon. The entire glenoid and labral attachment is inspected carefully. If a Bankart lesion is absent, but instead the capsule is lax or attenuated, the capsule is split from the deep surface of the subscapularis and left attached to the glenoid. Successful capsular separation from the deep surface of the subscapularis tendon is accomplished by developing the dissection plane at the inferior muscular border anterior to the capsule and splitting it superiorly. Capsular flaps are fashioned by making an incision in the midportion of the anterior capsule, which is directed medially toward four o'clock on the glenoid. The flaps are shifted, overlapped, and reattached to a groove in the proximal humerus. The subscapularis tendon is repaired anatomically.

When a Bankart (or Perthes) lesion is present, a Hohman retractor is placed upside down over the anterior lip of the glenoid through the capsular defect. The Hohman is then rotated 180 degrees, and the tip of the retractor is firmly fixed on the anterior glenoid by tapping the handle with a mallet (Fig. 3, *bottom*). The Fukuda and Hohman retractors must lean together medially or laterally to expose the anterior glenoid neck or the articular surface respectively. For a complete description of this technique, refer to Thomas and Matsen.[2]

Subscapularis Lengthening

When external rotation has been restricted significantly as a result of recalcitrant frozen shoulder or longstanding glenohumeral arthritis, the subscapularis tendon should be lengthened. Subscapularis lengthening is accomplished by incising the tendon insertion beginning adjacent to the medial wall of the bicipital groove. The upper and lower borders of the subscapularis are identified. The tendon is sharply elevated from the lesser tuberosity. The entire breadth of the tendon insertion is incised subperiosteally away from the lesser tuberosity.

We estimate that for every centimeter of lengthened subscapularis tendon, we gain approximately 20 degrees of additional external rotation. The tendon is split in the coronal plane superficial to the capsule from the rotator interval to within 1.5 cm of the anterior humeral circumflex vessels, the "three sisters." While splitting the subscapularis tendon, it is best to externally rotate the arm gradually to expose the deep layer of the articular capsule and deep subscapularis tendon.

After the desired length of the subscapularis tendon has been split coronally, the articular capsule is then incised vertically directly into the glenohumeral joint (Fig. 4). Generally, the tendon is lengthened approximately 2 cm. However, lengthening of the subscapularis can be tailored to accommodate a specific external rotation goal. It is imperative to free the subscapularis

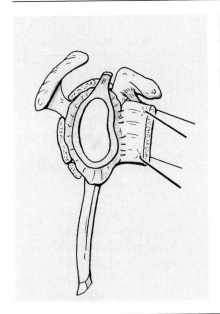 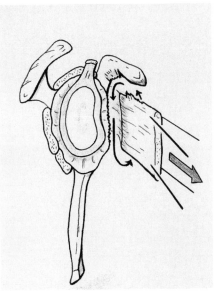

Fig. 5 Left, The subscapularis tendon is mobilized by releasing adhesions and all anterior capsule connecting the tendon to the glenoid. The superior and anterior border of the subscapularis tendon must be freed completely from the base of the coracoid. **Right,** A complete 360-degree release about the subscapularis tendon affords a good muscular "bounce" and functionally increases the length of the subscapularis.

tendon and muscle from all adhesions (Fig. 5, *left*). The muscle and tendon is mobilized using blunt and occasional sharp dissection 360 degrees about all surfaces until a good, muscular bounce is noted with manually applied repetitive traction (Fig. 5, *right*). For repairs, the arm is externally rotated until the lateral edge of the subscapularis tendon matches the medial edge of the incised capsule.

The Deltopectoral Approach

We primarily use the deltopectoral approach for shoulder arthroplasty. Because this approach does not violate the deltoid origin, we are able to encourage early active arm elevation. This approach can be extended both proximally and distally and is, therefore, well suited for traumatic injuries. All anterior surgical procedures can be accomplished using the deltopectoral exposure, but for the sake of cosmesis we recommend the axillary approach. Neither approach, however, provides optimal access for procedures in the subacromial space, such as acromioplasty and repairs to the rotator cuff.

If extended at both ends, the deltopectoral incision would bisect the clavicle and humerus. The incision begins below the middle third of the clavicle, crosses the coracoid tip, and continues distally in an oblique lateral projection to the anterior aspect of the humerus (Fig. 6, *left*). Continuation of the incision laterally would intersect the deltoid tuberosity. Placement of the deltopectoral incision does not follow Langer's lines, but instead parallels the anterior medial border of the deltoid. The incision is positioned with the intent of avoiding the axilla.

Gelpi retractors are used to retract the skin over the deltopectoral interval. Because the deltoid branch of the thoracoacromial artery lies parallel and lateral to the cephalic vein and supplies blood to the deltoid, and the cephalic vein drains the venous blood from the deltoid, we prefer to retract these vessels with the deltoid. The split in the deltopectoral interval separates a true internervous plane between the axillary innervation to the deltoid and the lateral and medial pectoral innervation to the pectoralis major.

Access to the subdeltoid and subacromial space to release adhesions can be provided by applying manual traction and arm rotation. The rotator cuff can be examined using the same maneuver.

For many years, Frederick A. Matsen III, MD, has taught that the lateral side of the conjoined tendons is "the surgical side" and warned the unwary that the medial aspect should be respected as "the suicide" (personal communication). Dissection medial to the conjoined tendons is rarely indicated unless there is a need to expose the brachial plexus or major vessels. The tip of the coracoid, which provides the surgeon with deep structural orientation, has been called the "lighthouse of the shoulder." It is especially helpful for orientation during repeat surgical exposures unless a Bristow coracoid transfer has preceded.

Blunt dissection and mobilization on the anterior subscapularis should begin by placing the digit deep to the coracoid and posterior to the conjoined musculature. Adhesions that need to be released are frequently found in this location. The musculocutaneous nerve can usually be palpated on the deep surface of the coracobrachialis. This nerve, which is a branch of the lateral cord of the brachial plexus, generally enters the posterior muscular aspect of the coracobrachialis about

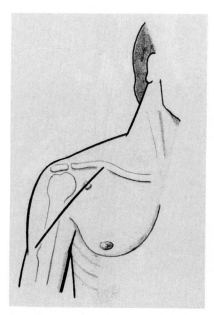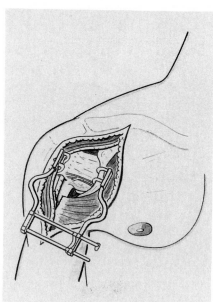

Fig. 6 **Left**, The deltopectoral incision does not follow Langer's lines but preserves the deltoid attachments and is extensile at both ends. **Right**, The Balfour retractor is especially useful during exposure of the proximal third of the humerus for arthroplasty or fracture fixation. It helps protect the cephalic vein and when placed properly will not contact the musculocutaneous or axillary nerves. Notice the release of the falciform border of the pectoralis tendon.

5 cm distal to the coracoid tip but can be as close as 1 to 2 cm.[3] The axillary nerve and circumflex vessels are identified and protected as described in the axillary approach.

Frequently, we release the upper 1 cm of the pectoralis insertion to gain additional exposure. Release of this falciform border increases humeral external rotation and abduction and allows greater access for glenohumeral arthroplasty (Fig. 6, *right*).

The Balfour retractor is placed in the proper orientation to expose the anterior aspect of the proximal humerus. The Joker elevator is inserted through the rotator interval deep to the anterior capsule and subscapularis tendon, 1 cm medial to their insertion into the lesser tuberosity. The remaining deep exposure of the glenohumeral joint proceeds in the same manner as described previously.

Superior Subacromial Approach

The superior subacromial approach can be used for (1) coracoacromial ligament release; (2) acromioplasty and bursectomy; (3) excision of calcareous deposits in the rotator cuff or biceps tendon; (4) rotator cuff repair; (5) tuberosity fixation, osteotomy, or transfer; (6) distal clavicle excision (in conjunction with any of the above procedures); and (7) tenodesis of the biceps long head.

The incision to access the subacromial space is made obliquely across the anterolateral corner of the acromion (Fig. 7, *top left*). This corner is identified easily by pulling traction on the arm to create a sulcus. Rotation of the extremity confirms the distinction between the acromion and the greater tuberosity.

The incision begins lateral and superior to the coracoid tip and courses superolaterally across the anterolateral corner of the acromion, with care being taken to stay in Langer's lines. Even in the largest of patients, 6 to 8 cm is usually plenty of length.

Once the superficial fascia overlying the deltoid has been exposed, skin flaps are elevated superiorly on the acromion and inferiorly down along the fibrous raphe that divides the anterior and middle thirds of the deltoid. It is important to expose the anterior acromion from the lateral corner to the acromioclavicular joint. The surgeon will notice that the fibers of the deltoid course perpendicular to the skin incision. The tendinous raphe is best visualized by pulling traction on the arm to form a sulcus. The greatest indention in the muscle is normally along the tendinous raphe separating the anterior and middle thirds of the deltoid.

The incision in the deltoid proceeds in line with the tendinous raphe. When this incision is extended superiorly on the acromion, it should cross the middle third of the acromioclavicular joint. A full thickness deltoid incision is made at the anterolateral corner of the acromion. A Joker elevator is inserted into the subacromial space through the deep deltoid fascia (Fig. 7, *top right*). The anterior acromial lip is exposed by careful anteromedial subperiosteal dissection, and the deltoid origin is lifted as an intact flap medially over to the acromioclavicular joint.

A Senn retractor used to elevate the deep fascia of the anterior deltoid affords exposure for release or resection of the coracoacromial ligament. Because the deltoid origin remains in continuity, attaching proximally over the acromion, this approach is referred to as the "deltoid-on" approach (Frederick A. Matsen III, personal communication). Usually only a few millimeters of the lateral deltoid are elevated to provide excellent visualization of the entire anterior acromion.

The Joker elevator is then rotated 180 degrees in line with the tendinous raphe and directed distally towards the deltoid tuberosity. Denervation of the anterior deltoid is prevented by limiting the maximum length of full thickness muscle incision to 3 cm.

Digital examination of the subacromial space and blunt release of bursal curtains and adhesions before the Darrach retractor is inserted will help to open the space and ease insertion. The tip of a midsized Darrach retractor is placed to lock behind the posterior lip of the acromion on top of the rotator cuff. Placement of the Darrach retractor behind the acromion exposes the bone, any remaining coracoacromial ligament, and the acromioclavicular joint.

Leverage on the rotator cuff and humeral head stabilizes the Darrach retractor to allow anterior and inferior acromioplasty. The acromioplasty augments exposure of the rotator interval, the coracohumeral ligament, and the rotator cuff (Fig. 7, *bottom*).

The acromial osteotomy is performed with a flexible AO osteotome oriented in line with the posterolateral corner of the acromion. The bevel of the osteotome is directed superiorly, causing the osteotome to exit the bone in the subacromial space adjacent to the Darrach retractor, protecting the cuff.

Once the acromial osteotomy is complete, the osteotome is removed and the bone wedge is grasped in a Kocher clamp. The soft-tissue attachments are released from the fragment. After excision of the bone, the undersurface of the acromion is smoothed with a pine cone bur.

Army-navy retractors are inserted to elevate the medial and lateral flaps of the deltoid to allow examination of the subacromial space and to facilitate complete bursectomy. Arm rotation helps to differentiate the bursa from the rotator cuff using the "roll-no-roll" test. Rotation of the arm enhances visualization not only of the bursal surface overlying the rotator cuff tendons, but also of the rotator interval, and the coracohumeral ligament.

If the acromioclavicular joint is arthritic and painful, the superior incision can be extended proximally over the middle of the acromioclavicular joint for resection of the distal clavicle. The anterior deltoid origin should be elevated subperiosteally, leaving a full thickness anterior flap. The articular capsule is released anteriorly and posteriorly around the distal clavicle. The acromioclavicular joint capsule and the deltotrapezius fascia are dissected sharply away from the distal 2 cm of the clavicle. Hohman retractors are placed anterior and

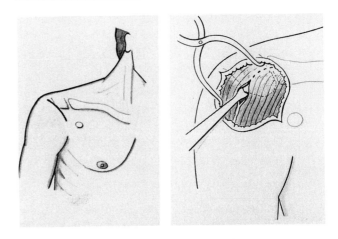

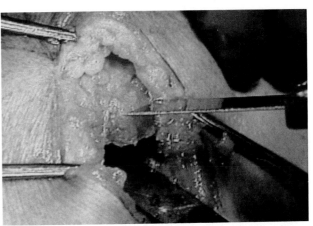

Fig. 7 **Top left**, The superior subacromial incision courses in Langer's lines. The incision crosses directly over the anterolateral corner of the acromion. The fibers of the deltoid are nearly perpendicular to the direction of the skin incision. **Top right**, The deltoid is split in line with the raphe separating the anterior and middle third of the deltoid. The Joker elevator is inserted through the posterior deltoid fascia passing into the subacromial space. Deltoid splitting can be extended across the acromioclavicular joint for distal clavicle resection. **Bottom**, The deltoid flaps have been elevated subperiosteally to maintain their continuity for repair. The mid-sized Darrach retractor protects the rotator cuff during acromial osteotomy with the AO osteotome.

posterior to the distal clavicle for osteotomy and resection.

Surgical Approach for Acromioclavicular Repair or Reconstruction

The surgical approach to the distal third of the clavicle is useful for acute and chronic reconstructions. We use the posterior half of this surgical incision for isolated distal clavicular resection. Reconstruction or repair of the coracoclavicular ligaments, as in the procedure of Weaver and Dunn,[4] requires anterior extension of the incision.

The surgical approach to the distal clavicle begins at

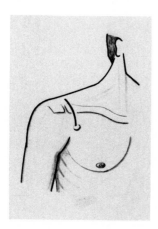
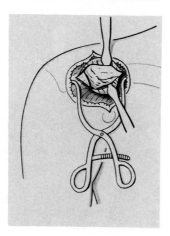
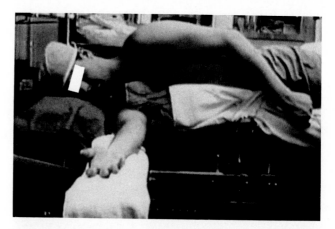

Fig. 8 **Left,** The incision to access the distal clavicle begins posterior to the posterolateral corner of the clavicle and continues anteriorly in Langer's lines toward the coracoid. **Right,** The anterior deltoid and the trapezius must be elevated subperiosteally as an intact flap to expose the distal 2 cm of the clavicle. Hohman retractors ease access for clavicular osteotomy.

the posterior aspect of the clavicle, approximately 1 cm medial to the acromioclavicular joint, and courses anteromedially in Langer's lines toward the coracoid (Fig. 8, *left*). If only the distal clavicle is to be resected, then the incision is no longer than 4 cm. If repair or reconstruction of the coracoclavicular ligaments is also necessary, then the incision must be extended anteromedially to gain access to the coracoid.

After dividing the skin and subcutaneous tissue, the medial and lateral skin flaps are elevated, exposing the fascia overlying the trapezius, clavicle, and deltoid. The acromioclavicular joint is identified by palpation. An incision is made on the clavicle, splitting the deltotrapezius fascia laterally to the middle of the acromioclavicular joint. Occasionally, the deltoid origin has been disrupted. This disruption is commonly seen with acute third-degree acromioclavicular and coracoclavicular ligament tears. After subperiosteal deltotrapezius dissection and acromioclavicular capsular release, spiked Hohman retractors are placed anterior and posterior to the distal clavicle for bone resection (Fig. 8, *right*). The deltoid can then be retracted anteriorly to expose the coracoid and coracoclavicular ligaments for repair.

Draping for Posterior Shoulder Surgery

In preparation for a posterior surgical approach to the shoulder, the patient is placed in the anterolateral decubitus position on a regular operating room table. A bean bag with a U-shaped recess for the bottom shoulder is positioned to brace the patient and to help provide decompression of the axilla. The patient is supported by kidney rests and bean bag, with pillows between the legs (Fig. 9, *top*). The forequarter and ex-

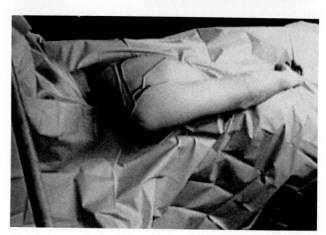

Fig. 9 **Top,** The axillary relief pad is placed under the edge of the U-shaped recess in the bean bag to provide additional space for the bottom shoulder. The bean bag provides firm support to the sternum anteriorly and the spine posteriorly. **Bottom,** The anterior, superior, and posterior aspects of the shoulder and scapular borders can be approached using this position and draping technique. It provides the best visibility to the posterior glenohumeral joint.

tremity are prepped and draped free to provide full mobility and access to the shoulder.

The draping steps for the shoulder are as follows: A Bose bar is connected transversely above the patient for drape attachment. A U-shaped barrier drape is sealed around the shoulder, and the medial scapular border is left free. A border barrier drape closes the gap across the base of the neck. It is important to triangulate the forequarter without compromising exposure. The incision and surgical anatomy are then outlined on the skin (Fig. 9, *bottom*). A sterile sponge is placed in the axillary fossa and a surgical incision drape is sealed to the patient and drapes. Finally, a lap drape is placed over the extremity and positioned about the forequarter. This draping technique allows the shoulder a full range of motion and provides access to the posterior and superior aspect of the shoulder.

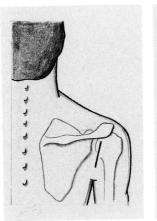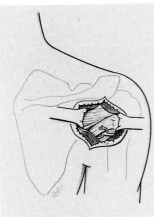

Fig. 10 **Left**, The vertical posterior incision follows Langer's lines toward the posterior axillary skin crease. The deltoid can be split safely 7 cm down toward the axillary nerve bifurcation. **Right**, The internervous plane separating the infraspinatus and teres minor allows direct access to the posterior glenohumeral joint. The axillary nerve should be identified and protected.

Posterior Approach

The posterior shoulder can be approached through either a vertical or a horizontal incision. The preferred vertical incision is directed toward the posterior axillary skin crease following Langer's lines (Fig. 10, *left*). We use the vertical posterior incision for (1) septic joint drainage; (2) posterior capsulorrhaphy; (3) posterior glenoid osteotomy; (4) fixation of scapular neck or glenoid fractures; and (5) axillary nerve grafting.

The vertical posterior incision is made adjacent to the division between the lateral and posterior third of the deltoid near the posterior lateral corner of the acromion. The incision begins just inferior and medial to the posterior corner of the acromion and extends 6 to 7 cm toward the axillary skin crease. The skin flaps are elevated superficial to the deltoid fascia. The division of the deltoid is made in line with the deltoid fibers parallel to the tendinous raphe.

The deep surface of the deltoid is freed using blunt dissection. Retractors are placed to elevate the deltoid. Alternatively, the deltoid may be retracted using the self-retaining Balfour. The interval between the infraspinatus and teres minor is located (Fig. 10, *right*). This true internervous plane between the suprascapular and axillary nerves is split down to the thin posterior capsule of the glenohumeral joint.

The joint capsule can be opened directly for glenohumeral joint access, or the tendons can be incised and split as for a posterior capsulorrhaphy. When the tendons are incised away from their attachment to the greater tuberosity, the capsule and deeper layers of the

external rotator tendons are left intact. After the external rotators and capsule have been split transversly to access the joint, the posterior capsule can then be incised vertically near the greater tuberosity tailoring flaps for a capsular shift.

The axillary nerve lies adjacent to the inferior margin of the teres minor. It is important to identify and protect the axillary nerve and posterior humeral vessels branching to the teres minor and deltoid (Fig. 10, *right*). The posterior branches of the axillary nerve, which innervate the posterior third of the deltoid and the teres minor, are located 7 to 9 cm distal to the acromion. The horizontal incision along the spine of the scapula (although it may not leave a cosmetically acceptable scar) does provide exposure of the posterior scapula, the infraspinatus, and supraspinatus fossa and notch. If access to the posterior scapula, glenoid neck, or infraspinatus fossa is necessary, the posterior third of the deltoid muscle is incised subperiosteally away from the scapular spine. Careful reflection of the infraspinatus from its fossa allows visualization of the scapular neck, spinoglenoid notch, and scapular body. It is important to remember the close proximity of the suprascapular nerve and artery to the posterior lip of the glenoid immediately branching to the infraspinatus.

Comments

The goals of these surgical approaches are to afford rapid recovery from surgical trauma and to optimize rehabilitation of the extremity. If the surgeon preserves essential anatomy and maintains deltoid integrity, early postoperative range of motion can be encouraged.

Individual circumstances, especially after previous surgery, can make it necessary for the surgeon to modify or adapt the approaches presented here. There are many surgical approaches to the shoulder, but I rarely use other incisions for common procedures.

References

1. Leslie JT, Ryan TJ: The anterior axillary incision to approach the shoulder joint. *J Bone Joint Surg* 1962;44A:1193–1196.
2. Thomas SC, Matsen FA III: An approach to the repair of avulsion of the glenohumeral ligaments in the management of traumatic anterior glenohumeral instability. *J Bone Joint Surg* 1989;71A:506–513.
3. Flatow EL, Bigliani LU, April EW: An anatomic study of the musculocutaneous nerve and its relationship to the coracoid process. *Clin Orthop* 1989;244:166–171.
4. Weaver JK, Dunn HK: Treatment of acromioclavicular injuries, especially complete acromioclavicular separation. *J Bone Joint Surg* 1972;54A:1187–1194.

Fractures of the Distal Radius

Jesse B. Jupiter, MD

Introduction

Fractures of the distal radius are among the most common injuries treated by the orthopaedic surgeon. These fractures have been estimated to account for one sixth of all fractures seen and treated in emergency rooms.[1-4] In an epidemiologic survey of all forearm fractures treated over a five-year period in Malmö, Sweden, a city with an urban population of slightly more than 200,000 during the time of study, Alffram and associates[5] recorded nearly 2,000 fractures of the distal radius. This equaled 74.5% of all forearm fractures. The greatest frequency of distal radius fractures occurred in two age groups—children aged 6 to 10 and adults aged 60 to 69 years. Most of these fractures were the result of low energy trauma, and, in patients 60 years or older, women significantly outnumbered men.

It is remarkable that this common fracture remains one of the most challenging of all fractures treated nonsurgically. There is no consensus regarding description, treatment, or even anticipated outcome. It is still commonly believed that there is no real need for special treatment, because deformity is rarely a functional concern.[1,6-7] This belief, however, is being challenged, as interest is directed toward the surgical treatment of complex, intra-articular fractures of the distal radius.[8-13]

Classification

It is remarkable that eponymic descriptions have enjoyed such longevity with fractures of the distal radius.[14] Classification of these injuries as Colles', Smith's, or Barton's fractures continues not only in fracture education and management, but also in the contemporary literature.

To be useful, any classification system must consider the type and severity of the fractures and must serve as a basis for treatment and the evaluation of the outcome of treatment.[15] Over the past quarter century, a number of classifications have been developed in an attempt to represent more accurately the variety and extent of fracture patterns of the distal radius.[16-19] Frykman[20] in 1967 established a classification that identified both radiocarpal and radioulnar joint involvement as well as the presence or absence of an ulnar styloid fracture. Although this classification is now well accepted by many authors, it fails to identify the extent or direction of the initial displacement, dorsal comminution, or shortening of the distal fragment. Because

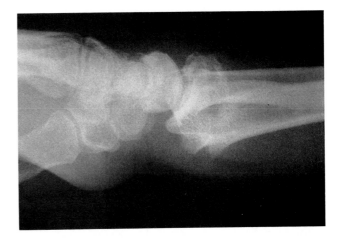

Fig. 1 A lateral radiograph demonstrates an unstable distal radius fracture. Comminution is seen to extend volar to the mid-axial plane of the radius.

of this, it has less prognostic value in evaluating the outcome of treatment.

In an attempt to further define the unstable distal radius fracture, Cooney and associates[21] considered widely displaced fractures, with extensive dorsal comminution, a dorsal angulation of 20 degrees or more, and/or extensive intra-articular involvement, to have a significant chance of redisplacement following reduction. Weber[22] extended this group to include any fracture in which the dorsal comminution extends volar to the mid-axial plane of the radius when seen on the lateral radiograph (Fig. 1).

Fernandez[23] developed a more useful classification, based in part on the mechanism of injury. His classification, which reflects an expanded understanding of the various fracture patterns, includes five groups: (1) Bending, in which the metaphysis fails to tensile stress (Colles, Smith); (2) Compression, which involves fracture of the joint surface with impaction of subchondral and metaphyseal bone (die-punch); (3) Shearing, which includes fractures of the joint surface (Barton's, radial styloid); (4) Avulsion, which are fractures of ligament attachments (ulna, radial styloid); and (5) Combinations of the other four types, resulting from high velocity injuries.

The identification and classification of intra-articular involvement in the distal radius has also been expanded. McMurtry[24] defined intra-articular fractures based on the number of fracture parts, as follows: (1) Two-part, in which the opposite portion of the radiocarpal joint remains intact (dorsal/palmar Barton's, Chauffeur, die-punch); (2) Three-part, in which the lunate and scaphoid facets separate from each other and from the proximal radius; (3) Four-part, which is the same as three-part, except that the lunate facet is further fractured into dorsal and volar fragments; and (4) Five-part (or more), which includes a wide variety of comminuted fragments. Melone[11] further defined the four-part fracture into four subgroups based on the extent of the separation and displacement of the articular fragments (Fig. 2).

The most detailed classification, to date, is the AO, which is organized in order of increasing severity of the bony and articular lesion.[15] This classification divides these fractures into extra-articular (type A), partial articular (type B), and complete articular (type C). Each type is subdivided into three subgroups. Type C, for example, can be divided into C_1 (simple articular and metaphyseal fracture); C_2 (simple articular with complex metaphyseal fracture); and C_3 (complex articular and metaphyseal fractures). These, in turn, can be further subdivided to reflect the morphologic complexity, difficulty of treatment, and prognosis. In addition, fractures of the distal ulna can be identified.

Radiographic Anatomy

Three radiographic measurements are accepted in the anatomic evaluation of the distal radius.[7,16,17,25–30] All three are recorded in relation to the longitudinal axis of the radius. In the lateral view the palmar slope of the distal radius averages between 11 and 12 degrees.[31] Radial inclination, measured on the anteroposterior radiograph, is represented by the angle between a line that joins the tip of the radial styloid and the ulnar corner of the distal articular surface of the radius and a line that is perpendicular to the longitudinal axis of the radius. The average radial inclination is 22 to 23 degrees.[26,29,31] Lastly, radial length, also measured on the anteroposterior radiograph, is represented by the distance between the two perpendiculars to the long axis of the radius—one at the tip of the radial styloid and the other at the distal articular surface of the ulnar head.[16,18,28] Normal radial length averages 11 to 12 mm.

A fourth radiologic measurement that has prognostic value in assessing fractures is that of radial width or shift.[30] The distance between the longitudinal axis through the center of the radius and the most lateral tip of the radial styloid is measured on the anteroposterior radiograph and is compared with the same measurement on the contralateral side.

Functional Anatomy

The metaphyseal flare of the distal end of the radius has a large bi-concave surface that articulates with the proximal carpal row. In addition, the distal radius articulates with the convex articular surface of the distal ulna at the sigmoid notch. This latter articulation plays an integral role in the functional anatomy of the hand and wrist, as the radius and hand rotate about the fixed ulna. Instability of this articulation must be considered in the assessment and management of some unstable fractures of the distal radius.[32,33]

Reversal of the normal palmar tilt of the distal radius has deleterious effects. In mechanical studies using pressure-sensitive film, Short and associates[34] noted a marked transfer of load onto the ulna with progressive dorsal angulation of the distal radius. With a 45-degree dorsal angulation deformity, 65% of the axial load across the carpus is directed into the ulna. The remaining loads on the radius were observed to be eccentric and concentrated on the dorsal aspect of the scaphoid fossa. Clinically, this can result in pain at the radiocarpal articulation as well as limitation in grip strength if this angulation is not reduced.

In some patients, especially those under 25 years of age, a midcarpal instability pattern has been described in association with loss of normal palmar tilt. Pain, decreased grip strength, and a midcarpal instability pattern seen on lateral radiographs are the hallmarks of this dynamic, intercarpal instability, which can be corrected by a correctional osteotomy that restores the palmar tilt of the distal radius.[3,35,36]

Finally, loss of volar tilt, when associated with shortening of the distal radial fracture fragment, can result in dysfunction of the distal radioulnar joint manifested by limitation of forearm rotation and ulnar impingement.[17]

Evaluation of Outcome

The variability in outcome reported in a number of clinical studies can be explained in large part by the wide variation in fracture patterns, the numerous methods of radiographic and clinical evaluation, and the duration of time from injury to final follow-up.

Radiographic Evaluation Studies of radiographic outcome have varied from those measuring only residual dorsal angulation,[37] those measuring dorsal angulation combined with either radial inclination[29] or radial shortening,[17] and those combining all three of these standard measurements.[16,18,20] In a prospective study, van der Linden and Ericsson[30] evaluated the applicability of these three measurements as well as that of radial shift. They observed that only radial shift and dorsal angulation were independent of each other and concluded that residual displacement could accurately be measured with these two criteria alone.

The radiographic outcome of intra-articular fractures has been subjected to more recent evaluation, with Knirk and Jupiter[38] developing criteria to identify residual articular incongruity within the radiocarpal ar-

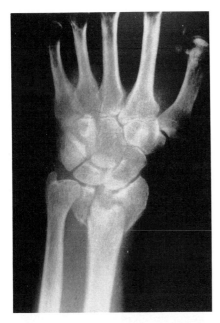

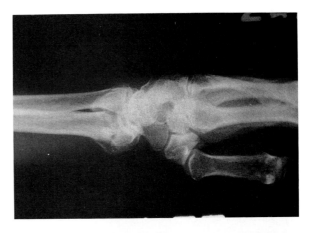

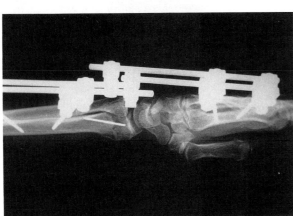

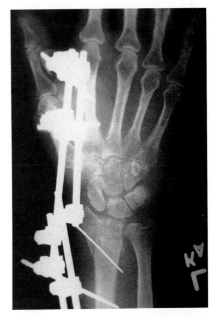

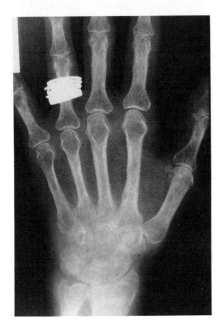

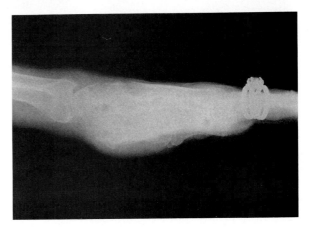

Fig. 2   A complex, three-part intraarticular fracture in a 62-year-old woman treated by longitudinal traction, manipulative reduction of the articular fragments, percutaneous Kirschner wires, and external skeletal fixation. **Top left** and **right,** Anteroposterior and lateral radiographs demonstrate a displaced three-part fracture. **Center left** and **right,** Lateral and anteroposterior radiographs following closed reduction, percutaneous pins, and external skeletal fixation. **Bottom left** and **right,** Anteroposterior and lateral radiographs 4 months post treatment.

ticulation. Four grades were established ranging from excellent (0 mm to 1 mm of residual stepoff) to poor (greater than 3 mm).

Anatomy and Function

Extra-articular Anatomy Despite the inclusion of a variety of fracture types and the use of different methods for evaluation, a number of retrospective studies have suggested a direct relationship between residual deformity and disability.[16,17,19,21,25,27–30,39–50]

Several prospective studies have highlighted the relationship of anatomy to function. Howard and associates,[43] comparing external fixation and plaster immobilization, found that functional results were related more to the quality of the anatomic restoration than to the method of immobilization. These findings were supported by van der Linden and Ericsson,[30] Porter and Stockley,[27] and Jenkins and associates.[44]

In each of these studies, function, as reflected in grip strength and endurance, was impaired if the fracture healed with dorsal angulation greater than 20 degrees, less than 10 degrees of radial inclination, and a radial shift beyond 2 mm. Radial shortening was associated with disruption of the distal radioulnar joint in some cases.

Intra-articular Anatomy Involvement of the radiocarpal, radioulnar, or both articulations is commonplace with distal radius fractures. Fortunately, articular involvement in low energy fractures in postmenopausal women has little effect on the generally favorable outcome found with these patients.[17,20] In contrast, higher energy, shearing, two-part radiocarpal fracture-dislocations require restoration of the articular anatomy to assure hand and wrist function and prevent posttraumatic arthritis.[51–54]

Impacted intra-articular fractures have generated interest in recent years, because failure to reduce these fractures to within 2 mm of articular congruity, especially in young adults, can lead to symptomatic, posttraumatic arthritis.[9–13,38,55–58] Coined "die-punch" injuries by Scheck,[29] these fractures are a result of compressive force delivered through the carpus into the end of the radius. When seen in younger patients, these fractures are often the result of high energy trauma and can be associated with a spectrum of injuries, including carpal instability,[11,38,59] disruption of the distal radioulnar joint, and local soft-tissue injury. With a greater understanding of the pathomechanics of these fractures has come the recognition that conventional manipulation or reduction by traction may not adequately reduce many of these impacted or rotated articular fractures and may not restore intercarpal ligament dissociations.

Treatment

The therapeutic approach to fractures of the distal radius is still influenced today by the observations of Abraham Colles,[60] who noted 176 years ago "one consolation only remains, that the limb will, at some remote period, again enjoy perfect freedom in all its motions, and be completely exempt from pain; the deformity, however, will remain undiminished through life." The fact that some patients function well despite obvious deformity has been supported in the literature.[7,61] The majority of cases occur either in the young, who have the potential for remodeling, or in older patients with generally lower functional demands, and it is not surprising that the majority of patients do relatively well, although not uniformly well.[7,16–18,20,21,25–28,30,37,40–42,44,48,61–68]

In addition to the fracture pattern seen on the anteroposterior, lateral, and oblique radiographs, local factors, including the quality of the bone, associated comminution, extent of fracture displacement, and energy of injury must be taken into account when formulating a treatment plan, because all of these factors can contribute to the inherent instability of the fracture and, thus, may influence the choice of immobilization.[18,21,24,43,47,48,69] Individual patient factors, including lifestyle, psychological outlook, associated medical conditions, and compliance must also be considered in establishing a management plan. The functional loading anticipated should have a greater influence on the method of fracture stabilization than does the chronological age of the patient.[24]

Stable Fractures Closed reduction and plaster immobilization remains the accepted method of treatment for 75% to 80% of fractures of the distal radius and for extra-articular fractures that are minimally displaced or impacted and are thus judged inherently stable.[16,17,69] The manipulative method of reduction suggested by Sir Robert Jones[70] requires increasing the deformity, followed by the application of traction and the subsequent positioning of the hand and wrist in the reduced position. Positioning the hand and wrist in too much flexion in the so-called "Cotton-Loder position" led to such complications as median nerve compression and stiffness of the digits. This method has largely been supplanted by the techniques of Böhler,[71] who advocated longitudinal traction followed by extension and realignment.

There remain questions regarding plaster immobilization, including the optimal position, the duration of immobilization, and the need to extend the cast above the elbow. Several studies have addressed these issues in a prospective manner,[30,37,47] looking at different positions of the hand and wrist,[30] functional bracing with the forearm in supination versus short-arm splints,[47] and above-the-elbow versus below-the-elbow casts.[37] Neither the position of immobilization nor the extension of the cast above the elbow appears to influence the anatomic outcome to any noteworthy degree. However, immobilization of the fracture with the forearm in supination, as advocated by Sarmiento and associates,[67,72] offers the advantages of holding the distal radioulnar joint in a reduced position and minimizing the tendency of the brachioradialis to cause the distal fragment to displace in a radial direction.[30]

Redisplacement of fractures during cast or splint immobilization can occur, and remanipulation is common practice. Little has been written, however, about the ultimate fate of the fracture that has undergone remanipulation. Two retrospective studies found lasting improvement in 33%[73] and 54% of cases following remanipulation.[74] There was a greater likelihood of retaining the reduction in younger patients and in those fractures remanipulated between 7 and 15 days after the initial reduction.[17,73] Unstable fractures with displacement or extensive dorsal comminution tended to lose reduction even following remanipulation, especially in elderly patients.

Unstable Fractures A number of treatment options can offset the loss of reduction in an unstable distal radius fracture in patients for whom the maintenance of anatomy is considered important for functional demands. These techniques include percutaneous pinning of the distal fracture,[26,40,62,68] immobilization of the limb with pins incorporated in plaster,[25,29,42,61,75,76] metal external skeletal fixation devices,[21,43,44,56,77–81] limited open reduction with or without bone graft,[55,65] and extensive open reduction and internal fixation.[8–13,58]

Percutaneous Pinning Extra-articular fractures with extensive comminution or fractures that involve no more than two articular fragments, in which anatomic reduction is obtainable, are amenable to percutaneous pinning of the fracture fragments and application of a plaster cast. This treatment was advocated as early as 1952 by De Palma,[40] and Clancy[62] recently reported on 30 consecutive patients with displaced unstable fractures treated by percutaneous pinning. Anatomic reduction was maintained in 28 with minimal complications in the series. This technique does not work as well with high-energy, complex fractures or fractures associated with soft-tissue problems that preclude the use of a circular cast. However, the technique can be effectively combined with metal external fixation in these situations (Fig. 3).

Pins and Plaster Pins placed in the metacarpals and forearm bones, initially advocated by Böhler in 1929, reached widespread popularity following the report of Green[42] in 1975, who documented good to excellent results in 86% of patients. Green, however, noted a high incidence of both minor and major complications, with one third of the patients having pin-related problems. Other studies have supported the prevalence of complications with this technique. Chapman and associates[75] noted one third of the complications were pin-related and 16% required re-operation for the com-

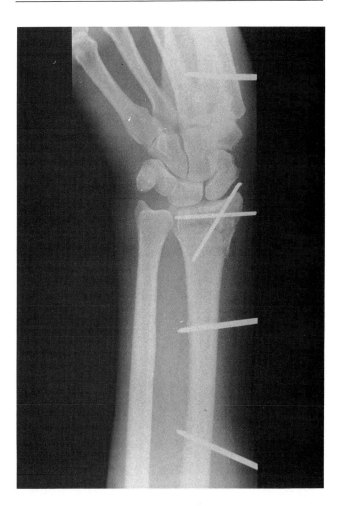

Fig. 3 A 56-year-old woman had a displaced intra-articular fracture treated with a limited open technique. Through a small dorsal incision, the displaced lunate facet fragment was manipulated and pinned. An external fixator maintained axial length.

plication. Weber and Szabo,[76] in a series that featured fractures caused by high energy trauma, reported a complication rate of 53%. Carrozzella and Stern[82] also reported a high number of complications, which resulted in the premature termination of the treatment in over 30% of patients. Although pins and plaster offer a method of maintaining reduction of many unstable fractures at a limited expense, the complications associated with the use of pins incorporated into circumferential plaster has led to a reevaluation of this technique.

External Skeletal Fixation External skeletal fixation has become increasingly popular in the management of complex fractures of the distal radius. This popularity can be attributed, in part, to the improvements in design of the frame and methods of pin insertion.[78,80,83] Although a number of studies have reported favorable results with external fixation, most have been retrospective in nature and are difficult to interpret because of the heterogeneous groups of patients and the variety of skeletal and soft-tissue injury patterns.[21,76-78,83] The prevalence of complications in these series is also high, ranging from 20% to 60%. These complications include pin-tract infection, radial sensory neuritis, reflex sympathetic dystrophy, stiffness of the wrist, and fracture through the pin sites. However, two prospective, randomized studies that compared external fixation with plaster immobilization for unstable fractures showed external fixation to be significantly more effective in maintaining the fracture reduction, with resultant improved function of the hand.[43,44] The overall complication rate in these two series was markedly lower.

Improved pin application techniques, including predrilling, open pin placement, and more strategic pin placement, have diminished the prevalence of problems related to the pins,[80,83] but the potential for permanent loss of wrist motion remains a concern. Although a study by Cooney and associates,[21] in 1979, reported minimal loss of motion in patients followed for two years or more, other authors have recommended decreasing the amount of traction applied by the external fixation frame across the radiocarpal ligaments after three weeks, limiting the duration of treatment by adding percutaneous pins or autogenous bone graft to permit earlier removal of the external frame without loss of fracture reduction,[55,65,80] or using hinged fixators to afford wrist motion while traction is maintained.[56] Interest in the concept of dynamic external fixation has been tempered by the complexity of the surgical protocol, the difficulty in controlling the position of the impacted "die punch" fragments, and the difficulty in controlling the reduction of an unstable distal radioulnar joint. The range of wrist motion reported by Clyburn,[56] who used a mobile external fixation device, showed little, if any, improvement over Cooney and associates'[21] series, although it must be pointed out that many of Clyburn's patients were in a younger age group with high-energy fractures.

While radial length and radial inclination are usually reestablished and maintained with traction (ligamentotaxis), the palmar tilt of the radius is not commonly restored to normal. An anatomic study by Bartosh and Saldaña[84] suggested that this may be caused by the fact that the stout palmar radiocarpal ligaments reach maximum length before the z-shaped dorsal ligaments do, which prevents the latter from pulling the dorsal aspect of the distal radius into its normal palmar inclination.

Limited Open Reduction In certain displaced intra-articular fractures, incongruity of the radiocarpal joint may exist following closed reduction. This usually involves the lunate facet of the distal radius, because the radial styloid and scaphoid facet are more amenable to reduction through ligamentotaxis or by manipulation and reduction with a large pointed bone clamp. Both anteroposterior and lateral tomography are helpful in ac-

curately defining the nature and extent of the articular injury.

Axelrod and associates[55] reported on their technique, which combines external skeletal fixation with open reduction of the displaced lunate facet through a small, longitudinal, dorsal incision, and elevation of the impacted fragment without directly visualizing the joint surface. They detailed the surgical steps based on two different patterns of fracture (impaction or shear) previously identified by Saito and Shibata[57] and recommended that the reduction be supported with transverse or oblique Kirschner wires (K-wires) and autogenous iliac crest graft. In this way, settling of the elevated articular fragments is avoided, and the external fixation frame can be removed by six weeks after application. Leung and associates[65] reported on 100 cases of complex, distal radial fractures in which the fracture reduction was supported with autogenous iliac crest graft, which allowed removal of the external fixation frame at three weeks, followed by use of a functional brace for an additional three weeks. These authors noted few complications and maintenance of the reduction with good to excellent function in nearly all cases.

Open Reduction and Internal Fixation Despite the complex skeletal and articular anatomy of the distal radius and the limited surgical access, there are two groups of fractures for which open reduction and internal fixation may be advisable. The first group includes the two-part shearing fractures (Barton's, reverse Barton's), which actually represent radiocarpal fracture-dislocations. Although anatomic reduction is possible by closed means in some cases, these fractures are extremely unstable and difficult to control in plaster. Several studies have specifically addressed these fractures, noting the anterior fracture-dislocation to be far more common than its dorsal counterpart, and that these fracture-dislocations often occur in younger adults whose stronger bone is amenable to supporting the reduction with a small buttress plate (Fig. 4).[51-54]

The second group includes complex articular fractures in which the articular fragments are displaced, rotated, or impacted and are not amenable to reduction, even through a limited surgical exposure. Often, these fractures are caused by high-energy trauma in younger adults and are associated with concomitant skeletal or soft-tissue injury.[8-10,13,38,74] Several studies have suggested that the restoration of the articular anatomy is the most critical factor in obtaining a good functional result and preventing late posttraumatic arthritis.[8,9,11,13,38,74]

The surgical management of these fractures is difficult and is associated with significant early and late morbidity.[8] Preoperative planning, including anteroposterior and lateral tomography, is exceptionally helpful. Before making the incision, distraction and the tem-

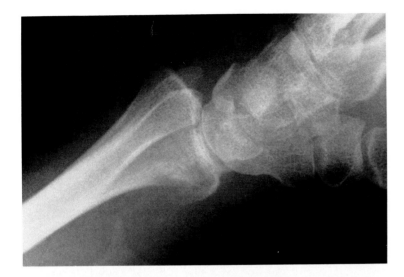

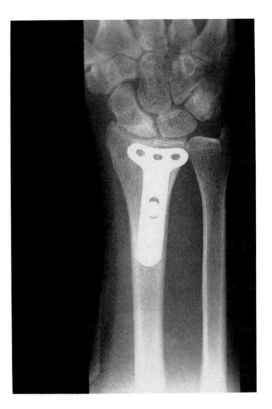

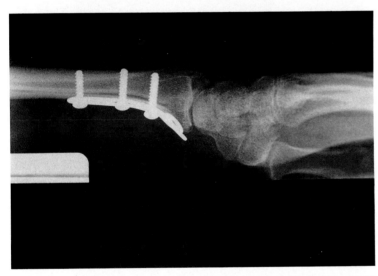

Fig. 4 A 28-year-old woman with an anterior fracture-dislocation. **Top left,** Lateral radiograph demonstrates an unstable shearing, two-part fracture-dislocation. **Top right** and **bottom left,** Open reduction and internal fixation was preferred through an anterior approach. Full function resulted.

porary application of an external fixator will make it easier to manipulate the small articular fragments and will minimize soft-tissue dissection. The anterior approach is helpful for fractures with anterior displacement or rotation of the articular fragments. By approaching the radius ulnarward to the flexor tendons, trauma to the median nerve and its palmar cutaneous branch is minimized. When exposing the articular fragments anteriorly, the surgeon must be aware of the critical anterior radiocarpal ligaments. Disruption of these ligaments can result in subsequent intercarpal instability. In most cases, the articular reconstruction should be supported both by autogenous cancellous bone graft and by a small buttress plate. In some cases involving multiple, small articular fragments, the use of a plate may not be possible. In these instances, definitive fixation is accomplished with K-wires along with external skeletal fixation (Fig. 5).[10]

The severity of these injuries is reflected in the fact that most patients will have some residual limitation in wrist mobility as well as in grip strength.[8–10,12,13] While enthusiasm is growing for the surgical approach for the complex, articular, distal radial fractures, the surgeon must be mindful that serious complications, including loss of fixation, median nerve neuritis, reflex sympathetic dystrophy, wound infection, and late, posttraumatic arthritis, can occur even though the surgeon is an experienced one.[8,10,13]

Complications

Despite Colles' optimistic outlook, the management of fractures of the distal radius is fraught with complications. In a large retrospective series of 565 fractures, Cooney and associates[85] reported a complication rate of more than 31%, including median nerve dysfunction, malposition, radiocarpal or radioulnar joint arthritis, stiffness of the digits, tendon rupture, causalgia, and even Volkmann's ischemic contracture.

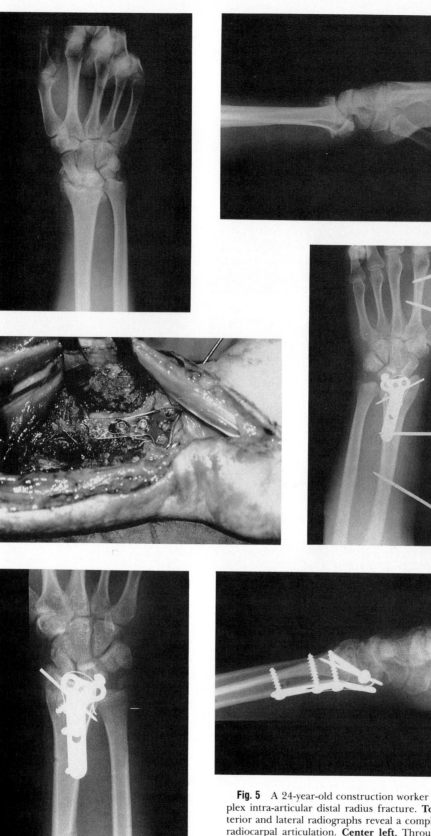

Fig. 5   A 24-year-old construction worker fell 20 feet, sustaining a complex intra-articular distal radius fracture. **Top left** and **right,** Anteroposterior and lateral radiographs reveal a complex fracture-dislocation of the radiocarpal articulation. **Center left,** Through an anterior approach the fracture was reduced by longitudinal traction and direct manipulation of the fracture fragments. Internal fixation was provided by a combination of wires, plates, and screws. **Center right,** The postoperative radiograph demonstrates the combined internal and external fixation. **Bottom left** and **right,** Anteroposterior and lateral radiographs 12 weeks postoperatively reveal maintenance of the anatomy. Excellent hand and wrist function resulted.

Some of these complications result from treatment rather than from the original fracture. Colles[60] himself admonished his colleagues against the use of constricting bandages. Even so, the end of the 19th century saw widespread use of standardized splints and overzealous immobilization, which all too often resulted in permanent disability. Recognition of this problem led many authors at the turn of the 20th century to recommend limited duration of immobilization (one to three weeks) followed by an active therapy program.[86]

Median nerve dysfunction is the most commonly observed complication in most series.[20,37,49,87-90] Several studies note that the transient neuropathy associated with the injury did not appear to be related to the type of fracture, the extent of the initial displacement, or the accuracy of the primary reduction. On the other hand, persistent median nerve compression did appear to be more prevalent with malunited fractures.[20,49,87,91]

McCarroll[89] established a series of sound guidelines for the management of median nerve compression associated with a fracture of the distal radius. If no improvement is noted in a complete nerve lesion following reduction of the fracture, surgical exploration is justified. Lewis[91] stressed that decompression of the median nerve should include not only the transverse retinacular ligament but, more importantly, the antebrachial fascia over the anterior aspect of the distal forearm. When faced with a partial lesion of the nerve, the fracture is reduced and the patient observed for a minimum of seven days. If no change is noted and some motor weakness exists, McCarroll recommended that exploration be considered. If the nerve lesion develops following reduction of the fracture or worsens despite the reduction, the cast or splints should be released and the wrist placed in a neutral position. Carpal tunnel pressures can be measured.[92] Should sensory abnormality or motor weakness persist despite change of wrist position, exploration is indicated. When a nerve lesion, even an incomplete one, is present with a fracture that requires surgical intervention, McCarroll,[89] as well as Axelrod and McMurtry,[8] recommend release of the nerve at the same time.

When increasing pain, swelling, loss of joint mobility, or paresthesias are present, an impeding causalgia should be considered. Atkins and associates[93] observed some or all of these to be more common than previously thought in association with distal radial fractures. Lynch[88] and Stein[94] both noted the strong possibility that median nerve compression is a common precursor of major causalgia (reflex sympathetic dystrophy) in these patients. Stein, in fact, observed marked improvement following median nerve decompression in four patients with causalgia following a distal radius fracture.

A number of studies have highlighted the importance of the distal radioulnar joint in the functional outcome after distal radial fracture.[1,20,85,95] This joint can be involved either by diastasis as a result of direct injury or by residual deformity of the distal radius. Pain, instability, and loss of forearm rotation can be disabling.[20] Although distal ulnar excision has been widely used, the outcome is unpredictable,[96] because the procedure may result in distal ulnar instability[97,98] as well as weakness.[36,98]

While there are numerous reports of posttraumatic arthritis following intra-articular fractures of the distal radius,[8,9,11-13,38,55,56,58] the frequency of osteoarthritis following Colles' type fractures has been investigated in only a few studies.[7,16,17,20,85,99] Smaill[7] noted that, of 41 patients followed between five to six years postfracture, ten had radiographic changes of osteoarthrosis, but only three had symptoms. Overgaard and Solgaard,[99] with a seven-year followup, found 17 of 56 patients (30%) had radiographic evidence of osteophytes, and eight patients (14%) had advanced radiographic changes. The occurrence of osteoarthrosis in their series was not related to residual dorsal angulation or radial shortening but rather to the initial displacement and to advanced age at the time of injury. Frykman[20] found a high rate (19%) of distal radioulnar joint arthrosis which was frequently symptomatic.

Complications involving tendons include peritendinous adhesions, involving both the extensor and flexor tendons, as well as tendon rupture. The most frequently observed ruptured tendon is the extensor pollicis longus.[75,100] Rupture of this tendon after a minimally displaced fracture suggests an ischemic etiology rather than attritional rupture over a bony spike. In most cases, tendon transfer, using the adjacent extensor indicis proprius, provides a predictable outcome.

References

1. Golden GN: Treatment and programs of Colles' fracture. *Lancet* 1963;1(7280):511–515.
2. Hollingsworth R, Morris J: The importance of the ulnar side of the wrist in fractures of the distal end of the radius. *Injury* 1976;7:263–266.
3. Jupiter JB, Masem M: Reconstruction of post-traumatic deformity of the distal radius and ulna. *Hand Clin* 1988;4:377–390.
4. Owen RA, Melton LJ, Johnson KA, et al: Incidence of a Colles' fracture in a North American community. *Am J Public Health* 1982;72:605–613.
5. Alffram PA, Goran CH, Bauer GCH: Epidemiology of fractures of the forearm: A biomechanical investigation of bone strength. *J Bone Joint Surg* 1962;44A:105–114.
6. Altissimi M, Antenucci R, Fiacca C, et al: Long-term results of conservative treatment of fractures of the distal radius. *Clin Orthop* 1986;206:202–210.
7. Smaill GB: Long-term follow-up of Colles' fracture. *J Bone Joint Surg* 1965;47B:80–85.
8. Axelrod TS, McMurtry RY: Open reduction and internal fixation of comminuted intraarticular fractures of the distal radius. *J Hand Surg* 1990;15A:1–11.
9. Bradway JK, Amadio PC, Cooney WP: Open reduction and internal fixation of displaced, comminuted intraarticular frac-

tures of the distal end of the radius. *J Bone Joint Surg* 1989; 71A:839–847.

10. Jupiter JB, Lipton H: Operative treatment of intraarticular fractures of the distal radius. *Clin Orthop*, in press.

11. Melone CP Jr: Articular fractures of the distal radius. *Orthop Clin North Am* 1984;15:217–236.

12. Melone CP Jr: Open treatment for displaced articular fractures of the distal radius. *Clin Orthop* 1986;202:103–111.

13. Porter ML: Pilon fractures of the wrist: Displaced intraarticular fractures of the distal radius, in press.

14. Peltier LF: Fractures of the distal end of the radius: An historical account. *Clin Orthop* 1984;187:18–22.

15. Müller ME, Nazarian S, Koch P: Classification AO des fractures, in *Les Os Longs*. Berlin, Heidelberg, New York, Springer-Verlag, 1987.

16. Gartland JJ Jr, Werley CW: Evaluation of healed Colles' fractures. *J Bone Joint Surg* 1951;33A:895–907.

17. Lidström A: Fractures of the distal radius: A clinical and statistical study of end results. *Acta Orthop Scand Suppl* 1959;41: 1–118.

18. Older TM, Stabler EV, Cassebaum WH: Colles fracture: Evaluation of selection of therapy. *J Trauma* 1965;5:469–476.

19. Solgaard S: Classification of distal radius fractures. *Acta Orthop Scand* 1985;56:249–252.

20. Frykman G: Fracture of the distal radius including sequelae: Shoulder-hand-finger syndrome, disturbance in the distal radioulnar joint and impairment of nerve function: A clinical and experimental study. *Acta Orthop Scand Suppl* 1967;108:1–155.

21. Cooney WP III, Linscheid RL, Dobyns JH: External pin fixation for unstable Colles' fractures. *J Bone Joint Surg* 1979;61A:840–845.

22. Weber ER: A rational approach for the recognition and treatment of Colles' fractures. *Hand Clin* 1987;3:13–21.

23. Fernandez DL: Avant-bras segment distal, in Mueller ME, Nazarian S, Koch P (eds): *Classification AO Des Fractures. Les Os Longs*. Berlin, Heidelberg, New York, Springer-Verlag, 1987, pp 106–115.

24. McMurtry RY, Jupiter JB: Fractures of the distal radius, in Browner B, Jupiter J, Levine A, Trafton P (eds): *Skeletal Trauma*. Philadelphia, WB Saunders, in press.

25. Cole JM, Obletz BE: Comminuted fractures of the distal end of the radius treated by skeletal transfixion in plaster cast: An end-result study of thirty-three cases. *J Bone Joint Surg* 1966; 48A:931–945.

26. Dowling JJ, Sawyer B Jr: Comminuted Colles' fractures: Evaluation of a method of treatment. *J Bone Joint Surg* 1961;43A: 657–668.

27. Porter M, Stockley I: Fractures of the distal radius: Intermediate and end results in relation to radiologic parameters. *Clin Orthop* 1987;220:241–252.

28. Rubinovich RM, Rennie WR: Colles' fracture: End results in relation to radiologic parameters. *Can J Surg* 1983;26:361–363.

29. Scheck M: Long-term follow-up of treatment of comminuted fractures of the distal end of the radius by transfixation with Kirschner wires and cast. *J Bone Joint Surg* 1962;44A:337–351.

30. van der Linden W, Ericson R: Colles' fracture: How should its displacement be measured and how should it be immobilized? *J Bone Joint Surg* 1981;63A:1285–1288.

31. Friberg S, Lindström B: Radiographic measurements of the radio-carpal joint in normal adults. *Acta Radiol (Stockholm)*, 1976;17:249–256.

32. Palmer AK: Fractures of the distal radius, in Green DP (ed): *Operative Hand Surg*, ed 2. Philadelphia, JB Lippincott, 1988, pp 991–1026.

33. Palmer AK: The distal radioulnar joint: Anatomy, biomechanics, and triangular fibrocartilage complex abnormalities. *Hand Clin* 1987;3:31–40.

34. Short WH, Palmer AK, Werner FW, et al: A biomechanical study of distal radial fractures. *J Hand Surg* 1987;12A:529–534.

35. Taleisnik J, Watson HK: Midcarpal instability caused by malunited fractures of the distal radius. *J Hand Surg* 1984;9A:350–357.

36. Fernandez DL: Correction of post-traumatic wrist deformity in adults by osteotomy, bone-grafting and internal fixation. *J Bone Joint Surg* 1982;64A:1164–1178.

37. Pool C: Colles's fracture: A prospective study of treatment. *J Bone Joint Surg* 1973;55B:540–544.

38. Knirk JL, Jupiter JB: Intra-articular fractures of the distal end of the radius in young adults. *J Bone Joint Surg* 1986;68A:647–659.

39. Bacorn RW, Kurtzke JF: Colles' fracture: A study of two thousand cases from the New York State Workmen's Compensation Board. *J Bone Joint Surg* 1953;35A:643–658.

40. De Palma AF: Comminuted fractures of the distal end of the radius treated by ulnar pinning. *J Bone Joint Surg* 1952;34A: 651–662.

41. Edwards H, Clayton EB: Fractures of the lower end of the radius in adults (Colles' fracture and backfire fracture). *Br Med J* 1929;1:61–65.

42. Green DP: Pins and plaster treatment of comminuted fractures of the distal end of the radius. *J Bone Joint Surg* 1975;57A:304–310.

43. Howard PW, Stewart HD, Hind RE, et al: External fixation or plaster for severely displaced comminuted Colles' fractures? A prospective study of anatomical functional results. *J Bone Joint Surg* 1989;71B:68–73.

44. Jenkins NH, Jones DG, Johnson SR, et al: External fixation of Colles' fractures: An anatomical study. *J Bone Joint Surg* 1987; 69B:207–211.

45. McBride ED: *Disability Evaluation*, ed 4. Philadelphia, JB Lippincott, 1948.

46. McQueen M, Caspers J: Colles' fracture: Does the anatomical result affect the final function? *J Bone Joint Surg* 1988;70B:649–651.

47. Solgaard S, Bünger C, Sølund K: Displaced distal radius fractures: A comparative study of early results following external fixation, functional bracing in supination, or dorsal plaster immobilization. *Arch Orthop Trauma Surg* 1989;109:34–38.

48. Stewart HD, Innes AR, Burke FD: Factors affecting the outcome of Colles' fracture: An anatomical and functional study. *Injury* 1985;16:289–295.

49. Stewart HD, Innes AR, Burke FD: The hand complications of Colles' fractures. *J Hand Surg* 1985;10B:103–106.

50. Villar RN, Marsh D, Rushton N, et al: Three years after Colles' fracture: A prospective review. *J Bone Joint Surg* 1987;69B:635–638.

51. de Oliveira JC: Barton's fractures. *J Bone Joint Surg* 1973;55A: 586–594.

52. Ellis J: Smith's and Barton's fractures: A method of treatment. *J Bone Joint Surg* 1965;47B:724–727.

53. Pattee GA, Thompson GH: Anterior and posterior marginal fracture-dislocations of the distal radius: An analysis of the results of treatment. *Clin Orthop* 1988;231:183–195.

54. Thompson GH, Grant TT: Barton's fractures - reverse Barton's fractures: Confusing eponyms. *Clin Orthop* 1977;122:210–221.

55. Axelrod T, Paley D, Green J, et al: Limited open reduction of the lunate facet in comminuted intraarticular fractures of the distal radius. *J Hand Surg* 1988;13A:372–377.

56. Clyburn TA: Dynamic external fixation for comminuted intraarticular fractures of the distal end of the radius. *J Bone Joint Surg* 1987;69A:248–254.

57. Saito H, Shibata M: Classification of fractures at the distal end of the radius with reference to treatment of comminuted fractures, in Boswick JA Jr (ed): *Current Concepts in Hand Surgery*. Philadelphia, Lea & Febiger, 1983, pp 129–145.

58. Szabo RM, Weber SC: Comminuted intraarticular fractures of the distal radius. *Clin Orthop* 1988;230:39–48.

59. Bickerstaff DR, Bell MJ: Carpal malalignment in Colles' fractures. *J Hand Surg* 1989;14B:155–160.

60. Colles A: On the fracture of the carpal extremity of the radius. *Edinburgh Med Surg J* 1814;10:182–186.

61. Cassebaum WH: Colles' fracture: A study of end results. *JAMA* 1950;143:963–965.

62. Clancey GJ: Percutaneous Kirschner-wire fixation of Colles' fractures: A prospective study of thirty cases. *J Bone Joint Surg* 1984;66A:1008–1014.

63. Dias JJ, Wray CC, Jones JM, et al: The value of early mobilization in the treatment of Colles' fractures. *J Bone Joint Surg* 1987;69B:463–467.

64. Jenkins NH: The unstable Colles' fracture. *J Hand Surg* 1989;14B:149–154.

65. Leung KS, Shen WY, Tsang HK, et al: An effective treatment of comminuted fractures of the distal radius. *J Hand Surg* 1990;15A:11–17.

66. Lucas GL, Sachtjen KM: An analysis of hand function in patients with Colles' fracture treated by Rush rod fixation. *Clin Orthop* 1981;155:172–179.

67. Sarmiento A, Zagorski JB, Sinclair WF: Functional bracing of Colles' fractures: A prospective study of immobilization in supination vs. pronation. *Clin Orthop* 1980;146:175–183.

68. Stein AH Jr, Katz SF: Stabilization of comminuted fractures of the distal inch of the radius: Percutaneous pinning. *Clin Orthop* 1975;108:174–181.

69. Cooney WP: Management of Colles' fractures: Editorial. *J Hand Surg* 1989;14B:137–139.

70. Jones R: *Injuries of Joints.* London, Henry Frowde and Hodder & Stoughton, 1915, p 110.

71. Böhler LB: Funktionelle bewegungsbehandlung der "Typischen Radiusbruche." *Med Wochenschr* (Munchen) 1923;20:387–.

72. Sarmiento A, Pratt GW, Berry NC, et al: Colles' fracture: Functional bracing in supination. *J Bone Joint Surg* 1975;57A:311–317.

73. Collert S, Isacson J: Management of redislocated Colles' fractures. *Clin Orthop* 1978;135:183–186.

74. McQueen MM, MacLaren A, Chalmers J: The value of remanipulating Colles' fractures. *J Bone Joint Surg* 1986;68B:232–233.

75. Chapman DR, Bennett JB, Bryan WJ, et al: Complications of distal radius fractures: Pins and plaster treatment. *J Hand Surg* 1982;7:509–512.

76. Weber SC, Szabo RM: Severely comminuted distal radial fracture as an unsolved problem: Complications associated with external fixation and pins and plaster techniques. *J Hand Surg* 1986;11A:157–165.

77. Anderson R, O'Neill G: Comminuted fractures of the distal end of the radius. *Surg Gynecol Obstet* 1944;78:434–440.

78. Jakob RP, Fernandez DL: The treatment of wrist fractures with the small AO external fixation device, in Uhthoff HK (ed): *Current Concepts of External Fixation of Fractures.* Berlin, Heidelberg, New York, Springer-Verlag, 1982, pp 307–314.

79. Riis J, Fruensgaard S: Treatment of unstable Colles' fractures by external fixation. *J Hand Surg* 1989;14B:145–148.

80. Seitz WH Jr, Putnam MD, Dick HM: Limited open surgical approach for external fixation of distal radius fractures. *J Hand Surg* 1990;15A:288–293.

81. Vaughan PA, Lui SM, Harrington IJ, et al: Treatment of unstable fractures of the distal radius by external fixation. *J Bone Joint Surg* 1985;67B:385–389.

82. Carrozzella J, Stern PJ: Treatment of comminuted distal radius fractures with pins and plaster. *Hand Clin* 1988;4:391–397.

83. Nakata RY, Chand Y, Matiko JD, et al: External fixators for wrist fractures: A biomechanical and clinical study. *J Hand Surg* 1985;10A:845–851.

84. Bartosh RA, Saldaña MJ: Intraarticular fractures of the distal radius: A cadaveric study to determine if ligamentotaxis restores radiopalmar tilt. *J Hand Surg* 1990;15A:18–21.

85. Cooney WP III, Dobyns JH, Linscheid RL: Complications of Colles' fractures. *J Bone Joint Surg* 1980;62A:613–619.

86. Linscheid RL: Kinematic considerations of the wrist. *Clin Orthop* 1986;202:27–39.

87. Aro H, Koivunen T, Katevuo K, et al: Late compression neuropathies after Colles' fractures. *Clin Orthop* 1988;233:217–225.

88. Lynch AC, Lipscomb PR: The carpal tunnel syndrome and Colles' fractures. *JAMA* 1963;185:363–366.

89. McCarroll HR Jr: Nerve injuries associated with wrist trauma. *Orthop Clin North Am* 1984;15:279–287.

90. Sponsel KH, Palm ET: Carpal tunnel syndrome following Colles' fracture. *Surg Gynec Obstet* 1965;121:1252–1256.

91. Lewis MH: Median nerve decompression after Colles' fracture. *J Bone Joint Surg* 1978;60B:195–196.

92. Gelberman RH, Szabo RM, Mortensen WW: Carpal tunnel pressures and wrist position in patients with Colles' fractures. *J Trauma* 1984;24:747–749.

93. Atkins RM, Duckworth J, Kanis JA: Algodystrophy following Colles' fracture. *J Hand Surg* 1989;14B:161–164.

94. Stein AH Jr: The relation of median nerve compression to Sudek's syndrome. *Surg Gynec Obstet* 1962;115:713–720.

95. Mohanti RC, Kar N: Study of triangular fibrocartilage of the wrist joint in Colles' fracture. *Injury* 1980;11:321–324.

96. Ekenstam F, Engkvist O, Wadin K: Results from resection of the distal end of the ulna after fractures of the lower end of the radius. *Scand J Plast Recon Surg* 1982;16:177–181.

97. Bell MJ, Hill RJ, McMurtry RY: Ulnar impingement syndrome. *J Bone Joint Surg* 1985;67B:126–129.

98. Bower WH: The distal radioulnar joint, in Green DP (ed): *Operative Hand Surgery,* ed 2. Philadelphia, JB Lippincott, 1988, pp 939–989.

99. Overgaard S, Solgaard S: Osteoarthritis after Colles' fracture. *Orthopedics* 1989;12:413–416.

100. Dobyns JH, Linscheid RL: Complications of treatment of fractures and dislocations of the wrist, in Epps CH Jr (ed): *Complications in Orthopaedic Surgery.* Philadelphia, JB Lippincott, 1978, pp 271–352.

Wrist Biomechanics

Leonard K. Ruby, MD

Introduction

Although wrist anatomy and function have been studied since medieval times, the current intense interest dates from the classic 1972 paper of Linscheid and associates,[1] which brought traumatic instability of the wrist and its pathomechanics to the clinicians' attention. As they pointed out, their studies were based on the works of several authors, including Destot,[2] Navarro,[3] Gifford and associates,[4] and Fisk.[5] The discovery of X-rays in 1895 by Roentgen had allowed earlier authors to study normal and abnormal wrist anatomy and function in the living subject. With the advent of computer technology, more accurate and detailed information is now available. This chapter attempts to describe some recent advances in our understanding of how the wrist is structured and its function in relation to certain clinical situations.

Anatomy

Bones

The carpus includes four sets of joints. These are from proximal to distal the distal radioulnar joint (DRUJ), the radiocarpal joint (RC), the midcarpal joint (MC), and the carpal metacarpal joints (CMC). We will consider only the radiocarpal and midcarpal joints. The carpus can be thought of as lying in two rows. The proximal row consists of the scaphoid, lunate, and triquetrum. The pisiform is a sesamoid bone in the tendon of the flexor carpi ulnaris and, as such, is not a functional part of the proximal carpal row. The distal row is composed of the trapezium, trapezoid, capitate, and hamate. The scaphoid occupies a unique position, as it spans the midcarpal joint and links the proximal and distal rows[6].

Ligaments

Each bone in each row is relatively tightly and strongly bound to its neighbor by strong interosseous ligaments. The distal row interosseous ligaments seldom fail clinically. The ligaments between the scaphoid and lunate (scapholunate interosseous ligament-SLIL) and the triquetrum and lunate (triquetrolunate interosseous ligament-TLIL) are C-shaped and attach the dorsal, palmar, and proximal edges of these three bones to each other. These ligaments open distally into the midcarpal joint. They are thickened dorsally and pal-

marly with relatively thin membranous portions centrally (Fig. 1). Mayfield and associates[7] and Logan and associates[8] have measured failure strengths and stress/strain behavior of these structures in cadaver specimens. They found that the scapholunate interosseous ligament failed at 232.6 ± 10.9 N (about 45 lbs) and the triquetrolunate interosseous ligament failed at 353.7 ± 69.2 N (about 70 lbs). Further, both these ligaments elongated (strain) from 50% to 100% of their original length before failure.

In addition to the interosseous ligaments, there are dorsal and palmar capsular ligaments, which are thickenings of the wrist capsule. These, too, have been well described by several authors, including Taleisnik,[9] Mayfield and associates,[7] and others.[10] The dorsal ligaments consist of the dorsal radiotriquetral and dorsal intercarpal ligaments. The former may be important as an accessory stabilizer of the lunate triquetral joint and the radiocarpal joint.[11] The palmar ligaments have recently been redescribed by Berger and Landsmeer.[10] According to Taleisnik[9] the palmar ligaments consist of the radioscaphocapitate (RSC), the radiolunate (RL), the radioscapholunate (RSL), the ulnalunate (UL), and the ulnatriquetral (UT) ligaments. In addition, the scaphocapitate and triquetral capitate ligaments cross the midcarpal joint and together form the "V," "deltoid," or "arcuate" ligaments (Fig. 2). According to Berger and Landsmeer,[10] the radioscaphocapitate ligament inserts strongly into the scaphoid and weakly into the capitate. They feel that the radiolunate ligament should be renamed the long radiolunate ligament (LRL) to distinguish it from the short radiolunate ligament (SRL), which originates from the palmar edge off the distal radius at its lunate facet and inserts into the palmar pole of the lunate (Fig. 3). This last ligament has not been previously described and should not be confused with the radioscapholunate ligament of Taleisnik.[9] It is probable that the radioscapholunate is less important as a ligament than as a vascular bundle.[10,12] The same loading to failure and stress/strain testing has been applied to some of the palmar radiocarpal ligaments and these studies have shown that the radioscaphocapitate ligament fails at 151 ± 30 N (30 lbs) and the long radiolunate ligament fails at $107.2 + 14.8$ N (21 lbs). These ligaments elongated approximately 30% before failure. Therefore, the proximal row interosseous ligaments are significantly stronger and more elastic than any of the capsular ligaments that have been tested.

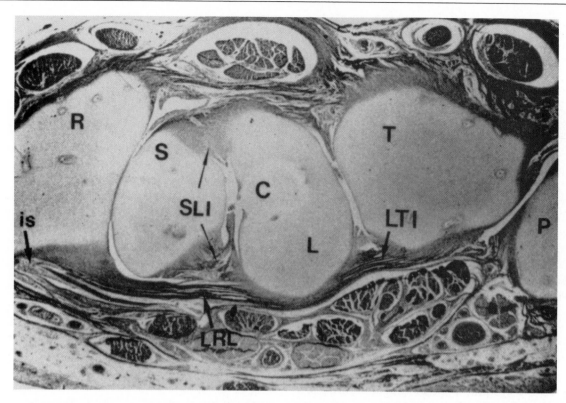

Fig. 1 Cross section of cadaveric wrist through proximal carpal row. R - Radius; S - Scaphoid; C - Capitate; L - Lunate; T - Triquetrum; P - Pisiform; SLI - Scapholunate interosseous ligament; LTI - Lunate triquetral interosseous ligament; and LRL - Long radiolunate ligament. (Reproduced with permission from Berger RA, Landsmeer JMF: The palmar radiocarpal ligaments: A study of adult and fetal human wrist joints. *J Hand Surg* 1990;15A:847–854.)

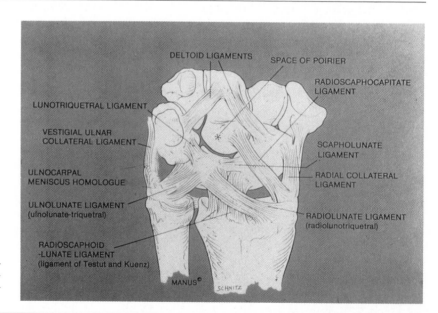

Fig. 2 The palmar wrist ligaments. (Reproduced with permission from Taleisnik J: The ligaments of the wrist. *J Hand Surg* 1976;1A:110–118.)

Tendons

The musculotendinous units that move the wrist originate at the elbow and insert on the metacarpals. The prime flexors are the flexor carpi radialis (FCR) and flexor carpi ulnaris (FCU). The prime extensors are the extensor carpi radialis longus (ECRL) and extensor carpi radialis brevis (ECRB). The primary radial deviator is the abductor pollicis longus (APL), and the ulnar deviator is the extensor carpi ulnaris (ECU). Because all these tendons insert on the metacarpal bases and

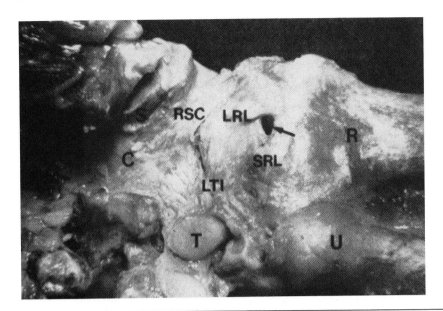

Fig. 3 The palmar ligaments. R - Radius U - Ulna; C - Capitate; T - Triquetrum; RSC - Radio scaphocapitate ligament; LRL - Long radiolunate ligament; SRL - Short radiolunate ligament; LTI - Lunate triquetral interosseous ligament; and (arrow) - Interligament sulcus. (Reproduced with permission from Berger RA, Landsmeer JMF: The palmar radiocarpal ligaments: A study of adult and fetal human wrist joints. *J Hand Surg* 1990;15A:847–854.)

because the carpal metacarpal joints are relatively immobile, the entire proximal row functions as an intercalated segment. No motors are attached to the proximal row of carpals, which is completely controlled by its surrounding structures. The wrist motors are also arranged peripherally, which places them as far from the center of motion (the head of the capitate) as possible. This arrangement allows for a maximum lever arm[6] at the wrist. Conversely, the digital motors are more centrally located (closer to the capitate head), which diminishes their effect on wrist motion. Furthermore, it is likely that the musculotendinous units in their fibro-osseous canals have a dynamic effect on wrist stability, but this has not yet been defined.

Kinematics

There have been two rival theories of wrist function over the last 70 years—the row theory and the column theory. The row theory considers the wrist as two carpal rows; proximal and distal. The column theory, as originally stated by Navarro,[3] considers that the wrist is composed of a radial column, a central column, and an ulnar column. The first of these columns is composed of the scaphoid, trapezium, and trapezoid. The second includes the lunate and capitate and the third, the triquetrum and hamate. The published evidence supports the row theory as being the correct view.[13]

Normal total wrist motion averages 150 degrees, of which 70 degrees is extension and 80 degrees is flexion.[14] Of this total, approximately half occurs at the midcarpal and half at the radiocarpal joint. From neutral to extension, 66% is radiocarpal and 33% is midcarpal. From neutral to flexion, 60% occurs at the mid-

carpal joint (lunate capitate) and 40% at the radiocarpal joint.[15] Total radial ulnar deviation is 50 degrees, of which 20 degrees is radial and 30 degrees ulnar deviation. Of the total, 60% occurs at the midcarpal joint and 40% at the radiocarpal joint.[13]

Not only do the midcarpal and radiocarpal joints contribute different amounts of motion to the total arc, but they also move in different directions when the wrist is moving in radial and ulnar deviation. As the wrist moves from radial to ulnar deviation, the entire proximal row rotates from a position of flexion to extension. As the wrist moves from ulnar to radial deviation, the entire proximal row rotates from extension into flexion. Although the mechanism by which this occurs is not completely understood, most authors agree that it is a combination of the interaction of the geometry of the carpal bones, their ligamentous constraints, and wrist motors acting through the distal row that causes this conjoined synchronous motion (Fig. 4). Linscheid and Dobyns[6] feel that pressure on the distal pole of the scaphoid by the trapezium and trapezoid in radial deviation causes the scaphoid to flex. This flexion is transmitted through the scapholunate interosseous ligament to the lunate and through the triquetrolunate interosseous ligament to the triquetrum, which thereby causes the entire proximal row to flex. The reverse occurs in ulnar deviation with the scaphoid being extended through the scaphotrapezial ligament. Weber[16] has an alternative theory. His impression is that the helicoidal shape of the triquetrohamate articulate causes the distal row to translate dorsally in ulnar deviation, which puts pressure on the dorsal aspect of the proximal row and causes it to extend. In radial deviation, the distal row translates palmarly, which puts pressure on the palmar aspect of the proximal row and

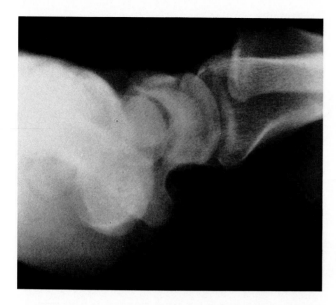
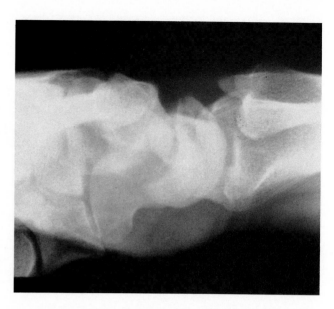

Fig. 4 **Left,** Lateral view of author's wrist in radial deviation. Note flexion of proximal row (lunate and scaphoid). **Right,** Lateral view of author's wrist in ulnar deviation. Note extension of proximal row (lunate and scaphoid) and dorsal translation of distal row.

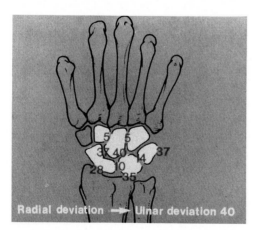
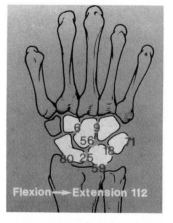

Fig. 5 **Left,** Relative motion of selected carpi bones with respect to each other and the radius as wrist moves from radial to ulnar deviation. (Reproduced with permission from Ruby LK, Cooney WP, An KN, et al: Relative motion of selected carpal bones: A kinematic analysis of the normal wrist. *J Hand Surg* 1988;13A:1–10.) **Right,** Relative motion of selected carpi bones with respect to each other and the radius as wrist moves from flexion to extension.

causes it to flex. Whatever the exact mechanism, there is normally a predictable amount of smooth synchronous motion between and within the two rows. There is less than 9 degrees of motion between the capitate, trapezoid, and hamate in all wrist motions. There are 10 ± 3 degrees of scaphoid-to-lunate motion and 14 ± 6 degrees of triquetrum-to-lunate motion as the wrist moves from radial to ulnar deviation. There are 25 ± 15 degrees of scaphoid-to-lunate motion and 18 ± 2 degrees of triquetrum-to-lunate motion as the wrist moves from flexion to extension.[13] These data are derived from cadaver studies, and it is possible that the actual numbers are greater (Fig. 5).

Force Transmission

The quantitative assessment of force transmission through the carpus has recently been the subject of several papers.[17-21] For technical reasons this has been and continues to be a difficult area to study. Nevertheless, using load cells, pressure sensitive film, and

11 DEGREES OF PALMAR TILT (ORIGINAL POSITION)

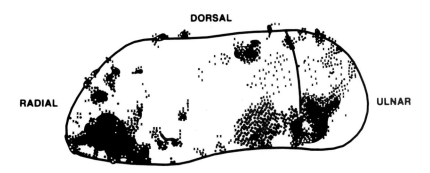

- ■ PRESSURE: >3.2 N/mm² (>460 PSI)
- ▦ PRESSURE: 1.9 TO 3.2 N/mm²
- ▤ PRESSURE: 1.1 TO 1.9 N/mm²

Fig. 6 End-on view of distal radius and triangular fibrocartilage showing contact areas and relative pressures in the normal wrist. Darker areas = higher pressures. (Reproduced with permission from Palmer AK, Werner FW: Biomechanics of the distal radioulnar joint. *Clin Orthop* 1984; 187: 26–35.)

cadaver specimens, data have been generated that describe the magnitude and location of forces at the radiocarpal joint in "normal" cadavers and in simulated abnormal conditions. Palmer and Werner[17] have shown that in the neutral position, in the intact cadaver wrist, 81% of the total load is carried by the radius and 18% by the ulna (Fig. 6). If the ulnar head is resected or the triangular fibrocartilage complex removed, the load borne by the ulna is drastically reduced toward 0%. These findings were confirmed by Trumble and associates[20] who found 83% of the load borne by the radius and 17% by the ulna in intact specimens. Viegas and associates[21] studied contact areas of the radius-triangular fibrocartilage articular surface in loaded cadaver wrist. They concluded that at light loads (23 lbs) only 20% of the available articular surface of the radius was in contact with the proximal row bones. With heavier loads (46 lbs and above) this area increased to a 40% maximum and did not increase further even if the load was doubled. They concluded that there is normally a great deal of incongruity at the radiocarpal joint. They further found that normally the load distribution on the radius is 60% scaphoid facet and 40% lunate facet.[21] The distribution of load at the midcarpal joint has been calculated by Horii and associates[22] as 31% of the total force through the scaphotrapezial trapezoid joint; 19% through the scaphocapitate joint; 29% through the lunate capitate, and 21% through the triquetrohamate joint. These are the areas in which arthritis is most likely to develop.

Clinical Correlations

Scapholunate Dissociation

In a wrist afflicted with this instability, the scaphoid assumes a more flexed position, by 60 degrees or more, with respect to the radius; the lunate becomes more extended by 25 degrees or more; the gap between them exceeds 2 mm to 3 mm; and the distal row migrates proximally (Fig. 7). Most studies confirm the clinical impression[23,24] that at least the entire scapholunate interosseous ligament must be completely disrupted to allow these displacements to occur. It is also probable that other ligaments are injured, although there is some controversy about which are most critical.[23-25] These secondary stabilizers include the long radiolunate ligament, the radioscaphocapitate ligament, and the radioscapholunate ligament. It is my impression that the long radiolunate ligament, which is also known as the radiolunate triquetral ligament, is the most important of these three.[23] Some of the more popular treatment methods for scapholunate dissociation have been analyzed in the laboratory. Garcia-Elias and associates[26] analyzed the changes in wrist kinematics that occur with simulated scaphotrapezial trapezoid fusion and scaphocapitate fusion. They found that both fusions significantly decreased global wrist motion and, perhaps more importantly, they caused articular incongruity by preventing the scaphoid from adapting to the "always changing space between the distal carpal row and the radius."[26] For this and other reasons, I prefer scapholunate linkage procedures in contrast to scaphoid "alignment" procedures.

Triquetrolunate Dissociation

The instability pattern seen in this condition consists of a palmar-flexed lunate and scaphoid, extended triquetrum, and proximal migration of the triquetrum with respect to the lunate. The distal row also migrates proximally but is palmarly displaced as opposed to dorsally displaced in scapholunate dissociation (Fig. 8). Viegas and associates[11] and Trumbel and associates[27] have both studied this problem in the laboratory setting.

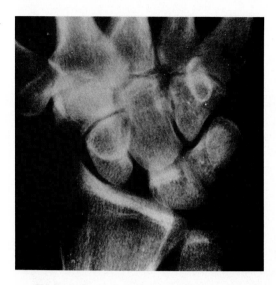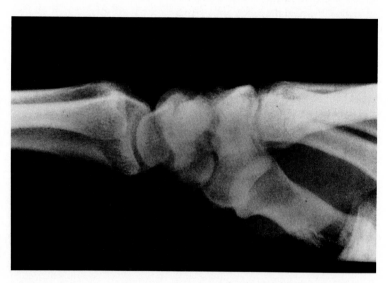

Fig. 7 **Left**, Anteroposterior view of a wrist with scapholunate dissociation showing scapholunate gap, palmar-flexed scaphoid, and extended lunate. (Reproduced with permission from Taleisnik J: *The Wrist*. New York, Churchill-Livingstone, 1985, p. 249.) **Right**, Lateral view of wrist with scapholunate dissociation showing palmar-flexed scaphoid, with dorsal subluxation of the proximal pole and extended lunate.

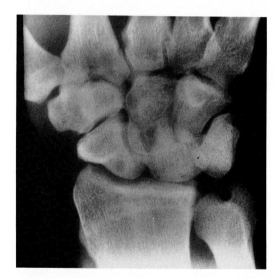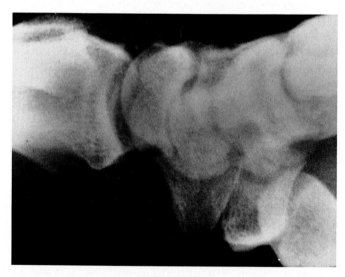

Fig. 8 **Left**, Anteroposterior view of wrist and triquetrolunate dissociation showing T-L step off and palmar-flexed scaphoid and lunate. **Right**, Lateral view of wrist with triquetrolunate dissociation showing palmar-flexed scaphoid and lunate.

These authors concluded that the triquetrolunate interosseous ligament and the palmar and dorsal radiotriquetral ligaments had to be completely disrupted. Trumbel also felt that the triquetrocapitate ligament was compromised.[27] Clinically, triquetrolunate linkage procedures are popular, but there is no laboratory data on their efficacy.

Kienböck's Disease

In the late stages of osteonecrosis of the lunate—stages III and IV—(Fig. 9) the carpus collapses into a dorsal intercalary segment instability pattern, with the scaphoid assuming a palmar-flexed position and the distal row migrating proximally. Laboratory studies have focused on the effect of various surgical procedures on lunate unloading, because increased force may be causing the lunate to become avascular and to collapse. Furthermore, some authors feel that unloading the bone may allow it to heal. Trumble and associates[18] studied capitolunate fusion, scaphoid trapezium trapezoid fusion, ulnar lengthening, and radial shortening. They concluded that only capitohamate arthrodesis failed to relieve lunate load. Horii and associates[22] studied scaphotrapezial trapezoid arthrodesis, scaphocapitate arthrodesis, capitohamate arthrodesis, capitate shortening plus capitohamate arthrodesis, ulnar lengthening, and radial shortening. They found that both ulnar lengthening and radial shortening decreased the force at the lunate radial joint by 45% without adversely affecting other intercarpal joints. However, ulnalunate and ulnatriquetral loads were increased by 50% and 78%, respectively. Of the other procedures, scaphotrapezial trapezoid fusion unloaded the lunate by 5% and scaphocapitate fusion unloaded it by 12%. Capitohamate fusion had no effect. Capitate shortening had the greatest effect on lunate unloading—60%—but dramatically overloaded the triquetrohamate and scaphotriquetral joints—14% and 69%, respectively. These authors concluded that joint leveling procedures were the least disruptive to normal carpal loading and the most effective at lunate unloading.

Scaphoid Fracture

Weber and Chao[28] were able to produce scaphoid fractures in cadaver wrists by subjecting them to between 460 and 960 lbs of force applied to the radial palmar aspect of the hand with the wrist in between 95 and 100 degrees of extension. They felt that the radial collateral ligament was lax in this position and that the scaphoid fractured because its unsupported distal portion was subject to bending stress over the dorsal lip of the radius. If less wrist extension was used in the cadavers, fractures of the radius were produced instead. For this reason, these researchers recommended a position of slight radial deviation and palmar flexion of the wrist to immobilize scaphoid waist fractures. Burgess[29] has shown, in cadavers, that with 15 degrees

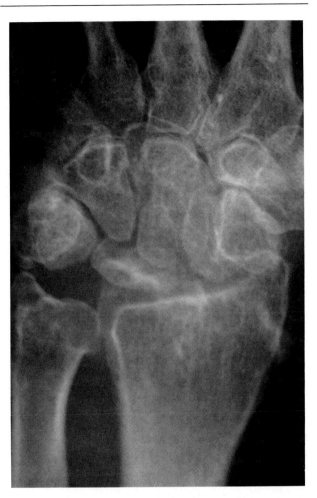

Fig. 9 Anteroposterior view of wrist with advanced lunate collapse secondary to Kienböck's disease. Note palmar-flexed scaphoid.

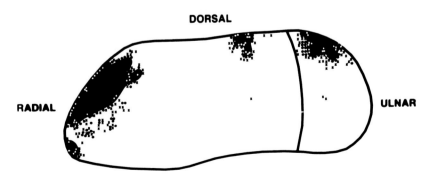

28 DEGREES OF DORSAL TILT

DORSAL

RADIAL

ULNAR

■ PRESSURE: >3.2 N/mm² (>460 PSI)

▦ PRESSURE: 1.9 TO 3.2 N/mm²

▥ PRESSURE: 1.1 TO 1.9 N/mm²

Fig. 10 End-on view of distal radius and triangular fibrocartilage with 28 degrees dorsal tilt showing high pressure on dorsal rim of radius and ulna. (Reproduced with permission from Palmer, AK, Werner FW: Biomechanics of the distal radioulnar joint. *Clin Orthop* 1984; 187: 26–35.)

of palmar angulation in simulated scaphoid waist fractures, all radiocarpal contribution to wrist extension would be lost. With 30 degrees of angulation, all midcarpal extension would also be lost. This implies, as clinical studies have shown, that union alone is not enough; accurate reduction is also necessary in scaphoid fractures. Smith and associates[30] simulated scaphoid fractures in loaded cadaver wrists and used an accurate computer analysis to measure the effect on wrist kinematics. They demonstrated increased motion and angulation between the proximal and distal rows in all specimens, which duplicates the clinical situation of dorsal intercalary segment instability in scaphoid nonunions. This is the best evidence yet that the scaphoid is a bony link between the distal and proximal rows, and that it must be aligned and stabilized to restore normal carpal kinematics.

Distal Radius Fracture

Short and associates[31] performed osteotomies on cadaver radii and simulated increasing dorsal tilt of the radial articular surface. They concluded that as angulation changed from a normal 10 degrees of palmar tilt to 45 degrees of dorsal tilt, contact areas shifted to the dorsal lip of the radius and the load on the ulna increased from a normal 21% to 67% of the total load (Fig. 10). This fits well with the clinical finding that distal radius malunion patients often present with ulna wrist pain from ulna carpal impingement.

Conclusion

As more sophisticated quantitative analysis of normal and abnormal wrist function becomes available, clinicians are making greater efforts to restore wrist injuries more nearly to anatomic configuration. Treatment techniques are being guided to some extent by information provided by these analyses. As clinical studies corroborate these laboratory studies, our approach to wrist problems should continue to improve.

References

1. Linscheid RL, Dobyns JH, Beabout JW, et al: Traumatic instability of the wrist: Diagnosis, classification, and pathomechanics. *J Bone Joint Surg* 1972;54A:1612–1632.
2. Destot E: *Injuries of the Wrist and Radiological Study.* London, Ernest Benn, 1925.
3. Navarro A: *Anales de Instituto de Clinica Quirurgica y Cirugia Experimental.* Montevideo, Imprenta Artistica de Dornaleche Hnos, 1935.
4. Gifford WW, Bolton RH, Lambrinudi C: The mechanisn of the wrist area with special reference to fractures of the scaphoid. *Guys Hosp Rep* 1943;92:52–59.
5. Fisk GR: Carpal instability and the fractured scaphoid: Hunterian lecture delivered at the Royal College of Surgeons of England. *Ann R Coll Surg, Engl* 1970;46:63–76.
6. Linscheid RL, Dobyns JH: Carpal instability. *Curr Orthop* 1989; 3:106–114.
7. Mayfield JK, Johnson RP, Kilcoyne RF: The ligaments of the human wrist and their functional significance. *Anat Rec* 1976; 186:417–428.
8. Logan SE, Nowak MD, Gould PL, et al: Biomechanical behavior of the scapholunate ligament. *Biomed Sci Instrum* 1986;22:81–85.
9. Taleisnik J: The ligaments of the wrist. *J Hand Surg* 1976;1A: 110–118.
10. Berger RA, Landsmeer JMF: The palmar radiocarpal ligaments: A study of adult and fetal human wrist joints. *J Hand Surg* 1990; 15A:847–854.
11. Viegas SF, Patterson RM, Patterson PD, et al: Ulnar sided perilunate instability: An anatomic and biomechanical study. *J Hand Surg* 1990;15A:268–278.
12. Hixson ML, Stuart C: Microvascular anatomy of the radioscapholunate ligament of the wrist. *J Hand Surg* 1990;15A:279–282.
13. Ruby LK, Cooney WP, An KN, et al: Relative motion of selected carpal bones: A kinematic analysis of the normal wrist. *J Hand Surg* 1988;13A:1–10.
14. Heck CV, Hendryson IE, Carter RR: *Joint Motion: Method of Measuring and Recording.* Chicago, American Academy of Orthopaedic Surgeons, 1965, p 14.
15. Sarrafian SK, Melamed JL, Goshgarian GM: Study of wrist motion in flexion and extension. *Clin Orthop* 1977;126:153–159.
16. Weber ER: Concepts governing the rotational shift of the intercalated segment of the carpus. *Orthop Clin North Am* 1984;15: 193–207.
17. Palmer AK, Werner FW: Biomechanics of the distal radioulnar joint. *Clin Orthop* 1984;187:26–35.
18. Trumble T, Glisson RR, Seaber AV, et al: A biomechanical comparison of the methods for treating Kienböck's disease. *J Hand Surg* 1986;11A:88–93.
19. Viegas SF, Tencer AF, Cantrell J, et al: Load transfer characteristics of the wrist: Part I. The normal joint. *J Hand Surg* 1987; 12A:971–978.
20. Trumble T, Glisson RR, Seaber AV, et al: Forearm force transmission after surgical treatment of distal radio ulnar joint disorders. *J Hand Surg* 1987;12A:196–202.
21. Viegas SF, Patterson R, Petterson P, et al: The effects of various load paths and different loads on the load transfer characteristics of the wrist. *J Hand Surg* 1989;14A:458–465.
22. Horii E, Garcia-Elias M, An KN, et al: Effect on force transmission across the carpus in procedures used to treat Kienbock's disease. *J Hand Surg* 1990;15A:393–400.
23. Ruby LK, An KN, Linscheid RL, et al: The effect of scapholunate ligament section on scapholunate motion. *J Hand Surg* 1987; 12A:767–771.
24. Meade TD, Schneider LA, Cherry K: Radiographic analysis of selective ligament sectioning at the carpal scaphoid: A cadaver study. *J Hand Surg* 1990;15A:855–862.
25. Berger RA, Blair WF, Crowninshield RD, et al: The scapholunate ligament. *J Hand Surg* 1982;7A:87–91.
26. Garcia-Elias M, Cooney WP, An KN, et al: Wrist kinematics after limited intercarpal arthrodesis. *J Hand Surg* 1989;14A:791–799.
27. Trumble TE, Bour CJ, Smith RJ, et al: Kinematics of the ulnar carpus related to the volar intercalated segment instability pattern. *J Hand Surg* 1990;15A:384–392.
28. Weber ER, Chao EY: An experimental approach to the mechanism of scaphoid waist fractures. *J Hand Surg* 1978;3A:142–148.
29. Burgess RC: The effect of a simulated scaphoid malunion on wrist motion. *J Hand Surg* 1987;12A:774–776.
30. Smith DK, Cooney WP III, An KN, et al: The effects of simulated unstable scaphoid fractures on carpal motion. *J Hand Surg* 1989; 14A:283–291.
31. Short WH, Palmer AK, Werner FW, et al: A biomechanical study of distal radial fractures. *J Hand Surg* 1987;12A:529–534.

Carpal Instability: Treatment of Ligament Injuries of the Wrist

William P. Cooney III, MD

Ronald L. Linscheid, MD

James H. Dobyns, MD

Introduction

Understanding the optimum treatment of ligament injuries about the wrist is difficult, particularly in view of new complex information about these injuries.[1] Since the classic description of posttraumatic carpal instability in 1972,[2] a number of different recommendations have been made regarding direct ligament repair,[3,4] ligament construction,[5-9] and stabilization by intercarpal fusion.[10-13] The controversy over which reconstructive procedures are most appropriate and easiest to adapt to different clinical presentations has been recently clarified.[4] The purpose of this chapter is to review the current concepts regarding management of carpal instabilities with respect to the time of presentation, the degree of ligament damage, and the presence or absence of associated arthritis. Because lasting knowledge requires a clear understanding of underlying principles, a brief review of the anatomy, physiology, and classification of carpal instability is included, and precedes the presentation of diagnostic criteria and specific treatment alternatives.

Anatomy and Physiology

The carpus is a complex unit of two carpal rows, the bony articulations of which are closely integrated to provide a wide range of motion with a framework of unparalleled stability.[14] Using the concept of Landsmeer,[15] the proximal carpal row may be described as an intercalated segment within a linked kinematic chain, to which no muscles or tendon attachments are attached (Fig. 1). Control of position of the two rows and of the individual carpal bones depends on carpal bone surface anatomy and positions of both intrinsic and extrinsic ligaments.[16-19] The extrinsic ligaments are specifically aligned to constrain rotational displacement of the proximal carpal row by closely binding the scaphoid, lunate, and triquetrum to the distal radius by a proximal inverted V-shaped ligament.[17,19] A second stabilizing group of extrinsic ligaments, which extends from the distal radius, attaches distally to the capitate and hamate, and then returns to the base of the ulnar styloid, provides the main anchor of the distal carpal row.[19,20] Nomenclature relating to the origin and insertion of the radiocarpal ligaments has recently been reviewed by Berger and associates.[16] The articular surfaces contribute to carpal stability by forming an acetabulum-shaped midcarpal joint, which constrains radial and ulnar deviation. The extrinsic ligaments mainly

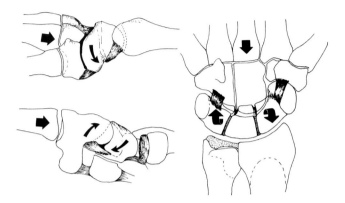

Fig. 1   Normal carpal kinematics. Under normal compressive loads across the wrist, (**top left**) the scaphoid will tend to palmar flex while the triquetrum (**bottom left**) is pushed into extension. The capitate and hamate linked as part of the distal carpal row influence the direction of proximal carpal bone rotation. The integrity of the scapholunate and lunotriquetral interosseous ligaments is crucial to balance (**right**) the two opposite rotational motions. (Reproduced with permission from Cooney WP III, Garcia-Elias M, Dobyns JH, et al: Anatomy and mechanics of carpal instability. *Surg Rounds Orthop* 1989;9:15–24).

limit flexion and extension. Displacement or a change in alignment of the proximal carpal row results primarily from compressive loads induced through the capitate and hamate across the carpal or acetabulum-shaped midcarpal joint. Any break in the stabilizing ligaments (intrinsic, extrinsic, or a combination of both) disrupts the smooth transition of compressive forces and results in carpal instability (Fig. 2).[21]

Motions of the wrist are centered on the head of the capitate in both flexion and extension as well as in radioulnar deviation.[22-24] The proximal carpal row is controlled radially by the "slider crank" effect of the scaphoid[25] and ulnarly by the helicoidal shape of the triquetrohamate articulation.[26] In radial deviation, the scaphoid flexes to clear the radiostyloid and the attachments of the intercarpal ligaments between the scaphoid-to-lunate and lunate-to-triquetrum cause the entire proximal row to follow.[27] In ulnar deviation, the scaphoid extends, bringing the lunate and triquetrum synchronously with it as the pull of the ulnar wrist tendons (extensor carpi ulnaris and flexor carpi ulnaris) forces the hamate down the inclined slope of the triquetrum. With a loss of intrinsic or extrinsic intercarpal ligament stability, this synchronous motion is lost, leading characteristically to a dorsi-angulated lunate insta-

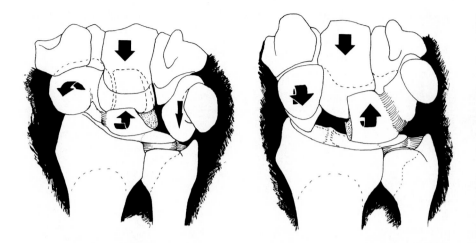

Fig. 2 Carpal instability. **Left**, Scapho-lunate dissociation (from a palmar view) demonstrating the gap between the scaphoid, which is palmar-flexed (down-ward arrow), and the lunate, which is dor-siflexed (upward arrow), and the capitate, which compresses the scapholunate in-terval contributing to the diastasis. **Right**, Lunotriquetral dissociation (palmar view) demonstrating palmar-flexion of the scaphoid and lunate and rotational dis-placement with extension and supination of the triquetrum. A mild diastasis (gap) between the lunate and triquetrum can be observed. (Reproduced with permis-sion from Cooney WP III, Garcia-Elias M, Dobyns JH, et al: Anatomy and mechanics of carpal instability. *Surg Rounds Orthop* 1989;9:15–24).

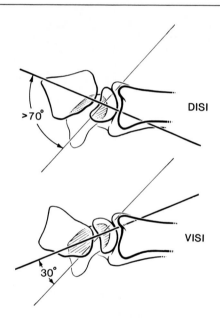

Fig. 3 **Top**, In dorsiflexion-intercalated segment instability, the lunate extends and the scaphoid flexes, resulting in a scapholunate angle of greater than 70 degrees. **Bottom**, In volar flexion-interca-lated segment instability, the lunate is flexed and the scaphoid remains neutral to slight flexion resulting in a scapholunate angle of 30 de-grees or less.

bility (dorsal intercalary segment instability) with scaph-oid-lunate dissociation or to a volar-angulated lunate instability (volar intercalary segment instability) with lunate-triquetrum dissociation (Fig. 3).[1,21,28,29] Under-standing the physiologic basis of wrist motion requires a knowledge of the complexity of the intrinsic and ex-trinsic carpal ligaments as well as a comprehension of the kinematics of the wrist during both normal and pathologic situations.

Classification of Carpal Instability

Carpal instability results in the loss of normal liga-mentous and bony constraints that control the wrist.[30] Under compressive loads there is a loss of normal sta-bility, so that forces of pinch and grasp are not directed across the distal radius and ulna in a uniform manner. In a practical sense, carpal instability results from injury to either the intrinsic or the extrinsic ligaments of the wrist (or from a fracture through the bony stabilizing elements, such as the scaphoid).[31] Two types of carpal instability have been identified by Dobyns: carpal in-stability dissociative (CID) and carpal instability non-dissociative (CIND).[32,33] Loss of intrinsic ligament sup-port results in a dissociation of the bones of the proximal carpal row, a condition classically character-ized as carpal instability dissociative (CID). In the sec-ond type, loss of the extrinsic ligaments that support the wrist can result in a carpal instability with rotational deformity of the proximal carpal row (but intact inter-osseous ligaments), referred to as carpal instability non-dissociative (CIND). Intrinsic ligaments are intercarpal ligaments that connect carpal bones in the same row. The scapholunate and lunotriquetral ligaments are the most familiar intercarpal ligaments.[19,30]

Carpal instability dissociative can be separated from carpal instability nondissociative (CIND) by the pres-ence of contrast dye on arthrography[34–36] across the ra-diocarpal and midcarpal joint (Fig. 4, *right*).[32,37] Dis-sociative carpal instability is characterized by disruption of the intercarpal ligaments between the scaphoid and lunate or lunate and triquetrum. It has been recognized that there also exist fairly strong interosseous ligaments that connect the scaphoid and capitate and the capitate and hamate.[16] It is important to note that no intercarpal ligaments cross between the proximal and distal carpal rows. By definition, in a nondissociative carpal insta-bility, the intercarpal ligaments are not torn, and, there-

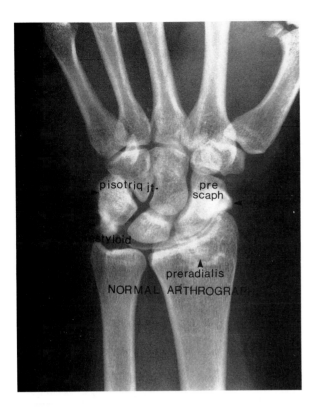
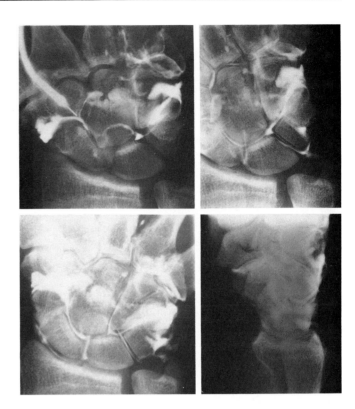

Fig. 4 Wrist arthrography. **Left,** Normal arthrogram demonstrating a dye column in the radiocarpal joint without filling of the midcarpal joint. Note normal prescaphoid recess, preradialis recess, prestyloid recess and filling of the pisotriquetral joint. **Right,** Abnormal midcarpal arthrogram sequentially showing dye (contrast) fill across the lunotriquetral joint (top right) and scapholunate joint (lower left). A positive arthrogram is indicative of carpal instability, dissociative. (Reproduced with permission from Cooney WP III, Linscheid RL, Dobyns JH: Fractures and dislocations of the wrist, in Rockwood CA Jr, Green DP (eds): *Fractures in Adults*, ed 3. Philadelphia, JB Lippincott, 1991, p 613.)

fore, the arthrogram is normal (Fig. 5).[33] These injuries result from damage to the extrinsic capsular ligaments that pass from the distal radius and ulna to the proximal or distal carpal row. Although most investigators believe that the volar radiocarpal ligaments are most involved in CIND deformities,[38-40] two recent studies indicate that the dorsal radiotriquetral ligament also provides important control in ulnar carpal instability.[41,42] Primary extrinsic ligament damage can lead to radiocarpal or midcarpal instability. An example of radiocarpal instability is dorsal dislocation of the radiocarpal joint secondary to disruption of the volar extrinsic ligaments. Midcarpal instability[38] can be more subtle and consists of either ligament attenuation between the scaphoid and capitate[43] and/or the triquetrum and capitate.[39] This is sometimes called capitolunate instability pattern (CLIP),[40,44] ulnocarpal, or dynamic instability, and it is usually seen with a volar intercalary segment instability (VISI) pattern. Midcarpal instability can also be associated with malalignment of distal radius fractures leading to secondary midcarpal instability, in which the lunate rides up dorsally on the distal radius.[45] The volar flex position of the lunate in CIND deformities, however, can also be associated

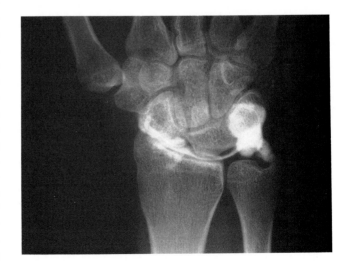

Fig. 5 A normal radiocarpal arthrogram in a patient with midcarpal instability; the scaphoid, lunate, and triquetrum are palmarflexed. A negative arthrogram with radiographic appearance of deformity is indicative of carpal instability, nondissociative.

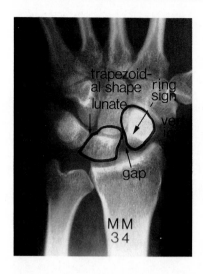

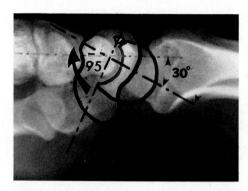

Fig. 6   Radiographic appearance of scapholunate disassociation. **Left**, The scaphoid is palmar flexed (vertical) and separated from the lunate, which is extended. This produces a scaphoid ring sign and scapholunate gap along with a trapezoidal shaped lunate. **Right**, Lateral radiograph demonstrates dorsiflexed position of the lunate and palmar flexed position of the scaphoid, resulting in a scapholunate angle of 95 degrees and radiolunate angle of 30 degrees. (Reproduced with permission from Cooney WP III, Linscheid RL, Dobyns JH: Fractures and dislocations of the wrist, in Rockwood CA Jr, Green DP (eds): *Fractures in Adults*, ed 3. Philadelphia, JB Lippincott, 1991, p 613.)

with rupture of the dorsal radiocarpal ligaments.[42] These are just several examples of nondissociative carpal instability.

Classification by Position

Carpal instability has also been previously classified based on the position of mechanical instability. Loss of lateral carpal support usually results in a pattern of instability in which the lunate faces dorsally from its normal position.[1,32] This dorsiflexion instability (dorsal intercalary segment instability deformity)[6,21] results from intercarpal ligament injury between the scaphoid and lunate (Fig. 2, *left*) or from a displaced fracture of the scaphoid.[25] Because the scaphoid has a strong tendency to rotate into flexion with respect to the longitudinal axis of the wrist[46,47] and the triquetrum has a tendency to extend at the hamatotriquetral joint,[26] a rotational malalignment occurs between the scaphoid and the lunate, resulting in scapholunate dissociation. This deformity is recognized clinically and radiographically as a scapholunate gap with a palmar rotated scaphoid[47,48] and an extended lunate (Fig. 6). The capitate usually is displaced proximally into the scapholunate gap. In reference to the general classification (above) this deformity is classified as a carpal instability dissociative, dorsal intercalary segment instability type, with the primary injury involving the scapholunate interosseous ligaments.[21,32,37] Secondary extrinsic carpal ligament injury is believed to play a role in controlling the degree of carpal collapse that results from scapholunate instability as well as the degree of rotational displacement of both the scaphoid and lunate. Such secondary injury results in a progression toward advanced collapse of the scaphoid, leading to radiocarpal arthrosis.[4]

Carpal instability on the ulnar side of the wrist[49,50] results from the loss of stability between the lunate and the triquetrum.[42,51] This presents as a pattern of instability in which the triquetrum extends and the lunate (Fig. 7), influenced by the scaphoid, flexes. The result is a volar flexion or volar intercalary segment instability pattern of carpal instability. Clinically and radiographically, the signs of instability are more subtle and more difficult to recognize than those of scapholunate dissociation.[52] The gap between the lunate and the triquetrum is not commonly observed, although occasionally the smooth arc of articular surfaces across the proximal carpal row may be disrupted (Fig. 7).[53,54] Excessive volar flexion of the lunate in the volar intercalary segment instability deformity is commonly seen on the lateral radiographic view (and is diagnostic) but a triangular rather than a rectangular appearance of the lunate may also be seen in the posteroanterior view. On careful examination, one can also see a triquetrum that appears to be extended on the triquetrohamate articulation. Lunotriquetral dissociation is classified as a carpal instability dissociative, volar intercalary segment instability type, with the primary injury to the lunotriquetral interosseous ligaments.[32,50] Progression to the volar intercalary segment instability deformity actually requires attenuation or rupture of dorsal or volar extrinsic carpal ligaments.[42]

Diagnosis of Carpal Instability

Patients with carpal instability have a history of pain, weakness, and giving away, with occasional snapping or clicking associated with single or repetitive use of the wrist. There is tenderness over the area of ligament injury, such as tenderness over the scapholunate articulation, which is located just distal to Lister's tubercle, or tenderness over the lunotriquetral articulation, which is just distal to the head of the ulna. Marked

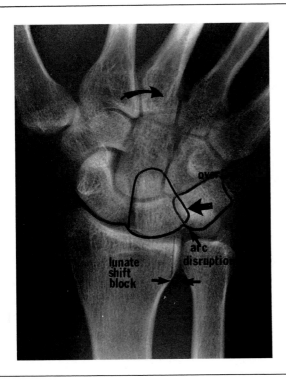

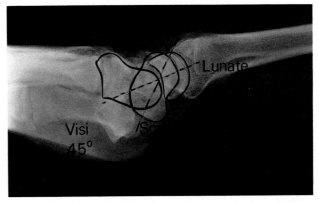

Fig. 7 Radiographic appearance of lunotriquetral instability. **Left,** In this posteroanterior radiograph, the lunate is palmar-flexed and triangular in shape; it overlaps the triquetrum. The triquetrum is extended and rotated, both of these contribute to disruption of the normal smooth arc of the proximal carpal row. **Right,** In this lateral radiograph, the lunate and scaphoid are palmar flexed and the capitate and triquetrum are extended, producing a volar-flexed (volar intercalary segment instability) appearance. (Reproduced with permission from Reagan DS, Linscheid RL, Dobyns JH: Lunotriquetral sprains. *J Hand Surg* 1984;9A:508.)

swelling of the wrist is unusual except immediately after an acute injury. Pain is usually present at the extremes of motion, and a characteristic click or snap may be elicited during repetitive radioulnar deviation. Dynamic stress testing of the wrist may be diagnostic.[52] This is particularly true in scapholunate dissociation, where a snap or painful catch may be elicited as the wrist is brought from ulnar to radial deviation with the examiner's thumb blocking flexion of the distal scaphoid by application of pressure over the scaphoid tubercle (Watson's test). Other stress tests include dorsal volar displacement of the scaphoid on the lunate, scapholunate ballottement, and radial compression of the scaphoid against the lunate or distal radius by exerting pressure just distal to the radial styloid. Excessive laxity of the distal scaphoid is indicated by volar prominence of the vertically aligned scaphoid.

Similarly, on the ulnar side of the wrist, lunotriquetral stress loading by a dorsal volar ballottement (attributed to Linscheid)[55] or ulnar to radial compression of the triquetrum against the lunate (attributed to Kleinman)[56] can also be diagnostic. Lunotriquetral dissociation must be differentiated from injury to the triangular fibrocartilage by discrete palpation. Pain at the extremes of forearm pronation-supination indicates primarily pathology related to the distal radioulnar joint. It may be intensified by ballottement of the head of the ulna. Occasionally, lunotriquetral and triangular fibrocartilage tears are seen in the same patient.

The definitive diagnosis of intercarpal scapholunate or lunotriquetral injury is by invasive examination: wrist

arthrography[34–36,53] and/or wrist arthroscopy.[57,58] Midcarpal arthrography is less likely to result in a false negative examination.[35] A video radiographic recording is used to replay the injection of contrast media and to record the location of contrast crossing from the midcarpal to the radiocarpal joint. A second injection of contrast media into the distal radioulnar joint is helpful to assess triangular fibrocartilage damage. A radiocarpal arthrogram has also been recommended, when the pathology appears primarily within the radiocarpal or distal radioulnar joint.[34,53] Each of these techniques should be diagnostic, but Zinberg and associates[59] suggest that a triple-phase injection arthrogram is best to avoid false negative studies. Many interosseous ligament tears of the wrist (incomplete or chronic tears) may require more detailed study, including stress roentgenographic views, gripping or wrist motion views, or distraction-compression studies.[52]

Wrist arthroscopy[57,58] is an appropriate alternative to wrist arthrography, because it can determine more accurately the location and extent of pathology in the diagnosis of internal derangement of the wrist. Combining multiple portals with triangulation probes, the specific location and size of ligament tears can be diagnosed more accurately with arthroscopy than with arthrography, which usually indicates only that some ligament damage has occurred. Wrist arthroscopy can assess the tautness of volar carpal ligaments, the degree of ligament damage, and the presence of more than one area of pathology. Arthrography and arthroscopy are preferred procedures to assess carpal instability and provide better information than can be gained by other diagnostic studies, including bone scan, cineradiographic stress testing, and ultrasound.[60] Magnetic resonance imaging enhanced by gadolinium or saline can be quite specific in the identification of ligament tears of the wrist and can help to accurately separate extrinsic from intrinsic carpal ligament damage. The full potential of magnetic resonance imaging as a noninvasive method of diagnosing intra-articular carpal ligament injuries awaits further study.

Treatment of Carpal Instabilities

The treatment of carpal instabilities must be considered based on factors related to the following: (1) the time of presentation (acute or chronic); (2) the degree of pathology; and (3) the presence of associated carpal injuries.[4] With respect to acute injuries, the wrist, much like other joint systems (the knee joint, ankle or shoulder), is quite capable of healing by ligament repair, particularly if the diagnosis is made early. For recent injuries of the wrist in which the routine radiograph is normal, immediate joint aspiration combined with wrist arthrography is recommended. The aspirate is inspected for blood or for fat globules, which can indicate an occult fracture. The arthrogram is examined for dye leakage between the proximal and distal carpal rows. If these studies are positive, wrist arthroscopy should be considered to determine the extent or seriousness of the potential ligament injury. These techniques are used to distinguish a strain or partial ligament tear from a complete ligament tear, in which carpal instability can be anticipated. Based on the degree of ligament damage, treatment can proceed with either: (1) arthroscopically controlled reduction and pinning of a scapholunate or lunotriquetral dissociation, or (2) open reduction and direct scapholunate or lunotriquetral ligament repair. If closed pinning techniques are to be used, arthroscopic and imaging control are essential for accurate placement of internal fixation Kirschner-wires (K-wires). Arthroscopy can also be used to determine the preferred approach for open reduction and internal ligament repair. For example, a radial incision is preferred for repair of scapholunate dissociation, and an ulnar incision is preferred for a lunotriquetral dissociation. In our experience, the scapholunate ligament can be torn either through the dorsal third along with an intramembranous extension or through the volar third with primary extrinsic ligament involvement. For the former injury, a dorsal approach is preferred, with ligament repair (Fig. 8). For the latter, a volar approach is recommended for volar radiocarpal ligament advancement and scapholunate ligament repair. Most recent laboratory studies have shown that the dorsal one third and volar one third of both the scapholunate and lunotriquetral ligaments are the key support structures, and that the membranous portion is probably less essential structurally, because it is fibrocartilaginous and not ligamentous.

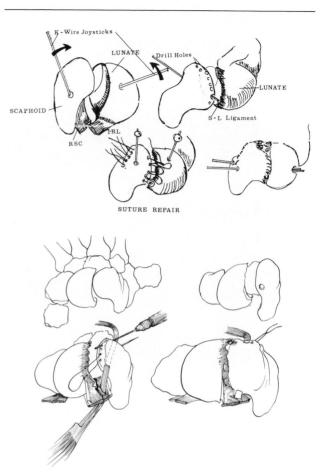

Fig. 8 Techniques for scapholunate ligament repair. **Top**, Acute (subacute) ligament tear. K-wire joysticks assist in reducing the scaphoid and lunate (**upper left**); retrograde drill holes are placed through the waist of the scaphoid into the scapholunate interval (**upper right**). After sutures are placed through the retained ligament attached to the lunate and brought through the scaphoid (**lower left**), the scapholunate ligament repair is completed and held with transfixing K-wires. **Bottom**, Alternative ligament repair techniques. A portion of the flexor carpi radialis (FCR) is drilled from a palmar to dorsal direction through the scaphoid to augment repair of the scapholunate ligament and support volar-carpal ligaments.

In the repair of acute ligament injuries of the wrist as well as subacute injuries of the wrist (those from four weeks to six months from the time of injury),[11] excellent results can be accomplished with open repair techniques that reattach intercarpal ligaments to the bone. Open repair is preferred to closed percutaneous pinning except in acute ligament injuries, because closed treatment has not been carefully studied in subacute carpal instabilities.

Chronic ligament tears of the wrist are defined as those that are first seen 12 months or more after the time of injury.[4,5] These usually have a more progressive change with respect to carpal instability beyond that of a simple intraosseous ligament injury. When rotational subluxation of the scaphoid is present, for example, more specific treatment techniques will be required to

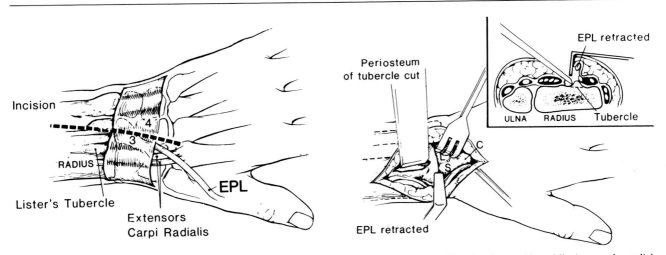

Fig. 9 Universal dorsal approach to the wrist. **Left,** The skin incision is made directly over Lister's tubercle (dotted line) or to the radial side of the third dorsal compartment. **Right,** With the skin flaps elevated, the periosteum is divided and Lister's tubercle is removed with an osteotome to increase exposure. (Reproduced with permission from Weil C, Ruby LK: The dorsal approach to the wrist revisited. *J Hand Surg* 1986;11A:911.)

reduce the carpal instability, followed by either a ligament reconstruction[20,37] or intercarpal fusion.[11,12] In these situations, it is important to differentiate between the treatment alternatives based on the second factor mentioned above, that is, the degree of ligament pathology. When chronic carpal instability is present, the surgeon has two alternatives to consider: (1) ligament repair with capsuloplasty, assuming carpal stability can be reduced,[1,3,4,32] or (2) intercarpal fusion.[11-13] For chronic scapholunate ligament tears with a scapholunate gap of 3 to 5 mm and a scapholunate angle of 60 to 80 degrees with reducible carpal instability, we generally recommend that ligament repair and/or reconstruction be strongly considered.[4,5] The techniques of this will be described later. However, if chronic instability is present, with a fixed deformity accompanied by difficulty in reducing the scaphoid, excessive lunate rotation, or a capitate that is proximally displaced into the scapholunate gap, an intercarpal fusion of the scaphoid either to the capitate[51] or to the trapeziotrapezoidal joint is preferred.[12] Intercarpal fusion is also the preferred technique for manual laborers or athletes who have excessive stress potential across the wrist. These concepts will continue to be valid until stronger, lasting methods of ligament reconstruction can be demonstrated. Finally, when there is evidence of cartilage damage or early signs of arthritis within the wrist, radiocarpal or midcarpal wrist fusions should be the treatment of choice, rather than ligament reconstruction or limited two-bone fusions.[61]

For lunotriquetral ligament tears, a similar treatment approach is recommended, because good results can be anticipated from direct repair of early lunotriquetral ligament injuries[50,55] Reconstruction or fusion should be reserved for late presentation of lunotriquetral ligament tears.[62] With late instability, in which a volar intercalary segment instability (VISI) deformity is well established, extrinsic ligament reconstruction may be required, in addition to interosseous ligament repair or lunotriquetral fusions.[42] Lunotriquetral-capitate-hamate fusions[38,63] have also been recommended for advanced lunotriquetral instability with volar intercalary segment instability deformity. If there is any associated ulnar carpal abutment, these procedures may require a simultaneous ulnar recessional osteotomy.[64]

Specific Treatment Techniques

Ligament Repair Local tissues that remain attached to the adjacent carpal bone can usually be used to repair scapholunate or lunotriquetral ligaments. We believe it is best to reattach these local tissues to fresh bone edges through drill holes with stout nonresorbable sutures of 2-0 or 3-0 Mersilene or Dacron. After ligament repair, the repair site should be stabilized for a minimum of eight weeks by transfixing K-wires. Local collagen tissue from an adjacent joint capsule or tendons can be used to augment repair of subacute or chronic injuries. Previous techniques that involved drilling large holes in the lunate, scaphoid, and triquetrum to pass tendons have been largely revised or abandoned.[8]

Scapholunate Ligament Repair Scapholunate ligament repair is usually performed through a dorsal exposure aligned with Lister's tubercle. Arthroscopy or arthrography should have demonstrated that a tear involved the dorsal one third to one half of the scapholunate ligament. A universal dorsal approach described by Weil and Ruby[23] is recommended (Fig. 9). The dissection is between the third and fourth extensor compartments, and Lister's tubercle is detached in a subperiosteal fashion with the extensor retinaculum. The extensor pollicis longus and wrist extensor tendons are retracted radially and the extensor digitorum communis is retracted ulnarly. The joint capsule is exposed by self-retaining retractors. It is important to divide the capsule incision in line with the dorsal radiotriquetral ligament and dorsal intercarpal ligament, because these structures may be needed later for ligament reconstruction. For better exposure of the radiocarpal joint, a Jones elevator placed between the lunate and distal radius can be used to distract the carpal joint for inspection of the scapholunate ligament region. Palpation with a dental probe or nerve hook confirms the area of scapholunate ligament tear. To improve exposure, K-wires, inserted dorsally into both the scaphoid and the lunate, are used as "joysticks" to assist in manipulating the carpal bones for ligament repair and to assist in eventual reduction of the carpal instability.[20] The K-wire "joysticks" are often essential to reach the middle to volar third of the scapholunate ligament region. As the initial step in the scapholunate ligament repair, drill holes are placed across the waist of the scaphoid from a distal to proximal (or proximal to distal) direction with the drill exiting (or entering) at the scapholunate cartilage interface (Fig. 8). The proximal edge of the scaphoid is usually freshened to bleeding bone with a burr, small osteotome, or rongeur. To assist in suture placement, a 4-0 nylon suture wedged onto a straight needle is inserted retrograde through the drill holes to exit at the proximal pole of the scaphoid. Sutures of 2-0 or 3-0 Mersilene or Dacron are placed in the free edge of the scapholunate ligament in a horizontal mattress fashion (Fig. 8, *top*). They are then brought through the scaphoid drill holes, and the loop of 4-0 nylon is used to retrieve the free end of the suture. The sutures placed through the free edge of the scapholunate ligament are reinforced by suture repair imbricating the dorsal third of the scapholunate ligament with the dorsal wrist capsule. With the ligament repair in place, the scapholunate gap is reduced and cross-pinned with 0.045 K-wires. The scapholunate sutures are then tightened at the waist of the scaphoid to snug together the scapholunate ligament repair.

In some patients it is necessary to augment the scapholunate ligament repair by developing a carefully constructed dorsal capsuloligamentous flap as described by Blatt.[3] We have used the dorsal intercarpal ligament and the dorsal radiotriquetral ligament to provide the additional collagen tissue to the repair site. Others have used these ligament capsule flaps and tendons as check reins to prevent or control hyperflexion of the scaphoid (Fig. 8, *bottom*). When the dorsal radiotriquetral ligament is used for this purpose, it is left attached proximally on the radius to retain some innervation and blood supply. For suture repair, the ligament flap is rotated to the dorsal portion of the scapholunate interval (as mentioned above), or it can be

sutured distally to the scaphoid in order to hold it in an extended rather than a flexed position. Alternatively, the dorsal intercarpal ligament (dorsal scaphotrapezoidal ligament) can be used as a check rein. It is left attached distally to the scaphoid and is sutured proximally to the distal radius. This method lifts the scaphoid from a vertical to a horizontal position.

Intercarpal Fusion for Late Scapholunate Instability When there is chronic carpal instability without potential for ligament repair, intercarpal fusion can be used to stabilize the scaphoid alignment. Both scaphotrapeziotrapezoidal[12] or scaphocapitate fusions[51] are reliable techniques. Fusion is done through a dorsal incision made transversely over the area of the scaphotrapeziotrapezoidal joint[12] or a curvilinear incision over the dorsal radial scaphocapitate joint. The latter, longitudinal incision allows inspection of the proximal scapholunate area and full exposure of the scaphocapitate joint. The transverse incision is recommended in cases in which arthroscopy has demonstrated an irreparable scapholunate interval and a scaphotrapeziotrapezoidal fusion is selected.

For intercarpal fusion, a bone graft from the distal radius (or iliac crest) is needed. The dorsal wrist incision is centered over Lister's tubercle and the extensor retinaculum is reflected (Fig. 9). Bone graft can be harvested by removing Lister's tubercle. The scapholunate ligament and scaphocapitate joint can be visualized through the distal portion of the same incision. With the transverse incision, the scaphotrapeziotrapezoidal joint is identified with a needle or a dental probe and can be verified by imaging. Articular cartilage is removed with a combination of small burrs, curettes, and an osteotome. Only the joint cartilage needs to be removed along with a small amount of subchondral bone. Excessive removal of bone from the fusion site can cause deformity and abnormal carpal bone alignment.

With rotatory subluxation of the scaphoid, it is necessary to reduce the scaphoid from its vertically rotated displacement. We prefer a temporary pin fixation with biplanar radiographic control to confirm that malalignment of the scaphoid has been corrected. It is also possible to judge radial styloid to scaphoid impingement radiographically at this stage and determine if a radial styloidectomy is to be performed.

Bone graft harvested from the iliac crest or the distal radius is packed between the distal scaphoid and the trapeziotrapezoid joint or between the scaphoid and capitate. K-wires temporarily placed across the fusion site are reinserted. Alternative techniques include internal fixation with staples or selfcompressing Herbert or AO bone screws.

Aftercare Immobilization in a thumb spica for an average of eight weeks is recommended after either ligament repair or intercarpal fusion. With a compression screw device, mobilization at five to six weeks can be

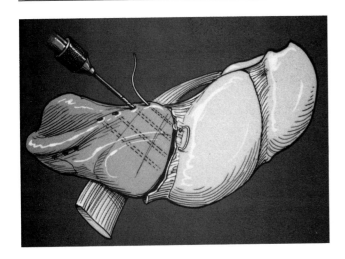

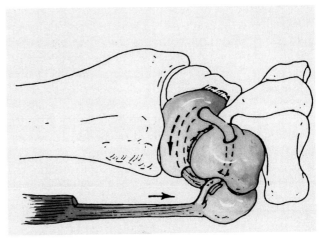

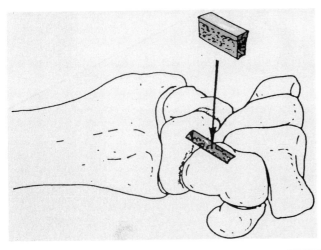

Fig. 10 Lunotriquetral ligament repair. **Top left**, Technique of repair with sutures involves drill holes placed through the triquetrum to the triquetrolunate junction and repair of the lunotriquetral ligament with nonresorbable sutures. **Top right**, An alternative technique involves ligament reconstruction through drill holes placed dorsally and palmarly in both lunate and triquetrum. **Bottom left**, Lunotriquetral fusion is performed with an inlay corticocancellous bone graft after removing the opposing articular cartilage surfaces of both bones. (Reproduced with permission from Reagan DS, Linscheid RL, Dobyns JH: Lunotriquetral sprains. *J Hand Surg* 1984;9A:506.)

considered. Following cast removal, we recommend a thumb spica splint for an additional four to six weeks. Return of wrist motion is assisted by methods of physical therapy, and only occasionally is it necessary to add dynamic wrist flexion or extension support splints. Before immobilization is discontinued, tomograms are recommended to evaluate healing of the intercarpal fusion and to determine when the patient can return to work or sports without restrictions. Ligament repair should be protected for a minimum of three months before allowing individuals to return to work or sporting activities. Repeat radiographs, to judge malalignment of the carpus are essential following ligament repair.

Lunotriquetral Repair

Repair of the lunotriquetral ligament is generally recommended when there is a complete tear demonstrated by arthrography or arthroscopy without associated carpal instability (a volar intercalary segment instability deformity).[50,55] The surgical procedure involves a dorsal ulnar incision centered over the distal radioulnar joint.

The extensor retinaculum is divided between the fourth and fifth extensor compartments, and the dorsal radiotriquetral ligament is preserved. The dorsal ulnar cutaneous nerve and its transverse branches must be protected. With distraction and radial deviation of the wrist, the lunotriquetral joint can be well visualized. Tears through the lunotriquetral ligament are examined with a dental probe to confirm their extent and location. K-wires placed in the lunate and the triquetrum can be used to manipulate the proximal carpal row from a flexed position and to provide sufficient visualization for lunotriquetral ligament repair. Repair techniques generally involve drill holes placed through the dorsal ulnar aspect of the triquetrum across the lunotriquetral joint (Fig. 10). The radial border of the triquetrum is freshened with an osteotome through the articular cartilage to provide an area for ligament reattachment. Horizontal mattress sutures of 3-0 Dacron or Mersilene are placed in the ligament remnant and brought through drill holes in the triquetrum to be tied on the dorsal ulnar aspect of the triquetrum. Immobilization with intraosseous K-wires is performed after the lunotriquetral joint is snugly reduced using the previously placed dorsal "joysticks."

When there is insufficient ligament remaining for repair and the ligament injury involves the dorsal third of the lunotriquetral joint, which is the most common involvement, the dorsal intercarpal ligament or one half of the extensor or flexor carpi ulnaris can be detached and rotated to be used as a ligament substitute. If the dorsal ligament is chosen, it passes through a trench or drill holes in the dorsal third of the lunate and triquetrum. If extensor or flexor tendon is harvested, it is placed through drill holes in the dorsal lunate and triquetrum. If a complete dissociation of the lunotriquetral ligament is present, a tendon (or capsular) loop repair of both dorsal and volar thirds is recommended (Fig. 10). Use of dorsal intermetacarpal ligament for augmented repair has become a reliable method of stabilization, particularly in combination with repair of the radiotriquetral ligament to the triquetrum. Partial or complete repair of the lunotriquetral ligament can be achieved by the use of local tissue alone, or it can be augmented by the addition of a dorsal ligament reconstruction.

Following ligament repair and/or reconstruction, K-wires are left in place across the lunotriquetral joint for a period of six to eight weeks followed by four to six weeks of splint immobilization. When there is associated ulnar carpal abutment, the ulnar aspect of the wrist should be decompressed by ulnar resection at the same time.

Lunotriquetral Fusion or Ligament Reconstruction for Late Instability When patients have ulnar wrist pain over the lunotriquetral joint in association with a volar flexion deformity of the lunate (the volar intercalary segment instability deformity), more advanced reconstructive procedures, including ligament reconstruction with half the extensor carpi ulnaris (or flexor carpi ulnaris) or lunotriquetral fusion may be indicated (Fig. 10, *top right* and *bottom left*).[55] In general, when the lunotriquetral dissociation can be reduced and there are no associated extrinsic ligament injuries, lunotriquetral reconstruction appears to be the procedure of choice.[50] Lunotriquetral fusion is an acceptable alternative, although recent studies show a success rate of only 70% to 80%, with a 20% incidence of nonunion. In most circumstances, the extrinsic ligaments (dorsal radiotriquetral and dorsal intercarpal) should be reattached to the triquetrum, because loss of the extrinsic dorsal ligaments can contribute to the volar flexion deformity of the lunate in association with the lunotriquetral tear.[42] The dorsal ligaments must be reattached to help control flexion of the proximal carpal row. Lunotriquetral fusion alone, without associated dorsal extrinsic ligament plication, can leave a persistent volar intercalary segment instability (VISI) deformity. The technique of lunotriquetral fusion or ligament reconstruction involves a dorsal ulnar incision in the interval between the fifth and sixth extensor compartments. Retraction of the extensor carpi ulnaris and release of a portion of its tendon sheath distally may be necessary to completely expose the dorsal surface of the lunotriquetral joint. Often more exposure is necessary for lunotriquetral reconstruction or fusion than is required for lunotriquetral ligament repair. When performing a fusion, all articular cartilage must be removed from the lunotriquetral interface. In most circumstances, an inlay bone grafting procedure of the dorsal surface of the lunate and triquetrum is recommended (Fig. 10, *bottom left*). With ligament reconstruction, half of the extensor carpi ulnaris or flexor carpi ulnaris is detached and rotated to bridge the lunotriquetral interval. In dorsal ligament reconstruction, the tendon graft is placed horizontally through the lunate and triquetrum. This procedure is combined with fixation using a combination of K-wires. As noted previously, any volar flexion deformity of the lunate must be corrected before attempting the lunotriquetral fusion. Appropriate anteroposterior and lateral radiographs taken after temporary fixation of the reconstruction or fusion site will ensure correction of the volar flexion deformity. For fusion, the bone graft is countersunk into the lunotriquetral joint, and internal fixation is performed with the K-wires or with a Herbert screw in conjunction with a single K-wire.

Aftercare involves immobilization in an ulnar wrist support cast for a period of eight to ten weeks. After fusion, cast immobilization is maintained until tomograms demonstrate solid union of the lunotriquetral area. As with lunotriquetral ligament repair or reconstruction, ulnar resection may be necessary if ulnar carpal abutment is present.[63] Lunotriquetral reconstruction or fusion is often combined with ulnar resection in the treatment of ulnar wrist pain in our patients.

Conclusions

Knowledge of the basic anatomy, kinematics, and biomechanics of the wrist as expressed in this chapter and in Chapter 3 provides the background for knowledgeable treatment of carpal instability. To make recommendations to the patient regarding the best methods of treatment, the surgeon must have important diagnostic clinical information including knowledge of clinical symptoms, signs, and roentgenographic findings that can demonstrate the location and extent of internal ligament tears. We have found recently that arthroscopy of the wrist is a helpful adjuvant to determine precisely the appearance, size, and location of ligament disruption associated with intercarpal pathology. It can be quite helpful in planning the surgical approach. With respect to general guidelines, when a patient is seen within four weeks from the time of injury, we prefer to repair both the scapholunate and lunotriquetral ligaments. In subacute injuries between four weeks and six months from the time of ligament injury, repair, often augmented by ligament reconstruction techniques, is usually still possible. A gray period exists between six months and 12 months after injury, during which ligament repair or reconstruction can be performed in carefully selected patients. For others in this group, intercarpal fusion may be preferable based on the patient's work, the extent of pathology, or the personal preference of the patient or surgeon.

Chronic ligament instability is defined as that instability for which treatment commences more than 12 months after the time of injury. In the majority of the patients, intercarpal fusion remains the treatment of choice. In comparing scaphotrapeziotrapezoidal and scaphocapitate fusions, results appear to be equal. On the ulnar side of the wrist, our results have been quite satisfactory with lunotriquetral ligament repair and reconstruction. Lunotriquetral fusion is less predictable, so for late instability associated with volar flexion of the lunate, repair of the dorsal radiolunotriquetral ligament may be necessary in addition to lunotriquetral repair or fusion in order to prevent a chronic volar intercalary segment instability deformity. Preoperative assessment of the patients, including not only history, physical examination, and invasive arthrographic or arthroscopic studies, but also their work environment and sport activities, is essential in making recommendations regarding the alternatives for surgical treatment of acute and chronic carpal instability.

References

1. Taleisnik J: Current concepts review: Carpal instability. *J Bone Joint Surg* 1988;70A:1262–1268.
2. Linscheid RL, Dobyns JH, Beabout JW, et al: Traumatic instability of the wrist: Diagnosis, classification and pathomechanics. *J Bone Joint Surg* 1972;54A:1612–1632.
3. Blatt G: Capsulodesis in reconstructive hand surgery: Dorsal capsulodesis for the unstable scaphoid and volar capsulodesis following excision of the distal ulna. *Hand Cl* 1987;3:81–102.
4. Cooney WP III, Linscheid RL, Dobyns JH: Ligament repair and reconstruction, in Neviaser RJ (ed): *Controversies in Hand Surgery*. New York, Churchill Livingstone, 1990, chap 14, pp 125–145.
5. Dobyns JH: Invited comment. *J Hand Surg* 1984;9A:526–527.
6. Dobyns JH, Linscheid RL: Injuries to the wrist, in Lamb DW, Kuczynski K (eds): *The Practice of Hand Surgery*. Oxford, England, Blackwell Scientific Publications, 1981, pp 221–237.
7. Glickel SZ, Millender LH: Ligamentous reconstruction for chronic intercarpal instability. *J Hand Surg* 1984;9A:514–525.
8. Palmer AK, Dobyns JH, Linscheid RL: Management of posttraumatic instability of the wrist secondary to ligament rupture. *J Hand Surg* 1978;3A:507–532.
9. Taleisnik J: Post-traumatic carpal instability. *Clin Orthop* 1980;149:73–82.
10. Goldner JL: Treatment of carpal instability without joint fusion—Current assessment. *J Hand Surg* 1982;7A:325–326.
11. Kleinman WB: Management of chronic rotary subluxation of the scaphoid by scapho-trapezial-trapezoid arthrodesis: Rationale

12. Watson HK, Hempton RF: Limited wrist arthrodeses: I. The triscaphoid joint. *J Hand Surg* 1980;5A:320–327.
13. Watson HK, Goodman ML, Johnson TR: Limited wrist arthrodesis: II. Intercarpal and radiocarpal combinations *J Hand Surg* 1981;6A:223–233.
14. MacConaill MA: The mechanical anatomy of the carpus and its bearing on some surgical problems. *J Anat* 1941;75:166–175.
15. Landsmeer JMF: Study on anatomy of articulation: I. The equilibrium of the "intercalated" bone. *Acta Morphol Neer Scand* 1961;3:287–303.
16. Berger RA, Kauer JMG, Landsmeer JML: Radioscapholunate ligament: A gross anatomic and histologic study of fetal and adult wrist. *J Hand Surg* 1991;16A:350–355.
17. Mayfield JK: Wrist ligamentous anatomy and pathogenesis of carpal instability. *Orthop Clin North Am* 1984;15:209–216.
18. Ruby LK, An KN, Linscheid RL, et al: The effect of scapholunate ligament section on scapholunate motion. *J Hand Surg* 1987;12A:767–771.
19. Taleisnik J: The ligaments of the wrist. *J Hand Surg* 1976;1A:110–118.
20. Taleisnik J: *The Wrist*. New York, Churchill Livingstone, 1985.
21. Linscheid RL, Dobyns JH, Beckenbaugh RD, et al: Instability patterns of the wrist. *J Hand Surg* 1983;8A:682–686.
22. McMurtry RY, Youm Y, Flatt AE, et al: Kinematics of the wrist. II. Clinical applications. *J Bone Joint Surg* 1978;60A:955–961.
23. Weil C, Ruby LK: The dorsal approach to the wrist revisited. *J Hand Surg* 1986;11A:911–912.
24. Youm Y, McMurtry RY, Flatt AE, et al: The kinematics of the wrist: I. An experimental study of radial-ulnar deviation and flexion-extension. *J Bone Joint Surg* 1978;60A:423–431.
25. Gilford WW, Bolton RH, Lambrinudi C: The mechanism of the wrist joint with special reference to fractures of the scaphoid. *Guy Hosp Rep* 1943;92:52–59.
26. Weber ER: Wrist mechanics and its association with ligamentous instability, in Lichtman DM (ed): *The Wrist and Its Disorders*. Philadelphia, WB Saunders, 1988, pp 41–52.
27. Dobyns JH, Linscheid RL: Fractures and dislocations of the wrist, in Rockwood CA Jr, Green DP (eds): *Fractures*, ed 1. Philadelphia, JB Lippincott, 1975.
28. Adelaar RS: Traumatic wrist instabilities. *Contemp Orthop* 1982;4:309–324.
29. Dobyns JH, Linscheid RL, Chao E-Y, et al: Traumatic instability of the wrist. American Academy of Orthopaedic Surgeons *Instructional Course Lectures, XXIV*. St. Louis, CV Mosby, 1975, pp 182–199.
30. Linscheid RL, Dobyns JH: The unified concept of carpal injuries. *Ann Chir Main* 1984;3:35–42.
31. Fisk GR: Carpal instability and the fractured scaphoid: Hunterian lecture delivered at the Royal College of Surgeons of England. *Ann R Coll Surg Engl* 1970;46:63–76.
32. Cooney WP III, Garcia-Elias M, Dobyns JH, et al: Anatomy and mechanics of carpal instability. *Surg Rounds Orthop* 1989;9:15–24.
33. Dobyns JH, Linscheid RL, Macksoud WS, et al: Carpal instability, nondissociative. Presented at the 54th Annual Meeting of the American Academy of Orthopaedic Surgeons, San Francisco, CA, Jan 24, 1987.
34. Gilula LA, Totty WG, Weeks PM: Wrist arthrography: The value of fluoroscopic spot viewing. *Radiology* 1983;146:555–556.
35. Levinsohn EM, Palmer AK: Arthrography of the traumatized wrist. *Radiology* 1983;146:647–651.
36. Palmer AK, Levinsohn EM, Kuzma GR: Arthrography of the wrist. *J Hand Surg* 1983;8A:15–23.
37. Cooney WP III, Dobyns JH, Linscheid RL: Fractures and dislocations of the wrist, in Rockwood CA Jr, Green DP (eds): *Fractures*, ed 3. Philadelphia, JB Lippincott, 1991, pp 563–579.

38. Alexander CE, Lichtman DM: Triquetrolunate and midcarpal instability, in Lichtman DM (ed): *The Wrist and Its Disorders*. Philadelphia, WB Saunders, 1988, pp 274–285.

39. Garth WP Jr, Hofamann DY, Rooks MD: Volar intercalated segment instability secondary to medial carpal ligamental laxity. *Clin Orthop* 1985;201:94–105.

40. Lichtman DM, Schneider JR, Swafford AR, et al: Ulnar midcarpal instability—Clinical and laboratory analysis. *J Hand Surg* 1981;6A:515–523.

41. Horii E, Ani KN, Garcia-Elias M, et al: A kinematic study of lunotriquetral dissociation. *J Hand Surg* 1991;16A:355–362.

42. Viegas SF, Patterson RM, Peterson PD, et al: Ulnar-sided perilunate instability: An anatomic and biomechanic study. *J Hand Surg* 1990;15A:268–278.

43. Johnson RP, Carrera GF: Chronic capitolunate instability. *J Bone Joint Surg* 1986;68A:1164–1176.

44. Lichtman DM: *The Wrist and Its Disorders*. Philadelphia, WB Saunders, 1988, pp 53, 54, 91–95, 244, 245, 249, 250, 274, 275.

45. Taleisnik J, Watson HK: Midcarpal instability caused by malunited fractures of the distal radius. *J Hand Surg* 1984;9A:350–357.

46. Gordon WD, Armstrong GWD, Armstrong MD: Rotational subluxation of the scaphoid. *Can J Surg* 1968;11:306–314.

47. Howard F, Fahey T, Wojcik E: Rotatory subluxation of the navicular. *Clin Orthop* 1974;104:134–139.

48. Jackson WT, Protas JM: Snapping scapholunate subluxation. *J Hand Surg* 1981;6A:590–594.

49. Alexander CE, Lichtman DM: Ulnar carpal instabilities. *Orthop Clin North Am* 1984;15:307–320.

50. Favero KJ, Bishop AT, Linscheid RL: Lunotriquetral ligament disruption: A comparative study of treatment methods. *J Hand Surg*, in press.

51. Pisano SM, Peimer CA, Wheeler DR, et al: Scaphocapitate intercarpal arthrodesis. *J Hand Surg* 1991;16A:328–333.

52. Beckenbaugh RD: Accurate evaluation and management of the painful wrist following injury: An approach to carpal instability. *Orthop Clin North Am* 1984;15:289–306.

53. Destouet JM, Gilula LA, Reinus WR: Roentgenographic diagnosis of wrist pain and instability, in Lichtman DM (ed): *The Wrist and Its Disorders*. Philadelphia, WB Saunders, 1988, pp 82–95.

54. Gilula LA, Destouet JM, Weeks PM, et al: Roentgenographic diagnosis of the painful wrist. *Clin Orthop* 1984;187:52–64.

55. Reagan DS, Linscheid RL, Dobyns JH: Lunotriquetral sprains. *J Hand Surg* 1984;9A:502–514.

56. Kleinman WB: Diagnostic Exam for Ligamentous Injuries—Shear, Shuck, and Compression. American Society for Surgery of the Hand Correspondence Club Newsletter No. 51, 1985.

57. Botte MJ, Cooney WP III, Linscheid RL: Arthroscopy of the wrist: Anatomy and technique. *J Hand Surg* 1989;14A:313–316.

58. Roth JH, Haddad RG: Radiocarpal arthroscopy and arthrography in the diagnosis of ulnar wrist pain. *J Arthroscopy* 1986;2:234–243.

59. Zinberg EM, Coren AB, Levinsohn EM, et al: The triple injection wrist arthrogram. *J Hand Surg* 1988;13A:308.

60. Belsole RJ, Eikman EA, Muroff LR: Bone scintigraphy in trauma of the hand and wrist. *J Trauma* 1981;21:163–166.

61. Watson HK, Ballett FL: The SLAC wrist: Scapholunate advanced collapse pattern of degenerative arthritis. *J Hand Surg* 1984;9A:358–365.

62. Pin PG, Young VL, Gilula LA, et al: Management of chronic lunotriquetral ligament tears. *J Hand Surg* 1989;14A:77–83.

63. Trumble T, Bour CJ, Smith RJ, et al: Intercarpal arthrodesis for static and dynamic volar intercalated segment instability. *J Hand Surg* 1988;13A:384–390.

64. Bell MJ, Hill RJ, McMurty RY: Ulnar impingement syndrome. *J Bone Joint Surg* 1985;67B:126–129.

Kienböck's Disease

Ronald L. Linscheid, MD

In 1910 Kienböck[1] described the progressive deterioration of the lunate bone as seen by x-ray as lunatomalacia and suggested that the etiology was injury to the blood supply of the bone. The next important observation was that of Hultén[2] who, in 1928, noted that in patients with Kienböck's disease there was more likely to be a discrepancy in length between the ulna and radius than there was in the general population. This discrepancy was for the ulna to be shorter than the radius as measured at the dense cortical line of the lunate fossa perpendicular to the longitudinal axis of the forearm. This observation suggested the possibility of a mechanical susceptibility to this problem. It also suggested a mechanical solution, for which he proposed radial shortening. Persson[3] described an ulnar lengthening procedure in 1945, and others soon followed with reports of radial shortening procedures. The aims of both procedures were to redistribute the forces from the injured lunate towards the triquetrum.

The vascular supply to the bone was also of obvious importance. In 1963, Lee[4] proceeded beyond the observation of the foraminal openings in the dorsal and palmar poles of the lunate to study the intraosseous vascular distribution within the bone. This suggested an increased susceptibility to avascular necrosis in those individuals with deficient anastomotic patterns. A number of authors have made significant advancements in the study of the natural history of this problem. Antuna-Zapico,[5] in a brilliant monograph in 1966, looked at the morphologic variations of the lunate and the stress concentration considerations this posed for the injured lunate. More recently, the carpal collapse aspect of the problem has suggested additional treatment plans, but before proceeding further a look at the natural history of the problem may be in order.

Natural History

The incidence of Kienböck's disease is greatest in the active young adult population but it can occur in childhood and well into the later decades of life. It affects a higher proportion of men than of women. The initial symptom, aching in the wrist with activity, progresses to increasing limitation of motion, weakness, and sharp pain with movement. Some patients may tolerate these symptoms for years, and, occasionally, the symptoms slowly ameliorate to where function is not severely impaired. It is partly for this reason that the various treatments of this condition are difficult to compare objectively.[6,7]

The pathologic changes that occur vary somewhat, depending on the etiology, the shape of the lunate, and the configuration of the radioulnar articulation.[6,8-10] Sclerosis of the bone secondary to avascularity renders the bone susceptible to shear stress fractures in the subcortical trabeculae. These fractures usually occur parallel to the proximal articular surface and are similar to those seen in avascular necrosis of the hip and similar osteochondroses.[11] Collapse of the trabeculae leads to compressive shortening of the lunate. If there are transverse fractures in the coronal plane, these same forces acting through the capitate tend to extrude the two fragments of the lunate dorsopalmarly. There is usually more involvement on the proximal convex aspect than on the distal concave surface, and flattening of the former is evident. The articular cartilage generally remains in good condition, but it is pliable because of the collapsed bone beneath. Collapse progresses until the joint compressive forces are attenuated by redistribution to the proximal scaphoid and triquetrum.[12,13] The ulnar aspect of the lunate, which overlies the triangular fibrocartilage, is usually less involved in the collapse than is the portion that articulates with the lunate fossa of the radius. This variation is most readily explained by the difference in compliance between the two surfaces, especially in those with greater ulna minus variance. Shortening of the lunate may lead the scaphoid to adapt a progressively more flexed attitude as it supports more of the joint compressive load, and this flexion is used to justify the method of treatment in which the scaphotrapeziotrapezoidal joint is arthrodesed.[14] For the most part, the scapholunate and lunotriquetral ligaments remain intact, helping to provide transverse stability to the carpus. There are exceptions to this, however, in which there appears to be concomitant scapholunate dissociation and lunatomalacia.[15] Recent evidence suggests that the former condition is also more likely to occur with ulna minus variance.[16] Therefore, it is not surprising to see the simultaneous expression of both conditions.

Diagnosis

A history of injury is elicited in over 50% of patients. Even though the injury may have occurred months or even years earlier, there is reason to believe that the

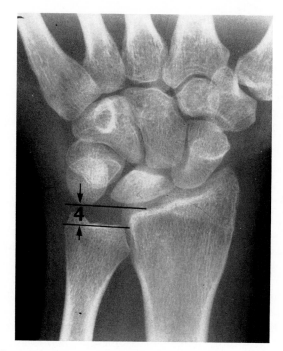

Fig. 1 Anteroposterior radiograph shows increased radiodensity of the lunate. Ulnar variance −4 mm.

expression of osteonecrosis is often delayed, as will be explained later. The injury is usually a fall on the extended hand.

The physical findings are limitation of motion, weakness, and point tenderness over the dorsal central aspect of the wrist. Palmar flexion is more likely to be limited than dorsiflexion because of extrusion of the palmar pole of the lunate. Grip strength is often reduced to 50% of the opposite hand.

Radiographic findings are based primarily on plain films of the wrist taken in the anteroposterior and sagittal planes. The earliest finding is usually an increased radiodensity of the lunate as compared with the adjacent bones (Fig. 1). This increase is followed by a radiolucent line parallel to the articular surface through the subcortical area. Flattening of the articular surface, particularly over the lunate fossa, occurs with resorption of trabecular bone, and the height of the lunate becomes noticeably reduced (Fig. 2). Further fragmentation is followed by increasing signs of degenerative arthritis. This sequence of change is formalized in the staging plans of Stahl,[7] DeCoulx and associates,[17] and Lichtman and associates.[18] Surprisingly little attention is paid to the sagittal views in most reports, which is unfortunate because these often provide important information. The superimposition of the radial styloid, scaphoid, triquetrum, and ulnar styloid make interpretation difficult. Transverse fractures in the coronal

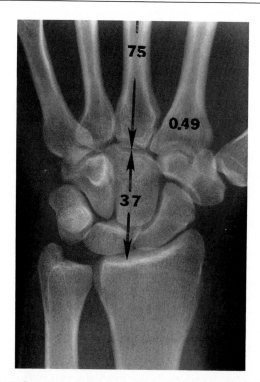
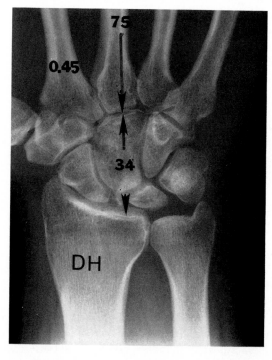

Fig. 2 **Left**, Anteroposterior comparison views right and left wrists. Right lunate shows collapse of proximal articular surface. **Right**, Carpal height and the carpal index ratio are reduced as compared with the left.

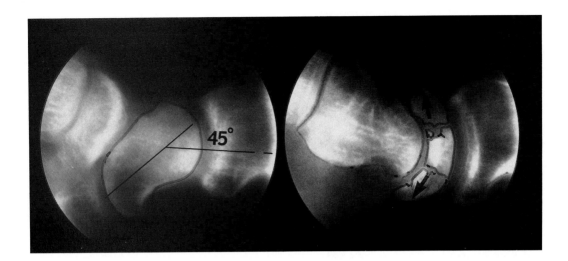

Fig. 3   **Left**, The radioscaphoid angle is 45 degrees, which suggests that no compensatory collapse of the radial stabilizing column has occurred. **Right**, The sagittal view shows two fractures transversely through the sagittal plane. Both the dorsal and palmar poles are extruding. The central portion of the body of the lunate is sclerotic and is collapsing.

plane, dorsopalmar extrusion, midcarpal angulation, and scaphoid angulation, however, may be seen with careful inspection.[19]

Polyaxial tomograms are even more informative, especially when taken at intervals of 2 to 3 mm.[19] I find that the stage of the disease is often upgraded when tomography and plain films are compared (Fig. 3). Fractures are much more apparent, and so are the degree of flattening, the displacement of fragments, and carpal alignments. Although it is difficult to be certain unless an unequivocal fracture is seen in the lunate radiographs shortly after an injury, I believe that the coronal fractures are generally responsible for initiating the avascular changes. These coronal fractures may be subtle fractures at the palmar or dorsal poles or more obvious fractures through the body of the bone. The subcortical fractures in the sagittal or transverse planes appear to be more likely the result of shear fractures through avascular bone.[20] Widening of the transverse fracture gaps by intrusion of the capitate is readily appreciated on these films, and it can also be seen on computed tomographic or magnetic resonance imaging scans.[21] It is not unusual to see the palmar pole displaced so that it impinges against the palmar rim of the radius, which helps explain the loss of palmar flexion.

The stance of the scaphoid is also easier to appreciate on trispiral tomograms.[19] In the neutral position of the wrist, the radioscaphoid angle is usually between 40 degrees and 60 degrees. Angulation much beyond this suggests some collapse of the carpus (Fig. 4).[14] This carpal collapse may be caused by collapse of the lunate, by midcarpal angulation, or, as is sometimes noted, by fragmentation of the palmar aspect of the lunate with

proximal displacement and palmar subluxation of the capitate. To be sure, the scaphoid may also undergo angulatory displacement under dynamic loading, but unloaded static films suggest that only a small percentage of scaphoids are abnormally flexed.

Because ulnar variance measurement is important in assessing the status of lunatomalacia and in its treatment, it should be done in a standard and reproducible manner.[22-26] The wrist should be in a neutral position flat on the x-ray plate with the elbow flexed to 90 degrees and the shoulder abducted 90 degrees. A line perpendicular to the longitudinal axis of the forearm is drawn from the proximal cortical line of the lunate fossa over the ulnar head. The distance to the cortical surface of the ulnar pole is measured (Fig. 1). If available, the concentric circle template recommended by Palmer is desirable, but the method must be consistent.[26]

Flattening or abnormal enchondral bony growth of the lunate fossa as a result of the lunate collapse has been noted minimally only in late cases.

Technetium 99 bone scans may provide an early indication of lunate injury, but localization may be imprecise and, if the scan is positive, it is best followed by tomography or magnetic resonance image scanning.[27,28] The latter has the unique advantage of suggesting avascular changes in the bone long before they can be seen by radiograph. There is also the advantage of detecting articular effusion as well as fractures and the status of the adjacent carpus. This is likely to be an increasingly important tool both for diagnosis and followup, particularly if such examinations become less expensive (Fig. 5).

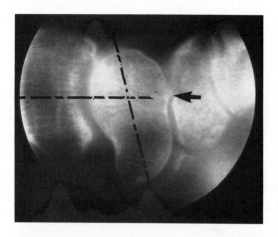
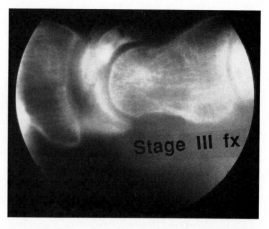

Fig. 4   Left, Radioscaphoid angle is 80 degrees, which indicates collapse of the support of the radial column (compare with Fig. 3, *left*). This is apparent in about 20% of stage III and IV cases. **Right,** The lunate shows an oblique fracture through the body and collapse of the proximal articular surface of the dorsal fragment. The palmar pole impinges against the palmar rim.

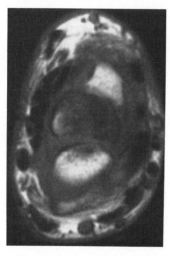

Fig. 5   Magnetic resonance imaging, transverse section. Note lack of signal in the most affected portions of the lunate but the suggestion of viability of the palmar pole.

Etiology

The mechanism of injury to the vascular supply of the lunate is not well understood. The vessels can enter the bone only at the dorsal and palmar poles, because the bone is otherwise covered by articular cartilage except at the attachment of the interosseous membranes. The entering vessels execute a sharp bend as they come off the proximal carpal arcades.[30] The studies of Lee[4] and, more recently, of Gelberman and associates[29] have shown three general categories of vascularity. These categories, described as Y, X, and I patterns, are marked by a decreasing intraosseous anastomotic network (Fig. 6).

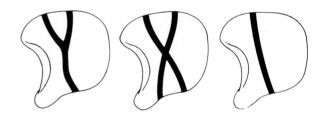

Fig. 6   Schematic representation of Y, X, and I intraosseous vascular patterns. (Reproduced with permission from Gelberman RH, Bauman TD, Menon J, et al: The vascularity of the lunate bone and Kienböck's disease. *J Hand Surg* 1980;5A:272–278.)

At both extreme extension and flexion the foraminal areas may impinge against the radial rims. There seems no doubt that interference with these vessels accounts for many cases of Kienböck's disease, because, in my experience, at least 40% of patients show no evidence of prior fracture.[6,31] In this group of patients, sclerosis and proximal shear fracture or collapse of the convex surface are less likely to show extrusion lengthening of the lunate.

There is evidence of transverse lunate fractures occurring at the time of injury and progressing to fragmentation in a matter of several weeks. In other instances, however, a known fracture has not resulted in the secondary changes for several years or has persisted as a nonunion.

It is interesting to speculate why, when the lunate and scaphoid undergo essentially similar lesions, only a small percentage of scaphoid proximal poles undergo necrotic fragmentation but a large percentage of frac-

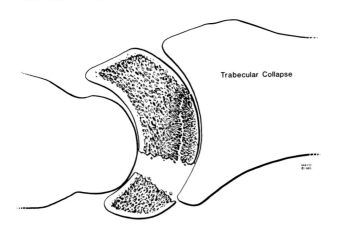

Fig. 7 A fractured lunate allows the compressive force exerted by the capitate to markedly increase the stress at the apex of the articular surface and fracture surface. (Reproduced with permission from Mayo Foundation.)

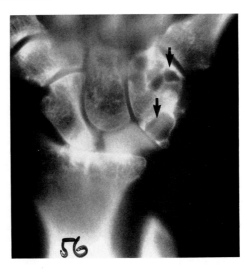

Fig. 8 Failed ulnar lengthening in 40-year-old man resulted in Darrach resection of the ulna and silicone rubber replacement of the lunate. Trispiral tomograms 10 years postoperatively show an ulnar translation of the carpus, cystic degeneration of the capitate, cold flow deformity of the prosthesis, and particulate synovitis of the triquetrohamate joint.

tured lunates do. One answer may be that the stress concentration caused by the direct pressure of the capitate becomes much higher at the acute angle between the articular surface and fracture facet in the lunate than at the corresponding situation in the scaphoid. The more closed convex configuration of the cortical envelope of the scaphoid may also be much more resistant to compression.

Treatment

The ideal treatment is either to prevent deformity or to restore the lunate to normal appearance and function. The latter has been an elusive goal. To accomplish this task in a stage III or IV situation would require restoring the height of the bone proximodistally, reducing the length dorsopalmarly, restoring the proximal spherical convexity, re-establishing the vascular circulation, and preventing recollapse of the bone during the soft healing period. Some attempts to accomplish this using external distraction apparatuses, bone grafting of the trabecular defects, and introduction of a pedicled artery and its venae communicante have met with limited success.[32-35] The healing period may readily extend beyond the wrist's tolerance for mechanical distraction, anatomic reduction is difficult, and ligated vessels may not maintain a flow capacity especially within the confines of trabecular bone graft fragments. If the initial susceptible condition is not corrected, the problem can recur. Continued research in this area is, however, to be encouraged.[36,37]

Prevention of Kienböck's disease can be accomplished only when there is early suspicion after injury, with demonstration of a lunate fracture through the body of the bone. Unfortunately this opportunity is usually missed because the wrist is placed in a cast. Why this eminently sensible approach is likely to fail is explained by the propensity of the capitate to force the fracture facets apart even with the wrist limited in motion. This problem is caused by the persistent joint compressive forces induced by the tension of the wrist and finger tendons still intermittently contracting within the cylindrical confines of a cast. If these forces can be removed from their impingement on the lunate, the stress risers at the sharply angled fracture edge will be reduced and the fracture facets are more likely to coapt (Fig. 7).

The inability of the subcortical trabeculae to sustain the increased stress, especially when devascularized, can lead to collapse. The lunate fracture may heal even with a reduced vascularity and improve the late results. Even in that group in which no initial fracture exists, the earlier the lunate is unloaded, the less collapse is to be anticipated. For this reason, early decompression should be considered rather than conservative observation in plaster.

Excision of the fragmented lunate, the oldest surgical treatment, has been effective in reducing pain at least initially. However, over time, the capitate intrudes into the open space and displaces the scaphoid and triquetrum, which leads to progressive degenerative arthritis.[7,38] To prevent this collapse, a variety of lunate replacements have been used, including metal spheres, acrylic, silicone, and titanium models of prosthetic lunates.[39-45] Biologic replacements have included capsular suspension, coiled tendons ("anchovies"), carved chondral cartilage, and pedicle pisiform bones.[34,46] The dis-

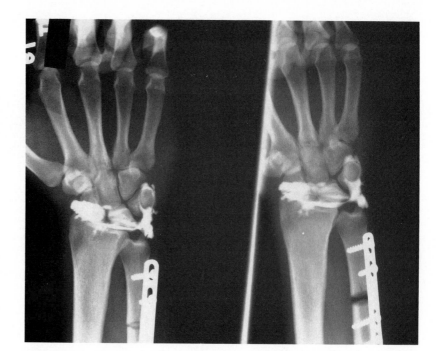

Fig. 9 Ulnar lengthening for lunatomalacia. **Left**, Radiocarpal arthrogram shows a thin layer of dye beneath the lunate. A slotted plate is in place over the distal ulna where an osteotomy cut has been made. **Right**, The ulna has been distracted 3 mm and the screws tightened before insertion of the graft. The height of the dye layer under the lunate is now thicker, which suggests that the lunate has been elevated from the lunate fossa. (Reproduced with permission from Armistead RB, Linscheid RL, Dobyns JH, et al: Ulnar lengthening in the treatment of Kienböck's Disease. *J Bone Joint Surg* 1982;64A:170–178.)

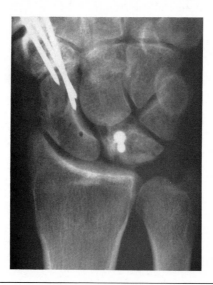
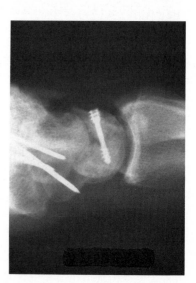

Fig. 10 Left, Stage III Kienböck's disease with ulna zero variance. Anteroposterior intraoperative radiograph during scaphotrapeziotrapezoidal arthrodesis (Watson technique). The lunate was compressed dorsopalmarly to close the fracture gap, and a Herbert screw was used for internal fixation. **Right**, Lateral view shows an approximate 45-degree radioscaphoid angle and reduction of the lunate.

advantage of lunate excision is the disruption of the perilunate ligamentous supports, which favors displacement of the scaphoid, ulnar translation of the carpus, and instability of the prosthesis. Dislocation of the prosthesis through the floor of the capsule is common unless integrity is maintained by retention of a bony remnant of the palmar pole.[45] Harder materials have a tendency to erode into the radius. Softer materials often deform or degrade to produce inflammation-exciting microfragments.[47-49] All of the above treatments, however, have enjoyed a measure of success for varying periods (Fig. 8).

So-called leveling procedures date from the early attempts of Persson[3] to decompress the lunate by lengthening the ulna.[50-56] Some patients treated by the early methods had followups as long as 30 years with generally satisfactory results.[57] Better internal fixation devices, which allowed distraction lengthening with greater precision, used an inserted wafer of iliac crest or a grafted step-cut extension (Fig. 9).

The obvious disadvantage of requiring a bone graft, along with the occasional nonunion, led others to adopt radial shortening as the preferred procedure. Both ulnar lengthening and radial shortening are based on the

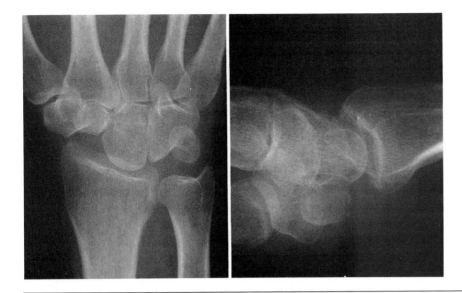

Fig. 11 Snap in wrist occurred 12 months previously while lifting. Recurrent injury with radiographic findings of a sclerotic lunate with a central cyst and ulna positive variance. **Left,** After proximal row carpectomy, the capitate head shows a large radius of curvature, satisfactory joint space, and good position. **Right,** Sagittal view shows good alignment of capitate with radial articular surface.

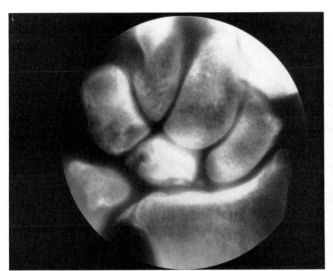 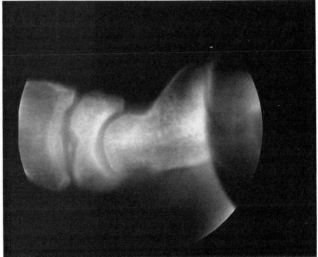

Fig. 12 Sixteen-year followup of an ulnar lengthening procedure. **Left,** The ulnar variance was changed from a −2 mm to +3 mm. There is evidence of ulnar impingement with a small fragment free from the ulnar margin of the lunate and small cystic changes in the triquetrum. The lunate is less radiodense than it was originally. The contour of the sigmoid notch of the radius has reversed its obliquity as a result of enchondral new bone formation proximally. **Right,** The ratio of height to width of the lunate is abnormal and the proximal contour is flattened with a small central free fragment evident. The patient has worked full time at a moderately stressful job and is seldom bothered with discomfort. He has mild limitation of motion, which is most apparent on ulnar deviation.

premise that the ulnar head and the triangular fibrocartilage are able to distribute more of the compressive force through the triquetrum and ulnar aspect of the lunate.[58-62] The latter was generally less affected than that part residing on the lunate fossa. Relative lengthening of the tendons also diminishes the overall joint compressive force. Another premise, later generally confirmed, was that the triangular fibrocartilage was thicker and usually unperforated in patients with an ulna minus variance. Thus, this fibrocartilage provides

a compliant pad that supports the ulnar carpus. Fortunately, the distal radioulnar joint is quite forgiving to longitudinal displacement, except in those instances when it lies at a markedly oblique angle. Correction to an ulna 0 or +1 variance is usually satisfactory. This technique may be used with a zero variant as well, but the correction should be small, or the patient is likely to complain of ulnar impingement symptoms.[60]

Other methods of decompressing the lunate include scaphotrapeziotrapezoidal arthrodesis,[14] capitohamate arthrodesis,[63] and capitate recession.[64] The first of these three methods depends on extending the scaphoid to its normal static position of about 45 degrees of radioscaphoid obliquity so that the proximal pole accepts the primary joint compressive load (Fig. 10). The second method assumes that the proximal migration of the capitate will be prevented by fusion to the hamate. The third method decreases the central loading through the wrist directly by shortening the capitate. All three methods have been afforded encouraging clinical reports.

Biomechanical studies suggest that the forces are redistributed more evenly with forearm leveling procedures, and that scaphotrapeziotrapezoidal fusion is more effective than capitohamate fusion.[12,65-67] Alterating the slope of the radial articular surface may also help levitate the lunate.

Salvage procedures, such as proximal row carpectomy, are occasionally warranted, especially when the distal surface of the lunate has collapsed or there is advanced collapse of the lunate as in the late stage III and IV (Fig. 11).[68]

The contact area for the radiocapite is considerably smaller than that of the radiocarpal because of the smaller radius of curvature; therefore, the compressive loading is high. The stability of the joint, however, is surprisingly good with an intact radiocapite ligament. Isolated radiolunate fusion has not been effective, because the avascular lunate does not heal to a graft.

Discussion

Long-term followups of the various methods of treatment are few and are not comparable in most instances. As noted, good results are reported by most techniques, a fact that may be explained in part by the tendency of the carpus to seek a state where further collapse has stopped and the wrist has stabilized. Little mention is made of the long-term status of the lunate or the carpus. Healing with apparent revascularization may be seen in children and adolescents, but the proximal convexity of the bone does not reconstitute. In adults, free avascular fragments may be seen between healed portions of the lunate after as long as 17 years. The degree of original fragmentation and displacement may be a significant factor in this.

Most treatment algorithms are based on the staging of Kienböck's disease as seen on the anteroposterior radiographs of the wrist.[17] This cookbook type of approach is better supplemented by a careful assessment of the multiple factors that may be involved. If polyaxial tomograms are not available, computed tomographic scans or a magnetic resonance image will give additional information. Study of the sagittal projections can often be more important than the anteroposterior view in assessing the lunate. Radial recession or ulnar length-

ening to a 0 or +2 mm variance, depending on the degree of initial variance, has the advantage of not destroying a normal carpal joint or interfering with intracarpal relationships. These treatments, which allow other methods to be employed later without compromise if the initial procedure is ineffective, may be combined with revascularization, bone grafting or fracture reduction. For this reason, this procedure appears to be the current benchmark against which other treatments are evaluated (Fig. 12).

References

1. Kienböck R: Veber Traumatische Malazie des Mondbeins und Ihre Folgezustände: Entartungsformen und Kompressionsfrakturen. *Fortschr Geb Rontgenstr* 1910;16:77–103.
2. Hultén O: Uber Anatomische Variationen der Handgelenknochen. Ein Beitrag zur Kenntnis der Genese zwei verschiedener Mondbeinveranderungen. *Acta Radiol* 1928;9:155–168.
3. Persson M: Pathogeneses und Behandlung der Kienböckschen Lunatummalazia: Der Frakturtheorie Im Lichte der Erfolge Operativer Radiusverkurzung (Hultén) und Einer Neuen Operationsmethode-Ulnaverlangerung. *Acta Chir Scand* 1945;(suppl 98):68.
4. Lee MLH: The intraosseous arterial pattern of the carpal lunate bone and its relation to avascular necrosis. *Acta Orthop Scand* 1963;33:43–55.
5. Antuna-Zapico JM: Malacia del Semilunar. Tesis Doctoral, Monograph, Universidad de Valladolid, Industrias y Editorial Severe-Cuesta, Valladolid, 1966, pp 343.
6. Beckenbaugh RD, Shives TC, Dobyns JH, et al: Kienböck's disease: The natural history of Kienböck's disease and consideration of lunate fractures. *Clin Orthop* 1980;149:98–106.
7. Stahl F: Lunatomalacia (Kienböck's Disease): A clinical and roentgenological study, especially on its pathogenesis and the late results of immobilization treatment. *Acta Chir Scand* 1947:5(suppl 126):1–133.
8. Bar P, Labourdette P: A clinical and radiological study of Kienböck's disease. *Ann Chir Main* 1982;1:239.
9. Mirabello SC, Rosenthal DI, Smith RJ: Correlation of clinical and radiographic findings in Kienböck's disease. *J Hand Surg* 1987;12A:1049–1054.
10. Razemon JP: Pathogenic study of Kienböck's disease. *Ann Chir Main* 1982;1:240–242.
11. Kenzora JE, Steele RE, Yosipovitch ZH, et al: Experimental osteonecrosis of the femoral head in adult rabbits. *Clin Orthop* 1978;130:8–46.
12. Horii E, Garcia-Elias M, An KN, et al: Effect on force transmission across the carpus in procedures used to treat Kienböck's disease. *J Hand Surg* 1990;15A:393–400.
13. Kashiwagi D, Fujiwara A, Inoue T, et al: An experimental and clinical study of lunatomalacia. *Orthop Trans* 1977;1:7.
14. Watson HK, Ryu J, DiBella A: An approach to Kienböck's disease: Triscaphe arthrodesis. *J Hand Surg* 1985;10A:179–187.
15. Bourne MH, Linscheid RL, Dobyns JH: Concomitant scapholunate dissociation and Kienböck's disease. *J Hand Surg* 1991;16A:460–464.
16. Czitrom AA, Dobyns JH, Linscheid RL: Ulnar variance in carpal instability. *J Hand Surg* 1987;12A:205–208.
17. DeCoulx P, Marchand M, Minet P, et al: La Maladie de Kienböck Chez le Mineur. Etude Clinique et Pathogenique (avec analyse de 1330 radios du poignet). *Lille Chir* 1957;12:65–81.
18. Lichtman DM, Alexander AH, Mack GR, et al: Kienböck's disease: Update on silicone replacement arthroplasty. *J Hand Surg* 1982;7A:343–347.

19. Linscheid RL, Dobyns JH, Younge DK: Trispiral tomography in the evaluation of wrist injury. *Bull Hosp Joint Dis Orthop Inst* 1984; 44:297–308.

20. Lesire MR, Allieu Y: Traumatic etiology of Kienböck's disease. (Perilunate luxations and necrosis of the lunate.) *Ann Chir Main* 1982;1:242–246.

21. Nakamura R, Horii E, Tanaka Y, et al: Three-dimensional CT imaging for wrist disorders. *J Hand Surg* 1989;14B:53–58.

22. Chan KP, Huang P: Anatomic variations in radial and ulnar lengths in the wrists of Chinese. *Clin Orthop* 1971;80:17–20.

23. Chen WS, Shih CH: Ulnar variance and Kienböck's disease: An investigation in Taiwan. *Clin Orthop* 1990;255:124–127.

24. Epner RA, Bowers WH, Guilford WB: Ulnar variance: The effect of wrist positioning and roentgen filming technique. *J Hand Surg* 1982;7A:298–305.

25. Gelberman RH, Salamon PB, Jurist JM, et al: Ulnar variance in Kienböck's disease. *J Bone Joint Surg* 1975;57A:674–676.

26. Palmer AK, Glisson RR, Werner FW: Ulnar variance determination. *J Hand Surg* 1982;7A:376–379.

27. Sowa DT, Holder LE, Patt PG, et al: Application of magnetic resonance imaging to ischemic necrosis of the lunate. *J Hand Surg* 1989;14A:1008–1016.

28. Trumble TE, Irving J: Histologic and magnetic resonance imaging correlations in Kienböck's disease. *J Hand Surg* 1990;15A: 879–884.

29. Gelberman RH, Bauman TD, Menon J, et al: The vascularity of the lunate bone and Kienböck's disease. *J Hand Surg* 1980;5A: 272–278.

30. Hori Y, Tamai S, Okuda H, et al: Blood vessel transplantation to bone. *J Hand Surg* 1979;4A:23–33.

31. Amadio PC, Hanssen AD, Berquist TH: The genesis of Kienböck's disease: Evaluation of a case by magnetic resonance imaging. *J Hand Surg* 1987;12A:1044–1049.

32. Braun RM: Pronator pedicle bone grafting in the forearm and proximal carpal row. *Orthop Trans* 1983;7:35.

33. Foucher G, Saffar PL: Revascularization of the necrosed lunate, stages I and II, with a dorsal intermetacarpal arteriovenous pedicle. *J Chir Main* 1982;1:259.

34. Saffar P: Replacement of the lunate by the pisiform bone. *Ann Chir Main* 1982;1:276–279.

35. Yazema H, Tamai S, Hori Y: A vascular bundle implantation for the treatment of Kienböck's disease. *J Jpn Orthop Assoc* 1988;62: 973.

36. Benz HJ, Blencke BA: Restitution Einer Lunatumnekrose beim bind. *Z Orthop* 1976;114:819–821.

37. Linscheid RL: Kienböck's disease, editorial. *J Hand Surg* 1985; 10A:1–3.

38. Blanco RH: Excision of the lunate in Kienböck's disease: Long-term results. *J Hand Surg* 1985;10A:1008–1013.

39. Agerholm JC, Goodfellow JW: Avascular necrosis of the lunate bone treated by excision and prosthetic replacement. *J Bone Joint Surg* 1963;45B:110–116.

40. Alexander AH, Turner MA, Alexander CE, et al: Lunate silicone replacement arthroplasty in Kienböck's disease: A long-term follow-up. *J Hand Surg* 1990;15A:401–407.

41. Barber HM, Goodfellow JW: Acrylic lunate prosthesis: A long-term follow-up. *J Bone Joint Surg* 1974;56B:706–711.

42. Carroll RE: Fascial arthroplasty in the treatment of Kienböck's disease. *Orthop Trans* 1977;1:36.

43. Evans G, Burke FD, Barton NH: A comparison of conservative treatment and silicone replacement arthroplasty in Kienböck's disease. *J Hand Surg* 1986;11B:98–102.

44. Kato H, Usui M, Minami A: Long-term results of Kienböck's disease treated by excisional arthroplasty with a silicone implant or coiled palmaris longus tendon. *J Hand Surg* 1986;11A:645–653.

45. Swanson AB, Maupin BK, de Groot Swanson G, et al: Lunate implant resection arthroplasty: Long-term results. *J Hand Surg* 1985;10A:1013–1024.

46. Nahigian SH, Li CS, Richey DG, et al: The dorsal flap arthroplasty in the treatment of Kienböck's disease. *J Bone Joint Surg* 1970;52A:245–252.

47. Carter PR, Benton LJ, Dysert PA: Silicone rubber carpal implants: A study of the incidence of late osseous complications. *J Hand Surg* 1986;11A:639–644.

48. Peimer CA, Medige J, Eckert BS, et al: Reactive synovitis after silicone arthroplasty. *J Hand Surg* 1986;11A:624–638.

49. Smith RJ, Atkinson RE, Jupiter JB: Silicone synovitis of the wrist. *J Hand Surg* 1985;10A:47–60.

50. Armistead RB, Linscheid RL, Dobyns JH, et al: Ulnar lengthening in the treatment of Kienböck's disease. *J Bone Joint Surg* 1982;64A:170–178.

51. Axelsson R, Moberg E: Le Traitement de la Maladie de Kienböck et le role des Interventions de Reequilibration Radio-Cubitale, in Razemon J-P, Fisk GR (eds): *Monographies du Groupe d'Etude de la Main*. Paris, le Poignat, 1983, chap 12, pp 210–217.

52. Linscheid RL: Kienböck's disease: Ulnar lengthening, in Robert J. Neviaser (ed): *Controversies in Hand Surgery*. New York, Churchill Livingstone, 1990, pp 159–166.

53. Soeur R, Navarre M, DeRacker CH: L'Allongement de Cubitus Respectant l'Articulation Radio-Cubitale Inferieure dans la Maladie de Kienböck. *Ann Chir Main* 1982;1:261.

54. Sundberg SB, Linscheid RL: Kienböck's disease: Results of treatment with ulnar lengthening. *Clin Orthop* 1984;187:43–51.

55. Tillberg B: Kienböck's disease treated with osteotomy to lengthen ulna. *Acta Orthop Scand* 1968;39:359–368.

56. Verbrugge J, Verjans H: L'Allongement du Cubitus Comme Traitement de Choix de la Maladie de Kienböck. *Rev Chir Orthop* 1963;49:563–576.

57. Moberg E: Treatment of Kienböck's disease by surgical correction of the length of the radius or ulna, in Tubiana R (ed): *The Hand*. Philadelphia, WB Saunders, 1985, vol 2, pp 1117–1120.

58. Almquist EE, Burns JF Jr: Radial shortening for the treatment of Kienböck's disease: A 5- to 10-ten year follow-up. *J Hand Surg* 1982;7A:348–352.

59. Eiekn O, Neichajev I: Radius shortening in malacia of the lunate. *Scand J Plast Reconstr Surg* 1980;14:191–196.

60. Nakamura R, Imaeda T, Miura T : Radial shortening for Kienböck's disease: Factors affecting the operative result. *J Hand Surg* 1990;15B:40–45.

61. Razemon JP: Shortening of the radius. *Ann Chir Main* 1982;1: 261–265.

62. Tajima T: Shortening osteotomy of forearm bone or bones in Kienböck's disease with minus, zero or plus variant. Presented at the combined meeting of the American and British Societies for Surgery of the Hand, Edinburgh, Scotland, May, 1977.

63. Chuinard RG: Kienböck's disease: Capitate-hamate arthrodesis, in Neviaser RJ (ed): *Controversies in Hand Surgery*. New York, Churchill Livingstone, 1990, pp 167–178.

64. Almquist EE: Kienböck's disease. *Hand Clin* 1987;3:141–148.

65. Trumble T, Glisson RR, Seaber AV, et al: A biomechanical comparison of the methods for treating Kienböck's disease. *J Hand Surg* 1986;11A:88–93.

66. Viegas SF, Patterson R, Peterson P, et al: The effects of various load paths and different loads on the load transfer characteristics of the wrist. *J Hand Surg* 1989;14A:458–465.

67. Werner FW, Murphy DJ, Palmer AK: Pressures in the distal radioulnar joint: Effect of surgical procedures used for Kienböck's disease. *J Orthop Res* 1989;7:445–450.

68. Inoue G, Miura T: Proximal row carpectomy in perilunate dislocations and lunatomalacia. *Acta Orthop Scand* 1990;61:449–452.

Lower Extremity

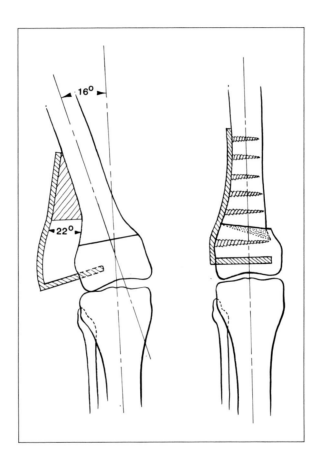

Patellofemoral Pain

John P. Fulkerson, MD

Alexander Kalenak, MD

Thomas D. Rosenberg, MD

Jay S. Cox, MD

Introduction

Patellofemoral (PF) pain is often attributed to chondromalacia. Cadaver studies,[1] however, have demonstrated clearly that chondromalacia is present commonly as an incidental finding. Also, McGinty and McCarthy,[2] Metcalf,[3] Bentley and Dowd,[4] and others have noted that many patients with anterior knee pain have completely normal patellar articular cartilage at the time of arthroscopy.

One must differentiate anterior knee pain caused by retinacular or articular trauma from pain that occurs as a result of chronic patellar malalignment. Also, one must look for signs of less common causes of anterior knee pain, such as saphenous neuropathy, reflex sympathetic dystrophy, plica, hemangioma,[5] or referred pain.

The most frequent cause of anterior knee pain is retinacular stress associated with PF malalignment. Biopsies of the lateral retinaculum done at the time of lateral release have shown that small nerves in the retinaculum can sustain injury, presumably related to chronic patellar imbalance.[6] Gomori trichrome stains of painful retinacular segments will confirm traumatic neuroma as a cause of peripatellar pain in patients with chronic patellar malalignment. It is also important to recognize that many patients with persistent anterior knee pain after surgery have neuromas and retinacular injury, which can be treated by therapy directed specifically to this area rather than to the patella.

Over long periods of time, however, patellar imbalance can cause articular breakdown because of increased focal stress or diminished normal loading of patellar articular cartilage. This is particularly true when normal cartilage function has already been altered as a result of age, injury, or increased water content. In many cases, therefore, patients who manifest retinacular pain early in the course of PF malalignment[7] will eventually begin to show signs of articular breakdown. For this reason, progression from early retinacular pain to eventual articular breakdown is not surprising.

Patellar Subluxation

As an isolated entity, patellar subluxation can lead to problems of extensor mechanism instability, increased risk of dislocation, apprehension, patellar hypermobility (often associated with patella alta), and some risk of articular or retinacular damage. Fre-

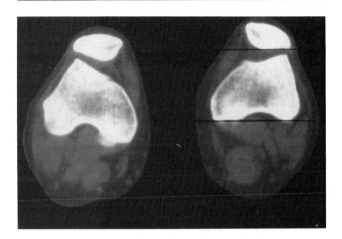

Fig. 1 Computed tomographic image with knees flexed 15 degrees. Patellar tilt as determined using mid-patellar transverse images of the PF joint with posterior condyles of the femur fully imaged.

quently, when the extensor mechanism is lateralized, subluxation can also be associated with tilt.[8] The five vowels aid in remembering the problems associated with subluxation: A-apprehension; E-excessive lateral glide; I-instability; O-often associated with tilt; U-unpredictable response to lateral release.

Abnormal Patellar Tilt

Abnormal patellar tilt (Fig. 1) differs from subluxation in that it creates a pattern of increased lateral facet loading, adaptive shortening of the lateral retinaculum, and increased risk of patellar articular breakdown and retinacular strain. The mnemonic for tilt is TOPER: Tight lateral retinaculum; Occasionally with subluxation; Positive patellar tilt test (cannot raise the lateral patellar past the horizontal plane); Excessive lateral pressure syndrome; Responds favorably to lateral release.

Clinical Examination

The differentiation between subluxation and tilt is quite important (Fig. 2). Subluxation leads to instability; tilt leads to excessive compressive loads and more rapid progression of patellar arthrosis. When the two are combined, both problems, instability and accelerated articular breakdown, can occur. Although differ-

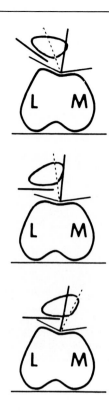

Fig. 2 The different patellar alignment patterns; from top to bottom: 1) subluxation alone 2) subluxation and tilt 3) tilt without subluxation. (Reproduced with permission from Schutzer S, Ramsby G, Fulkerson J: Computed tomographic classification of patellofemoral pain patients. *Orthop Clin North Am* 1986;17:235–248.)

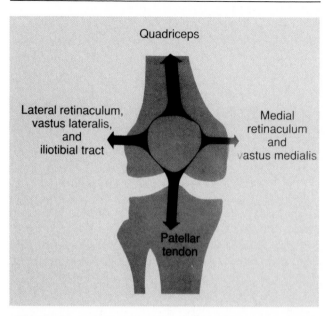

Fig. 3 The cardinal restraints of the patella must be examined independently to determine if there is excessive tightness, laxity, or pain superiorly, inferiorly, medially, and laterally. (Reproduced with permission from Fulkerson J, Hungerford D: *Disorders of the Patellofemoral Joint.* Baltimore, William and Wilkins, 1990, p 14.)

entiation of these patterns is possible through clinical examination, appropriate radiographs are very helpful in confirming or uncovering these patterns.

Some patients with no evidence of malalignment experience patellar articular breakdown. Frequently this occurs as a result of trauma, obesity, inflammatory disease in the joints, congenital malformation of the patella or trochlea, or overuse. Such patients should be differentiated from those who have extensor mechanism malalignment.

Finally, there are patients who have no evidence of extensor mechanism malalignment or patellar articular damage, but who complain of pain. It is particularly important to avoid surgery in the treatment of such patients. Surgical treatment should be reserved for patients shown by clinical and radiographic evidence to have a clearly definable mechanical disorder, which can be predicted to respond to an appropriate surgical procedure.[8] The predominant abnormal restraint or alignment should be the focus of surgical correction.

Examination of the patient with PF pain starts with a complete history. Note particularly whether the onset of pain was spontaneous or was related to trauma. This can provide evidence of some underlying structural malalignment. The patient should be asked specifically if the problem is one of instability, pain, or a combination of the two.

Observation of the patient both standing and supine will reveal structural problems, such as excessive knee valgus, excessive hip anteversion, or pronation, that can cause or aggravate patellar maltracking. The active and passive tracking of the patella should be noted, and tightness of hamstrings, iliotibial band, or quadriceps should be documented.

Examination of the Peripatellar Retinaculum

The complete PF examination must include a meticulous examination of the peripatellar retinaculum, including the patellar tendon origin and distal quadriceps. Abnormal tightness or laxity of any restraint—proximal, distal, medial, or lateral (Fig. 3)—should be noted. If there has been previous surgery or arthroscopy, it is extremely important that all scars and portals be examined for evidence of tender scar or neuroma. Many patients with anterior knee pain have a soft-tissue (usually tendon or retinaculum) source of pain. After examining the retinaculum, the clinician should determine also if there is a painful plica, saphenous neuropathy, effusion, reflex sympathetic dystrophy, or referred pattern of pain (usually from either the back or hip).

Crepitation and Articular Pain

Flexing and extending the knee while compressing the patella will reveal if true articular pain can be elicited. The clinician will note at which degree of knee flexion pain occurs, and will see if pain is related specifically to the crepitation noted on clinical examination. Unless PF pain is related directly to articular compression and/or crepitation, the clinician should not attribute pain to the articular surface.

Passive Patellar Tilt

The passive patellar tilt test evaluates tension of the lateral restraint, which includes the lateral capsule and retinaculum, the iliotibial tract, and the vastus lateralis tendon. Passive elevation of the lateral margin of the patella is restricted by these structures, which are often incised in lateral release.

Passive patellar tilt is performed with the patient supine on the examination table and the knees fully extended, relaxing the quadriceps. The examiner stands at the foot of the table and positions the limb so that the palpated transepicondylar axis is parallel to the table. The examiner grasps the patella with thumb and forefinger and elevates the lateral side of the patella while depressing the medial side (Fig. 4). The coronal patellar axis is referenced to the horizontal plane and assigned positive degrees of tilt if the lateral side can be elevated above the medial side. Negative degrees are assigned if the lateral side cannot be elevated above the horizontal plane.

Kolowich and associates,[9] using a gravitational inclinometer, tested 100 patents with normal patellae. A range of 0 to +20 degrees was found. A passive patellar tilt of less than 0 degrees indicates a significant tightness of the lateral restraint and correlates with a successful outcome in patients who have undergone a lateral release.

Medial and Lateral Patellar Glides

The glide tests indicate the integrity and tightness of the medial and lateral restraints. Lateral patellar glide, which tests the medial capsule, the medial retinaculum, and the vastus medialis obliquus is performed in a manner similar to that used for the qualitative patellar apprehension test described by Hughston.[10] Lateral patellar glide, however, measures the distance that the patella can be manually translated laterally from its passive resting position in the femora trochlea. McConnell[11] also emphasized the importance of evaluating patellar glide. The use of a position bump or the examiner's leg maintains the 30-degree angle and helps the patient relax (Fig. 5, *left*). Medial patellar glide, which tests the lateral restraint, is performed in a similar fashion and measures translation of the patella in the medial direction (Fig. 5, *right*). In order to standardize for patient knee and size variations, translations are recorded as the number of quarter-widths that the patella is displaceable. Complete dislocation of the patella by the examiner would be recorded as four quadrants of lateral glide.

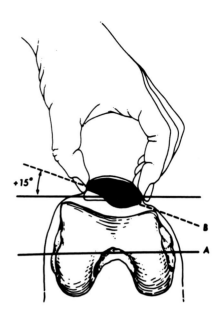

Fig. 4 Evaluation of patellar tilt.

In their study of 100 normal patients, Kolowich and associates[9] also tested medial and lateral glides. The range of lateral glide at 30 degrees of knee flexion was .05 to 2.5 quadrants; the range of medial glide at 30 degrees was 1 to 2.5 quadrants. A lateral glide of 3 quadrants suggests an incompetent medial restraint, while 0.5 to 2 quadrants is considered normal. A medial glide of 1 quadrant or less is generally indicative of a tight lateral restraint and will often be found with a negative passive patellar tilt. A medial glide of 3 or 4 quadrants suggests a hypermobile patella and "subluxability," but not necessarily "subluxation."

Quadriceps Angle at 90 Degrees

The quadriceps (Q) angle at 90 degrees of knee flexion is a modification of the quadriceps angle measured at full extension. The quadriceps angle at extension was meant to describe the degree of lateral pull exerted on the patella by vectors created by the patellar tendon and the action of the quadriceps muscle. However, this angle can be falsely reduced or even negated by lateral subluxation of the patella that occurs when the knee is extended as the patella rides superior to the trochlea. To avoid inadvertent underestimation of the quadriceps angle, the patella must be seated within the trochlear notch, which can be accomplished by flexing the knee to 90 degrees.

A more accurate representation of the distal vector of pull on the patella is obtained by measuring the quadriceps angle with the knee flexed 90 degrees. The reference points are as follows: (1) A line from the anterior inferior iliac spine to the center of the patella defines the proximal (anatomic) vector, and (2) A line

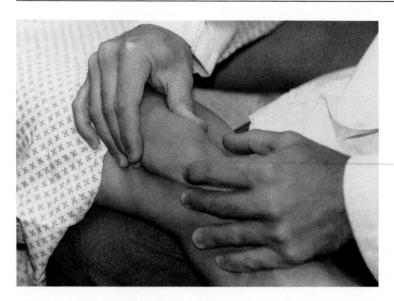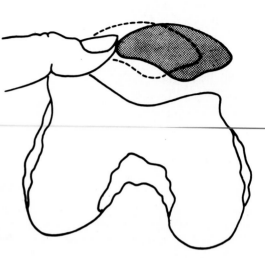

Fig. 5 **Left**, The knee should be relaxed and maintained at a 30-degree knee flexion to evaluate patellar glide. **Right**, Medial glide should be checked as well as lateral glide, particularly in the patient who notes patellar instability after surgery.

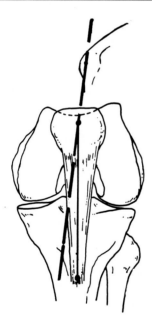

Fig. 6 Quadriceps angle measured at 90 degrees of knee flexion.

from the center of the patella to the mid-tibial tubercle defines the distal vector (Fig. 6).

The patient is positioned supine with both the hip and the knee flexed to 90 degrees. Measuring with a goniometer has established a normal range of −4 to +6 degrees. Angles greater than 8 degrees are strongly indicative of an abnormally lateralized distal patella vector.

Putting the Clinical Findings Together

Complete clinical examination of the patient with PF pain requires meticulous attention to detail. As outlined above, the clinician must differentiate between articular and retinacular pain. Also required is a clear concept of whether the patient has subluxation, subluxation and tilt, tilt alone, or no malalignment. A clear understanding of which restraints were either too loose or too tight (including muscle restraints around the knee) is necessary, and other causes of pain, including neuroma, plica, and referred pain, must be noted. With this information, the clinician will be better able to prescribe appropriate nonsurgical treatment, directed specifically at the source of pain, tightness, or instability.

Nonsurgical Treatment

Once a definitive or firm diagnosis is made, one may embark on a nonsurgical treatment plan. The vast majority of patients with a PF disorder will not require immediate surgical intervention. All patients need counseling in order to understand their disorder and start a program of home therapy. The specific program will vary somewhat depending on the patient's exact source of pain. A course of nonsteroidal anti-inflammatory medication will be started in most cases, either to reduce a defined inflammation, or to control pain. The home therapy portion of a program for PF disorders is designed to alter PF biomechanics. Any athlete who has had to rest because of this sort of problem

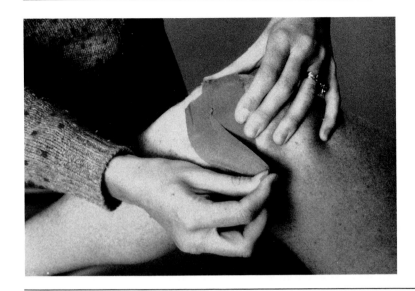

Fig. 7 The McConnell taping technique gives support of the patella to help control patellar instability (excessive medial/lateral glide, tilt, or rotation).

appreciates the fact that rest alleviates pain by diminishing the load.

In PF disorders, the pain usually emanates from one of two places, either the subchondral bone or the synovial/capsular and retinacular soft tissues. Stresses on these areas can be reduced somewhat by strengthening exercises and supporting devices. Strengthening is accomplished through specific exercises chosen to strengthen the quadriceps and hamstring muscles. Resultant changes in the PF mechanics may alter the load at the PF joint. Support in the form of an elastic or neoprene knee sleeve (with or without an open patella and with or without buttresses) may help. With excessively tight hamstrings, the quadriceps must pull harder across the PF joint, and stretching exercises to relieve tight hamstring and calf musculature can diminish the load transmitted across the PF joint.

The first phase of nonsurgical treatment, four to six weeks of home therapy, is performed by the patient, who uses simple equipment that is readily available. This program usually involves simple quadriceps strengthening, stretching, and graduated exercise. After this first phase, the patient is sent to a physical therapist only if symptoms are not significantly improved or if no definitive progress has been made.

The physical therapist assures steady progress in rehabilitation not only by evaluating and treating PF disorders, but also by helping to educate the patient in the particulars of the PF disorder and in the proper treatment regimen, by encouraging the patient on a regular basis, and by making sure that the exercise program is followed.

During the second four to six weeks, various physical therapy modalities, such as electrical stimulation of the quadriceps and hamstrings, may be tried. Ultrasound, phonophoresis, or iontophoresis may be used to treat localized painful areas. The therapist can add cautious isokinetic progressive resistive exercises, usually at higher speeds, or the exercise bicycle. Orthotic devices for the foot, by changing the mechanics of the entire lower extremity, can alter PF mechanics.

If significant pain persists after four to six weeks of physical therapy, nonsteroidal anti-inflammatory medication can be changed or discontinued. The orthotic device for the shoe may be altered in a further attempt to change mechanical loading. A custom-fitted rigid orthotic device should be fabricated to determine whether or not this change will alleviate pain in the PF articulation. Gait analysis and precise computed tomography (CT) or magnetic resonance imaging (MRI) can help at this stage by providing PF alignment pattern information.

At this point a closed-chain exercise program[11] should be considered, although some may wish to use such a program earlier. Jenny McConnell, a physical therapist in Australia, has formulated such a treatment protocol for PF disorders. This treatment, which includes taping the patella to support it in an improved alignment (Fig. 7), has been reported to have a 96% success rate. Her method of managing PF pain involves assessing orientation of the patella, determining which components need to be corrected, training the vastus medialis obliquus, and taping the patella.

McConnell first considers factors that affect patellar alignment, such as quadriceps angle, muscle tightness, excessive pronation, patella alta, and vastus medialis obliquus insufficiency. Factors to consider when embarking on this program include the position of the femur, alignment of the vastus medialis obliquus fibers, the effect of pain on muscle contraction, and specific training and biofeedback measurements to overcome this pain. Three components to be considered in patellar orientation are glide, tilt, and rotation.

The nonsurgical treatment protocol begins with stretching of quadriceps, hamstrings, and calf muscles. Medial patellar glide, especially with the patient lying on one side, is quite effective in stretching tight lateral structures.

A second thrust of the McConnell program is enhancement of the vastus medialis obliquus activity by muscle strengthening and taping. Taping may alter PF tracking. For training to be effective, the patient must not experience pain, because pain has a strong inhibitory effect on muscle function. Therefore, in order to enhance vastus medialis obliquus activity, the patella must be firmly taped to stabilize it and to reduce pain. Vastus medialis obliquus training involves tightening the medial quadriceps and using the adductors isometrically without activating the vastus lateralis. Specific strengthening exercises for the vastus medialis obliquus in order to tighten the medial quadriceps by using the adductors isometrically is a concept that is not universally appreciated. Vastus medialis obliquus training should be done in the standard fashion and also in the weightbearing position, which is a walk-stance position with the symptomatic leg forward and the knee flexed 30 degrees. Pronation and supination of the foot are also valuable assets in rehabilitation. In the McConnell program, the patient is instructed to contract the vastus medialis obliquus and to relax the lateral hamstrings and the vastus lateralis. This position is held for ten seconds while the patient supinates the foot just past mid-position. Then the patient allows the foot to return to a pronated position, but still keeping it more supinated than it is at resting. This is repeated a number of times. The exercise is repeated with the knee flexed to 75 degrees.

The next objective is to train the foot so that pronation is decreased in standing, and to increase awareness of foot positioning. Training in the weightbearing position, such as doing a plié, also facilitates vastus medialis obliquus contraction. Supination and pronation movements are repeated also. The exercise is repeated in half-squat or three-quarter squat position if pain permits. McConnell further states that eccentric muscle training must be included. The patient steps down from a step with one foot and then back up while the quadriceps of the leg remaining on the step contracts eccentrically and then concentrically. The central aspects of the program are stretching of tight peripatellar structures, retraining the vastus medialis obliquus musculature, and taping the patella to relieve pressure and pain.

Patient education is crucial to the successful treatment of PF disorders. The patient should have a thorough understanding of the mechanism of pain and of the role exercise plays in rehabilitation and pain relief. A skilled physical therapist is extremely helpful in this process. Some patients may be referred to a pain management service for evaluation and treatment, particularly if there is no specific, identifiable mechanical abnormality to correct. A patient with saphenous nerve entrapment may require injections of the saphenous nerve in the adductor canal. Other patients may require sympathetic blocks for reflex sympathetic dystrophy. The formation of a PF pain support group may be helpful, just as support groups can help patients with other chronic pain disorders or with such problems as eating disorders and substance abuse.

Radiographic and Arthroscopic Evaluation of the PF Joint

The different alignment patterns can be differentiated by careful clinical examination, but well-done radiographs add considerably to the understanding and confirmation of these patterns. Radiographs can help the clinician to avoid unnecessary operations when there is no specific alignment disorder to correct. Detailed radiographic evaluation, other than simple anteroposterior, lateral, and axial radiographs, is usually not necessary unless surgery is a serious possibility.

It is important to recognize that none of the available diagnostic tests are perfect. Examining a nonweight-bearing, supine knee clinically, radiographically, or arthroscopically cannot reveal all the intricacies of day-to-day PF function. For this reason, the authors recommend high quality studies emphasizing normal standing alignment.

Radiographic Studies

Because tangential radiographs of the patella can have distorted images, there is some risk of misinterpretation. The use of axial radiography to evaluate tilt (as opposed to subluxation) is also difficult, because the anatomy of the anterior trochlea varies considerably. Nonetheless, a good tangential axial radiograph can be very helpful in screening patients with complaints of anterior knee pain. The Merchant[12] view, in which the knee is flexed 45 degrees in the Merchant frame, or a patellar axial radiograph taken at an angle of 30 degrees from the upper leg, can be satisfactory for this purpose. The Laurin 20-degree knee flexion view[13] is also helpful in obtaining an overview of patellar alignment. CT, properly performed, can also add greatly to the understanding of PF mechanics.[5,14] Three-dimensional CT offers even greater versatility.

Mid-patellar transverse CT cuts through progressive knee flexion in the 15- to 30-degree range will give excellent knowledge of patellar tracking when mid-patellar transverse images are taken in normal standing alignment as determined by the technician before the study (Fig. 8). The patient is positioned carefully in the scanner gantry using bolsters or blankets to maintain appropriate alignment, rotation, and flexion (Fig. 8,

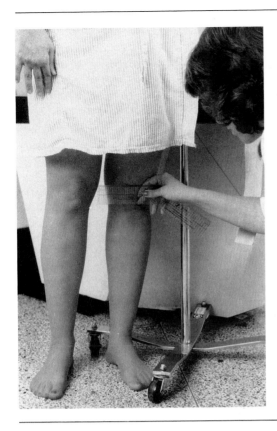

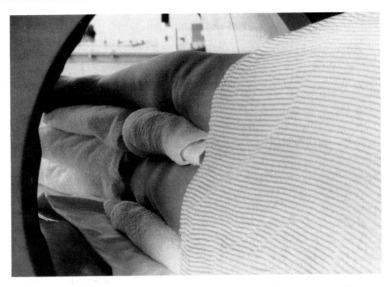

Fig. 8 Left, The CT technician will need to spend some time taking measurements between femoral condyles and malleoli adjacent to an upright (an IV pole works well) so that normal standing alignment can be reproduced in the scanner gantry. **Right**, CT of the PF joints requires attention to detail. The knees must be positioned so that precise mid- patellar tomographic images can be obtained while the patient's normal, standing varus/valgus, rotation, and lower extremity alignment are reproduced in the scanner gantry.

right). The knees are fully extended to start, and then are flexed at 15-degree increments to 45 or 60 degrees of knee flexion, and precise mid-patellar transverse images are taken at each increment of knee flexion. This series of images will simulate dynamic tracking of the patella. The angle formed by a line along the lateral patellar facet and a line along the posterior femoral condyles (Fig. 9) taken on a 15-degree knee-flexion CT cut (at the mid-patellar level) should be greater than 12 degrees in normal patellar alignment. MRI used in the same way will provide similar information, but flexion past 30 degrees may be difficult or impossible. Images that can be measured on a view box are preferable to cine studies, which, in our experience, require a more subjective interpretation. In any radiographic study, however, care must be taken to reproduce normal lower extremity alignment so that findings are not distorted. Also, gaining insight into the dynamic function of the patella by studying serial mid-patellar transverse images in progressive knee flexion is helpful.

Early studies indicate that CT or MRI can give the appearance of medial subluxation in patients who really have normal alignment or tilt. This occurs when tomographic cuts are taken distally on the patella, that is, distal to the articulating area of the patella. To avoid this problem, it is necessary to make sure that tomographic images are taken at the precise mid-patellar transverse plane. Also, it is important to be sure that what appears to be medial subluxation is not really pa-

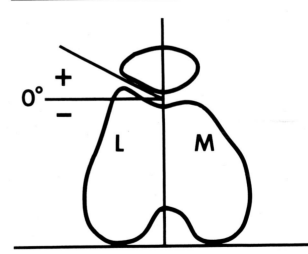

Fig. 9 To determine tilt, lines are drawn along the lateral patellar facet and along the posterior femoral condyles. The angle formed by these lines is the patellar tilt angle. Subluxation is determined best by noting medial or lateral deviation of the apex of the patella from a line perpendicular to the posterior condyle line and passing through the deepest point of the trochlea. (Reproduced with permission from Schutzer S, Ramsby G, Fulkerson J: The evaluation of patellofemoral pain using computerized tomography: A preliminary study. *Clin Orthop* 1986;204:283–286.)

tellar tilt, causing medial rotation of the central patellar ridge.

Radionuclide scans (bone scan) can be used to detect the presence or location of arthrosis.[15] At times a patient with PF joint pain may have a positive bone scan only on the trochlear side of the PF joint. Surgery on the patella of such a patient is less likely to achieve a satisfactory result.

Arthroscopy

Once the clinician understands a specific malalignment pattern, the best way to investigate patellar articular lesions is with an arthroscope. For each patient with anterior knee pain who is to undergo surgery, careful evaluation of the patella is essential. In general, the Outerbridge[16] classification has been most helpful in classifying patellar articular lesions. In determining treatment, classify each patient as to the specific malalignment pattern, and define the specific articular lesion, noting the exact location, size, and extent. Treatment when there is a lesion on the medial patella can differ from that used when there is one on the lateral facet.

In the Outerbridge classification, a grade 1 lesion is cartilage softening only; a grade 2 lesion is fibrillation less than $1/2$ inch in diameter; a grade 3 lesion is fibrillation more than $1/2$ inch in diameter; and a grade 4 lesion has exposed bone. If every articular lesion is classified and localized at the time of arthroscopy or open surgery, it is likely that the surgeon will make a better decision regarding subsequent surgery. In general, the aim is to unload a defective articular surface, particularly if there is good cartilage elsewhere on the patella that may be better able to accept contact stress.

The arthroscope may also be used to confirm the clinical and radiographic alignment pattern. Fluid distension, tourniquet pressure, instruments, anesthesia, muscle paralysis, and image distortion, however, can lead to errors regarding the alignment pattern. During arthroscopy, evaluation of tracking in the 0- to 60-degree range from a superior portal can help confirm findings before surgery. This part of the exam is most effective with low inflow pressure, without tourniquet, and under local anesthesia. A nerve stimulator can be used to cause quadriceps contraction under anesthesia, thereby simulating functional patellar tracking. Mark Friedman (personal communication, 1990) has suggested selective epidural anesthesia as another way to enable patients to contract the quadriceps while under anesthesia.

Why Is This Type of Differentiation Important?

Patients without significant objective findings of malalignment and/or arthrosis are less likely to respond favorably to treatment, particularly surgery, designed to alter alignment or contact stress. If the clinician can identify the specific disorder, it is more likely that treatment will be appropriate. For instance, lateral release will not be helpful if there is patellar arthrosis and normal alignment (lateral release is best suited for the patient with tilt and minimal arthrosis). If there is significant subluxation and recurrent dislocation, lateral release may not be enough. Similarly, if a patient has minimal arthrosis and tilt, there is no reason to do an anteromedial tibial tubercle transfer or Maquet procedure when lateral release may be very effective. It is important to know as much as possible about what is being treated before the treatment plan is selected. Careful clinical examination, followed by appropriate radiographs and arthroscopy (when surgery is necessary), will provide the needed information.

Surgical Treatment of PF Disorders

The use of surgery in the treatment of PF disorders is a last resort measure, to be undertaken only after all attempts at nonsurgical treatment have failed. Because the PF joint is highly complex in its mechanism, surgery must be carefully planned and accurately performed. The basic procedures are those directed at articular cartilage, soft-tissue surgical procedures, and realignment procedures involving movement of the anterior tibial tuberosity (Outline 1).

Surgical Procedures Directed at Articular Cartilage

Articular cartilage can undergo a repair process under certain conditions, but the repair tissue usually differs in molecular composition, organization, material properties, and durability from normal articular cartilage. The quantity, quality, and durability of the repair tissue following a specific cartilage injury cannot be reliably predicted. The success of cartilage repair will depend on the extent of the injury, the location of the injury, and whether the injury is limited to articular cartilage or extends into the subchondral bone.

If the injury involves the subchondral bone, the blood supply can induce a healing response of fibrocartilage. Obviously, healing of large defects is less satisfactory than healing of small defects. In regard to location, lesions that articulate with another cartilage surface heal less well than nonarticulating lesions.[17]

Laceration of articular cartilage perpendicular to the joint surface produces no inflammatory response. The chondrocytes at the site of the injury die, and there is no migration of chondrocytes into the injured area. The chondrocytes near the lesion will proliferate and make new matrix, but the new matrix does not fill the defect. Although there is no repair of the injury, the lesions seldom progress.

A laceration of the articular cartilage tangential or parallel to the surface will injure the chondrocytes, and

Outline 1
Cox/Kalenak recommendations for specific surgical treatment for various PF disorders.

I. PF Arthralgia
  A. No instability, malposition, chondrosis/arthrosis
     No surgery
  B. Malposition (static)
     1. Lateral—lateral release if symptomatic with tilt
     2. Medial (rare)—surgery usually not indicated
     3. Alta—no surgery
     4. Infera—proximal shift only if symptomatic
     5. Lateral compression with tilt—minimal arthrosis—lateral release
  C. Chondrosis/Arthrosis
     1. Surgery directed at diseased cartilage
        a. Debridement of fibrillated cartilage
        b. Removal of loose cartilage
        c. Subchondral bone abrasion or drilling to form some protective cartilage
     2. Surgery directed at change in forces
        a. Normal patellar position—anterior tibial tuberosity elevation to decrease PF pressures
        b. Abnormal patellar position
           1) anteromedial realignment for decompression and redistribution of forces
           2) three-dimensional surgery to also correct patella alta or patella infera
II. PF Instability
  A. General Principles
     1. Arthralgia may or may not be present
     2. Chondrosis/arthrosis may or may not be present
  B. Subluxation/Dislocation
     1. Normal PF position
        a. Medial subluxation/dislocation
           1) very rare
           2) occasionally traumatic and usually associated with ligamentous injuries of the knee
           3) usually iatrogenic
              (a) follows a lateral retinacular release, particularly when vastus lateralis tendon insertion is detached
              (b) may follow extensor mechanism realignment if anterior tibial tuberosity is shifted too far medially
           4) associated occasionally with muscle paralysis (poliomyelitis)
           5) surgical treatment for medial subluxation/dislocation of patella
              (a) difficult problem to correct surgically; get CT or MR scan to determine tracking
              (b) determine degree of knee flexion at which medial subluxation occurs
              (c) surgical realignment with use of femoral nerve stimulation to determine dynamic tracking
        b. Lateral subluxation/dislocation—normal PF position
           1) almost always an underlying malalignment problem and/or tight lateral retinaculum
           2) watch for ligamentous laxity of the knee, particularly if there is anterior cruciate ligament laxity
           3) when patella is in normal position, in regard to alta or infera, a realignment procedure in itself will usually correct problem
           4) if chondrosis/arthrosis is present, may also require anterior transfer of anterior tibial tuberosity to decompress forces
     2. Abnormal PF position—try to correct existing problems, such as patella alta, which may be associated with lateral or medial dislocation
        a. When two malalignment factors are present, such as patella alta and in increased quadriceps angle, it may be more difficult to recognize these factors than when the variation appears alone, because in combination each finding is less pronounced
        b. Medial dislocation (rare)—try to correct all existing abnormal problems
        c. Lateral subluxation/dislocation—correct all malalignment problems
        d. Abnormal PF position may require correction of patella infera and patella alta along with medial realignment (three-dimensional tuberosity shift)

they will die. The adjacent chondrocytes will synthesize matrix, and a layer of new matrix may form. However, the durability of this layer cannot be predicted.

A full-thickness cartilage injury involving bone will expose the marrow, and the marrow blood cells will produce an inflammatory response. A reparative tissue is produced and the defect will heal with a form of fibrocartilage, which is not the same as normal articular cartilage. The composition is abnormal, the structure is imperfect, and the integrity of the repair tissue is not maintained. Furukawa and associates[18] studied the amounts of type I and type II collagen in reparative cartilage tissue in rabbits. This tissue contains large amounts of type I collagen and some type II collagen, but not in normal amounts. Type II collagen makes up 90 to 95% of the total collagen in normal cartilage. However, in this repair cartilage, the type II collagen was less than 40% of the total collagen three to four weeks after the defects were created. Even at one year after injury, approximately 20% of the collagen in the reparative tissue was type I.[18] The problem is that type I collagen contains large amounts of small proteoglycans with feeble elastic properties, instead of the normal large proteoglycans seen in type II collagen. The feeble elastic properties result in fibrillation and breakdown of the repair cartilage. Also, the repair tissue cells are not normal chondrocytes.

In the treatment of cartilage lesions, superficial lesions are sometimes treated by simple debridement, such as shaving of the fibrillated cartilage. This may relieve symptoms by removing some of the irritating effect on the synovium of the breakdown products of the cartilage. There is really no evidence of significant cartilage repair. When swelling of articular cartilage or blister formation is encountered, it is probably best to leave this alone, because any type of surgical treatment would expose the cartilage matrix and perhaps hasten the breakdown process. If treatment is necessary, it is better to alter the loading forces.

Perpendicular lacerations of the articular cartilage are best left alone. Although the lesions will not heal, they seldom progress. Larger penetrating defects that involve only articular cartilage may be debrided, but care must be taken to debride only the fibrillated cartilage without beveling the edges, because such beveling damages normal cartilage.

In treating penetrating defects to subchondral bone, abrasion or drilling of the cortex produces an inflammatory response and the formation of reparative tissue. Johnson[19] has shown that irrigation of the cartilage defect with saline will extract proteoglycans and allow fibrin clot formation. Matrix proteoglycans inhibit platelet aggregation and clot formation in these defects, so extraction of the proteoglycans will improve the repair. Because the repair cartilage produced will contain a large amount of type I collagen and insufficient type II collagen, it may be necessary to change the loads that will be applied to this repair cartilage to preserve the reparative material. An appropriate osteotomy or realignment may relieve the loading forces.

Realignment Procedures—Soft-tissue Surgical Procedures

Lateral Retinacular Release This operation was originally described by Pollard[20] in 1891. Lateral release, first recommended for symptomatic patellar subluxation and dislocation, was later advocated for treatment of any PF pain. Merchant and Mercer,[21] who prepared one of the first papers in the American literature, reported 85% good or excellent results in an early series of lateral retinacular releases. However, they recommended the procedure for patients with incongruence of the PF mechanism, as visualized on axial roentgenograms. They stated that the outcome of surgery could not be predicted in patients with normal roentgenograms whose only complaint was patellar pain. In 1978, Larson and associates[22] reported good or excellent results for pain relief in patellar compression syndrome with lateral retinacular release. They used a Z-plasty technique to lengthen the lateral patellar retinaculum. In

a further report, Ceder and Larson[23] found 81% good or excellent results from the Z-plasty technique of lateral retinacular release. Micheli and Stanitski[24] performed a series of 100 retinacular releases in 33 patients over a period of 27 months, and reported this in 1981. Their results assessed functional and anatomic criteria, and 76.7% of the patients had excellent or good results following surgery.

The next stage in lateral retinacular release involved using the arthroscope to perform releases. McGinty and McCarthy[2] obtained 82% good or excellent results with endoscopic lateral retinacular release. Although they stated that the release must extend through the substance of the vastus lateralis, more recent experiences have shown that care must be taken in releasing the insertion of the vastus lateralis.[25] In 1984, Bigos and McBride[26] reported good or excellent results in 95 of 102 cases. These were performed for chondromalacia patellae, patellar compression syndrome, and subluxations and dislocations of the patella. Dzioba,[27] in a 1985 report on open lateral release, found good to excellent results with the open procedure. In 1986, Henry, Goletz, and Williamson[28] reported on 100 lateral retinacular releases performed percutaneously with a Smillie knife. They recommended that the patella be able to be tilted to 90 degrees after release and reported 88% good results in relieving pain and instability. However, they did report that 4% of their patients developed reflex sympathetic dystrophy. In 1987, Bray, Roth, and Jacobsen[29] reported on arthroscopic lateral releases performed in workers' compensation and noncompensation cases. They stated that, judged by objective criteria, only 46% in each group had satisfactory results, and that poor outcome was related to advancing age, obesity, and poor quadriceps function. They found no relation to the outcome in those that developed hemarthrosis, those that already had chondromalacia, and whether an open versus a closed technique was used. In 1987, Schonholtz, Zahn, and Magee[30] reported on 22 patients that had undergone arthroscopic lateral release. Fifteen of the procedures had been done to correct subluxation or dislocation, and only 67% were improved. Among the seven patients who underwent the procedure for PF pain, only one had a satisfactory result. The conclusion was that lateral retinacular release performed for pain without instability was not successful. Betz, Magill, and Lonergan[31] reported on lateral retinacular release in 39 cases. They found that only 29% of those performed for recurrent subluxation and dislocation had no instability symptoms and that the results deteriorated with time. In 1987, Fulkerson and associates[8] reported on the correlation of a CT scan with lateral retinacular release. They stated that lateral retinacular release does reduce abnormal patellar tilt and a good clinical result was obtained when there was tilt without subluxation and with minimal arthrosis. They also noted that lateral release was much less consistent in relieving subluxation.

Therefore, a review of the literature suggests that the current indications for lateral release should consist of: (1) PF pain with lateral tilt; (2) lateral retinacular pain with lateral tilt or lateral patellar position; and (3) tight lateral retinaculum - excessive lateral pressure syndrome. In cases of patellar instability, when there is significant subluxation or dislocation, a more extensive procedure should probably be performed, either a procedure that combines the lateral release with medial capsular reefing or a complete realignment involving the anterior tibial tuberosity.

Contraindications for lateral retinacular release are: (1) PF pain syndrome (anterior knee pain of adolescence); (2) advanced PF arthrosis; and (3) normal tracking patella.

The types of surgical lateral retinacular release include the open techniques of incision of the lateral retinaculum, excision of a small strip of retinaculum, or a Z-plasty performed on the transverse fibers. Closed methods are percutaneous release, arthroscopic incision, and arthroscopic electrosurgical release. The general principles of the surgical technique involve first a diagnostic arthroscopic evaluation of the chondral surfaces and treatment of the articular pathology if necessary. For observation of the patellar position and tracking, a superior medial or superior lateral portal is best. When possible, it is wise to evaluate the dynamic tracking by femoral nerve stimulation under general anesthesia, by selective epidural anesthesia to allow active quadriceps contraction, or by local anesthesia. The principles of the release involve severing the lateral retinaculum within 1 cm of the patella, where it is less vascular. The superior lateral geniculate vessels should be identified and cauterized. The vastus lateralis tendon must be avoided. If severed, it can retract and cause weakness and can lead to medial subluxation. Disruption of the tendon also decreases the overall strength of the extensor mechanism, and the tendon is very hard to identify for a successful late repair. After a lateral retinacular release has been performed, if there is no improvement in the patellar tracking, consider cautious imbrication of the medial capsule. As a final step in performing the surgery, the tourniquet, if used, should be released and bleeding controlled. The author's preferred method is an open Z-plasty procedure performed through a very small longitudinal incision 2 to 3 cm in length. The Z-plasty of the transverse fibers of the lateral retinaculum allows 1 to 1.5 cm of lengthening. It is also easy to identify and coagulate the superior lateral geniculate vessels through this incision, and suturing the Z-plasty prevents medial dislocation.

Postoperative management includes the use of ice for 48 hours and early gentle active range-of-motion exercises. It is wise at some point after surgery to re-evaluate PF tracking with a CT scan to confirm the results of the lateral retinacular release.

Of the complications reported, hemarthrosis has been the most common.[32] The incidence of hemarthrosis is higher when a tourniquet is used and when a drain is used. Other complications reported include medial subluxation, ankylosis, infection, and reflex sympathetic dystrophy.

The other soft-tissue procedure—a medial imbrication of the medial capsule—is seldom indicated as an isolated procedure. It is usually used in conjunction with a lateral retinacular release and other bony procedures.

Bone and Soft-tissue Procedures

Medial Realignment A medial realignment of the extensor mechanism was first reported in 1888 by Roux.[33] It was later performed by Hauser[34] and subsequently by Trillat and associates.[35] Trillat attributed his knowledge of the procedure to Elmslie from England, who had never published the surgical technique. The Roux-Elmslie-Trillat procedure involves a lateral retinacular release, medial capsular reefing, and medial transfer of the anterior tibial tuberosity. The indications for this procedure are recurrent lateral patellar subluxation or dislocation with an increased quadriceps angle. It is also performed in certain cases of PF arthrosis with lateral patellar position, lateral patellar tilt, and increased quadriceps angle. This realignment relieves the pain from the arthrosis by redistributing the forces on the PF joint. The contraindications for the procedure are open epiphyseal plates or a normal quadriceps angle.

The surgical technique involves a lateral longitudinal incision, lateral retinacular release by Z-plasty, medial capsular reefing to take up the slack medially, and a medial transposition of the anterior tibial tuberosity. The tuberosity is moved medially only enough to correct the quadriceps angle to within normal limits. It is important to avoid moving the tuberosity too far medially, which could result in medial subluxation or dislocation. Also, moving the tuberosity posteriorly on the tibia, as was done in the Hauser procedure, must be avoided, because to do so causes increased PF pressure (Fig. 10, *left*).

The advantages of the Roux-Elmslie-Trillat procedure (Fig. 10, *right*) are that it realigns the extensor mechanism without placing the tibial tuberosity posteriorly. These realignment efforts can be evaluated at the time of surgery. A longitudinal lateral incision avoids the infrapatellar branch of the saphenous nerve, and the long-term results have been quite satisfactory.[36]

The disadvantage of this procedure is that it does not in itself correct all patellar malposition problems, such as patella alta or patella infera. There is also no decompression of the PF forces.

Complications, which usually occur when the procedure is performed in patients with open epiphyseal

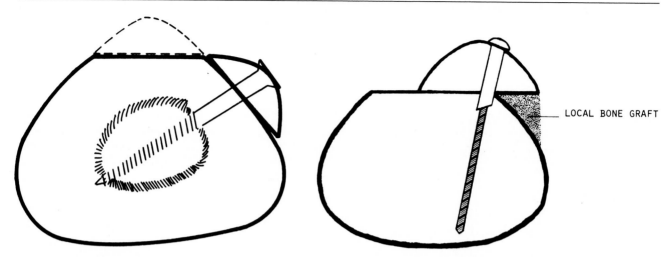

Fig. 10   **Left,** The Hauser procedure, as well as some other medial tibial tubercle transfer procedures, will "posteriorize" the tibial tubercle, potentially resulting in increased pressure on the patellar articular surface. **Right,** The Trillat procedure, as depicted by Cox, allows straight medial transfer of the tibial tubercle. (Reproduced with permission from Cox J: Evaluation of the Roux-Elmslie-Trillat procedure for knee extensor realignment. *Am J Sports Med* 1982;10:303–310.)

plates, can result in growth abnormalities, such as patella infera and external tibial rotation. When done in acute traumatic cases of subluxation or dislocation of the patella, fibrous ankylosis is common.[36] It is also necessary to avoid extensor mechanism realignment if there is anterior cruciate ligament laxity, because such cases have a high failure rate.[36]

An alternative to the Roux-Elmslie-Trillat procedure in young patients with recurrent subluxation of the patella and open epiphyseal plates is the transfer medially of the medial one-half of the patellar tendon as described by Slocum and associates.[37]

Anterior Realignment Elevation of the anterior tibial tuberosity to reduce PF joint force was described by Maquet in 1976.[38] His recommended elevation, at least 2 cm, was accompanied by many complications. In 1979, Ferguson and associates[39] stated that a 1.25-cm elevation was adequate to reduce the PF joint force and also to reduce the incidence of complications. Nakamura and associates,[40] in studying the contact areas with various elevations of anterior tibial tuberosity, showed that with a 1-cm elevation there was minimal change in the contact area. With 2 cm of elevation there was marked change in the contact area, with concentration of forces on the proximal part of the patellar surface. This concentration of force was increased by any further anterior advancement of the tibial tuberosity. They found the PF joint force was reduced through all angles of flexion of the knee by an elevation of only 1 cm of the anterior tibial tuberosity. There is minimal disturbance of patterns of contact and minimal reduction in the size of the area of the contact.

The primary indication for anterior realignment is PF pain secondary to chondrosis, particularly if the chondrosis is on the distal articular surface of the patella. A contraindication is advanced, diffuse PF arthrosis, particularly arthrosis that involves the proximal patella.

The surgical technique involves a long incision, preferably lateral, to avoid the infrapatellar branch of the saphenous nerve. A long osteotomy of at least 10 cm is necessary to reduce the distal displacement of the patella. The elevation of the tibial tuberosity should be at least 1 cm and probably no more than 1.5 cm. The bone graft can be obtained from the adjacent tibia or from the iliac crest. A modification of this procedure uses an oblique osteotomy and local bone graft. This results in anteriorization with less bone graft (Fig. 11). There should be adequate fixation, with one or more bicortical screws to allow immediate motion of the knee joint. The complications following this procedure have been reported as anterior compartment syndrome and skin necrosis, but with attention to detail these can be avoided. Again, the purpose of this procedure is to relieve pain by decompressing the PF forces.

Anteromedial Realignment A combination of transfer of the tibial tubercle medially as well as anteriorly was described in 1983.[41] Variations of this technique were published by Brown and associates[42] in 1984 and Miller and associates[43] in 1986. The principle involved is extensor mechanism realignment by shifting the tibial tuberosity medially, and elevation of the tuberosity by shifting it forward. This not only provides a redistribution of force by realigning the extensor mechanism, it also reduces force concentration by elevating the tibial tuberosity. The procedure is most effective when there is chondrosis or arthrosis of the lateral and/or distal patellar surface associated with malalignment.

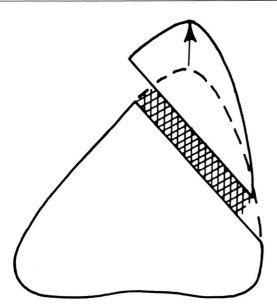

Fig. 11 Local graft behind oblique osteotomy deep to the tibial tubercle will allow anteriorization of the tibial tubercle with less bone graft.

The procedure is very similar to the Roux-Elmslie-Trillat procedure, and involves a lateral retinacular release, as well as anterior and medial displacement of the anterior tibial tuberosity. The procedure of choice (Fig. 12) results in a very stable displacement of the anterior tibial tuberosity.[44] Fixation with two or more bicortical screws allows immediate mobilization of the knee joint. The maximum anterior transfer that can be obtained

with this technique is approximately 17 mm.[44] The amount of anterior shift can be controlled by the angle of the osteotomy. The medial shift should be only enough to correct the patellar tracking to within the limits of normal.

Distal Shift of the Patella This procedure is indicated in cases of subluxation or dislocation of the patella accompanied by patella alta. Usually, a combination of malalignment problems is present, such as external tibial torsion, excessive femoral anteversion, an increase in the quadriceps angle, or genu varum or genu valgum. When two or more malalignment factors are present, each is more difficult to recognize in itself. Therefore, one must look for patella alta in these cases of recurrent subluxation of the patella. The surgical procedure consists of realignment of the extensor mechanism, with a distal shift of the anterior tibial tuberosity to correct the patella alta. The correction should not be excessive, and it should allow the patella to be within the normal ratio of the length of the patella to the length of the patellar tendon. Usually, the tibial tuberosity can be shifted distally 1 to 1.5 cm without putting excessive pressure on the PF mechanism. However, if a more distal transfer is necessary, a Z-Y-plasty of the quadriceps mechanism may be necessary[45].

Proximal Shift of the Patella This procedure may be necessary in cases of patella infera. Patella infera is usually a patellar tendon contracture syndrome secondary to quadriceps loss of tone from longstanding knee problems. When the patella is displaced distally, there is excess PF pressure accompanied by pain. The proce-

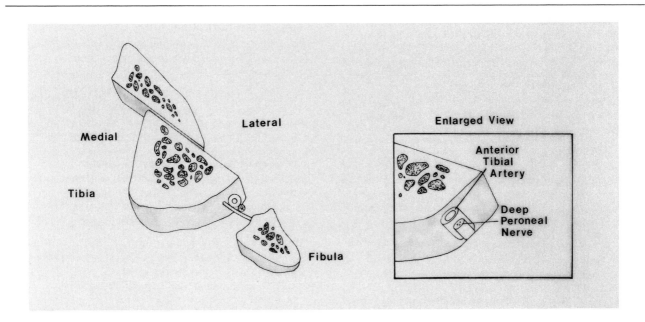

Fig. 12 Anteromedial transfer of the tibial tubercle. (Reproduced with permission from Fulkerson JP: Anteromedial tibial tubercle transfer without bone graft. *Am J Sports Med* 1990;18:490–497.)

dure requires the proximal shift of the anterior tibial tuberosity. This can be accomplished either by a simple superior shift or in combination with realignment, techniques previously described. Lengthening the patellar tendon is not recommended.

Three-Dimensional Shift This has become much more common in our practice, because of the variety of malalignment problems that frequently accompany PF arthrosis or instability. Anteromedialization of the tibial tuberosity can be performed, and if there is also patella alta the tuberosity can be shifted distally. Also, in cases of patella infera, the anteromedialization can be accompanied by a proximal shift of the tuberosity to compensate for the inferior position of the patella. Three-dimensional shift is accompanied by lateral retinacular release and medial capsular reefing. The tuberosity is fixed with two or more bicortical screws to allow early mobilization, just as in two-dimensional realignment. Finally, when performing extensor mechanism realignment, dynamic tracking should be evaluated whenever possible. This can be accomplished by femoral nerve stimulation when the patient is under general anesthesia, or by using selective epidural anesthesia or local anesthesia to allow quadriceps contraction.

References

1. Casscells W: Gross pathological changes in the knee joint of the aged individual: A study of 300 cases. *J Bone Joint Surg* 1975; 57A:1033.
2. McGinty JB, McCarthy JC: Endoscopic lateral retinacular release: A preliminary report. *Clin Orthop* 1981;158:120–125.
3. Metcalf RW: An arthroscopic method for lateral release of the subluxating or dislocating patella. *Clin Orthop* 1982;167:9–18.
4. Bentley G, Dowd G: Current concepts of etiology and treatment of chondromalacia patellae. *Clin Orthop* 1984;189:209–228.
5. Fulkerson J, Hungerford D: *Disorders of the Patellofemoral Joint.* Baltimore, Williams and Wilkins, 1990.
6. Fulkerson JP, Tennant R, Jaivin JS, et al: Histologic evidence of retinacular nerve injury associated with patellofemoral malalignment. *Clin Orthop* 1985;197:196–205.
7. Fulkerson JP: Awareness of the retinaculum in evaluating patellofemoral pain. *Am J Sports Med* 1982;10:147–149.
8. Fulkerson JP, Schutzer SF, Ramsby GR, et al: Computerized tomography of the patellofemoral joint before and after lateral release or realignment. *Arthroscopy* 1987;3:19–24.
9. Kolowich PA, Paulos LE, Rosenberg TD, et al: Lateral release of the patella: Indications and contraindications. *Am J Sports Med* 1990;18:359–365.
10. Hughston JG: Subluxation of the patella. *J Bone Joint Surg* 1968; 50A:1003–1026.
11. McConnell J: The management of chondromalacia patella: A long term solution. *Aust J Physiotherapy* 1986;32:215–223.
12. Merchant AC, Mercer RL, Jacobsen RH, et al: Roentgenographic analysis of patellofemoral congruence. *J Bone Joint Surg* 1974; 56A:1391–1396.
13. Laurin CA, Dussault R, Levesque HP: The tangential x-ray investigation of the patellofemoral joint: X-ray technique, diagnostic criteria and their interpretation. *Clin Orthop* 1979;144: 16–26.

14. Schutzer SF, Ramsby GR, Fulkerson JP: The evaluation of patellofemoral pain using computerized tomography: A preliminary study. *Clin Orthop* 1986;204:286–293.
15. Dye SF, Boll DA: Radionuclide imaging of the patellofemoral joint in young adults with anterior knee pain. *Orthop Clin North Am* 1986;17:249–262.
16. Outerbridge R: The etiology of chondromalacia patella. *J Bone Joint Surg* 1961;43B:752–757.
17. Buckwalter JA, Hunziker E, Rosenberg LC, et al: Articular cartilage: Composition and structure, in Woo SL, Buckwalter JA (eds): *Injury and Repair of the Musculoskeletal Soft Tissues.* Park Ridge, American Academy of Orthopaedic Surgeons, 1988, pp 405–425.
18. Furukawa T, Eyre DR, Koide S, et al: Biochemical studies on repair cartilage resurfacing experimental defects in the rabbit knee. *J Bone Joint Surg* 1980;62A:79–89.
19. Johnson LL: Characteristics of the immediate postarthroscopic blood clot formation in the knee joint. *Arthroscopy* 1991;7:14–23.
20. Pollard B: Old dislocation of patella by intra-articular operation. *Lancet* 1891;1:988–989.
21. Merchant AC, Mercer RL: Lateral release of the patella: A preliminary report. *Clin Orthop* 1974;103:40–45.
22. Larson RL, Cabaud HE, Slocum DB, et al: The patellar compression syndrome: Surgical treatment by lateral retinacular release. *Clin Orthop* 1978;134:158–167.
23. Ceder LC, Larson RL: Z-plasty lateral retinacular release for the treatment of patellar compression syndrome. *Clin Orthop* 1979; 144:110–113.
24. Micheli LJ, Stanitski CL: Lateral patellar retinacular release. *Am J Sports Med* 1981;9:330–336.
25. Hughston JC, Deese M: Medial subluxation of the patella as a complication of lateral retinacular release. *Am J Sports Med* 1988: 16:383–388.
26. Bigos SJ, McBride GG: The isolated lateral retinacular release in the treatment of patellofemoral disorders. *Clin Orthop* 1984; 186:75–80.
27. Dzioba RB: Diagnostic arthroscopy and longitudinal open lateral release: A four year follow-up study to determine predictors of surgical outcome. *Am J Sports Med* 1990;18:343–348.
28. Henry JH, Goletz TH, Williamson B: Lateral retinacular release in patellofemoral subluxation. Indications, results, and comparison to open patellofemoral reconstruction. *Am J Sports Med* 1986;14:121–129.
29. Bray RC, Roth JH, Jacobsen RP: Arthroscopic lateral release for anterior knee pain: A study comparing patients who are claiming worker's compensation with those who are not. *Arthroscopy* 1987; 3:237–247.
30. Schonholtz GH, Zahn MG, Magee CM: Lateral retinacular release of the patella. *Arthroscopy* 1987;3:269–272.
31. Betz RR, Magill JT III, Lonergan RP: The percutaneous lateral retinacular release. *Am J Sports Med* 1987;15:477–482.
32. Small NC: An analysis of complications in lateral retinacular release procedures. *Arthroscopy* 1989;5:282–286.
33. Roux C: Luxation habituelle de la rotule: Traitement operatoire. *Rev Chir* 1888;8:682–689.
34. Hauser EDW: Total tendon transplant for slipping patella: A new operation for recurrent dislocation of the patella. *Surg Gynecol Obstet* 1938;66:199–214.
35. Trillat A, DeJour H, Couette A: Diagnostic et traitement des subluxation recidevantes de la rotule. *Rev Chir* 1864;50:813–823.
36. Cox JS: Evaluation of the Roux-Elmslie-Trillat procedure for knee extensor realignment. *Am J Sports Med* 1982;10:303–310.
37. Slocum DB, Larson RL, James SL: Late reconstruction of ligamentous injuries of the medial compartment of the knee. *Clin Orthop* 1974;100:23–55.

38. Maquet P: Advancement of the tibial tuberosity. *Clin Orthop* 1976;115:225–230.

39. Ferguson AB Jr, Brown TD, Fu FH, et al: Relief of patellofemoral contact stress by anterior displacement of the tibial tubercle. *J Bone Joint Surg* 1979;61A:159–166.

40. Nakamura N, Ellis M, Seedhom BB: Advancement of the tibial tuberosity: A biomechanical study. *J Bone Joint Surg* 1985;67B: 255–260.

41. Fulkerson JP: Anteromedialization of the tibial tuberosity for patellofemoral malalignment. *Clin Orthop* 1983;177:176–181.

42. Brown DE, Alexander AH, Lichtman DM: The Elmslie-Trillat procedure: Evaluation in patellar dislocation and subluxation. *Am J Sports Med* 1984;12:104–109.

43. Miller BJ, LaRochelle PJ: The treatment of patellofemoral pain by combined rotation and elevation of the tibial tubercle. *J Bone Joint Surg* 1986;68A:419–423.

44. Fulkerson JP, Meaney JA, Becker GJ, et al: Anteromedial tibial tubercle transfer without bone graft. *Am J Sports Med* 1990;18: 490- 497.

45. Scott RD, Siliski JM: The use of modified Z-Y quadricepsplasty during total knee replacement to gain exposure and improve flexion in the ankylosed knee. *Orthopaedics* 1985;8:45–48.

Unicompartmental Arthritis: Biomechanics and Treatment Alternatives

Donald L. Bartel, PhD

Introduction

Unicompartmental arthritis is associated with an increase in the force on the affected compartment of the knee. Usually, it is assumed that the increased force is secondary to malalignment. It is also possible, however, that the increase in force could cause the supporting bone to fail and lead to subsequent malalignment of the joint. In either case, realignment must be introduced as part of the surgical treatment in order to decrease the force on the affected compartment. Detailed and somewhat complex procedures have been introduced and implemented to determine the amount of realignment required and to ascertain whether corrections should be made on the femoral or the tibial side of the joint.[1-4] However, the underlying principle in all of these procedures is simple. The lower extremity must be reconstructed so that the mechanical axis of the leg passes through or near the center of the knee joint. If the mechanical axis does not pass near the center of the knee, the functional loads on the foot will produce large moments about the knee. These moments will result in a large medial compartment force in the varus knee or a large lateral compartment force in the valgus knee.

The purpose of this chapter is to describe how alignment affects the loads on the medial and lateral compartments of the knee and to use this information to understand suggested alignment procedures and clinical observations. We will first look at the forces in the normal knee and then consider the effects of malalignment on these forces. The numerical examples presented in this chapter are consistent with those developed by Burstein[5] for the normal knee.

The Normal Knee

The major voluntary function of the knee is flexion and extension in the sagittal plane. The peak functional force on the foot during gait occurs just after heel strike, and its line of action is behind the knee joint (Fig. 1). The primary loads at the knee may be reduced to two: a joint contact force and a force in the patellar ligament. The three forces acting on the lower leg—the force on the foot, the joint contact force, and the ligament force—must pass through a single point. Thus, the direction of the joint contact force can be determined readily, because the direction of the ligament

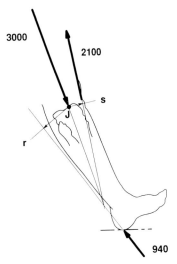

Fig. 1 The maximum forces on the knee during normal gait for a 700 N individual. The forces at the knee may be reduced to a joint contact force (3,000 N) and a patellar ligament force (2,100 N). (Adapted with permission from Burstein AH: Biomechanics of the knee, in Insall JN (ed): *Surgery of the Knee*. New York, Churchill Livingstone, 1984, pp 21–39.)

force is known from the anatomy. When the directions of the forces and the magnitude of the force on the foot are known, the equations of equilibrium can be solved to determine magnitudes of the joint contact force and the ligament force.

The joint contact force (3,000 N) and the ligament force (2,100 N) are both quite large, as high as three to four times body weight (700 N), because the line of action of the ligament force passes so close to the joint. The counterclockwise moment produced by the ligament force about the contact point, shown as point J, in Figure 1, must equal the clockwise moment produced by the force on the foot. Because the moment arm of the ligament force, **s**, is much smaller than the moment arm of the functional force on the foot, **r**, equilibrium can only be achieved if the ligament force is much larger than the force on the foot.

The 940 N force on the foot shown in Figure 1 can be resolved into components (Fig. 2), which act in the vertical direction (900 N) and the medial direction (50 N). The 50 N force produces a varus moment at the knee joint, which is resisted by the moment produced by the contact forces on the medial and lateral plateaus and by the soft-tissue structures around the joint. The 3,000 N joint contact force is distributed unequally

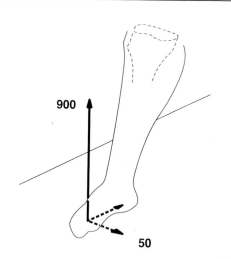

Fig. 2 Components of the force on the foot. The force on the foot during gait may be resolved into a vertical component (900 N) and a lateral-medial component (50 N). (Adapted with permission from Burstein AH: Biomechanics of the knee, in Insall JN (ed): *Surgery of the Knee.* New York, Churchill Livingstone, 1984, pp 21–39.)

between the lateral and medial plateaus of the tibia; the magnitude of the force carried by each plateau depends on the varus (or valgus) moment produced by the functional loading on the foot.

In the normal knee during normal gait, the varus

moment is caused almost entirely by the lateral-medial force on the foot, because the line of action of the vertical component of the foot force (900 N) passes through or near the center of the joint and, therefore, produces no moment about the center of the joint. The line of action of the ligament force also passes through the center of the joint. Consequently, the resisting moment at the knee joint must be produced by an appropriate distribution of the joint force between the lateral and medial plateaus (Fig. 3, *left*). This is possible because the articular cartilage deforms as a result of a very small varus rotation of the tibia, and this deformation allows the load on the medial plateau (1,950 N) to be larger than that on the lateral plateau (1,050 N). As a result, a clockwise moment is produced that counteracts the counterclockwise moment produced by the 50 N force. If the lateral component of the force on the foot is increased to 150 N, the varus moment is also increased (Fig. 3, *center left*). An additional small varus rotation of the tibia allows the medial force to increase to 2,850 N and the lateral force to decrease to 150 N (Fig. 3, *center left*) through additional small deformations of the articular cartilage on the two plateaus. Note that the lateral and medial forces on the plateau still add up to 3,000 N, the total joint force. Of course, this redistribution of force on the lateral and medial plateaus can only be maintained if contact continues on the lateral side. If the lateral-medial force on the foot gets large enough to separate the medial

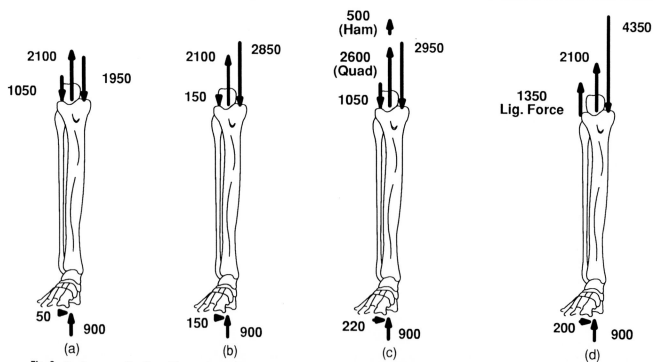

Fig. 3 In the normally aligned knee, the distribution of the forces on the lateral and medial plateaus depends on the magnitude of the lateral-medial force on the foot (**left**) and (**center left**) and for large lateral medial forces on whether or not there is co-contraction of the quadriceps and hamstrings (**center right**) or separation between the condyle and plateau on the lateral side (**right**).

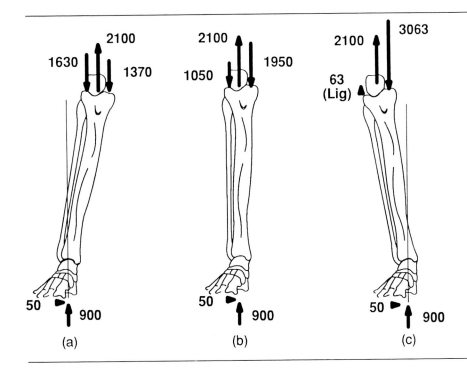

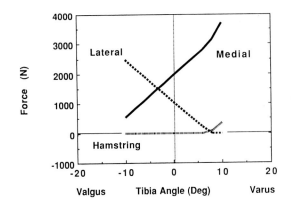

Fig. 4 Valgus (**left**) or varus (**right**) malalignment of the knee produces substantial changes in the force distributions between the two plateaus when compared to the knee with normal alignment (**center**).

condyle and the medial plateau, redistribution of force will require co-contraction of the quadriceps and hamstrings to increase the total joint force to maintain contact or, in the absence of co-contraction, a force in the lateral ligament (Fig. 3, *center right* and *right*). In the first case, the total joint force is increased because of co-contraction; in the second, the force on the medial plateau is increased substantially.

The Varus Knee

Any varus angulation of the knee results in the line of action of the 900 N force passing to the medial side of the joint center (Fig. 4, *right*). As a result, the varus moment caused by the 900 N force cannot be ignored, but must be added to the moment produced by the 50 N force that occurs during gait. As the varus angulation increases, the force on the medial plateau also increases and the force on the lateral plateau decreases (Fig. 5).

As the angulation of the tibia increases (to about 12 degrees in this example), contact can no longer be maintained without co-contraction of the flexors and extensors of the knee. As noted for the normal knee, co-contraction results in an increase in total joint contact force, which can be painful. The alternative is to minimize total joint contact force by allowing separation on the lateral side. In this case, the resisting moment at the knee joint cannot be supplied by compressive contact forces on the tibial plateaus alone. The additional moment required is supplied by tensile force in the lateral collateral ligament and increased compressive force on the medial plateau. This is consistent

Fig. 5 When a varus or valgus knee is corrected so that the mechanical axis of the tibia passes close to or through the center of the knee (tibia angle zero degrees), the plateau forces are made more equal and the force on the affected compartment is reduced. Overcorrecting a varus knee into valgus can further reduce the medial plateau force and the difference between the plateau forces.

with clinical observations of damage to the lateral ligament in varus knees.

The Valgus Knee

In the valgus knee, the line of action of the 900 N force is on the lateral side of the knee (Fig. 4, *left*). As a result, the 900 N force produces a valgus moment about the center of the knee joint. This moment is resisted by the varus moment of the 50 N lateral-medial force caused by gait and by the varus moment produced by the unequal components of the joint contact force on the lateral and medial plateaus. The contact forces on the plateaus are substantially different from those of the normal knee (Fig. 4, *center*) but are smaller in magnitude and more equally distributed than they are for the varus knee (Fig. 4, *right*) with the same degree of angulation. Therefore, the counteracting moment produced by the lateral-medial force on the foot in the valgus knee makes the abnormal contact force distribution somewhat less severe for the valgus knee than for the varus knee with the same degree of angulation.

Observations

By applying the principles presented here, the surgeon can choose the appropriate degree of correction needed to reduce the amount of force on the affected compartment and to equalize the contact forces on the tibial plateau. The clear goal of any realignment of the knee is to make the mechanical axis of the knee (the line of action of the functional force on the foot) pass as close to the center of the knee joint as possible. The benefits are obvious. If a valgus knee is corrected to a more normal alignment, the force on the lateral plateau decreases and the force on the medial plateau increases (Fig. 5). Similarly, when a varus knee is corrected, the medial force decreases and the lateral force increases.

It is interesting to note that in normal alignment, in which the tibia angle equals zero degrees, the forces on the two plateaus are not equal; the medial plateau force is about 50% larger than the lateral plateau force. The forces on the two plateaus are equal when the knee is in a small amount of valgus (Fig. 5). Therefore, some overcorrection of a varus knee, which is suggested in some cases, has two benefits. First, it equalizes the forces on the two plateaus and further reduces the force on the medial plateau. Second, by putting the knee in some valgus, the effect of the varus moment caused by the lateral-medial force (the 50 N force in these examples) is counteracted by the valgus moment

produced by the vertical force on the foot (the 900 N force).

These observations also provide insight into recently published long-term results of the influence of walking mechanics on the results of tibial osteotomies.[6] It was found that patients with low adduction moments (varus moments) at the knee had better results than those with higher adduction moments. The low adduction moment in the malaligned knee was achieved by a toe-out gait, which caused the line of action of the force on the foot to pass closer to the center of the joint. As in the examples presented here, the toe-out gait tends to equalize the force distributed on the two plateaus by reducing the magnitude of the force on the medial plateau and increasing the lateral plateau force.

Finally, it should be noted that malalignment of the knee can be caused by any of a number of different conditions and can involve abnormalities of the distal femur, the proximal tibia, or both. As stated previously, methods have been developed that use measurements taken from radiographs to determine how and where corrections should be made.[1-4] The common goal of all these procedures is to move the line of action of the force on the foot (the mechanical axis of the knee) so that it once again passes through or close to the center of the knee joint.

References

1. Cooke TD, Pichora D, Siu D, et al: Surgical implications of varus deformity of the knee with obliquity of joint surfaces. *J Bone Joint Surg* 1989;71B:560–565.
2. Yoshioka Y, Siu DW, Scudamore RA, et al: Tibial anatomy and functional axes. *J Orthop Res* 1989;7:132–137.
3. Kettelkamp DB, Chao EYS: A method for quantitative analysis of medial and lateral compression forces at the knee during standing. *Clin Orthop* 1972;83:202–213.
4. Hsu RWW, Himeno S, Coventry MB, et al: Normal axial alignment of the lower extremity and load-bearing distribution at the knee. *Clin Orthop* 1990;255:215–227.
5. Burstein AH: Biomechanics of the knee, in Insall JN (ed): *Surgery of the Knee*. New York, Churchill Livingstone, 1984, pp 21–39.
6. Wang J-W, Kuo KN, Andriacchi TP, et al: The influence of walking mechanics and time on the results of proximal tibial osteotomy. *J Bone Joint Surg* 1990;72A:905–909.

Distal Femoral Osteotomy for Lateral Gonarthrosis

Bernard F. Morrey, MD

Bradley C. Edgerton, MD

Introduction

Proximal tibial osteotomy is generally associated with the treatment of a varus deformity and medial gonarthrosis. The short- and long-term value of upper tibial osteotomy in the management of medial gonarthrosis has been well documented to provide satisfactory results in as many as 85% to 90% of patients.[1-6] Valgus deformity of the knee is uncommon and may be due to a number of causes, the most frequent of which is primary arthrosis.[3,7-11] In contrast to its efficacy in the treatment of medial compartment disease, proximal tibial osteotomy for the treatment of lateral gonarthrosis with valgus deformity is more controversial.[3,11]

Some believe the results are too unpredictable and recommend that all varus correction be performed proximal to the joint.[11] Coventry[3] and Ranieri and associates,[6] however, have reported comparable results correcting either varus or valgus deformity with a proximal tibial osteotomy. Patients with valgus deformity of greater than 12 degrees are considered to have a less predictable outcome if corrected distal to the joint line.[3] The reason for these recommendations is that the tibial correction of such deformity leaves the joint line with a valgus orientation of more than 10 degrees. Furthermore, the size of the wedge that must be taken from the tibia to correct a more significant valgus angular deformity tends to be excessive, and can result in a

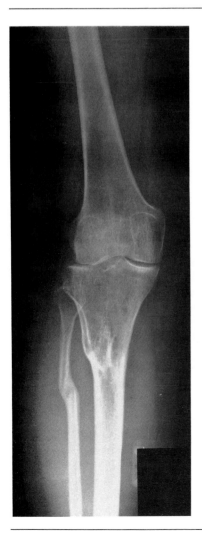 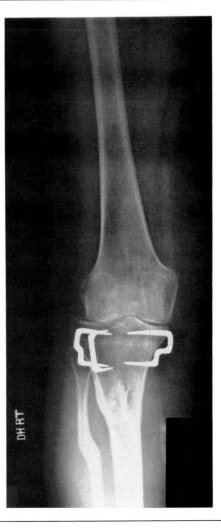

Fig. 1 A modest posttraumatic valgus deformity in a 25-year-old woman (**left**) is corrected to neutral (0 degrees) anatomic axis by proximal tibial osteotomy (**right**).

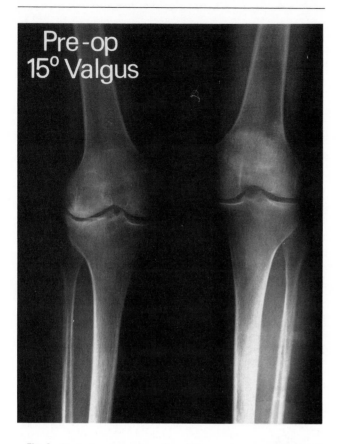

Fig. 2 Typical presentation of a middle-aged woman with significant cosmetic valgus deformity caused by a primary lateral gonarthrosis of the lateral compartment.

large step off and some instability of the osteotomy. In time, an excessive residual tilt of the joint line can cause medial subluxation of the femur referable to the tibia.[3,11] For these reasons, Coventry[3] recommends a distal femoral osteotomy if the valgus deformity exceeds 12 degrees or if the joint line exceeds 10 degrees valgus tilt. The problem is further compounded by the medial ligamentous laxity that occurs when the closing wedge osteotomy is placed between the origin and insertion of the medial collateral ligament.[11] Hence, although the tibial osteotomy is considered effective for some valgus knee deformities (Fig. 1),[3,5,6,11] limitations of angulation and articular tilt are imposed. Because the valgus deformity is uncommon, there is little discussion of the femoral osteotomy in the literature.

Presentation

The majority of patients with lateral knee deformity have primary lateral gonarthrosis[9,12]; however, traumatic, neurologic, congenital, and rheumatoid conditions can also cause a valgus alignment deformity.[7,8,10,11] The incidence of primary lateral gonarthrosis is 4 to 5

times higher in women than in men (Fig. 2).[7,8-10,12] The mean age of symptomatic degenerative lateral knee arthrosis is from 55 to 60 years but can range from 30 to 70 years of age.[8,10,12]

Although the valgus angulatory deformity can have significant cosmetic implications, cosmesis is rarely the primary goal of surgery in the adult. Motion, too, is not usually severely restricted. Pain, therefore, is the major indication for surgical intervention. Bilateral involvement occurs in approximately 10% of cases.[12]

Contraindications to femoral osteotomy to correct valgus deformity and gonarthrosis includes extension loss of greater than 15 degrees and flexion less than 90 degrees. Patellofemoral symptoms have not been specifically correlated with the prognosis of distal femoral osteotomy and, as with tibial osteotomy, such involvement is not considered a contraindication. Severe osteoporosis is not typical with lateral gonarthrosis but, if present, extra care must be taken with the osteotomy to assure rigid fixation.

Preparation Before Surgery

Careful preoperative planning is extremely important for any realignment procedure. Although the basic plan must assume that the desired angle of correction is known, this assumption has little scientific and only slightly greater clinical basis. The reason for this is the great amount of individual variation of pressure distribution even with the same tibial femoral angles. This is due to the individual differences in the orientation of the articular surface and of the angular relationship of the long bones. Furthermore, the desirable amount of correction as it relates to the distribution of forces across the joint is not known. It is, therefore, obvious that it is unwise to generalize and apply a single formula or relationship to all clinical instances. It is also important, however, to have some basis for determining the specified angular correction of the preoperative plan. The following relationships have been helpful and are used in our practice. (1) Normal alignment—Tibial femoral axis, 6 ± 2 degrees; mechanical axis, just medial to medial spine; pressure distribution, 60% through medial compartment (Fig. 3).[13] (2) Varus— Anatomic axis, 0 degrees; mechanical axis, medial to midportion of tibial plateau; force distribution, 80% through medial compartment. (3) Valgus alignment— Anatomic axis, 12 degrees; mechanical axis, midportion of lateral tibial plateau; force distribution, 80% through lateral compartment.

Clinically, the generally accepted recommendation is to correct the valgus knee to an anatomic (tibial femoral) angle of 0 degrees.[8-10,12] The high degree of individual variation does not assure that the same relative pressure distribution will be transmitted across the medial and lateral compartments in all patients. Nonetheless, this is a reasonable clinical guideline.

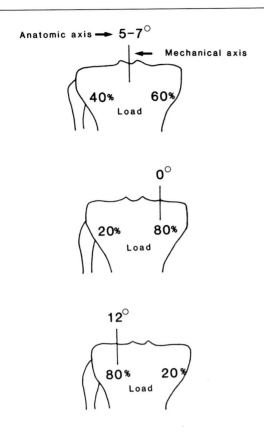

Load Distribution and Mechanical Axis

Fig. 3 General guidelines for the relationship of anatomic and mechanical axis with force distribution across the joint. From data by Johnson et al.[9] (By permission Mayo Foundation.)

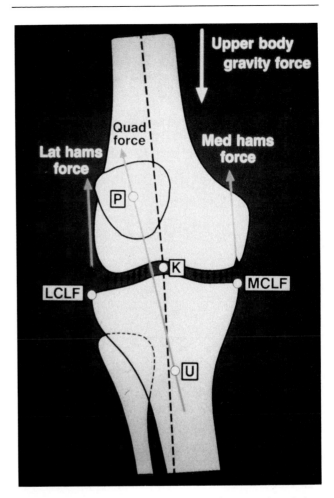

Fig. 4 Computer model considers articular and angular relationship as well as muscle ligament and articular surface contributions. (By permission Mayo Foundation.)

In an effort to incorporate a greater degree of scientific justification into the critical planning stage, a mathematical algorithm has been developed under the direction of E. Y. Chao to allow a more accurate prediction of the optimum axial alignment correction. This model considers the axial alignment of the extremity and the tilt of the joint line. Static and dynamic elements are incorporated, along with other more subtle features of the articular contact area (Fig. 4). While this approach does not define a unique optimum solution, the angular correction associated with different force distribution patterns is provided and has proven to be of great clinical value.

Without the advantage of a computer analysis for preoperative planning, we recommend a standing, full-length hip-to-ankle film to determine both mechanical axes, from the center of the femoral head to the center of the ankle. The anatomic or femoral tibial axis is also determined (Fig. 5). A calculation may then be performed to determine the angular correction at the femur required to place the mechanical axis just medial to the medial spine. This being done, the effect on the joint line orientation is also calculated. Typically, this correction is roughly equivalent to a 0 degree anatomic angle but, once again, there is significant individual variation. The use of tracings and simulated osteotomies with templates or cutouts is recommended to assure the proper preoperative plan is in place before the surgery is commenced.

Surgical Technique

There are several techniques available for the angular correction of valgus deformity at the femur. The prerequisites of each are to attain an accurate correction and rigid fixation. The most commonly performed surgical technique is that described by or modified from the AO group.[14] Two basic options are possible. The surgical procedure may be performed from a lateral approach employing a closing wedge osteotomy on the medial cortex (Fig. 6). However, a medial closing wedge design is the most commonly employed surgical procedure (Fig. 7). Just as several modifications of the AO

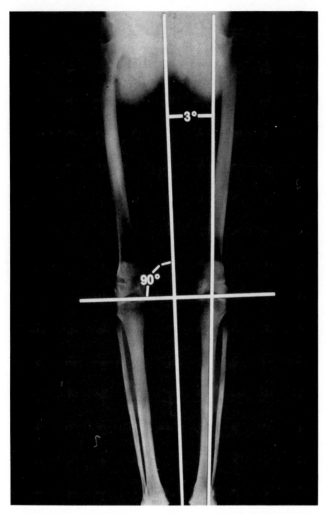

Fig. 5 The full-length standing radiograph to include the hip and ankle is essential in preoperative planning. Distinction between the mechanical and anatomic axes is essential as with any assessment of alignment deformity.

technique have been described,[8,10] we also perform this procedure with slight modifications.

The patient is placed supine on the operating table and the entire lower extremity is draped free. A medial incision, approximately 16 to 20 cm in length, is made with the distal extent just distal to the joint line. Proximally, the vastus medialis obliquus is retracted anteriorly. Dissection is carried distally to the joint capsule but the joint is not entered. Using fluoroscopy, the surgeon places a pin across the distal femoral metaphysis, approximately 2.5 cm proximal to the articular femoral condyles. This pin is directed slightly from anterior medial to posterior lateral in order to accommodate the geometry of the femoral condyles and to allow the plate to align along the shaft of the femur when the osteotomy is closed. A second pin is then placed perpendicular to the long axis of the femur and sufficiently proximal to allow the wedge to be removed

to be proximal to the adductor tubercle. The desired angular correction is determined and a second cut is made with the apex occurring at the lateral cortex. This is facilitated with the image intensifier but we also drive the proximal pin through the cortex so it may be palpated laterally, thus providing an additional three-dimensional reference source that facilitates orientation of the distal cut. An oscillating saw is used to perform the osteotomy. The precise orientation of this wedge, we believe, is of relatively little significance. It is of utmost importance to assure that there is adequate bone remaining distally and medially to accommodate the fixation device, and the distal aspect of the osteotomy must be proximal to the adductor tubercle. It is also of importance to assure that the apex of the removed wedge occurs just at or slightly medial to the lateral cortex. If an error is made it is much more acceptable to close the wedge several millimeters medial to the lateral cortex. This will provide a more stable osteotomy but also gives a slightly greater angular correction. A more parallel cut will result in greater instability and slightly less correction. The lateral cortex is cracked with an osteotome. Care is taken not to complete the osteotomy with the oscillating saw. If an error is made in the execution of the osteotomy, we prefer initially a thinner osteotomy than might ultimately be required. If a greater correction is necessary, this can usually be obtained by crushing the distal femur into the softer metaphyseal bone rather than by taking additional bone from the distal segment. Before the distal femur is destabilized by completion of the osteotomy, the blade plate is driven across the distal metaphysis along the line of the initially placed pin. The osteotomy plate is then employed to assist in closing the osteotomy, and the plate is secured to the femur with three to four screws. In this age group, three screws are usually adequate, but, if there is significant osteoporosis, more are used. The removed bone is sometimes used as a graft if there is concern about the rigidity or the healing potential of the osteotomy.

Results

It is of interest to note that there is more in the European than in the English literature with regard to the technique and anticipated results of distal femoral osteotomy for lateral gonarthrosis.[15,16] The procedure is technically demanding and the basis of correction, as noted, has not been well established. Because of the infrequent need to perform a distal femoral osteotomy, there are thus few reports that allow a clear estimation of the anticipated results (Table 1). In fact, there have only been four major reports of this procedure in the English literature and these have all occurred in the last several years.[8–10,12]

In addition to the excellent reviews by McDermott

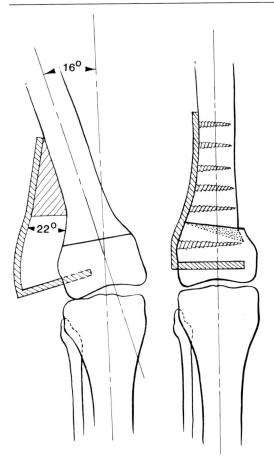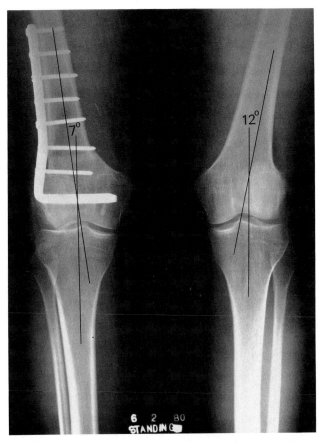

Fig. 6 **Left** and **right**, A lateral approach for a closing wedge osteotomy at the distal femur is one option for correcting valgus deformity.

and associates[10] and Healy and associates,[8] we have further assessed the experience of distal femoral osteotomy at the Mayo Clinic first reported by Johnson and Bodell.[9] Although more than 100 surgical procedures have been performed at the Mayo Clinic since 1978, the discussion will be based primarily on those patients with primary lateral gonarthrosis reviewed by Edgerton and associates.[12]

In the six years from 1978 to 1983, 28 patients underwent 30 distal femoral osteotomies for painful genu valgus caused by lateral compartment gonarthrosis. Twenty-three of these patients with 24 distal femoral osteotomies were followed a minimum of five years and up to 11 years with an average follow-up of 8.3 years. The mean age of patients at the time of osteotomy was 55 years, and 17 of the patients were women and five were men. This is similar to the age and sex distribution reported by McDermott and associates[10] and Healy and associates.[8]

A detailed chart review revealed intra- and postoperative complications, type of fixation used to secure the osteotomy, time to union, and need for subsequent procedures. Unfortunately, for the majority (20) of the knees, fixation was done with one or several staples,

which is clearly inadequate by today's standards. Nonetheless, the detailed long-term assessment of the consequences of the realignment is of value and may be considered somewhat independent of the technique used to secure the osteotomy.

The preoperative and postoperative clinical evaluation provided data that allowed the calculation of The Hospital for Special Surgery knee score in all instances.

The tibiofemoral angle was measured by the intersection of lines drawn down the center of the long axis of the femur and of the tibia before and after surgery. The average preoperative valgus alignment was eighteen degrees (range 10 to 27).

Subjectively, 75% of the patients were satisfied with or felt they had benefited from the procedure.

The Hospital for Special Surgery knee score improved 20 points from an average of 58 before surgery (range 27 to 82) to a mean of 78 after surgery (range 40 to 94). This improvement is comparable in all three studies (Table 1). Excellent results were obtained in eight knees (33%), good results in nine (38%), fair results in three (12%), and a poor result in one. Three knees had been subsequently treated by total knee replacement and must also thus be considered failures

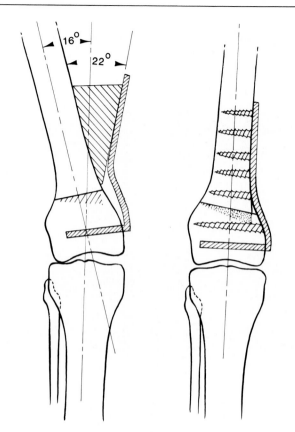

Fig. 7 The technique of choice employs a medial closing wedge distal femoral osteotomy for valgus deformity.

Radiographic Assessment

The preoperative tibiofemoral angle in our series (anatomic axis) was corrected to a mean of one degree valgus after surgery (range, 10 degrees varus to 18 degrees valgus). Of the 14 knees that were corrected to a tibiofemoral angle of zero degrees or were in varus, 77% had satisfactory results (Fig. 8). On the other hand, of the 10 knees left in some degree of valgus, only six had a satisfactory result. Because the numbers are so few, this difference is not statistically significant. However, of the four with at least 10 degrees remaining valgus, one was rated fair and two were rated as poor results. A mean correction to a zero-degree anatomic axis was also reported in the other two recent series.[8,10] Both these studies, however, had much less variation after surgery, ranging from 8 degrees varus to 6 degrees residual valgus. The wide range of final correction in our experience was due to the inadequate fixation afforded by the staples and the loss of correction associated with this. It is of interest to note, however, that McDermott and associates[10] were unable to correlate the degree of angular correction with the ultimate outcome. This, however, is in contrast to the majority of investigators who have considered this issue.[7,8,12,15,16]

One additional feature of interest was that satisfactory results were less common in those with the greatest medial and patellofemoral disease. Of the seven patients in our series with isolated lateral compartment disease, 86% had satisfactory results (Fig. 2). With mild, moderate, and severe disease of the medial and patellofemoral compartments, the satisfactory results were 80%, 33%, and 50%, respectively.

Complications

In the Mayo experience, considerable problems with delayed union or nonunion were encountered because of the poor fixation provided by the staples. However, nonunion or delayed union is not uncommon with a distal femoral osteotomy and has been reported in 5% to 12% of patients even with a more rigid AO type of

(17%). None of these patients felt that their initial results had deteriorated with time.

Not surprisingly, the probability of a satisfactory result according to the Hospital for Special Surgery knee score criteria with a distal femoral osteotomy is statistically greater in those with better scores before surgery (P < 0.04).

Satisfactory results were reported in 83% by Healy and associates,[8] which represented a mean improvement of 19 points in the objective index. McDermott and associates[10] recorded a satisfactory rate of 88% and a 28-point improvement in the knee index. Both these experiences averaged four years follow-up.

Table 1
Results of distal femoral osteotomy for lateral gonarthrosis

Author	Year	Number of Procedures	Femoral-Tibial Alignment Mean (Range)		The Hospital for Special Surgery Score		Follow-up (years)	Satisfactory (%)	Delayed Nonunion (%)
			Before	After	Before	After			
Edgerton et al[12]	1991	24	18 (10–27)	1 (−10, +18)	58	78	8.3	71	25†
Healy et al[8]	1988	23	18 (10–33)	2 (−7, +6)	65	86	4	83	9
McDermott et al[10]	1988	24	?	1 (−8, +6)*	48	76	4	88	4

*Approximations from data provided
†Staple fixation

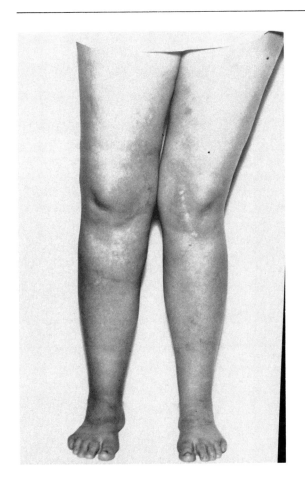

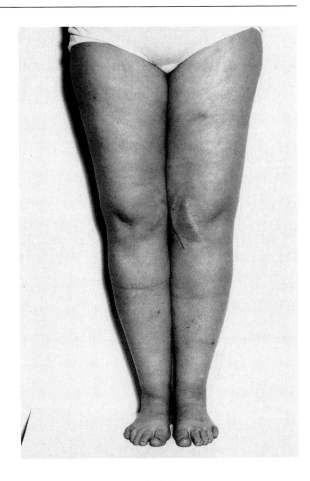

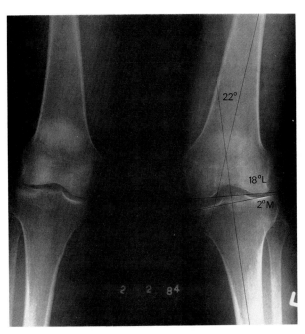

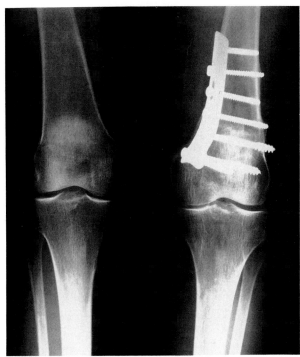

Fig. 8 Preoperative cosmetic (**top left**) and radiographic deformity (**bottom left**). Five years after medial closing wedge osteotomy with a mechanical axis of 0; patient has no symptoms (**top right** and **bottom right**).

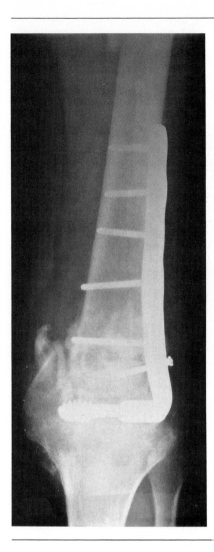

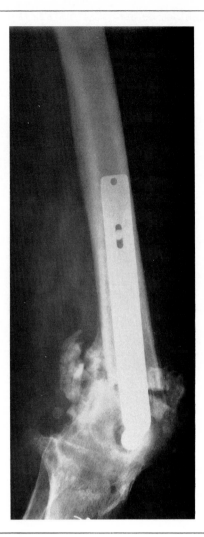

Fig. 9 **Left** and **right**, Nonunion is the most common complication of distal femoral osteotomy, reported in up to 12% of cases.

surgical technique (Fig. 9).[7,8,10] No deep infections were experienced in the Mayo series and no patients developed peroneal palsy or neurologic complications. Conrad and associates[7] reported the experience of 16 procedures from the Hospital for Special Surgery. Complications included two nonunions (12%), one femoral fracture, and one deep infection. After 24 procedures, Healy and associates[8] reported eight subsequent procedures, including arthroscopy assessment and knee replacement.

Conversion to Knee Replacement

Three of 24 knees (13%) in our sample were converted to total knee arthroplasty an average of five years after osteotomy. Of interest is that none of these patients were happy with the initial results after the osteotomy. This suggests that if the initial result is satisfactory, the long-term result might be, too. The 13% reported here is comparable to the two of 23 patients converted to knee replacement after distal femoral

osteotomy reported by Healy and associates[8] and is identical to the two of 16 reported by Conrad and associates.[7] Based on this information, if the patient does not realize a satisfactory result soon after surgery, consideration of a conversion to total knee arthroplasty might be considered sooner rather than later.

Conclusion

Valgus deformity is an uncommon problem, but one that is effectively treated by a realignment procedure. For angular deformities of less than 12 degrees and with lateral joint tilt of less than 10 degrees, proximal tibial osteotomy is effective and reliable, with up to 80% satisfactory results at long-term follow-up.[3,6] For deformities greater than this, distal femoral osteotomy is recommended. A satisfactory result between 70% and 80% may be expected for a period of five to 10 years. Unlike the proximal tibial osteotomy, these data suggest that a satisfactory result, if attained, does not significantly deteriorate with time. Prognostic features include the severity of the initial disease, the degree of angular deformity, and the ability to obtain an adequate correction (usually to 0 degrees anatomic axis). Complications are significant, with nonunion occurring in about 10% of cases. Conversion to knee replacement might be expected in 10% to 15% within five years.

References

1. Coventry MB: Upper tibial osteotomy for osteoarthritis. *J Bone Joint Surg* 1985;67A:1136–1140.
2. Coventry MB: Upper tibial osteotomy for gonarthrosis: The evolution of the operation in the last 18 years and long term results. *Orthop Clin North Am* 1979;10:191–210.
3. Coventry MB: Proximal tibial varus osteotomy for osteoarthritis of the lateral compartment of the knee. *J Bone Joint Surg* 1987;69A:32- 38.
4. Insall JN, Joseph DM, Msika C: High tibial osteotomy for varus gonarthrosis: A long-term follow-up study. *J Bone Joint Surg* 1984;66A:1040–1048.
5. Maquet P: The treatment of choice in osteoarthrosis of the knee. *Clin Orthop* 1985;192:108–112.
6. Ranieri L, Traina GC, Maci C: High tibial osteotomy in osteoarthritis of the knee: A long term clinical study of 187 knees. *Italian J Orthop Traumatol* 1977;3:289–300.
7. Conrad EU, Soundry M, Insall JN: Supracondylar femoral osteotomy for valgus knee deformities. *Orthop Transact* 1985;9:25–26.
8. Healy WL, Anglen JO, Wasilewski SA, et al: Distal femoral varus osteotomy. *J Bone Joint Surg* 1988;70A:102–109.
9. Johnson EW Jr, Bodell LS: Corrective supracondylar osteotomy for painful genu valgum. *Mayo Clin Proc* 1981;56:87–92.
10. McDermott AG, Finklestein JA, Farine I, et al: Distal femoral varus osteotomy for valgus deformity of the knee. *J Bone Joint Surg* 1988;70A:110–116.
11. Shoji H, Insall J: High tibial osteotomy for osteoarthritis of the knee with valgus deformity. *J Bone Joint Surg* 1973;55A:963–973.
12. Edgerton BC, Mariani M, Morrey BF: Distal femoral osteotomy for lateral gonarthrosis. *Clin Orthop*, in press.
13. Johnson F, Leitl S, Waugh W: The distribution of load across the knee: A comparison of static and dynamic measurements. *J Bone Joint Surg* 1980;62B:346–349.
14. Müller ME, Allgöwer M, Schneider R, et al: *Manual of Internal Fixation Techniques Recommended by the AO Group*, ed 2. New York, Springer-Verlag, 1979.
15. Baacke M, Legal H, Luther R: Grenzindikationen für die suprakondyläre Femurosteotomie zur Behandlung der Gonarthrose. *Z Orthop* 1974;112:221–229.
16. Nitsch R, Janssen G: Die Stellung der suprakondylären korrekturosteotomie in der behandlung der altersgonarthrose. *Z Orthop* 1976;114:226–232.

Tibial Osteotomy for Varus Gonarthrosis: Indication, Planning, and Operative Technique

Roland P. Jakob, MD

Stephen B. Murphy, MD

Introduction

While the role of tibial osteotomy in the management of varus gonarthrosis has become more refined, it remains the treatment of choice for a select group of patients. The ideal candidate for a lateral closing wedge valgus tibial osteotomy is the younger, more active, heavier patient with a good range of motion and a competent medial collateral ligament with unicompartmental osteoarthritis of mechanical cause. Although the long-term results of valgus osteotomy of the tibia are modest,[1-13] these are the very patients in whom unicompartmental and tricompartmental arthroplasty results are poor. Therefore, the delay of prosthetic reconstruction for five to eight critical years is a worthy goal, provided that the subsequent reconstruction is not compromised.

The results of tibial osteotomy are directly correlated with preoperative severity of the arthritis and maintenance of postoperative alignment.[1,3-6,8,10,12,14,15] Therefore, appropriate patient selection, preoperative planning, operative execution, and internal fixation must be combined to maximize the success rate of this procedure.

Radiographic Evaluation

Because not all varus knees are best treated by lateral closing wedge valgus tibial osteotomy, carefully executed preoperative functional radiographs are necessary to select the appropriate patient and plan the surgery. The first radiograph required is a one-leg standing film taken as a screening view. This radiograph is taken in slight flexion because full extension can hide the full extent of the deformity.[16,17] For planning of the osteotomy, an orthoradiogram (full-length radiograph) of the lower extremities is taken. This radiograph is taken with 90% of weightbearing on the involved side and 10% on the noninvolved side. Putting full weight on the affected knee can throw the patient off balance, which can result in an accidental varus or valgus stress view. Ninety percent weightbearing on the involved leg affords more reliability. The next two views to be taken are the anteroposterior varus and valgus stress views. A one-leg standing lateral view of the knee in 30 degrees of flexion is important to evaluate the tibial slope and an anterior tibial translation through active quadriceps contraction; lateral stress views can also be obtained if sagittal instability is a concern. Although patellofemoral arthritis is not a contraindication of osteotomy, the status of the patellofemoral joint should be evaluated.

Preoperative Planning

Not all varus knees are best treated by tibial osteotomy, and, for the wrong patient, this osteotomy will be unsuccessful even if perfectly performed. Several radiographic criteria must be met for the patient to be a candidate for this operation. First, the varus deformity must be located primarily in the tibia. Second, the valgus stress view must show both a competent medial collateral ligament and an adequate joint space in the lateral compartment. Third, varus stress films must show narrowing of the medial compartment. Finally, the long leg film must show that the mechanical axis passes through or medial to the medial compartment. If all of these criteria are met, the patient is a candidate for lateral closing wedge valgus tibial osteotomy.

Three specific patterns of varus knee deformity should not be treated with a lateral closing wedge valgus osteotomy. The first is the varus knee caused by femoral deformity. If such a varus knee is treated by lateral closing wedge valgus tibial osteotomy, the postoperative joint line will be oblique (Fig. 1). The resulting shear can lead to subluxation and will certainly complicate later prosthetic reconstruction. The second pattern is the patient with medial osteoarthritis, a varus tibia, and a lax medial collateral ligament. These patients usually have a history of trauma. If a lateral closing wedge tibial osteotomy is performed on a patient with medial collateral ligament laxity, the instability will be unmasked by the surgery. These patients are best treated by medial opening wedge tibial osteotomy (Fig. 2). The third pattern is the young patient with ligament laxity and intra-articular erosion. This is the so-called pagoda deformity (Fig. 3).[18] Preoperatively, these patients have such severe intra-articular instability that they walk with a closed medial compartment and a gapped lateral compartment. Postoperatively, these patients walk with a closed lateral compartment and gapped medial compartment. Thus, surgery can produce either undercorrection or overcorrection. This is a very difficult problem that can only be treated by prosthetic replacement.

Finally, consideration should be given to the sagittal

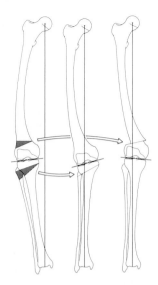

Fig. 1 Tibial osteotomy for a primary femoral deformity will produce an oblique joint line while femoral osteotomy will produce a horizontal joint line.

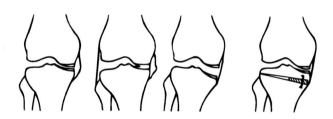

Fig. 2 The pattern of a varus tibia and medial ligament laxity is best treated by medial opening wedge valgus tibial osteotomy inserting tricortical grafts from the iliac crest and securing it with a T-plate. (Reproduced with permission from Jakob RP: Instabilitätsbedingte Gonarthrose—spezielle Indikationen für Osteotomien bei der Behandlung des instabilen Kniegelenkes, in Jakob RP, Stäubli HU (eds): *Kniegelenk und Kreuzbänder.* New York, Springer Verlag, 1991, pp 555–578.)

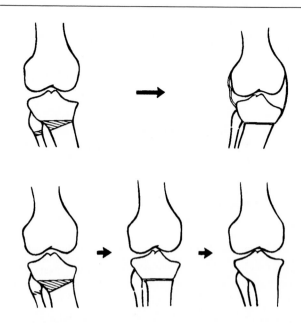

Fig. 3 The pagoda deformity. These patients have intra-articular erosion and weightbearing on one compartment or the other. This intra-articular problem is not readily solved by bony realignment, because of risk of overcorrection or undercorrection. (Reproduced with permission from Cartier P: Stellenwert der unikompartimentären Prothese bei der Femorotibialarthrose mit insuffizientem Zentralpfeiler, in Jakob RP, Stäubli HU (eds): *Kniegelenk und Kreuzbänder.* New York, Springer Verlag, 1991, pp 588–600.)

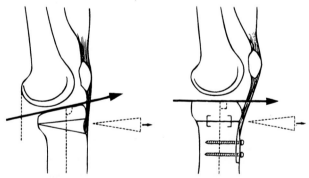

Fig. 4 If the candidate for a lateral closing wedge valgus tibial osteotomy has a posteriorly sloping tibia and anterior instability, a biplanar correction can be performed. The decrease in the posterior slope can decrease the horizontal shear forces. Staged ligament reconstruction can then be performed later if it is still necessary. This same theory applies to posterior instability. (Reproduced with permission from Dejour H, Neyret P: Der Einbeinstand bei chronischer Knieinstabilität, in Jakob RP, Stäubli HU (eds): *Kniegelenk und Kreuzbander.* New York, Springer Verlag, 1991, pp 579–587.)

plane and anteroposterior instability. If the candidate for lateral closing wedge valgus tibial osteotomy has a posteriorly sloping tibia and some anterior instability, a biplane correction can be performed to decrease the posterior slope (Fig. 4).[19] If instability remains following full rehabilitation, staged ligament reconstruction can be performed. The same principles apply to posterior instability in the presence of decreased posterior or even anterior sloping.

Osteotomy Level and Orientation

Once it has been determined that a patient is a candidate for a lateral closing wedge valgus tibial osteotomy, the surgical technique must be selected. Osteot-

omy above the tibial tubercle is a time-honored technique familiar to many surgeons.[3,4,12] At this osteotomy level, however, the amount of angular correction is limited. Osteotomy above the tubercle can also lead to problems with intra-articular hardware, intra-articular fracture, and osteonecrosis of the subchondral

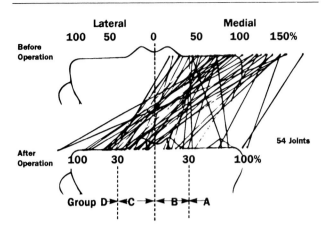

Fig. 5 Their best clinical results correlated with a postoperative mechanical axis that passes through the lateral compartment about one third of the way toward the periphery of the lateral tibial plateau. For this reason our preoperative plan is based on achieving a mechanical axis that passes through this region of the knee. (Reproduced with permission from Fujisawa Y, Masuhara K, Shiomi S: The effect of high tibial osteotomy on osteoarthritis of the knee: An arthroscopic study of 54 knee joints. *Orthop Clin North Am* 1979;10:585–608.)

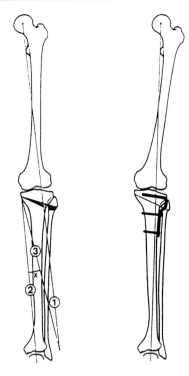

Fig. 6 After wedge removal, the osteotomy is fixed with an adolescent hip plate—(AO) 50 mm blade length, 15 mm displacement. This plate may have to be bent slightly to fit the bone and to achieve the desired angular correction. Small changes in angular correction can be achieved by placing washers under the proximal or distal part of the plate. (Reproduced with permission from Miniaci A, Ballmer FT, Ballmer PM, et al: Proximal tibial osteotomy: A new fixation technique. *Clin Orthop* 1989;246:250–259.)

bone. Osteonecrosis complicates prosthetic replacement because of bone-stock deficiency.

Osteotomy below the tibial tubercle produces a secondary deformity because of its long distance from the joint. This level is generally reserved for patients with open growth plates. The technique described in the following paragraphs—an oblique lateral closing wedge valgus tibial osteotomy behind the tibial tubercle—seeks to minimize the disadvantages of the other two operations while preserving their advantages. This technique allows for unlimited angular correction, stable fixation more than 1 cm from the joint, and does not create a secondary deformity.

Selection of Mechanical Axis

The ideal mechanical alignment following valgus osteotomy is not known. Studies that showed a femoral tibial valgus of five degrees to 13 degrees to be ideal were not based on full-length films and are, therefore, of limited validity.[1,3,10,20] Fujisawa and associates[6] have shown that good clinical results are correlated with the postoperative mechanical axis that passes through the lateral compartment about one third toward the periphery of the lateral tibia plateau (Fig. 5).[21]

Based on this information, as shown in Figure 6, a postoperative mechanical axis is drawn on the full-length anteroposterior radiograph from the center of the hip through a point one third of the way into the lateral compartment (line 1). Next, a second line is drawn from the medial hinge of the osteotomy through the center of the ankle (line 2). Finally, a third line is

drawn from the osteotomy hinge to intersect the postoperative mechanical axis at the level of the ankle joint (line 3). The angle between the second and third lines is the angle of the osteotomy wedge.

The valgus stress view is then carefully assessed to see if there is an intra-articular angular shift between the long-leg standing view and the valgus stress view as a result of gapping of the lateral compartment on the long-leg view caused by lateral collateral ligament deficiency. If there is an intra-articular shift, this small angle is subtracted from the planned angular correction. This angular shift must be accounted for in the preoperative planning, because the knee will fall into the valgus stress view position postoperatively. Failure to recognize this intra-articular angular shift will result in overcorrection.

Surgical Technique

The patient is positioned supine on a radiolucent table with a roll under the ipsilateral buttock. In general, arthroscopy is performed at the start of the procedure. Resection of medial meniscal tears and chon-

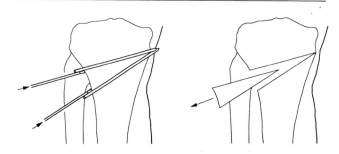

Fig. 7 Wedge resection is performed with the assistance of guide wires.

droplasty of the medial compartment and patellofemoral joint can be performed. The lateral compartment should be examined as well. Because arthroscopic findings do not correlate with results of tibial osteotomy,[22] they should not be used as a factor in the decision to perform an osteotomy. Instead, this decision is based on clinical and radiographic criteria, as previously described. Open arthrotomy should be avoided, if possible, because this complicates the postoperative course.

There are many popular incisions for the lateral closing wedge valgus tibial osteotomy. However, the effect the incision would have on a total knee replacement must always be considered. For this reason, a longitudinal incision is most appropriate. This incision can be in the midline, or just lateral to it, as long as a total knee replacement can be performed through the same incision without the need to raise large flaps.[23,24]

An anterolateral approach to the proximal tibia is performed, and the anterior compartment muscles are elevated to expose the tibia and proximal fibula. Small Kirschner wires (K-wires) are placed under the meniscus in the medial and lateral compartments to mark the position of the joint line. A 2.5-mm K-wire with threaded tip is passed across the tibia more than 1 cm below the joint line and parallel to it. The wire exits

the medial tibia and skin and is cut short on both sides so as not to interfere with later steps in the operation. The T-shaped chisel for the adolescent blade plate is then passed just under and along the K-wire. Radiographic information is not required, but may be of assistance during this part of the procedure. A point on the medial tibial cortex that is approximately 2 cm below the joint line is selected. A K-wire is then passed obliquely to meet this point (Fig. 7). Another K-wire is passed more obliquely to also meet this medial osteotomy hinge. The angle between these two K-wires should equal the desired angle of correction. This procedure can be performed with radiographic assistance and without the use of alignment jigs, or, if the alignment jigs are used, it can be performed without radiographic assistance.[25–27]

Involvement in the development and the clinical testing of the AO-ASIF tibial osteotomy jig has shown that it is possible to cut an osteotomy with an accuracy of 0.5 degrees. This jig works basically with the following technical points (Fig. 8): (1) It is used for doing wedge osteotomies; (2) The location of the apex of the osteotomy is at the level of the medial cortex or 5 to 10 mm inside or outside of it; and (3) The angle can be adjusted by 1-degree increments by moving the two arms of the jig. Three 2.5-mm threaded pins are advanced through the two guide plates. The jig is then removed and the osteotomy cuts are performed along the pins.

The osteotomy of the fibula is performed by removing a segment in the neck of the fibula. The proximal osteotomy is not completely transverse, but is cut in a way so that the posterior cortex remains intact. Following eventual closure of the osteotomy, the distal fibula then rests inside this cortical cage for additional stability. This technique also serves to protect the peroneal nerve.

Before tibial osteotomy, the tibial tubercle is elevated from proximal to distal, taking care to leave the extensor mechanism in bony continuity distally. The medial periosteum is left undisturbed to preserve additional

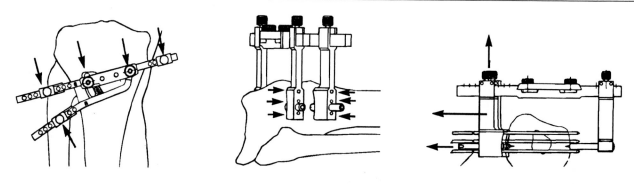

Fig. 8 For greater accuracy, a jig can be used. The AO osteotomy jig works with 2.5 mm wires between which the desired wedge resection can be performed accurately.

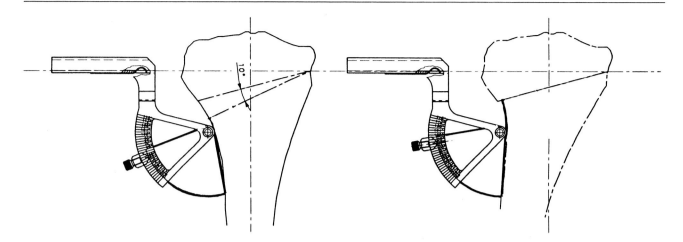

Fig. 9 A special ruler helps to determine the desired angular adaptation of the adolescent osteotomy plate so that the plate fits the bone once the osteotomy is closed.

blood supply to the tubercle. The two limbs of the wedge-shaped osteotomy are then cut with an oscillating saw, which glides along the guide wires. The sagittal plane deformities are corrected by flexing or extending the osteotomy appropriately. After the cut is completed to within a few millimeters of the medial hinge, the wedge is removed. A moderate varus stress is placed across the osteotomy site to check for flexibility. A valgus stress is not placed across the osteotomy site at this stage because the nutcracker effect of the remaining few millimeters of bone can produce enough tension on the medial hinge to break it. If the osteotomy is still rigid, the cut is extended a short distance toward the medial cortex, and the osteotomy flexibility is again checked until it can be closed. Now a special ruler is slid over the seating chisel, and the angle between the lateral cortex of the tibia and the ruler perpendicular to the blade is measured (Fig. 9). For example, if this angle is more or less equal to the desired correction, the adolescent blade plate is bent to the appropriate number of degrees prior to later insertion. If this angle measures 10 degrees and a correction of 10 degrees is desired, the plate has to be bent to 100 degrees to allow the appropriate closure of the osteotomy.

When the osteotomy is flexible, the guide wires are removed, the prebent adolescent blade plate is inserted, and the osteotomy is closed. Following fixation, an anteroposterior radiograph, with a large cassette, is taken. If the leg is slightly undercorrected, a screw washer is placed under the plate in line with the proximal screw to add a few degrees of valgus. If the leg is slightly overcorrected, the screw washer is placed under the plate in line with the distal screw to add a few degrees of varus. With this technique, it is not necessary to remove the plate, which could weaken the fixation. Because the tibial tubercle is intrinsically stable, no fixation is necessary. If there is concern about tibial tu-

bercle integrity, one or more 3.5-mm screws may be used for fixation.

The anterior compartment muscles are gently tacked back into position with a drain underneath. The anterior fascial incision is not closed. Clinical suspicion for compartment syndrome should always remain high, especially in the presence of postoperative epidural anesthesia. Continuous passive motion, if available, and active range-of-motion exercises are started early. Partial weightbearing, begun as soon as the patient can control the leg, is maintained for three months to promote chondroneogenesis.

Discussion

The success of tibial osteotomy in the treatment of varus gonarthrosis correlates directly with proper patient selection, and achievement and maintenance of adequate operative correction.[1,3–6,8,10,12,14,15,20] Patient selection criteria must include age, weight, activity, range of motion, patient expectation, severity of degenerative change, and, in particular, an appropriate interpretation of functional radiographs. Adequate correction depends on precise preoperative planning and intraoperative execution. Maintenance of correction requires adequate bony stability and internal fixation.

Large angular corrections, which are uncommon, require fracture of the medial hinge. In these cases, and in cases of inadvertent fracture of the medial hinge, the adolescent blade plate is especially useful, because it provides compression and intrinsic varus-valgus, flexion-extension, and axial rotational stability. In contrast, staples only provide a tension band, and a plate with screws provides no intrinsic varus-valgus stability. The use of the adolescent blade plate has solved problems that were occasionally encountered with a semitubular plate-and-screw fixation construct.[28,29] Adequate internal fixation is also particularly important when the osteotomy is combined with chondroplasty. In such cases, early motion is critical. Conversely, chondroplasty alone is never indicated in the treatment of medial compartment arthritis in the presence of mechanical malalignment. Chondroplasty, in these cases, must always be combined with mechanical realignment.[30-32]

The trend toward using the Ilizarov fixator and other external fixation devices instead of internal fixation reflects a reaction to prior problems with accurate surgical correction and fixation. These problems are not solved by abandoning these techniques, however, but by addressing the problems of surgical execution and fixation as previously described. The external fixator allows inexact preoperative planning and imprecise intraoperative execution because of the option of postoperative adjustment. In practice, the patient should never leave the operating room until the appropriate correction has been achieved. The apparatus is not as well tolerated by adults as by children, and it limits knee flexion, particularly in obese patients. The Ilizarov apparatus and other external fixators are best applied clinically in salvage situations where internal fixation has failed.

The tibial osteotomy is not an operation that competes directly with unicompartmental or tricompartmental knee replacement, but, rather, is a complementary procedure. In general, unicompartmental knee replacement is more appropriate for lesser degrees of varus, which are caused primarily by intra-articular erosion.[33,34] These patients are usually older, have more advanced medial compartment arthritis, and may have larger intra-articular angular shift. Patients with a depressed medial compartment and those with severe medial joint wear in the absence of varus deformity are more suitable candidates for hemiprostheses. Although tibia osteotomy, unicompartmental replacement, and total knee replacement have overlapping indications, most patients are clearly better suited to one of these three procedures.[35] In summary, with improved patient selection, preoperative planning, and intraoperative execution and fixation, the results of tibial osteotomy can be maximized.

References

1. Aglietti P, Rinonapoli E, Stringa G, et al: Tibial osteotomy for the varus osteoarthritic knee. *Clin Orthop* 1983;176:239–251.
2. Arnoldi CC, Lempberg RK, Linderholm H: Intraosseous hypertension and pain in the knee. *J Bone Joint Surg* 1975;57B:360–363.
3. Coventry MB: Osteotomy about the knee for degenerative and rheumatoid arthritis: Indications, operative techniques, and results. *J Bone Joint Surg* 1973;55A:23–48.
4. Coventry MB: Upper tibial osteotomy for gonarthrosis: The evolution of the operation in the last 18 years and long term results. *Orthop Clin North Am* 1979;10:191–210.
5. Engel GM, Lippert FG III: Valgus tibial osteotomy: Avoiding the pitfalls. *Clin Orthop* 1981;160:137–143.
6. Fujisawa Y, Masuhara K, Shiomi S: The effect of high tibial osteotomy on osteoarthritis of the knee: An arthroscopic study of 54 knee joints. *Orthop Clin North Am* 1979;10:585–608.
7. Insall JN, Joseph DM, Msika C: High tibial osteotomy for varus gonarthrosis: A long-term follow-up study. *J Bone Joint Surg* 1984;66A:1040–1048.
8. Insall JN, Shoji H, Mayer V: High tibial osteotomy: A five year evaluation. *J Bone Joint Surg* 1974;56A:1397–1405.
9. Jackson JP: Osteotomy for osteoarthritis of the knee. *J Bone Joint Surg* 1958;40B:826.
10. Kettelkamp DB, Wenger DR, Chao EYS, et al: Results of proximal tibial osteotomy: The effects of tibiofemoral angle, stance-phase flexion-extension, and medial-plateau force. *J Bone Joint Surg* 1976;58A:952–960.
11. Salter RB, Simmonds F, Malcom BW, et al: The biological effect of continuous passive motion on the healing of full-thickness defects in articular cartilage: An experimental investigation in the rabbit. *J Bone Joint Surg* 1980;62A:1232–1251.
12. Shoji H, Insall JN: High tibial osteotomy for osteoarthritis of the knee. *Int Surg* 1976;61:11–14.
13. Tjörnstrand BAE, Egund N, Hagstedt BV: High tibial osteotomy: A seven-year clinical and radiographic follow-up. *Clin Orthop* 1981;160:124–136.
14. Scott RD, Santore RF: Unicondylar unicompartmental replacement for osteoarthritis of the knee. *J Bone Joint Surg* 1981;63A:536–544.
15. Ziller R, Seyfarth H: Loss of correction following high tibial osteotomy. *Beitr Orthop Traumatol* 1974;21:358–363.
16. Maquet PGJ: *Biomécanique du Genou.* New York, Springer Verlag, 1977, p 135.
17. Maquet PGJ: *Biomécanique du Genou.* New York, Springer Verlag, 1977, p 194.
18. Cartier P: Stellenwert der unikompartimentären Prothese bei der Femorotibialarthrose mit insuffizientem Zentralpfeiler, in Jakob RP, Stäubli HU (eds): *Kniegelenk und Kreuzbänder.* New York, Springer Verlag, 1991, pp 588–600.
19. Dejour H, Neyret P: Der Einbeinstand bei chronischer Knieinstabilität, in Jakob RP, Stäubli HU (eds): *Kniegelenk und Kreuzbänder.* New York, Springer Verlag, 1991, pp 579–587.
20. Hernigou PH, Medevielle D, Debeyre J, et al: Proximal tibial osteotomy for osteoarthritis with varus deformity: A ten to thirteen-year follow-up study. *J Bone Joint Surg* 1987;69A:332–354.
21. Jakob RP: Instabilitätsbedingte Gonarthrose—spezielle Indikationen für Osteotomien bei der Behandlung des instabilen Kniegelenkes, in Jakob RP, Stäubli HU (eds): *Kniegelenk und Kreuzbänder.* New York, Springer Verlag, 1991, pp 555–578.
22. Keene JS, Dyreby JR Jr: High tibial osteotomy in the treatment of osteoarthritis of the knee: The role of preoperative arthroscopy. *J Bone Joint Surg* 1983;65A:36–42.
23. Katz MM, Hungerford DS, Krackow KA, et al: Results of total knee arthroplasty after failed proximal tibial osteotomy for osteoarthritis. *J Bone Joint Surg* 1976;69A:225–233.
24. Staheli JW, Cass JR, Morrey BF: Condylar total knee arthroplasty after failed proximal tibial osteotomy. *J Bone Joint Surg* 1987;69A:28–31.
25. Jiang C-C, Hang Y-S, Liu T-K: A new jig for proximal tibial osteotomy. *Clin Orthop* 1988;226:118–123.
26. Myrnerts R: Clinical results with the Saab jig in high tibial osteotomy for medial gonarthrosis. *Acta Orthop Scand* 1980;51:565–567.
27. Myrnerts R: Failure of the correction of varus deformity obtained by high tibial osteotomy. *Acta Orthop Scand* 1980;51:569–573.
28. Miniaci A, Ballmer FT, Ballmer PM, et al: Proximal tibial osteotomy: A new fixation technique. *Clin Orthop* 1989;246:250–259.
29. Weber BG, Brunner CF: *Special Techniques in Internal Fixation.* New York, Springer-Verlag, 1982.

30. Dandy DJ: Abrasion chondroplasty. *Arthroscopy* 1986;2:51–53.

31. Friedman MJ, Berasi CC, Fox JM, et al: Preliminary results with abrasion arthroplasty in the osteoarthritic knee. *Clin Orthop* 1984;182:200–205.

32. Johnson LL: Arthroscopic abrasion arthroplasty historical and pathologic perspective: Present status. *Arthroscopy* 1986;2:54–69.

33. Jackson RW, Burdick W: Unicompartmental knee arthroplasty. *Clin Orthop* 1984;190:182–185.

34. MacIntosh DL, Welsh RP: Joint debridement: A complement to high tibial osteotomy in the treatment of degenerative arthritis of the knee. *J Bone Joint Surg* 1977;59A:1094–1097.

35. Insall JN, Hood RW, Flawn LB, et al: The total condylar knee prosthesis in gonarthrosis: A five to nine-year follow up of the first one hundred consecutive replacements. *J Bone Joint Surg* 1983;65A:619–628.

Unicompartmental Knee Arthroplasty

Kurt J. Kitziger, MD

Paul A. Lotke, MD

Unicompartmental knee arthroplasty (UKA) has been a controversial procedure for the past 20 years. While there has been general agreement that the young, active patient with unicompartmental arthritis is best served by osteotomy and that the elderly patient with more extensive disease should undergo total knee arthroplasty (TKA), the dispute has been over the treatment of the older patient with moderate disease confined to one compartment. The consensus of opinion is that the advantages of UKA, compared with osteotomy and TKA, are quicker rehabilitation time, preservation of normal soft tissue and bone in uninvolved compartments, and improved proprioception in joint kinematics, leading to superior functional results. Several specific areas of controversy persist: (1) conflicting results regarding the efficacy of UKA; (2) conflicting rates of deterioration of good results; and (3) conflicting opinions regarding the ease with which UKA can be converted to total knee arthroplasty. This chapter reviews the indications, techniques, results, and reasons for failure of UKA and balances the advantages and disadvantages of the procedure.

Indications for UKA

As experience with UKA accumulates, its indications have become better defined. The primary indication for UKA is osteoarthritis of either the medial or lateral compartment (Fig. 1). Large series have revealed that medial replacement is about seven times more common than lateral replacement.[1,2] UKA can also be indicated for the treatment of posttraumatic degenerative arthritis and osteonecrosis, although the depth of damage that occurs in osteonecrosis may preclude UKA.[3] Clinically, the pain should be confined to the involved compartment.

What constitutes unicompartmental arthritis may be difficult to define precisely. Minimal radiographic changes of osteoarthritis may be allowed in the opposite compartment, but the final assessment is made at surgery when the entire knee is closely inspected. Most authors allow asymptomatic changes of chondromalacia patellae as well as small erosions in the nonweight-bearing portion of the opposite compartment.[2,4,5] Interesting experimental data provided by Brocklehurst and associates[6] have shown that areas of visually normal articular cartilage in the osteoarthritic knee are normal histologically, chemically, and metabolically. The inference is that normal-appearing cartilage found in the opposite compartment of a knee being evaluated for UKA is biomechanically sound. Their report suggests that visual assessment of articular cartilage in the "uninvolved" compartment is adequate.

The patient should be elderly, usually older than 60

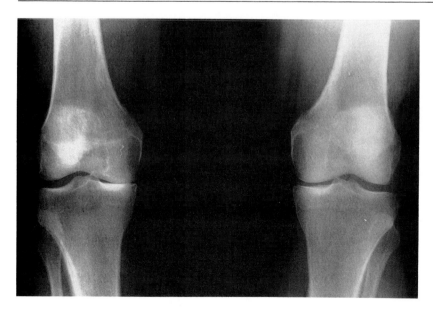

Fig. 1 This 63-year-old man with moderate medial compartment osteoarthritis of the right knee is a candidate for UKA.

years of age, and overall level of activity should be moderate. The average age in successful series of UKA is 65 to 70 years.[4,7-11] A high failure rate has been reported in patients younger than 50 years of age, in whom an increased level of activity was felt to lead to excessive wear and loosening.[11] The patient should not be overweight, because obesity also has been associated with high rates of UKA failure.[2,4,12]

Other important clinical prerequisites include a range of motion of at least 90 degrees, less than 5 degrees flexion contracture, minimal joint laxity, and malalignment less than 15 degrees (varus deformity up to 10 degrees or valgus deformity up to 15 degrees). In general, UKA is indicated in patients with a moderate level of osseous and soft-tissue disease, and TKA is preferred for those with more extensive involvement.

Contraindications to UKA include young or obese patients; active patients with high functional demands; knees with greater than 20 degrees of deformity; deformity of either the tibial or femoral shaft; excessive joint laxity, including absence or degeneration of the cruciate ligaments; inflammatory arthropathies, especially rheumatoid arthritis; chondrocalcinosis; significant opposite compartment or patellofemoral arthritis as determined before or during surgery; and antecedent infection.[13] Other treatment alternatives, such as osteotomy or TKA, should be considered in cases where UKA is contraindicated.

Technique

The important technical points of UKA have been well-described,[1,5] and the following is a description of our technique. The patient considered for UKA should be selected according to the criteria described above. Physical examination should localize the patient's symptoms to either the medial or lateral compartment of the knee, and standing radiographs should be scrutinized for signs of opposite compartment involvement or of joint subluxation, which may contraindicate UKA.

A standard medial parapatellar incision can be used for either the medial or lateral prosthesis. Although a lateral parapatellar incision can be adequate for lateral unicompartmental replacement, TKA, if deemed necessary, can be difficult through this approach. The subvastus approach is an option for medial UKA. Care should be taken, during the dissection, to avoid injury to the uninvolved compartment or to either cruciate ligament. The medial arthrotomy should extend distally past the joint line, maintaining a continuous soft-tissue envelope, which folds away from the proximal tibial metaphysis to allow exposure for the osteotomies.

The surgeon inspects the entire joint to ensure that the primary pathology is in the involved compartment. If eburnated subchondral bone is discovered either in the patellofemoral joint or in the opposite femorotibial

joint, a TKA should be performed. Large hypertrophic peripheral osteophytes involving both compartments are a relative contraindication for UKA. Smaller osteophytes in the opposite compartment, however, should not preclude UKA. These osteophytes should be removed carefully down to the anatomic bone contour.

Proper positioning of the prosthesis is most important. The tibial component should be perpendicular to the mechanical axis of the tibia in the coronal plane and tilted 5 to 10 degrees posteriorly in the sagittal plane. Most UKA systems provide either an intra- or extramedullary tibial guide to aid in proper component orientation. Minimal bone should be removed from the tibia, and a tibial component thick enough to restore the anatomic joint line should be selected. Our goal is placement of a tibial component that is 8 mm thick. The tibial prosthesis should not overhang the cortical margin of the osteotomized tibia, although placement of the component close to the cortical edge is desirable for bone support.

The femoral component should be placed centrally on the condyle to allow congruent tracking between both components (Fig. 2). It is essential that the femoral component be parallel to the tibial component in both extension and flexion. We use the tibial cut to guide the orientation of the femoral osteotomy. The remaining articular cartilage and fibrocartilage on the distal femur is removed with a burr, and enough bone is resected to allow the component to lie flush against the femur and to restore the anatomic joint line. If, during the procedure, large subchondral cysts are discovered, or if either bone surface is deemed inadequate to support the UKA components, a TKA should be performed.

After insertion of the trial components, knee stability should be checked in both flexion and extension in order to simulate normal joint motion. One or two millimeters of laxity of the collateral ligament is desirable when the knee is stressed in a few degrees of flexion. There should be no tendency for the tibial component to lift off the osteotomy surface as the knee is flexed, nor should the patella impinge on the anterior portion of the femoral component. The goal is to restore extremity alignment to the premorbid state, avoiding either over- or undercorrection. Once the knee demonstrates adequate balance and stability, the components are cemented or press fit into place. Postoperative rehabilitation proceeds in a manner similar to that used for TKA. Early range of motion is begun and weightbearing is protected for six weeks.

Results of UKA

Marmor, a long-time proponent of UKA, has published extensively on the subject.[1,4,14-16] In 1979, he reported short-term results on 56 patients who under-

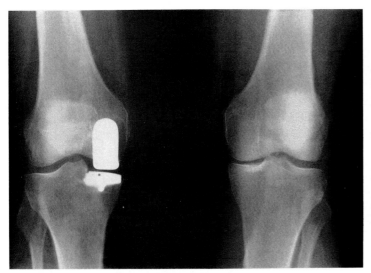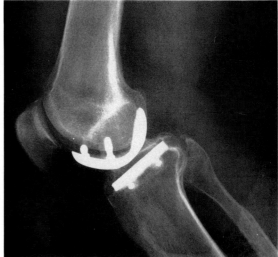

Fig. 2 **Left**, Excellent component position three years later of the same patient as in Figure 1. **Right**, A lateral radiograph of the same patient.

went UKA with his prosthesis.[1] Good to excellent results were found in 80% of patients. The range of motion averaged 112 degrees and the rate of revision was 20%. Most cases requiring revision were associated with the use of tibial components only 6 mm thick. Because patellar impingement on the femoral component was a cause of postoperative pain, the author recommended that the femoral component be recessed and that anterior placement be avoided. In 1988, reporting on the same group of patients plus others with a minimum 10-year follow-up, the author noted that satisfactory results had declined to 63% and reported a 30% revision rate.[4] Use of the thinner tibial component had accounted for additional failures over the interim, but degeneration of the uninvolved compartment was the cause for revision in only two cases, both at 9.5 years after surgery. It should be noted that these results concern the early experience with UKA (Fig. 3). Technical modifications recommended by Marmor include the use of a tibial guide to ensure accurate bone cuts and placement of the tibial component on the cortical rim to prevent early subsidence. Other investigators using the Marmor prosthesis have reported excellent results with shorter followup.[7]

Scott and associates have documented the evolution of UKA at their institution.[2,3,5,9,17] In 1981, Scott and Santore[2] reported satisfactory results in 92 of 100 patients 3.5 years after surgery in which all-polyethylene tibial components were used. Range of motion averaged 114 degrees. In three knees that were revised to TKA, failure was attributed to obesity and excessive deformity. Also, pes anserine bursitis was noted in 12% of patients. Radiologic assessment demonstrated that two femoral components had subsided and four tibial

components had complete radiolucent lines. The authors recommended central positioning of the components on each bone surface. In 1989, survivorship analysis revealed 91% UKA survival at 9 years. UKA survival decreased to 53% at 12 years.[3] The authors felt that the precipitous drop could be attributed to the small number of patients with a follow-up period of more than 10 years.

Kozinn and associates[9] reported on a series of patients who had undergone UKA with a metal-backed tibial component at least 8 mm thick. This modification of the Brigham prosthesis was intended to minimize the problem of tibial loosening. At an average of 5.5 years after surgery, 92% of these patients had good to excellent results. No signs of radiographic loosening were detected, and no revisions had been performed.

In addition, reports from Europe regarding the St. Georg Sledge unicompartmental prosthesis have been encouraging. Olsen and associates[10] described favorable results in 30 of 31 knees at 4.5 years after surgery. For osteoarthritic knees at 5 years after surgery, McKinnon and associates[8] reported excellent results in 90% of patients on the basis of pain relief and 70% of patients on the basis of function. Poor results were noted in patients with rheumatoid arthritis.

Failure of UKA

The causes of failed UKA include infection, improper patient selection, aseptic loosening, polyethylene wear, degeneration of the uninvolved compartment, patellofemoral symptoms, and pes anserine bursitis. In his original series, largely before the use of prophylactic

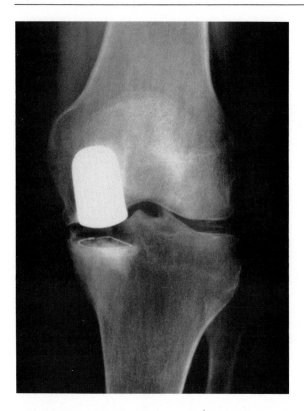
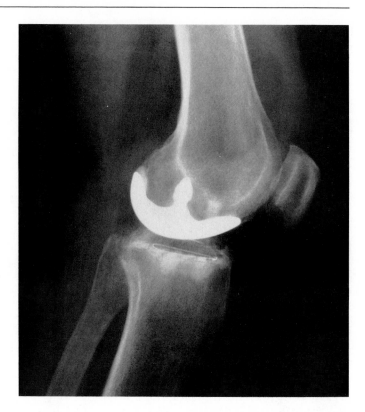

Fig. 3 **Left**, Eleven years after Marmor UKA, this 75-year-old woman has an excellent clinical result. **Right**, A lateral radiograph of the same patient.

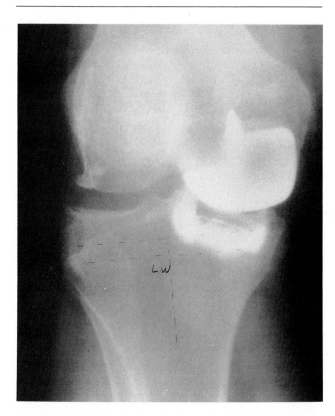

Fig. 4 This 68-year-old man has a painful UKA caused by malalignment and component malposition.

antibiotics, Marmor[14] reported 31% superficial and 4% deep infection rates. Recent series, however, demonstrate infectious complications in 0 to 1% of cases.[4,9]

Poor patient selection, particularly in the early experience with UKA, was an important cause of failure. Younger age, obesity, and the diagnosis of inflammatory arthropathy, all documented as predictors of failure, have been discussed above.[2,4,11,12] Poor results in two commonly cited series early in the development of UKA can be attributed in part to poor patient selection. In 1978 Laskin[12] reported dismal short-term results in 37 patients, 35 of whom were obese. In addition, in a majority of his patients signs of opposite compartment degeneration were noted at surgery. Insall and Aglietti[18] in 1980 reported a 31% rate of revision, and a 50% rate of progression of arthritis in 22 knees at 6 years after surgery. The fact that more than half of the patients underwent patellectomy for patellofemoral arthrosis at the time of UKA suggests that extensive disease was present in a majority of patients. Incidentally, both of the above series documented better results with lateral UKA.

Aseptic loosening and polyethylene wear, particularly of the tibial component, are the most common causes of failed UKA.[7,11,16,17,19–21] The causes of tibial component failure are multiple, and most involve technical errors. The use of too thin a tibial component leads to

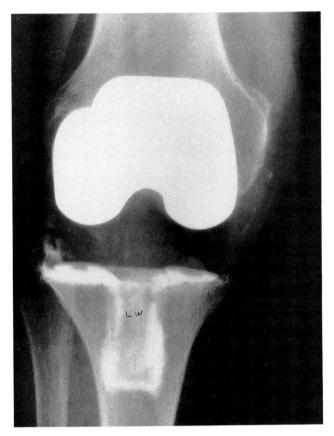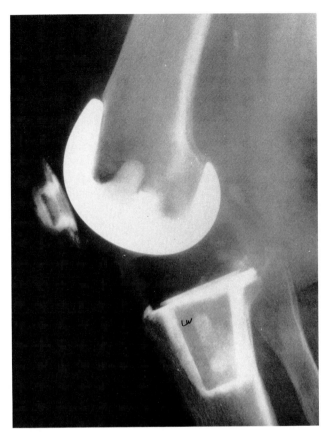

Fig. 5 **Left**, The same patient as in Figure 4, five years after successful revision to a total knee arthroplasty. A large tibial component was used to compensate for bone loss. **Right**, A lateral radiograph of the same patient.

accelerated polyethylene wear, deformity, and subsequent loosening.[1,4,21] The high contact stresses already present on the component may be increased by undercorrection of joint alignment. The use of metal backing in components at least 8 mm thick resulted in excellent clinical and radiologic scores at 5.5 years.[9] Another solution to tibial wear—the use of a meniscal-bearing prosthesis—has demonstrated promising short-term results.[22]

Malposition of either the femoral or the tibial component is associated with loosening. In particular, components should be parallel in flexion and extension and centered over the respective condyles (Fig. 4). Cementless fixation has also been associated with component loosening. Bernasek and associates[19] reported 39% failure rate with cementless UKA at a two-year follow-up examination. Fibrous ingrowth was predominant in the revised knees. Newer cementless devices may show better results, but long-term data on such prostheses are not yet available.

Degeneration of articular cartilage in the opposite compartment has been reported at varying rates in the literature.[4,8,11,12,18,23] Again, selection of patients with extensive pathology will predispose to this means of failure. In addition, overcorrection of joint alignment,

through the use of components that are too thick, transfers increased forces to the uninvolved compartment and may accelerate the progression of disease there.[1,12] Jones and associates[11] reported 207 knees at a maximum six-year follow-up and found that only 2.9% of cases had progression of radiographic disease and that only half of these were symptomatic. The decreased survivorship at ten years reported by Thornhill and Scott,[3] however, suggests that progression of osteoarthritis may be a later complication. The risk of such progression in untreated knees with unicompartmental osteoarthritis has been estimated at 25% at ten to 18 years.[24]

Finally, patellofemoral complications and pes anserine bursitis have already been discussed as reasons for failed UKA.

Revision of UKA

Although ease of revision to TKA has been listed as an advantage of UKA,[1,5,8] two recent reports indicate otherwise. Barrett and Scott[17] reviewed 29 cases of UKA revised to TKA. The most common cause of failure was loosening; the next most common was disease progression. Approximately one half of the knees required bone grafting and special components to reconstruct the osseous defects. Satisfactory results were reported in 66% of patients at two years (Fig. 5).

Padgett and associates,[25] reviewed 21 cases of UKA revised to TKA. The primary reason for failure of the UKA was progression of disease. Component loosening was the other frequent cause. Of these cases, 76% required reconstruction of major osseous defects, and satisfactory results were found in 84% of the revised knees. These researchers noted a particular problem with UKA, which we have termed the paradox of the tibial component. Although increasing the thickness of the tibial component reduces polyethylene wear, more tibial bone must be resected to avoid overcorrection of joint alignment when the thicker component is used. Thus, should the UKA eventually need to be revised to a TKA, a larger tibial defect will result. Empirically, we have used tibial components 8 to 10 mm thick.

Conclusions

(1) The best candidate for UKA is an elderly, sedentary, nonobese patient with unicompartmental osteoarthritis. (2) The final decision to proceed with UKA, rather than TKA, is made at surgery, after visual confirmation that the articular cartilage in the weight-bearing region of the opposite compartment is normal. (3) The goal of alignment should be restoration of the original joint line, because undercorrection leads to early component failure and overcorrection leads to accelerated degeneration of the uninvolved compartment. (4) Acceptable results can be expected in 80% to 90% of patients at 10 years. (5) The primary reason for revision of the UKA is failure of the tibial component, especially in cases where it is less than 7 mm thick. The thickness of polyethylene is limited by the presence of metal backing and by the amount of tibial bone that can be prudently resected. (6) In properly selected patients, degeneration of the opposite compartment is a rare reason for revision at present, but this problem may become more prevalent as UKA follow-up extends beyond 10 years. (7) Revision of UKA to TKA spans a wide range of technical difficulty and, in over half of the cases, will require tibial augmentation.

Although arguments regarding the best treatment for unicompartmental osteoarthritis persist, the role of UKA has become better defined over the past decade. With good technique and a well designed prosthesis, UKA provides excellent results for the properly selected patient. UKA occupies a specific niche in the treatment of unicompartmental osteoarthritis and supplements the techniques of tibial osteotomy and TKA.

References

1. Marmor L: Marmor modular knee in unicompartmental disease: Minimum four-year follow-up. *J Bone Joint Surg* 1979;61A:347–353.
2. Scott RD, Santore RF: Unicondylar unicompartmental replacement for osteoarthritis of the knee. *J Bone Joint Surg* 1981;63A:536–544.
3. Thornhill TS, Scott RD: Unicompartmental total knee arthroplasty. *Orthop Clin North Am* 1989;20:245–256.
4. Marmor L: Unicompartmental knee arthroplasty: Ten to 13 year follow-up study. *Clin Orthop* 1988;226:14–20.
5. Kozinn SC, Scott R: Unicondylar knee arthroplasty. *J Bone Joint Surg* 1989;71A:145–150.
6. Brocklehurst R, Bayliss MT, Maroudas A, et al: The composition of normal and osteoarthritic articular cartilage from human knee joints: With special reference to unicompartmental replacement and osteotomy of the knee. *J Bone Joint Surg* 1984;64A:95–106.
7. Bae DK, Guhl JF, Keane SP: Unicompartmental knee arthroplasty for single compartment disease: Clinical experience with an average four-year follow-up study. *Clin Orthop* 1983;176:233–238.
8. Mackinnon J, Young S, Baily RA: The St. Georg sledge for unicompartmental replacement of the knee A prospective study of 115 cases. *J Bone Joint Surg* 1988;70B:217–223.
9. Kozinn SC, Marx C, Scott RD: Unicompartmental knee arthroplasty: A 4.5 to 6 year follow-up study with a metalbacked tibial component. *J Arthroplasty* 1989;4(suppl):1–10.
10. Olsen NJ, Ejsted R, Krogh P: St. Georg modular knee prosthesis: A two-and-a-half to six-year follow-up. *J Bone Joint Surg* 1986;68B:787–790.
11. Jones WT, Bryan RS, Petersen LF, et al: Unicompartmental knee arthroplasty using polycentric and geometric hemicomponents. *J Bone Joint Surg* 1981;63A:946–954.
12. Laskin RS: Unicompartmental tibiofemoral resurfacing arthroplasty. *J Bone Joint Surg* 1978;60A:182–185.
13. Thornhill TS: Unicompartmental knee arthroplasty. *Clin Orthop* 1986;205:121–131.
14. Marmor L: The modular knee. *Clin Orthop* 1973;94:242–248.
15. Marmor L: Results of single compartment arthroplasty with acrylic cement fixation: A minimum follow-up of two years. *Clin Orthop* 1977;122:181–188.
16. Marmor L: Unicompartmental and total knee arthroplasty. *Clin Orthop* 1985;192:75–81.
17. Barrett WP, Scott RD: Revision of failed unicondylar unicompartmental knee arthroplasty. *J Bone Joint Surg* 1987;69A:1328–1335.
18. Insall J, Aglietti P: A five to seven-year follow-up of unicondylar arthroplasty. *J Bone Joint Surg* 1980;62A:1329–1337.
19. Bernasek TL, Rand JA, Bryan RS: Unicompartmental porous-coated anatomic total knee arthroplasty. *Clin Orthop* 1988;236:52–59.
20. Cameron HU, Hunter GA, Welsh RP, et al: Unicompartmental knee replacement. *Clin Orthop* 1981;160:109–113.
21. Mallory TH, Danyi J: Unicompartmental total knee arthroplasty: A five-to nine-year follow-up study of 42 procedures. *Clin Orthop* 1983;175:135–138.
22. Goodfellow J, Tibrewal S, Sherman K, et al: Unicompartmental Oxford meniscal knee arthroplasty. *J Arthroplasty* 1987;2:1–9.
23. Jackson RW, Burdick W: Unicompartmental knee arthroplasty. *Clin Orthop* 1984;190:182–185.
24. Hernborg JS, Nilsson BE: The natural course of untreated osteoarthritis of the knee. *Clin Orthop* 1977;123:130–137.
25. Padgett D, Stern S, Insall J: Revision total knee arthroplasty for failed unicompartmental replacement. *J Bone Joint Surg* 1991;73A:186–190.

Open Tibial Fractures: Current Orthopaedic Management

Robert J. Brumback, MD

Introduction

Although studies in recent years[1-7] have significantly improved the understanding and treatment of open fractures of the tibia, management of this injury remains one of the most controversial topics in orthopaedic trauma. This controversy is fueled by many factors. Foremost is the fact that, because most practicing orthopaedists do not encounter a significant number of these injuries on a yearly basis, they are forced to base their treatment decisions on past experience combined with what they believe to be the currently accepted treatment method. Secondly, the "treatment of choice" for an open tibial fracture depends largely on the individual characteristics of a given injury. Therefore, an open tibial fracture requires examination, judgment, and an individualized treatment plan. The multitude of variables inherent in open tibial fractures is conducive to a wide spectrum of chosen treatments, and thus, a wide spectrum of final results. Finally, in a surgical world of bone and soft-tissue transfers, replantation of amputated body parts, and lengthening of limbs, the constantly rising level of expectation evidenced by today's patient for an excellent clinical outcome increases the pressure to adopt improved treatment techniques.

Principles of Classification

Existing classification schemes for open fractures, most notably the widely accepted Gustilo and Anderson system, represent early attempts at grouping injuries by their severity.[8-11] Although the Gustilo and Anderson system remains the accepted "language" by which open fractures are described, the treating orthopaedist should initially be more concerned with identifying the amount of energy absorbed by the limb, and less concerned with assigning a specific grade to an injury. Although as yet not widely accepted, other recently proposed classification systems[12,13] may detail the components of injury more accurately than does the Gustilo and Anderson classification. Only after careful assessment can the injury be classified and an appropriate treatment plan formulated.

As the amount of energy exerted on the tibia increases, so does the severity of the multiple components of that injury. Although these components must be individually analyzed, together they represent the "personality" of the injury.

Components of Open Tibial Fractures

History/Mechanism of Injury The way that an accident occurs provides guidelines for assessing the amount of energy that created the injury and for treatment planning.[7,14-17] The length of time that has passed since the accident occurred is important, and knowledge of the environment in which it occurred is essential. Therefore, knowing whether the patient was a pedestrian struck by a car or a football player injured in a tackle helps the surgeon classify the severity of injury.

Vascular Status of the Extremity Any fracture, whether open or closed, that results in vascular damage and potential limb ischemia must be treated emergently. Even if the limb does not become necrotic, marginal tissue perfusion may lead to inadequate immune system response, infection, and/or muscular fibrosis. The functional outcome of open fractures associated with vascular injuries is often poor, and amputation may frequently be indicated.[18,19] Before assessing the local bony and soft-tissue damage associated with an open fracture, orthopaedists must be assured of adequate blood flow distal to the level of injury.

Size of the Soft-Tissue Wound Much emphasis has been placed on the size of the soft-tissue wound or laceration associated with an open fracture.[10,20] Certainly, leg wounds 1 cm in length usually represent the less severe open fractures, whereas larger wounds with or without soft-tissue flaps represent greater amounts of injury. However, orthopaedists should suspect the presence of high-energy injuries concealed by small open-fracture wounds. Overemphasis on classification of open fractures by the size of the wound is one of the most common errors in open-fracture management.

Soft-Tissue Crush or Loss Although there are no established criteria with which to quantify the magnitude of the soft-tissue crush or loss within an injury, an early estimate of the damage is provided by direct observation of the wound during debridement. Crushed tissue is usually poorly perfused and usually becomes necrotic within 36 hours of injury. At the initial debridement of an open fracture, it is not unusual to find bleeding skin edges or apparently viable, contractile muscle that requires further debridement a few days later.[21] Crushed soft-tissue or degloving injuries are indicative of high-energy open fractures and provide a clue to the future behavior of the open-fracture wound, regardless of its size.

Periosteal Stripping/Bone Necrosis Periosteal stripping of diaphyseal segments of bone can indicate the amount of displacement that occurred at the time of the fracture and is thus a measure of the amount of energy absorbed by the limb. Unfortunately, the outer surface of the cortex that has been denuded of its periosteal attachments has been devascularized.[22] This dead cortical bone presents a problem in the treatment of open tibial fractures, because it provides an avascular environment in which bacterial contamination can grow.[23] Comminuted cortical fragments with little or no soft-tissue attachments are undoubtedly necrotic.[24]

Fracture Pattern/Comminution/Bone Loss Because the amount of energy absorbed by the limb is reflected in the fracture pattern, even the initial radiographs, exclusive of the appearance of the wound, can provide clues into the "personality" of the fracture.[25] Low-energy fracture patterns, such as spiral fractures, usually are not associated with significant soft-tissue injuries. But as the energy of injury increases, so does the amount of fracture displacement, comminution, and bone devitalization and necrosis. Recognition of the fracture pattern and its relation to the magnitude of injury is a prerequisite for choosing the optimal open-fracture treatment method.

Contamination Regardless of the size of the open-fracture wound, contamination remains a key element in assessment of an open fracture. Fractures occurring in highly contaminated environments, such as barnyards or brackish water, should be treated with the utmost respect for the risk of infection. This consideration makes an accurate history of the accident an important piece of information before the start of treatment. Internal fixation of any type is generally contraindicated in significantly contaminated open fractures.[14,26,27]

Compartment Syndrome Although compartment syndrome may not be part of the initial injury evaluation, its development signals neuromuscular ischemia, which can occur within hours of the injurious event or after the completion of the initial orthopaedic management. High-energy open fractures are predisposed to compartment syndromes.[4] Regardless of the apparent lack of severity of an open tibial fracture, the development of a compartment syndrome increases the potential for infection, loss of function, or loss of limb. Extensive wounds associated with open fractures do not preclude the development of this complication.[4,28] A compartment syndrome that complicates an injury previously characterized as a low-energy injury changes the classification of that injury to high energy.

Assessing Components of Injury

Analysis of the various components of injury must be viewed as a progressive process. Some of the components, such as accident history, size of the soft-tissue wound, and fracture pattern, are known almost immediately. Others, such as the degree of periosteal stripping and bone necrosis or the magnitude of soft-tissue crush or loss, are identified at the time of initial wound debridement but may require reassessment at a later debridement. Therefore, no single assessment is adequate, and the orthopaedist's role is a process of continual identification and verification of the personality of the injury. It is impossible to classify an open fracture accurately before surgical debridement.

Treatment

The goals of treatment of an open tibial fracture, listed chronologically, are: (1) prevention of infection, (2) stabilization of bone and soft tissue, (3) wound closure or soft-tissue coverage, (4) maintenance of fracture alignment through fracture union, and (5) limb rehabilitation.

Many authors state that debridement is the key to preventing infection after open fracture.[29-32] Open wounds can be contaminated with three materials: foreign inert and organic debris, bacteria, and devitalized host tissue.[33] The goals of debridement include the removal of gross wound contamination, a reduction in the wound bacterial count, and the removal of all necrotic tissue.[34,35] Because bacterial contamination is present in all open-fracture wounds, it is imperative to perform the debridement as early as possible to prevent further colonization of the wound.[9,36,37] Regardless of the size or severity of an open tibial fracture, early surgical debridement is mandatory.

Unfortunately, although the principles of wound debridement have been established for decades,[31,38] the surgical process of debridement is anything but standardized. Physician-to-physician differences in the amount of debridement performed make this a widely variable procedure. Certain guidelines must be followed, because any divergence from these principles places the patient at an increased risk for the development of infection.

First, the entire zone of injury must be visualized. This requires surgical extension of the skin wounds, usually in a longitudinal fashion, for complete exposure of the soft-tissue and bony injury.[30,39] Many surgeons resist this tenet and merely excise the wound edges without undertaking further deep dissection. It is impossible to determine the vascularity of comminuted fracture fragments, the presence of foreign debris on the bone ends, or the viability of surrounding muscle without surgical extension of most open-fracture wounds. The debridement should proceed in an orderly manner, beginning with the skin and progressing to the depths of the wound. Exposed neurovascular structures should not undergo debridement, if possible, because their removal may significantly impair eventual limb function. Surgical extensions of open-fracture wounds are usually sutured closed at the end of the debridement.

Second, all necrotic tissue, including bone, should be removed from the wound. This portion of the debridement is controversial,[3,33,40–42] because the removal of large bone fragments or the creation of segmental gaps in the tibial diaphysis was associated, in the past, with a high rate of nonunion and eventual amputation. Surgeons, afraid of creating nonreconstructable problems, often performed inadequate debridements. Now that more aggressive bone-grafting,[3,43] reconstruction,[44–49] and bone-transport[50–53] techniques are available, concern for limb reconstruction plays a much less important role at the time of debridement. It is far better to have a tibia with a noninfected segmental gap than one in which bony apposition at the fracture site has been preserved, but which is complicated by an infected nonunion. To cure the latter problem, a large debridement of the infected necrotic bone would eventually be required, and months of treatment time would be lost.

Third, pulsatile-lavage irrigation has proved effective in removing particulate matter and in lowering bacterial counts from open wounds. All open fractures require a minimum of 9.0 liters of pulsatile-lavage irrigation. Bulb-syringe irrigation, which does not routinely generate sufficient pressure (15 psi) to remove particulate debris, is not a substitute for pulsatile lavage.[54–56]

Fourth, antibiotics should be given to help control the contamination remaining in the wound. All open wounds are contaminated, and the term "prophylactic antibiotics" is a misnomer.[32,57] For most low-energy open fractures, a broad-spectrum cephalosporin provides adequate microbiologic coverage. However, with increasing wound and/or fracture severity or contamination, an aminoglycoside is added. Finally, a penicillin is indicated if the accident occurred in an environment, such as soil, known to harbor *Clostridia*. Before 1985, the accepted duration of antibiotic therapy for open fractures was traditionally three to five days.[57–60] Recently, investigators have shown that shorter, 24- to 48-hour courses of antibiotics are equally effective and lessen the risk of the development of resistant bacterial strains.[61]

Although much has been written concerning wound cultures taken before, during, and after wound debridement,[37,57,62,63] this technique has not been found to be of significant clinical value. In a recent presentation, Lee and associates[64] demonstrated this process to be ineffective and pointed out its high ratio of cost to benefit. Wounds that appear infected or that have

significant drainage, erythema, or poor granulation should be cultured on an individual basis.

Finally, no open tibial fracture wound should undergo primary closure the day of injury, because closure only invites closed-space infection. Some surgeons seem unable to resist this temptation. No single debridement of a high-energy fracture wound can assure the surgeon that all necrotic tissue has been removed, because it is impossible to predict which tissues will become necrotic and which will remain viable. Wound closure inhibits the "second look" procedure, a planned procedure in which the patient is returned to the operating room 36 to 48 hours after initial debridement for a repeat debridement. Although this "second look" may be unnecessary in open fractures of lesser severity, it is required of any high-energy open fracture. Wound closure or coverage should be performed four to five days after injury. This delayed closure assures that viable host tissue defense mechanisms are allowed sufficient time to deal with wound contamination. Delayed wound closure has been shown to decrease significantly the incidence of wound infection.[33,58,65,66]

The surgeon must wait until after the initial debridement before deciding the type of stabilization procedure to be used. The surgeon who decides in the emergency room that a fracture is "perfect for an intramedullary nail" is depriving the patient of a treatment plan based on a total understanding of the injury. After the debridement has been completed, the fracture can then be classified. At this juncture, the next dilemma for the orthopaedist arises: the linkage between the grade of an open fracture and the optimal method of bony stabilization. Ideally, each type of open fracture would fit into a mutually exclusive classification system, which would provide the surgeon with the optimal form of treatment. Unfortunately, the world of trauma is imperfect, and each fracture must be individually analyzed and classified before the options for bony stabilization can be discussed. In general, a low-energy open fracture has a significant chance of progressing to uncomplicated fracture union without need for full-thickness flap coverage or bone-grafting procedures. A high-energy open fracture often requires extensive plastic surgical and orthopaedic reconstructive surgeries.

Fracture "Personality"

Low-Energy Open Fractures

In the classification system of Gustilo and Anderson, low-energy open fractures include the grade I and grade II classifications,[67] which are defined as follows: Grade I is an open fracture with a wound less than 1 cm in length; an "inside-out" injury with minimal soft-tissue damage or contamination. Grade II is an open fracture with a wound longer than 1 cm without extensive contamination, soft-tissue damage, flaps, or avulsions. The key to understanding this group of open fractures is to focus on the degree of soft-tissue disruption and not on the size of the open fracture wound. The majority of these open fractures are caused from the inside out, that is, the displaced bone lacerated or punctured the skin. Wounds shorter than 1 cm were probably caused by less energy than those longer than 1 cm. It is also likely that the contamination in an open fracture with a wound less than 1 cm in length is minimal, which greatly reduces the risk of infection. The surgeon, however, should conclude that these are low-energy injuries, not on the basis of wound size, but because the bone and its attached soft tissue are viable, without tissue crush, necrosis, periosteal stripping, severe comminution, or gross contamination. Therefore, because the host defense mechanisms are left intact for the most part, a healed, noninfected tibia is the predictable outcome from these less severe injuries. This predictable result has led to these injuries being treated with many and varying modalities. The rates of infection and nonunion for grade I and grade II open fractures are low. The incidence of infection in these injuries usually falls between 0% and 5% in most investigations.[20,33,59,68-76]

Nonsurgical skeletal stabilization with splints, casts, or skeletal traction was the accepted treatment before the era of surgical bony fixation.[77-83] As one would expect, most low-energy open tibial fractures healed, regardless of the method of treatment.[68] However, in addition to potentially inhibiting access to the open wound, these methods are plagued by the same complications reported with nonsurgical treatment of closed tibial fractures, namely, fracture shortening, angulation, and malrotation.[70,73,84-90] Although nonsurgical bone stabilization techniques are still used for open tibial fractures, they can be recommended only for the most stable of fracture patterns, where wound access would not be obstructed.[58] The multiply injured patient requires rigid long-bone fixation and should not be treated, unless unable to undergo anesthesia, with nonsurgical methods.[91,92]

Open reduction with plating of open tibial fractures was popularized in the 1970s and 1980s, but this technique never gained community-level acceptance. Because studies indicate that the incidence of infection increases after open reduction of open tibial fractures, this technique is rarely used today.[1,14,74,93-105] The dissection required to apply the plate causes further tissue devitalization, a definite disadvantage of this technique.[21,106-108] Historically, open reduction did, however, prevent fracture shortening and malalignment, and pioneered the doctrine of early range of motion of the joints of the lower extremity.[103,109] Open reduction and plating of open fractures is still common for injuries involving metaphyseal and intra-articular fractures, in which the restoration of anatomic alignment of the articular surfaces is required.[110,111]

Reamed intramedullary nailing of low-energy open tibial fractures has also been extensively studied. Although a recent review of reamed nailing of grade I and grade II open tibial fractures by Kaltenecker and associates[112] reported no infections, the incidence of infection reported in other studies ranged up to 20%.[113-120] Most authors feel that the obliteration of the endosteal blood supply to the diaphysis creates bone necrosis, hence, the predisposition for infection when this method is used for open tibial shaft fractures. Although debated by some authors,[121] reamed intramedullary nailing of the tibia has been reported to increase the risk of compartment syndrome of the leg.[122-124] As with open plating, most authors feel that this technique, although biomechanically attractive, creates too much iatrogenic damage to be recommended routinely for open tibial fractures.[114,117,125,126] It may be held in reserve as a second-line alternative if other methods of treatment are not available.

External fixation was initially heralded as the treatment of choice for open fractures, because it provided excellent bone stability, afforded excellent wound access, and caused minimal additional tissue or bone devitalization.[127-134] However, the rate of fracture union for open fractures treated with external fixation was questioned. The increased rates of delayed union and nonunion could have occurred because this type of stabilization limited axial loading of the fracture site, which decreased the propensity to heal.[135-144] Compounding this factor was the tendency by surgeons to use external fixation for more severe open fractures. These injuries have a natural history of delayed union and nonunion, and often require bone grafting to obtain fracture healing. The claims that external fixation created difficulties in obtaining fracture union may have been exaggerated when, in fact, the injuries themselves were predisposed to slower healing.

Unfortunately, external fixation pins were commonly complicated by pin-tract infection, which led to relatively poor acceptance of this treatment method by both patient and physicians.[130,131] The incidence of pin-tract infection has been reduced through the use of larger diameter blunt-tipped half-pin designs. Transfixion pins that impale the calf muscles are much more prone to pin-tract complications than are the newer designs.[2,145-148] Although external fixation may be used for low-energy open fractures, many believe that the complications associated with its application are not outweighed by its benefits, and newer methods of fixation are the current preferred treatment.

Some surgeons have used a combined internal/external fixation technique with cortical lag screws to improve alignment of the fracture fragments.[149] Despite the theoretical advantages of secure, anatomic fixation of large butterfly fragments in comminuted tibial fractures, the results reported using minimal internal fixation with external fixation have been suboptimal. The relatively poor results may have resulted from increased soft-tissue dissection for the insertion of the screws, the lack of bone grafting in these comminuted diaphyseal fractures, and early weightbearing after removal of the fixator six to eight weeks after injury. Although the technique is appropriate for stabilization of displaced intra-articular/metaphyseal open fractures, most authors do not recommend it for diaphyseal injuries. If used, bone grafting the fracture and delayed weightbearing are recommended.[43,149,150]

In the last five years, by far the greatest advance in open tibial-fracture care has been the development of nonreamed interlocking intramedullary nail stabilization. Nonreamed interlocking nailing has several advantages over previous methods: (1) because no reaming is performed, the endosteal blood supply is damaged as little as possible; (2) excellent bony stabilization and wound access are provided; and, (3) unstable, comminuted fractures from the proximal one third to the distal one third of the tibia can be treated. This technique has replaced the Lottes nail[75,151-153] and the multiple Ender nail methods,[154-158] because secure fixation of the proximal and distal fracture fragments is obtained, providing axial, angulatory, and rotational stability. Injuries that appear too comminuted to be treated by casting or previous intramedullary techniques are routinely stabilized by this method. Early results from several centers showed no increase in the incidence of infection with this technique, as compared with external fixation, in low-energy open tibial fractures.[154,159-161] Current thinking is that this technique has all the advantages of external fixation without the complications associated with percutaneous pin insertion. Conceptually, the nonreamed interlocking nail may be thought of as an internal fixator.

Several questions concerning nonreamed interlocking nailing of the tibia remain unanswered. These small-diameter nails (8.0 mm and 9.0 mm) use relatively small interlocking screws (4.0 mm and 4.5 mm). The ability of these smaller nails and interlocking screws to withstand the stresses of weightbearing during fracture healing must be further investigated. Several instances of breakage of the screws have occurred. This mechanical failure is extremely rare with reamed interlocking devices, as the larger diameter of these implants protects them against the cyclical loading of weightbearing. Further study on the durability of the nonreamed interlocking nails is required.

In open tibial fractures treated with nonreamed interlocking nails, delayed union or nonunion may still occur. This probably happens because of the severity of the open fracture and the general propensity of such fractures for slower fracture union. Surgeons may be forced into a treatment decision approximately 12 to 16 weeks after the initial injury and nailing, if satisfactory radiographic fracture union is not present (Figs. 1 through 3). The surgeon may elect to dynamize the statically interlocked nail to promote fracture union.[162] This simple outpatient surgical procedure involves removal of the proximal and/or distal interlocking screws. With smaller diameter nails, some unstable fractures may angulate after dynamization because the diameter of the intramedullary nail does not adequately fill the endosteal canal of the tibia. To avoid this complication, the surgeon may elect instead to perform an exchange nailing at this point, stimulating fracture union with a larger diameter, dynamically stabilized, reamed intramedullary nail. The optimal time and indications for dynamization or exchange nailing of open tibial fractures initially stabilized with nonreamed interlocking nails are unknown. However, as many as 20% of fractures treated with a statically interlocked nonreamed nail may require further surgical intervention (dynamization, exchange nailing, or bone grafting) to obtain union.[163]

There is little question, however, that the nonreamed interlocking tibial nail permits excellent bony stabilization with minimal iatrogenic damage to the fracture site. In low-energy open fractures, this technique permits the remaining host immune and healing systems to work relatively unimpeded by surgical interventions. Certainly enough evidence has been gathered to state that nonreamed interlocking nailing is the current treatment of choice for low-energy open fractures of the tibial shaft that are not amenable to nonsurgical methods.

Grade IIIA Open Fractures: The Gray Area

As the energy of injury increases, so does the spectrum of soft-tissue and bony damage. Some of these injuries have the personality of large low-energy open fractures. Others behave like severe open fractures, requiring a staged reconstruction approach. The surgeon's dilemma is in choosing which place along the spectrum of injury a certain fracture occupies. Grade IIIA open fractures, as defined by Gustilo and associates,[20,164] have adequate soft-tissue coverage of a fracture despite soft-tissue laceration or flaps, or are representative of high-energy trauma irrespective of the size of the wound. This imprecise definition permits a wide range of open fractures to be placed in this category.

Treatment of high-energy open fractures mandates a thorough initial debridement followed by a second debridement 36 to 48 hours later. Bone stabilization with casts, splints, and/or skeletal traction is contraindicated for these high-energy injuries. The majority of these open fractures are characterized by highly comminuted fracture patterns and severe open wounds, making optimal bony support and wound care impossible with circumferential plaster casts. Many of these injuries occur in patients with multiple organ system

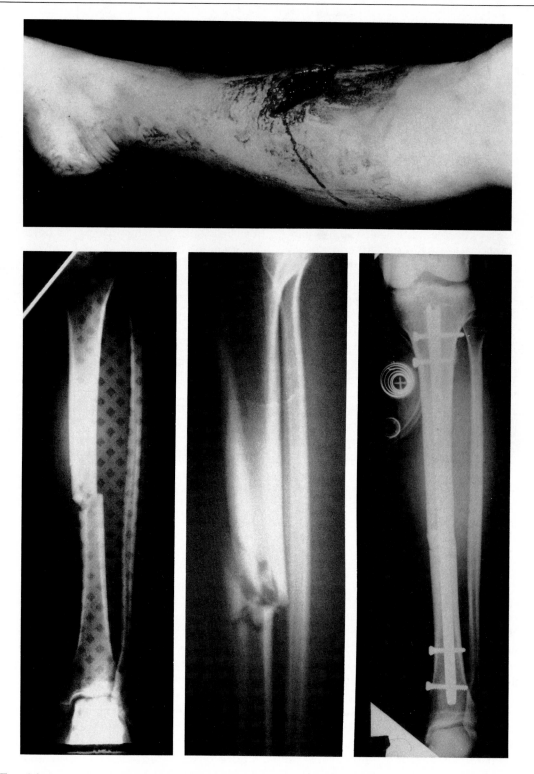

Fig. 1 **Top,** A low-energy (grade II) open tibial fracture occurred as a result of a motor vehicle accident. The patient sustained a closed intracranial injury as well as intra-abdominal trauma that required laparotomy. **Bottom left,** Anteroposterior radiograph demonstrated acceptable alignment with intact fibula and moderate comminution. **Bottom center,** Lateral radiograph showed degree of displacement and comminution. **Bottom right,** Anteroposterior radiograph after nonreamed static interlocking nailing. The multiple injured status of this patient warranted stabilization of the tibial fracture after surgical debridement.

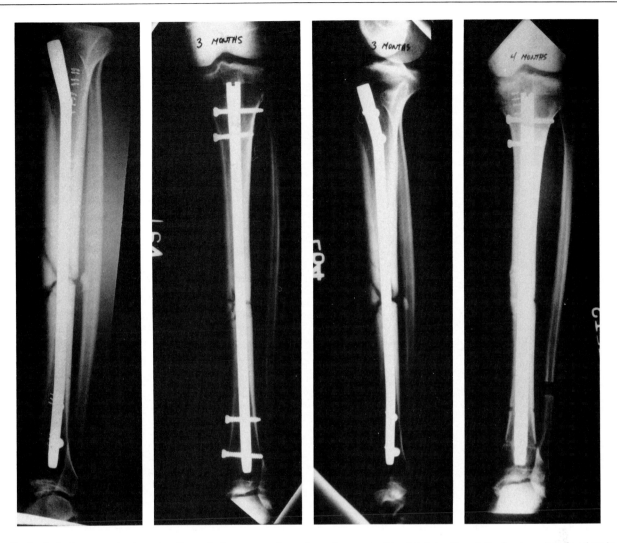

Fig. 2 **Left**, Postoperative lateral radiograph demonstrated excellent alignment with mild distraction at the fracture site of patient in Figure 1. **Left center**, Anteroposterior radiograph, taken 3 months postinjury, showed minimal healing response in the same patient. **Right center**, Lateral radiograph at 3 months showed persistent distraction of the fracture site without evidence of bridging callus. **Right**, Sixteen weeks postinjury, an exchange reamed nailing and fibulectomy were performed. This dynamic stabilization had only proximal interlocking. Due to the lack of healing response evident in this fracture, exchange nailing was selected instead of simple dynamization to stimulate fracture union.

injuries, who require rigid bony stabilization for increased patient mobility and decreased pulmonary compromise.[91]

Stabilization of the fracture also stabilizes the soft tissue of the limb. Nonsurgical methods of bony stabilization, which provide the least amount of bony support, also provide the least amount of soft-tissue stabilization. Stabilizing the injured soft tissues through rigid bony fixation may improve their ability to contain wound contamination.[93,104,125,165,166]

Open plating or reamed intramedullary nails are not recommended in the treatment of grade III open fractures. As discussed with low-energy open fractures, both of these techniques require further tissue dissection and can create further soft-tissue and bone necrosis. It is not surprising that the reported rate of

infection after open reduction or reamed intramedullary nailing of grade III open fractures is unacceptably high.[1,105,126,167–169]

External fixation was believed to be the ideal treatment for high energy open tibial fractures.[130,170,171] Surgeons were more accepting of the pin-tract problems and delayed union for high-energy fractures than they were for low-energy injuries. Recent studies, however, have demonstrated that selected high-energy open fractures can be safely managed with nonreamed interlocking nails.[159,160] According to a randomized study by Santoro and associates,[161] the infection rate for selected grade IIIA open fractures so treated, which were thoroughly debrided within eight hours of injury and had no gross contamination, no significant bone loss, and no need for full thickness soft-tissue flap wound cov-

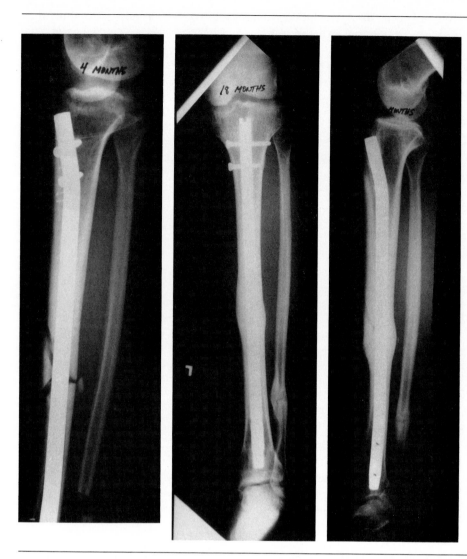

Fig. 3 **Left**, Lateral radiograph immediately after reamed interlocking exchange nailing of the fracture in patient in Figure 1. **Center**, Anteroposterior radiograph 18 months postinjury demonstrated healed tibial fracture in excellent alignment. **Right**, Anteroposterior radiograph at 18 months follow-up demonstrated healed tibial fracture in excellent alignment.

erage, was no higher than that of those treated with external fixation. Examples of grade IIIA open fractures that are excellent candidates for nonreamed interlocking nail stabilization include segmental fractures of the tibia with small open wounds, comminuted open fractures of the shaft without significant devitalized bone or soft tissue, and open fractures with relatively minor open wounds that develop compartment syndrome. Grade IIIA open fractures that have significant bone loss from either injury or debridement, have a delay in the time from injury to debridement, or will require rotational myoplasty or free flap coverage of the open fracture wound are currently believed to be poor candidates for nonreamed intramedullary nail fixation. These latter injuries should be treated with external fixation and the staged reconstruction protocol for grade IIIB open fractures (see below).

Recently, several investigators have studied the safety of secondarily placing intramedullary devices after external fixation has been applied as the initial stabilization for open tibial fractures.[49,162,172–174] Several facts have become clear. If an external fixator has been used for an extended period of time, or if pin-tract infection was present during the period of external fixation, regardless of its duration,[172] any internal fixation (intramedullary nails or plates) later used as a reconstructive tool will be accompanied by an increase in the rate of infection. However, Blachut and associates[49] have recently demonstrated that, if the external fixation is used as a planned temporary means of early fracture stabilization, to be changed to intramedullary nailing within three weeks of injury, the risk of infection may be lessened. Most authors suggest a period of cast immobilization or skeletal traction between the removal of the external fixation and the internal fixation to allow the immune system to control contamination at the pin insertion sites.[49] Simultaneous conversion from external fixation to intramedullary nailing should be viewed with extreme caution. Most investigators do not routinely recommend internal fixation after prolonged external fixation use.

In summary, a broad spectrum of injuries are classified as grade IIIA open fractures. Some of these injuries are best treated by nonreamed intramedullary nailing, some by external fixation. The best treatment method is chosen by determining whether or not this injury will require extensive soft-tissue and bony reconstruction. If not, the nonreamed intramedullary nail may be the treatment of choice. If multiple reconstructive planned procedures are necessary, external fixation should be used. Although conversion from external fixation to intramedullary nailing at some time after the injury has been investigated, this procedure may carry a significant risk of infection and should be considered controversial at this time. The surgeon must make the treatment decision based not on which treatment method appeals most to him, but on which is most appropriate for each individual injury.

Grade IIIB Open Tibial Fractures: Severe High-Energy Injuries

Grade IIIB open fractures are often characterized by extensive soft-tissue injury or loss with periosteal stripping and bone exposure and are commonly complicated by massive contamination. The goals of stabilization in these injuries are to provide adequate alignment and rigidity to the fracture and the soft tissues of the limb without further iatrogenic damage to the injury site. These goals are best accomplished by external fixation. Because these injuries are often highly comminuted or have bone gaps, acceptable alignment of the limb may be difficult to achieve at the time of initial application of the external fixator. External fixation frames that permit adjustment of the fracture after frame application are preferred for these injuries.

A logical, step-by-step protocol for limb salvage should be followed (Figs. 4 through 6).[5,6,171,175] The initial step is obviously surgical debridement. Aggressive removal of all devitalized and marginal soft tissue and bone is mandatory. Extension of the skin wound for visualization of the entire zone of injury, with visual inspection of the ends of the fragments, is routine. Reconstruction of the limb is of little concern at the initial debridement. Amputation, if performed at the initial debridement, should be thought of as removal of necrotic or dysfunctional tissue and not as a failure of limb salvage.

Amputation is indicated for a patient who has a grade IIIB open fracture with an insensate foot and documented disruption of the posterior tibial nerve. Amputation may also be indicated for severe grade IIIB injuries with extensive ipsilateral foot and ankle injuries. A patient with life-threatening multiple injuries, including a grade IIIB open tibial fracture requiring extensive limb surgery, may be forced to undergo limb ablation as a lifesaving measure.[30,50,176]

If amputation is not indicated, and the debridement is complete, then external fixation is applied.[2,146,177,178] Blunt, half-pin designs are used in the tibial diaphysis.

Including the foot (metatarsals) in this external fixator helps stabilize the soft tissue of the leg.[179] The longitudinal bars of the fixator must be positioned far enough from the level of the skin to avoid interfering with dressing changes. A second debridement is scheduled for 36 to 48 hours after the first, and at that time the wound is reexplored and all devitalized tissue is removed.

Unless neurovascular structures or tendons are denuded and exposed, soft-tissue coverage should be performed four to seven days after injury.[39,180–186] The experience of Godina[187] demonstrated that full-thickness coverage can safely be performed within 24 hours of injury after an aggressive surgical debridement. However, most authors agree that a second debridement should be performed on high-energy open fracture wounds before soft-tissue closure. Up to two thirds of grade IIIB open tibial fractures at the Shock Trauma Center require either local rotational myoplasty or a freely vascularized muscle transfer to fill local bony defects and provide full-thickness coverage of exposed bone.[3,7] The remaining grade IIIB open fractures require split-thickness skin grafting or delayed primary closure of the wound. Rarely is a large wound allowed to granulate closed by secondary intention, because this method has been associated with an increased rate of infection.[41,188]

After successful soft-tissue closure, the injury has been converted to a clean, nondraining fracture. A common pitfall at this time is to assume that the fracture should now be treated as if it had never been an open fracture at all. Inexperienced surgeons often remove the external fixator at this point, either placing the limb in a cast or performing an internal fixation procedure. Disregarding the extent of the initial injury after successful soft-tissue coverage of a severe open tibial fracture is a common, and often disastrous, mistake. The natural history of severe open tibial fractures is for delayed union or nonunion. Although a percentage heal without further surgical intervention, as many as 60% may need bone grafting to stimulate fracture healing.[7] Therefore, surgeons must remember the extent of the initial injury, which is an excellent predictor of the likelihood of eventual fracture union without further surgical intervention. In severe open tibial fractures, the external fixator should be continued for bony stabilization and alignment while healing of the fracture site is stimulated with bone graft.

Certain severe open tibial fractures have minimal bone loss. After wound coverage, these injuries may undergo a trial of weightbearing ambulation, usually while stabilized with an external fixator, to see if they will heal. Healing may be more likely to occur if the injury encompasses the metaphyseal region of the tibia. In general, the limb-salvage protocol assumes that all severe open tibial fractures, especially those with soft-tissue injuries requiring full-thickness closure or those

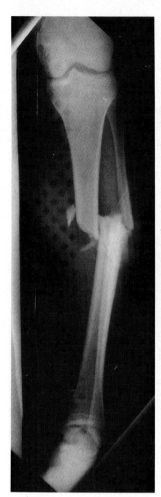
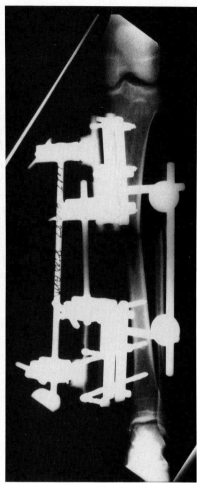
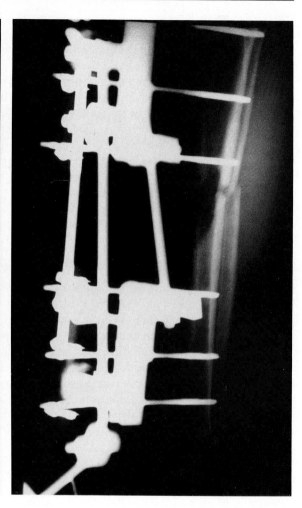

Fig. 4 **Left**, Anteroposterior radiograph of a grade IIIB open tibial fracture sustained in a motorcycle accident. Note the multiple comminuted fragments and the 100% displacement of the fracture. At the time of operative debridement, multiple devitalized comminuted fragments were removed. A large anteromedial defect remained. **Center**, Anteroposterior radiograph after the application of an anterior half-pin external fixator. Note the degree of bone loss due to debridement. **Right**, Lateral radiograph after external fixation of the fracture. The patient underwent repeat debridement 48 hours after injury and received soleus rotational myoplasty coverage at 5 days after injury. (Reprinted with permission from Brumback RJ: Orthopaedic follow-up, in Yaremchuck MJ, Brumback RJ (eds): *Lower Extremity Salvage and Reconstruction: Orthopedic and Plastic Surgical Management.* New York, Elsevier Science Publishing, 1989, chap 16, pp 221–235.)

with significant diaphyseal bone loss, require bone grafting as part of their staged reconstruction.[3,189] These fractures are bone-grafted two weeks after successful delayed primary closure or split-thickness skin grafting, or four to six weeks after local or freely vascularized flap closure. Bone grafting at the time of wound closure has been associated with an increase in the rate of postoperative infection.[189]

Tibial shaft fractures are most often grafted through the posterolateral approach, creating a tibia/fibula synostosis.[3,190-195] If the tibial fracture is accompanied by an ipsilateral fibular fracture at the same anatomic level, plating of the fibular fracture at the time of posterolateral bone grafting helps ensure union and helps prevent late deformation of the limb through the area of injury. Fractures in the proximal one-fifth of the

tibia may require anterolateral or posteromedial grafting, as the posterolateral approach places the anterior tibial artery in jeopardy.

In a study from the Shock Trauma Center, Blick and associates[3] reported that a planned, early "prophylactic" bone-grafting technique resulted in a union rate of up to 96% for high-energy open tibial fractures in an average of 40 to 52 weeks from injury. Although this time period may seem prolonged when compared with that for union of closed tibial shaft fracture, it is historically a relatively short time to fracture healing, given the extent of the bony and soft-tissue damage inherent in these injuries.[29,196] Repeat bone grafting was required in 13% of the fractures after this limb salvage protocol.

Bone transport techniques in limb reconstruction

have generated much enthusiasm over the reconstitution of bony gaps.[51-53,197-199] Injuries that previously required a massive cancellous bone-grafting procedure and that had the highest rates of failure and reoperation may now be treated by bone transport techniques.

The circular small-wire fixators currently used for limb lengthening and bone transport should be thought of as reconstructive tools, not external fixators for treatment of tibial shaft fractures the day of injury. These devices take longer than half-pin designs to apply, the access to the wound for dressing changes and repeat debridements is restricted, and the transfixion wires make soft-tissue flap procedures difficult to perform. Once a fracture has been debrided and stabilized and has received soft-tissue coverage, then the original external fixator can be electively exchanged for a circular fixator. Bone transport techniques do not, by any means, replace the need for all bone grafting procedures. A moderate percentage of these injuries may require bone grafting at the site of bony contact after the bone transport has been completed.[197,198,200] However, this grafting procedure is much less extensive than a large posterolateral grafting of a diaphyseal defect of the tibia.

Most grade IIIB open tibial fractures have loss of some devitalized comminuted fragments at the fracture site, but still retain some diaphyseal contact between the major fracture fragments. These fractures are best treated by direct cancellous posterolateral bone grafting and not bone transport. Bone transport techniques may replace freely vascularized fibular transfers as the treatment of choice for large diaphyseal defects of the tibia.

Grade IIIC Open Fractures: Fractures with Arterial Injury

Any open fracture with an associated arterial injury requiring repair is a grade IIIC injury.[164] Inherent in this definition is the component of time. The surgeon now has a limited time in which to restore blood flow to the distal extremity, or be faced with an increased risk of infection and amputation.

The extensive surgery required for vascular repair may be contraindicated in the life-threatened multiply injured patient, and amputation should be performed as a lifesaving maneuver. It is extremely difficult, and often impossible, to complete patient evaluation, resuscitation, and other lifesaving surgical procedures and still have enough time to restore vascular integrity to the limb within six to eight hours after injury. In the multiple trauma patient with a grade IIIC open tibial fracture who requires, for example, multiple preoperative radiographs and scans, followed by a laparotomy for a ruptured spleen, the leg should be sacrificed to ensure patient survival.[19]

For the patient with an isolated grade IIIC open tibial fracture, it is possible to reconstruct the vascularity of the distal limb within the allotted eight hours from in-

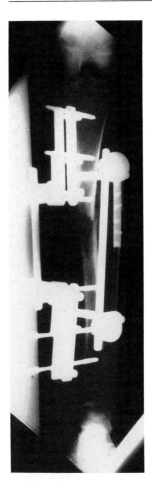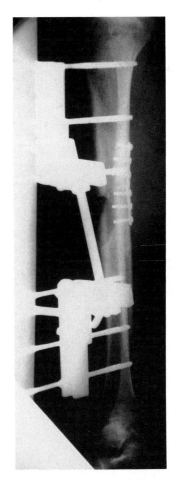

Fig. 5 Left, Anteroposterior radiograph after posterolateral bone grafting with fibular plating, which was performed 4 weeks after injury in patient in Figure 4. **Right**, Lateral radiograph after bone grafting and fibular plating. Note maintenance of alignment of the fracture. (Reprinted with permission from Brumback RJ: Orthopaedic follow-up, in Yaremchuck MJ, Brumback RJ (eds): *Lower Extremity Salvage and Reconstruction: Orthopedic and Plastic Surgical Management.* New York, Elsevier Science Publishing, 1989, chap 16, pp 221–235.)

jury. However, progressive muscle and nerve ischemia, as well as postischemic compartment syndrome, are persistent problems. I recommend an individualized approach to this injury for such patients. If the vascular assessment with arteriogram is not delayed, then revascularization may be attempted. Bone stabilization is best performed with an external fixator, which is quick, adjustable, and does not interfere with the surgical approach for vascular repair. Four compartment fasciotomies[201] should be performed on all emergency vascular repairs associated with fractures of the tibia. Postoperatively, the serum myoglobin and kidney function should be monitored to check for systemic signs of myonecrosis and organ failure.

Surgeons should be realistic in their outcome expectations for these injuries. Many will fail and result

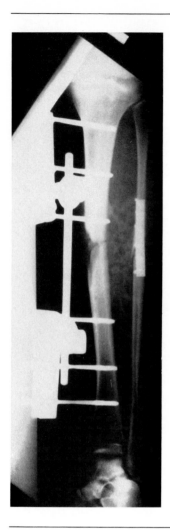
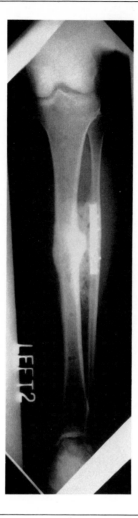
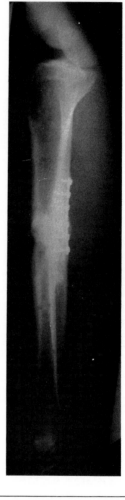

Fig. 6 **Left,** Internal rotation view of the tibia, which best demonstrates the status of the posterolateral bone graft, taken 10 weeks after grafting in patient in Figure 4. Early graft incorporation and synostosis were evident. The external fixator was removed at this time and partial weightbearing in a cast was begun. **Center,** Four months postinjury, the patient was fitted with a removable tibial orthosis and full weightbearing ambulation was begun. Anteroposterior radiograph 12 months after injury disclosed union of the fracture and tibia/fibula synostosis. **Right,** Lateral radiograph 12 months after injury disclosed a healed fracture with excellent alignment of the limb. (Reprinted with permission from Brumback RJ: Orthopaedic follow-up, in Yaremchuck MJ, Brumback RJ (eds): *Lower Extremity Salvage and Reconstruction: Orthopedic and Plastic Surgical Management.* New York, Elsevier Science Publishing, 1989, chap 16, pp 221–235.)

in eventual amputation.[18,19,202,203] This is a terrible situation for both patient and physician. After a grade IIIC open tibial fracture, a leg without functional ability, with an insensate foot, or with persistent infection and/or nonunion is better amputated early in the course of treatment.[50,204]

Summary

Treating the spectrum of bone and soft-tissue injuries that can accompany open fractures of the tibia requires experience and judgment. It appears that the non-reamed interlocking nail can safely and reproducibly stabilize most low-energy and selected high-energy open fractures of the leg. Severe open tibial fractures require a staged reconstructive protocol using external fixation as the method of bony stabilization. Differentiation between the requirements of individual injuries remains the key to successful treatment.

References

1. Bach AW, Hansen ST Jr: Plates versus external fixation in severe open tibial shaft fractures. *Clin Orthop* 1989;241:89–94.
2. Behrens F, Searls K: External fixation of the tibia. Basic concepts and prospective evaluation. *J Bone Joint Surg* 1986;68B:246–254.
3. Blick SS, Brumback RJ, Lakatos R, et al: Early prophylactic bone grafting of high-energy tibial fractures. *Clin Orthop* 1989;240:21–41.
4. Blick SS, Brumback RJ, Poka A, et al: Compartment syndrome in open tibial fractures. *J Bone Joint Surg* 1986;68A:1348–1353.
5. Bosse MJ, Burgess AR, Brumback RJ: Evaluation and treatment of the high-energy open tibia fracture. *Adv Orthop Surg* 1984;7:3–17.
6. Burgess AR, Poka A, Brumback RJ, et al: Management of open grade III tibial fractures. *Orthop Clin North Am* 1987;18:85–93.
7. Burgess AR, Poka A, Brumback RJ, et al: Pedestrian tibial injuries. *J Trauma* 1987;27:596–601.
8. Ash DC, Mercuri LG: External fixation of the unstable zygomatic arch fracture. *J Oral Maxillofac Surg* 1984;42:621–622.
9. Ashai F, Mam MK, Iqbal S: Ileal entrapment as a complication of fractured pelvis. *J Trauma* 1988;28:551–552.
10. Ashton H: The effect of increased tissue pressure on blood flow. *Clin Orthop* 1975;113:15–26.

11. Asko-Seljavaara S, Haajanen J: The exposed knee joint: Five case reports. *J Trauma* 1982;22:1021–1025.

12. Tscherne H, Gotzen L (eds): *Fractures with Soft Tissue Injuries*. Berlin, Springer-Verlag, 1984.

13. Muller ME, Allower M, Schneider R, et al: *Manual of Internal Fixation. Techniques Recommended by the AO-Group*, ed 2. Berlin, Springer-Verlag, 1979, pp 151–157.

14. Allum RL, Mowbray MA: A retrospective review of the healing of fractures of the shaft of the tibia with special reference to the mechanism of injury. *Injury* 1980;11:304–308.

15. Findlay JA: The motor-cycle tibia. *Injury* 1972;4:75–78.

16. Jackson RD: A characteristic type of motorcycle fracture of the tibia. *South Med J* 1970;63:222–225.

17. Van Der Linden W, Sunzel H, Larsson K: Fractures of the tibial shaft after skiing and other accidents. *J Bone Joint Surg* 1975;57A:321–327.

18. Caudle RJ, Stern PJ: Severe open fractures of the tibia. *J Bone Joint Surg* 1987;69A:801–807.

19. Hansen ST Jr: The type-IIIC tibial fracture. Salvage or amputation (editorial). *J Bone Joint Surg* 1987;69A:799–800.

20. Gustilo RB, Anderson JT: Prevention of infection in the treatment of one thousand and twenty-five open fractures of long bones: Retrospective and prospective analyses. *J Bone Joint Surg* 1976;58A:453–458.

21. Tønnesen PA, Heerfordt J, Pers M: 150 open fractures of the tibial shaft—the relationship between necrosis of the skin and delayed union. *Acta Orthop Scand* 1975;46:823–835.

22. Rhinelander FW: Tibial blood supply in relation to fracture healing. *Clin Orthop* 1974;105:34–81.

23. Van Winkle BA, Neustein J: Management of open fractures with sterilization of large, contaminated, extruded cortical fragments. *Clin Orthop* 1987;223:275–281.

24. Swiontkowski MF: Criteria for bone debridement in massive lower limb trauma. *Clin Orthop* 1989;243:41–47.

25. Johner R, Wruhs O: Classification of tibial shaft fractures and correlation with results after rigid internal fixation. *Clin Orthop* 1983;178:7–25.

26. Majeski JA, Gauto A: Management of peripheral arterial vascular injuries with a Javid shunt. *Am J Surg* 1979;138:324–325.

27. Sheikh MA: Respiratory changes after fractures and surgical skeletal injury. *Injury* 1982;13:489–494.

28. DeLee JC, Stiehl JB: Open tibia fracture with compartment syndrome. *Clin Orthop* 1981;160:175–184.

29. Gustilo RB: Management of infected fractures, in *Management of Open Fractures and Their Complications*. Philadelphia, WB Saunders, 1982, vol 4, pp 133–158.

30. Brumback RJ: Wound debridement, in Yaremchuk MJ, Burgess AR, Brumback RJ (eds): *Lower Extremity Salvage and Reconstruction: Orthopedic and Plastic Surgical Management*. New York, Elsevier Science Publishing, 1989, pp 71–80.

31. Committee on Surgery of the Division of Medical Sciences of the National Research Council: Traumatic wounds, in *Burns, Shock, Wound Healing and Vascular Injuries*. Philadelphia, WB Saunders, 1943, chap 2, pp 183–194.

32. Patzakis MJ, Wilkins J: Factors influencing infection rate in open fracture wounds. *Clin Orthop* 1989;243:36–40.

33. Burkhalter W: Open injuries of the lower extremity. *Surg Clin North Am* 1973;53:1439–1457.

34. Truetta J: *The Treatment of War Wounds and Fractures*. New York, Hoeber, 1940.

35. Witschi TH, Omer GE Jr: The treatment of open tibial shaft fractures from Vietnam War. *Trauma* 1970;10:105–111.

36. Robson MC, Duke WF, Krizek TJ: Rapid bacterial screening in the treatment of civilian wounds. *J Surg Res* 1973;14:426–430.

37. Robson MC, Heggers JP: Bacterial quantification of open wounds. *Milit Med* 1969;134:19–24.

38. Brown PW: The prevention of infection in open wounds. *Clin Orthop* 1973;96:42–50.

39. Yaremchuk MJ, Brumback RJ, Manson PN, et al: Acute and definitive management of traumatic osteocutaneous defects of the lower extremity. *Plast Reconstr Surg* 1987;80:1–12.

40. Gustilo RB: Principles of the management of open fractures, in *Management of Open Fractures and Their Complications*. Philadelphia, WB Saunders, 1982, vol 4, pp 15–54.

41. Ger R: The management of open fracture of the tibia with skin loss. *J Trauma* 1970;10:112–121.

42. Protzman RR: Open tibial shaft fractures: A study of 289 successive cases, in Moore TM (ed): American Academy of Orthopaedic Surgeons *Symposium on Trauma to the Leg and Its Sequelae*. St. Louis, CV Mosby, 1981, pp 131–140.

43. Christian EP, Bosse MJ, Robb G: Reconstruction of large diaphyseal defects without free fibular transfer in Grade IIIB tibial fractures. *J Bone Joint Surg* 1989;71A:994–1004.

44. Maurer RC, Dillin L: Multistaged surgical management of post-traumatic segmental tibial bone loss. *Clin Orthop* 1987;216:162–170.

45. Byrd HS, Cierny G III, Tebbetts JB: The management of open tibial fractures with associated soft-tissue loss: External pin fixation with early flap coverage. *Plast Reconstr Surg* 1981;68:73–82.

46. Buncke HJ, Furnas DW, Gordon L, et al: Free osteocutaneous flap from a rib to the tibia. *Plast Reconstr Surg* 1977;59:799–805.

47. Agiza AR : Treatment of tibial osteomyelitic defects and infected pseudarthroses by the Huntington fibular transference operation. *J Bone Joint Surg* 1981;63A:814–819.

48. Weinberg H, Roth VG, Robin GC, et al: Early fibular bypass procedures (tibiofibular synostosis) for massive bone loss in war injuries. *J Trauma* 1979;19:177–181.

49. Blachut PA, Meek RN, O'Brien PJ: External fixation and delayed intramedullary nailing of open fractures of the tibial shaft. *J Bone Joint Surg* 1990;72A:729–735.

50. Lange RH: Limb reconstruction versus amputation decision making in massive lower extremity trauma. *Clin Orthop* 1989;243:92–99.

51. Ilizarov GA: The tension-stress effect on the genesis and growth of tissues: Part I. The influence of stability of fixation and soft-tissue preservation. *Clin Orthop* 1989;238:249–281.

52. Ilizarov GA: The tension-stress effect on the genesis and growth of tissues: Part II. The influence of the rate and frequency of distraction. *Clin Orthop* 1989;239:263–285.

53. Aronson J, Johnson E, Harp JH: Local bone transportation for treatment of intercalary defects by the Ilizarov technique: Biomechanical and clinical considerations. *Clin Orthop* 1989;243:71–79.

54. Gross A, Cutright DE, Bhaskar SN: Effectiveness of pulsating water jet lavage in treatment of contaminated crushed wounds. *Am J Surg* 1972;124:373–377.

55. Madden J, Edlich RF, Schauerhamer R, et al: Application of principles of fluid dynamics to surgical wound irrigation. *Curr Top Surg Res* 1971;3:85–93.

56. Rodeheaver GT, Pettry D, Thacker JG, et al: Wound cleansing by high pressure irrigation. *Surg Gynecol Obstet* 1975;141:357–362.

57. Patzakis MJ, Harvey JP Jr, Ivler D: The role of antibiotics in the management of open fractures. *J Bone Joint Surg* 1974;56A:532–541.

58. Clancey GJ, Hansen ST Jr: Open fractures of the tibia: A review of one hundred and two cases. *J Bone Joint Surg* 1978;60A:118–122.

59. Patzakis MJ, Wilkins J, Moore TM: Considerations in reducing the infection rate in open tibial fractures. *Clin Orthop* 1983;178:36-41.

60. Patzakis MJ, Wilkins J, Moore TM: Use of antibiotics in open tibial fractures. *Clin Orthop* 1983;178:31–35.

61. Dellinger EP, Caplan ES, Weaver LD, et al: Duration of pre-

ventive antibiotic administration for open extremity fractures. *Arch Surg* 1988;123:333–339.

62. Levine NS, Lindberg RB, Mason AD Jr, et al: The quantitative swab culture and smear: A quick simple method for determining the number of viable aerobic bacteria on open wounds. *J Trauma* 1976;16:89–94.

63. Gustilo RB: Use of antimicrobials in the management of open fractures. *Arch Surg* 1979;114:805–808.

64. Lee J, Goldstein J, Madison M, et al: Value of pre and post-debridement cultures in the management of open fractures (abstract). Presented at the 58th Annual Meeting of the American Academy of Orthopaedic Surgeons, Anaheim, CA, March 7–12, 1991.

65. Patzakis MJ, Harvey JP, Moore TM: Comparing the incidence of infection in primary and delayed primary closure of open fracture wounds—a prospective study (abstract). *Orthop Trans* 1983;7:529.

66. Edlich RF, Rogers W, Kasper G, et al: Studies in the management of the contaminated wound: I. Optimal time for closure of contaminated open wounds. II. Comparison of resistance to infection of open and closed wounds during healing. *Am J Surg* 1969;117:323–329.

67. May JW Jr, Gallico GG III, Jupiter J, et al: Free latissimus dorsi muscle flap with skin graft for treatment of traumatic chronic bony wounds. *Plast Reconstr Surg* 1984;73:641–651.

68. Merchant TC, Dietz FR: Long-term follow-up after fractures of the tibial and fibular shafts. *J Bone Joint Surg* 1989;71A:599–606.

69. Benson DR, Riggins RS, Lawrence RM, et al: Treatment of open fractures: A prospective study. *J Trauma* 1983;23:25–30.

70. Brown PW, Urban JG: Early weight-bearing treatment of open fractures of the tibia: An end-result study of sixty-three cases. *J Bone Joint Surg* 1969;51A:59–75.

71. Gallinaro P, Crova M, Denicolai F: Complications in 64 open fractures of the tibia. *Injury* 1973;5:157–160.

72. Harvey JP Jr: Management of open tibial fractures. *Clin Orthop* 1974;105:154–166.

73. Nicoll EA: Closed and open management of tibial fractures. *Clin Orthop* 1974;105:144–153.

74. Rittmann WW, Schibli M, Matter P, et al: Open fractures. Long-term results in 200 consecutive cases. *Clin Orthop* 1979;138:132- 140.

75. Sladek EC, Kopta JA: Management of open fractures of the tibial shaft. *South Med J* 1977;70:662–665.

76. Velazco A, Whitesides TE Jr, Fleming LL: Open fractures of the tibia treated with the Lottes nail. *J Bone Joint Surg* 1983;65A:879–885.

77. Alexander JW, Hegg M, Alemeier WA: Neutrophil functions in selected surgical disorders. *Ann Surg* 1968;168:447–458.

78. Dehne E, Metz CW, Deffer PA, et al: Nonoperative treatment of the fractured tibia by immediate weight bearing. *Trauma* 1961;1:514- 535.

79. Sarmiento A: A functional below-the-knee cast for tibial fractures. *J Bone Joint Surg* 1967;49A:855–875.

80. Sarmiento A, Sobol PA, Sew Hoy AL, et al: Prefabricated functional braces for the treatment of fractures of the tibial diaphysis. *J Bone Joint Surg* 1984;66A:1328–1339.

81. Van Der Linden W, Larsson K: Plate fixation versus conservative treatment of tibial shaft fractures: A randomized trial. *J Bone Joint Surg* 1979;61A:873–878.

82. Watson-Jones R, Coltart WD: Slow union of fractures with a study of 804 fractures of the shafts of the tibia and femur. *Br J Surg* 1942;30:260–276.

83. Weissman SL, Herold HZ, Engelberg M: Fractures of the middle two- thirds of the tibial shaft. Results of treatment without internal fixation in one hundred and forty consecutive cases. *J Bone Joint Surg* 1966;48A:257–267.

84. Anderson LD, Hutchins WC, Wright PE, et al: Fractures of the tibia and fibula treated by casts and transfixing pins. *Clin Orthop* 1974;105:179–191.

85. Austin RT: The Sarmiento tibial plaster: A prospective study of 145 fractures. *Injury* 1981;13:10–22.

86. Bauer GCH, Edwards P, Widmark PH: Shaft fractures of the tibia. Etiology of poor results in a consecutive series of 173 fractures. *Acta Chir Scand* 1962;124:386–395.

87. Grosse A, Kempf I, Lafforgue D: Le traitement des fracas, pertes de substance ossuese et pseudarthroses du fémur et du tibia par l'enclouage verrouille (a propos de 40 cas). *Rev Chir Orthop* 1978;64(suppl):33–35.

88. Nicoll EA: Fractures of the tibial shaft. A survey of 705 cases. *J Bone Joint Surg* 1964;46B:373–387.

89. Puno RM, Teynor JT, Nagano J, et al: Critical analysis of results of treatment of 201 tibial shaft fractures. *Clin Orthop* 1986;212:113–121.

90. Welch MC, Miller EH: Complications of treatment of fractures and dislocations of the tibia and fibula, in Ettes C (ed): *Complications in Orthopedic Surgery*. Philadelphia, JB Lippincott, 1986, pp 585–597.

91. Bone LB, Johnson KD, Weigelt J, et al: Early versus delayed stabilization of femoral fractures. A prospective randomized study. *J Bone Joint Surg* 1989;71A:336–340.

92. Allgöwer M, Border JR: Management of open fractures in the multiple trauma patient. *World J Surg* 1983;7:88–95.

93. Chapman MW: The use of immediate internal fixation in open fractures. *Orthop Clin North Am* 1980;11:579–591.

94. Lewallen DG, Chao EYS, Kasman RA, et al: Comparison of the effects of compression plates and external fixators on early bone-healing. *J Bone Joint Surg* 1984;66A:1084–1091.

95. Schatzker J: Compression in the surgical treatment of fractures of the tibia. *Clin Orthop* 1974;105:220–239.

96. Rand JA, An KN, Chao EYS, et al: A comparison of the effect of open intramedullary nailing and compression-plate fixation on fracture-site blood flow and fracture union. *J Bone Joint Surg* 1981;63A:427–442.

97. Rüedi TP, Webb JK, Allgower M: Experience with the dynamic compression plate (DCP) in 418 recent fractures of the tibial shaft. *Injury* 1976;7:252–257.

98. Christensen J, Greiff J, Rosendahl S: Fractures of the shaft of the tibia treated with AO-compression osteosynthesis. *Injury* 1982;13:307–314.

99. Olerud S, Karlström G: Tibial fractures treated by AO compression osteosynthesis: Experiences from a five year material. *Acta Orthop Scand* 1972;140:1–104.

100. Anderson JT, Gustilo RB: Immediate internal fixation in open fractures. *Orthop Clin North Am* 1980;11:569–578.

101. Puranen J, Punto L: Osteomedulloangiography: A method of estimating the consolidation prognosis of tibial shaft fractures. *Clin Orthop* 1981;161:8–14.

102. Ali Kahn MA, Lucas HK: Plating of fractures of the middle third of the clavicle. *Injury* 1978;9:263–267.

103. Almond G, Vernon E: Iliac skeletal cross traction. A method of treatment of "oyster-shell" pelvis. *J Bone Joint Surg* 1959;41B:779–781.

104. Chapman MW, Mahoney M: The role of early internal fixation in the management of open fractures. *Clin Orthop* 1979;138:120–131.

105. Beauchamp CG, Clifford RP, Webb JK, et al: Functional results after immediate internal fixation of open tibial shaft fractures (abstract). *J Bone Joint Surg* 1985;67B:325.

106. Macnab I, de Haas WG: The role of periosteal blood supply in the healing of fractures of the tibia. *Clin Orthop* 1974;105:27–33.

107. Trueta J: Blood supply and the rate of healing of tibial fractures. *Clin Orthop* 1974;105:11–26.

108. Böstman O, Varjonen L, Vainionpää S, et al: Incidence of local complications after intramedullary nailing and after plate fixation of femoral shaft fractures. *J Trauma* 1989;29:639–645.

109. Marshall DV: Three-side plate fixation for fractures of the femoral and tibial shafts. *J Bone Joint Surg* 1958;40A:323–345.

110. Helpenstell TS, Hansen ST Jr: Review of 51 open distal femoral fractures treated with immediate open reduction and internal fixation (abstract). Presented at the 58th Annual Meeting of the American Academy of Orthopaedic Surgeons, Anaheim, CA, March 7–12, 1991.

111. Rüedi TP, Allgöwer M: The operative treatment of intra-articular fractures of the lower end of the tibia. *Clin Orthop* 1979;138:105- 110.

112. Kaltenecker G, Whurs O, Quaicoe S: Lower infection rate after interlocking nailing in open fractures of femur and tibia. *J Trauma* 1990;30:474–479.

113. Bone LB, Johnson KD: Treatment of tibial fractures by reaming and intramedullary nailing. *J Bone Joint Surg* 1986;68A:877–887.

114. Werry DG, Boyle MR, Meek RN, et al: Intramedullary fixation of tibial shaft fractures with AO and Grosse-Kempf locking nails: A review of 70 consecutive fractures (abstract). *J Bone Joint Surg* 1985;67B:325.

115. Alms M: Medullary nailing for fracture of the shaft of the tibia. *J Bone Joint Surg* 1962;44B:328–339.

116. Böstman O, Vainionpää S, Saikku K: Infra-isthmal longitudinal fractures of the tibial diaphysis: Results of treatment using closed intramedullary compression nailing. *J Trauma* 1984;24:964–969.

117. Ekeland A, Thoresen BO, Alho A, et al: Interlocking intramedullary nailing in the treatment of tibial fractures. A report of 45 cases. *Clin Orthop* 1988;231:205–215.

118. Hamza KN, Dunkerley GE, Murray CM: Fractures of the tibia. A report on fifty patients treated by intramedullary nailing. *J Bone Joint Surg* 1971;53B:696–700.

119. Klemm KW, Börner M: Interlocking nailing of complex fractures of the femur and tibia. *Clin Orthop* 1986;212:89–100.

120. Koval KJ, Clapper MF, Brumback RJ, et al: Complications of reamed intramedullary nailing of the tibia. *J Orthop Trauma* 1991;5:184–189.

121. McQueen MM, Christie J, Court-Brown CM: Compartment pressures after intramedullary nailing of the tibia. *J Bone Joint Surg* 1990;72B:395–397.

122. Tischenko GJ, Goodman SB: Compartment syndrome after intramedullary nailing of the tibia. *J Bone Joint Surg* 1990;72A:41–44.

123. Moed BR, Strom DE: Compartment syndrome after closed intramedullary nailing of the tibia: A canine model and report of two cases. *J Orthop Trauma* 1991;5:71–77.

124. Shakespeare DT, Henderson NJ: Compartmental pressure changes during calcaneal traction in tibial fractures. *J Bone Joint Surg* 1982;64B:498–499.

125. Chapman MW: The role of intramedullary fixation in open fractures. *Clin Orthop* 1986;212:26–34.

126. MacKenzie DA, Martimbeau C, Mudge K, et al: A prospective study of closed reamed locking intramedullary rods in the early management of open tibial fractures. Presented at the 6th Annual Meeting of the Orthopaedic Trauma Association, Toronto, Ontario, Canada, Nov 7–10, 1990.

127. Weis EB Jr, Roberts JB, Curtiss PH Jr: Salvage of complicated open fractures by transfixation. *J Trauma* 1976;16:266–272.

128. Burny F: Elastic external fixation of tibial fractures: Study of 1421 cases, in Brooker AF Jr, Edwards CC (eds): *External Fixation: The Current State of the Art. Proceedings of the 6th International Conference on Hoffmann External Fixation.* Baltimore, Williams & Wilkins, 1979, pp 55–73.

129. Edge AJ, Denham RA: External fixation for complicated tibial fractures. *J Bone Joint Surg* 1981;63B:92–97.

130. Edwards CC, Jaworski MF, Solana J, et al: Management of compound tibial fractures using external fixation. *Am Surg* 1979;45:190–203.

131. Edwards CC, Simmons SC, Browner BD, et al: 203 open tibial fractures treated with Hoffmann external fixation: Analysis of results (abstract). *Orthop Trans* 1984;8:383–384.

132. Emerson RH Jr, Grabias SL: A retrospective analysis of severe diaphyseal tibial fractures treated with external fixation. *Orthopedics* 1983;6:43–49.

133. Mears DC, Stone JP, Jarrett JN Jr: External fixation of tibial fractures, in Moore TM (ed): American Academy of Orthopaedic Surgeons *Symposium on Trauma to the Leg and Its Sequelae.* St. Louis, CV Mosby, 1981, pp 141–156.

134. Schrøder HA, Christoffersen H, Sørensen TS, et al: Fractures of the shaft of the tibia treated with Hoffmann external fixation. *Arch Orthop Trauma Surg* 1986;105:28–30.

135. Goodship AE, Kenwright J: The influence of induced micromovement upon the healing of experimental tibial fractures. *J Bone Joint Surg* 1985;67B:650–655.

136. Kenwright J, Goodship AE: Controlled mechanical stimulation in the treatment of tibial fractures. *Clin Orthop* 1989;241:36–47.

137. Kenwright J, Richardson JB, Goodship AE, et al: Effect of controlled axial micromovement on healing of tibial fractures. *Lancet* 1986;2:1185–1187.

138. Kimmell RB: Results of treatment using the Hoffmann external fixator for fractures of the tibial diaphysis. *J Trauma* 1982;22:960–965.

139. Meadows TH, Bronk JT, Chao EYS, et al: Effect of weight-bearing on healing of cortical defects in the canine tibia. *J Bone Joint Surg* 1990;72A:1074–1080.

140. Tencer AF, Claudi B, Pearce S, et al: Development of a variable stiffness external fixation system for stabilization of segmental defects of the tibia. *J Orthop Res* 1984;1:395–404.

141. Terjesen T: Healing of rabbit tibial fractures using external fixation. Effects of removal of the fixation device. *Acta Orthop Scand* 1984;55:192–196.

142. Terjesen T, Benum P: In vitro effects of external fixation on intact and osteotomized tibiae. A biomechanical study. *Acta Orthop Scand* 1983;54:212–219.

143. Terjesen T, Benum P: Stress-protection after external fixation on the intact rabbit tibia. *Acta Orthop Scand* 1983;54:648–654.

144. Sarmiento A, Schaeffer JF, Beckerman L, et al: Fracture healing in rat femora as affected by functional weight-bearing. *J Bone Joint Surg* 1977;59A:369–375.

145. Aho AJ, Nieminen SJ, Nylamo EI: External fixation by Hoffmann- Vidal-Adrey osteotaxis for severe tibial fractures. Treatment scheme and technical criticism. *Clin Orthop* 1983;181:154–164.

146. Behrens F, Comfort TH, Searls K, et al: Unilateral external fixation for severe open tibial fractures. Preliminary report of a prospective study *Clin Orthop* 1983;178:111–120.

147. Benum P, Svenningsen S: Tibial fractures treated with Hoffmann's external fixation. A comparative analysis of Hoffmann bilateral frames and the Vidal-Adrey double frame modification. *Acta Orthop Scand* 1982;53:471–476.

148. Young JWR, Burgess AR, Brumback RJ, et al: Pelvic fractures: Value of plain radiography in early assessment and management. *Radiology* 1986;160:445–451.

149. Spiegel PG, VanderSchilden JL: Minimal internal and external fixation in the treatment of open tibial fractures. *Clin Orthop* 1983;178:96–102.

150. Krettek C, Haas N, Tscherne H: Ninety-nine open tibial shaft fractures treated with external fixation: Advantages with supplemental lag screws. Presented at the 58th Annual Meeting of the American Academy of Orthopaedic Surgeons, Anaheim, CA, March 7–12, 1991.

151. Lottes JO: Intramedullary fixation for fractures of the shaft of the tibia. *South Med J* 1952;45:407–414.

152. Lottes JO: Medullary nailing of the tibia with the triflange nail. *Clin Orthop* 1974;105:253–266.

153. Sedlin ED, Zitner DT: The Lottes nail in the closed treatment of tibia fractures. *Clin Orthop* 1985;192:185–192.

154. Holbrook JL, Swiontkowski MF, Sanders R: Treatment of open fractures of the tibial shaft: Ender nailing versus external fixation: A randomized, prospective comparison. *J Bone Joint Surg* 1989;71A:1231–1238.

155. Wiss DA: Flexible medullary nailing of acute tibial shaft fractures. *Clin Orthop* 1986;212:122–132.

156. Dobozi WR, Saltzman M, Brash R: Ender nailing of problem tibial shaft fractures. *Orthopedics* 1982;5:1162–1171.

157. Mayer L, Werbie T, Schwab JP, et al: The use of Ender nails in fractures of the tibial shaft. *J Bone Joint Surg* 1985;67A:446–455.

158. Pankovich AM, Tarabishy IE, Yelda S: Flexible intramedullary nailing of tibial-shaft fractures. *Clin Orthop* 1981;160:185–195.

159. Henley M, Mayo K: Prospective comparison of unreamed interlocking IM nails and half-pin external fixation for grade II and III open tibia fractures. Presented at the Fifth Annual Meeting of the Orthopaedic Trauma Association, Philadelphia, PA, Oct 19–21, 1989.

160. DiPasquale T, Helfet D, Sanders R, et al: The treatment of open and/or unstable tibial fractures with an unreamed double-locked tibial nail. Presented at the Fifth Annual Meeting of the Orthopaedic Trauma Association, Philadelphia, PA, Oct 19–21, 1989.

161. Santoro V, Henley M, Benirschke S, et al: Prospective comparison of unreamed interlocking IM nails versus half-pin external fixation in open tibial fractures. Presented at the Sixth Annual Meeting of the Orthopaedic Trauma Association, Toronto, Ontario, Canada, Nov 7–10, 1990.

162. McGraw JM, Lim EV: Treatment of open tibial-shaft fractures: External fixation and secondary intramedullary nailing. *J Bone Joint Surg* 1988;70A:900–911.

163. Whittle AP, LaVelle DG, Taylor JC, et al: Treatment of open tibial shaft fractures with unreamed interlocking intramedullary nails (abstract). Presented at the 58th Annual Meeting of the American Academy of Orthopaedic Surgeons, Anaheim, CA, March 7–12, 1991.

164. Gustilo RB, Mendoza RM, Williams DN: Problems in the management of type III (severe) open fractures: A new classification of type III open fractures. *J Trauma* 1984;24:742–746.

165. Chapman MW: Part III: Role of bone stability in open fractures, in Frankel VH (ed): American Academy of Orthopaedic Surgeons *Instructional Course Lectures, XXXI*. St. Louis, CV Mosby, 1982, pp 75–87.

166. Trueta J, Barnes JM: The rationale of complete immobilization in treatment of infected wounds. *Br Med J* 1940;2:46–48.

167. Ketenjian AY, Shelton ML: Primary internal fixation of open fractures: A retrospective study of the use of metallic internal fixation in fresh open fractures. *J Trauma* 1972;12:756–763.

168. LaDuca JN, Bone LL, Seibel RW, et al: Primary open reduction and internal fixation of open fractures. *J Trauma* 1980;20:580–586.

169. McNeur JC: The management of open skeletal trauma with particular reference to internal fixation. *J Bone Joint Surg* 1970;52B:54–60.

170. Lawyer RB Jr, Lubbers LM: Use of the Hoffmann apparatus in the treatment of unstable tibial fractures. *J Bone Joint Surg* 1980;62A:1264–1273.

171. Edwards CC: Staged reconstruction of complex open tibial fractures using Hoffmann external fixation: Clinical decisions and dilemmas. *Clin Orthop* 1983;178:130–161.

172. Mauer DJ, Merkow RL, Gustilo RB: Infection after intramedullary nailing of severe open tibial fractures initially treated with external fixation. *J Bone Joint Surg* 1989;71A:835–838.

173. Fischer MD, Gustilo RB: Timing of flap coverage: Bone grafting and intramedullary nailing of tibial shaft fractures with extensive soft-tissue injury. Presented at the 58th Annual Meeting of the American Academy of Orthopaedic Surgeons, Anaheim, CA, March 7–12, 1991.

174. Benirschke SK, Santoro VM, Henley MB, et al: Secondary intramedullary nailing for delayed unions and nonunion after failed external fixation for open tibial shaft fractures. Presented at the 58th Annual Meeting of the American Academy of Orthopaedic Surgeons, Anaheim, CA, March 7–12, 1991.

175. Yaremchuk MJ, Burgess AR, Brumback RJ (eds): *Lower Extremity Salvage and Reconstruction: Orthopedic and Plastic Surgical Management*. New York, Elsevier Science Publishing, 1989.

176. Brotman S, Browner BD, Cowley RA: Proper timing of amputation for open fractures of the lower extremities. *Am Surg* 1982;48:484–486.

177. Karlström G, Olerud S: External fixation of severe open tibial fractures with the Hoffmann frame. *Clin Orthop* 1983;180:68–77.

178. Etter C, Burri C, Claes L, et al: Treatment by external fixation of open fractures associated with severe soft tissue damage of the leg. Biomechanical principles and clinical experience. *Clin Orthop* 1983;178:80–88.

179. Burgess AR: Fraction fixation, in Yaremchuk MH, Burgess AR, Brumback RJ (eds): *Lower Extremity Salvage and Reconstruction: Orthopedic and Plastic Surgical Management*. New York, Elsevier Science Publishing, 1989, pp 81–94.

180. Christensen NO: Technique, errors and safeguards in modern Küntscher nailing. *Clin Orthop* 1976;115:182–188.

181. Weiland AJ, Moore JR, Hotchkiss RN: Soft tissue procedures for reconstruction of tibial shaft fractures. *Clin Orthop* 1983;178:42–53.

182. Yaremchuk MJ: Acute management of severe soft-tissue damage accompanying open fractures of the lower extremity. *Clin Plast Surg* 1986;13:621–629.

183. Byrd HS, Spicer TE, Cierny G III: Management of open tibial fractures. *Plast Reconstr Surg* 1985;76:719–730.

184. Cierny G III, Byrd HS, Jones RE: Primary versus delayed soft tissue coverage for severe open tibial fractures. A comparison of results. *Clin Orthop* 1983;178:54–63.

185. Jones RE, Cierny GC III: Management of complex open tibial fractures with external skeletal fixation and early myoplasty or myocutaneous coverage. *Can J Surg* 1980;23:242–244.

186. Gorman PW, Barnes CL, Fischer TJ, et al: Soft-tissue reconstruction in severe lower extremity trauma: A review. *Clin Orthop* 1989;243:57–64.

187. Godina M: Early microsurgical reconstruction of complex trauma of the extremities. *Plast Reconstr Surg* 1986;78:285–292.

188. Ger R: Muscle transposition for treatment and prevention of chronic post-traumatic osteomyelitis of the tibia. *J Bone Joint Surg* 1977;59A:784–791.

189. Behrens F: Part E: Bone grafting: general principles and use in open fractures, in Murray DG (ed): American Academy of Orthopaedic Surgeons *Instructional Course Lectures, XXX*. St. Louis, CV Mosby, 1981, pp 152–156.

190. Harmon PH: A simplified surgical approach to the posterior tibia for bone-grafting and fibular transference. *J Bone Joint Surg* 1945;27A:496–498.

191. Fogdestam I, Hamilton R, Markhede G: Microvascular osteocutaneous groin flap in the treatment of an ununited tibial fracture with chronic osteitis. A case report. *Acta Orthop Scand* 1980;51:175–179.

192. Freeland AE, Mutz SB: Posterior bone-grafting for infected ununited fracture of the tibia. *J Bone Joint Surg* 1976;58A:653–657.

193. Hanson LW, Eppright RH: Posterior bone-grafting of the tibia for non-union. A review of twenty-four cases. *J Bone Joint Surg* 1966;48A:27–43.

194. Jones KG, Barnett HC: Cancellous-bone grafting for non-union of the tibia through the posterolateral approach. *J Bone Joint Surg* 1955;37A:1250–1260.

195. Lamb RH: Posterolateral bone graft for nonunion of the tibia. *Clin Orthop* 1969;64:114–120.

196. Urist MR, Mazet R Jr, McLean FC: The pathogenesis and treatment of delayed union and non-union. A survey of eighty-five ununited fractures of the shaft of the tibia and one hundred control cases with similar injuries. *J Bone Joint Surg* 1954;36A:931–968.

197. Tucker HL, Kendra JC, Kinnebrew TE: Tibial defects: Reconstruction using the method of Ilizarov as an alternative. *Orthop Clin North Am* 1990;21:629–637.

198. Alonso JE, Regazzonia P: The use of the Ilizarov concept with the AO/ASIF tubular fixateur in the treatment of segmental defects. *Orthop Clin North Am* 1990;21:655–665.

199. Paley D, Chaudray M, Pirone AM, et al: Treatment of malunions and mal-nonunions of the femur and tibia by detailed preoperative planning and the Ilizarov techniques. *Orthop Clin North Am* 1990;21:667–691.

200. Schwartsman V, Choi SH, Schwartsman R: Tibial nonunions: Treatment tactics with the Ilizarov method. *Orthop Clin North Am* 1990;21:639–653.

201. Mubarak SJ, Owen CA: Double-incision fasciotomy of the leg for decompression in compartment syndromes. *J Bone Joint Surg* 1977;59A:184–187.

202. Lange RH, Bach AW, Hansen ST Jr, et al: Open tibial fractures with associated vascular injuries: Prognosis for limb salvage. *J Trauma* 1985;25:203–208.

203. Ruoff AC III, Snider RK: Explosion fractures of the distal tibia with major articular involvement. *J Trauma* 1971;11:866–873.

204. Cone JB: Vascular injury associated with fracture-dislocations of the lower extremity. *Clin Orthop* 1989;243:30–35.

Local Response to Biomaterials: Bone Loss in Cementless Femoral Stems

Joshua J. Jacobs, MD

Jorge O. Galante, MD, DSc

Dale R. Sumner, PhD

Introduction

In the last few years we have gained increasing experience with the behavior of biomaterials as functioning elements of prosthetic devices. The concepts of biocompatibility established for bulk materials in isolated experimental models apply only partially to their behavior under functional conditions. Unexpected undesirable local tissue responses can cause an otherwise well functioning implant to fail.

The development and application of cementless technology has brought some of these problems to light. Issues of concern with cementless devices relate to fixation, bone loss, and long-term biocompatibility.

Bone loss with cementless total hip prostheses is a problem that can have severe deleterious effects. It can lead to loosening, failure of the host bone, and failure of the device and can present very serious problems for subsequent surgical reconstruction. Both mechanical and biologic effects can contribute to bone loss. In cementless total hip replacements, bone loss is generally attributable to one of two phenomena: adaptive bone remodeling and osteolysis.

Adaptive Bone Remodeling

Proximal cortical atrophy of varying severity has been reported with a number of cementless femoral stems.[1-4] Resorptive remodeling changes tend to appear sooner and to be more severe in cementless femoral stems than in cemented prostheses.

The basic hypothesis is that the implantation of the prosthesis alters the local mechanical environment and, thus, the bony architecture. In stress shielding, the stress that would normally be experienced by the host bone is diminished in magnitude, which leads to atrophy of the affected parts of the skeleton. In total hip arthroplasty, the phenomenon takes the form of proximal femoral cortical atrophy caused by the transfer of stresses to the distal femur through the implant rather than through the proximal cortical bone.

Experimental Models

Our laboratory has used a canine experimental model to study bone remodeling phenomena, particularly the specific influence exerted by design features of the femoral stem.[5-14] A unilateral total hip replacement was performed, and the contralateral hip served

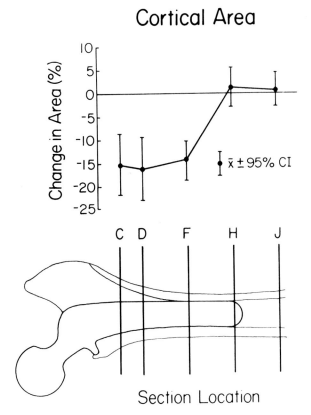

Fig. 1 Cortical area change two years after implantation of Ti6Al4V stems in the canine model. The stems were porous coated along their length. Proximally, cortical atrophy was observed and distally, cortical hypertrophy was apparent. (Reproduced with permission from Sumner DR, Turner TM, Urban RM, et al: Experimental studies of bone remodeling in total hip replacement. *Clin Orthop*, in press.)

as a control. The femoral stem was designed with a constant geometry. Variables investigated included the type of coating, the extent of coating, and the material from which the stem was made.

A consistent pattern of bone remodeling was observed with the use of titanium alloy (Ti6Al4V) stems. This pattern was characterized by the development of proximal cortical atrophy and distal cortical hypertrophy (Fig. 1). At two years there was a 15% reduction in cortical bone area adjacent to the porous-coated regions of the stem. Proximally, most bone loss was caused by subperiosteal resorption. At the distal and mid-stem levels bone was lost from the cortex through cancelization of the endosteal surface, effectively expanding the medullary cavity. Although there were increases in cortical porosity, this change in microstructure accounted for only a minor fraction of the bone loss. At the stem tip, the area of the cortex increased mainly because of the addition of bone at the subperiosteal surface. Within the medullary canal, the density of the cancellous bone increased proximally and, particularly, distally.

In these experimental studies, the remodeling pattern described was shown to be independent of the type of porous coating in titanium implants (plasma spray, bead, and fiber metal) and whether or not the coating was applied circumferentially or restricted to the anterior and posterior surfaces in stems coated along their entire length. Restricting the porous coating to the proximal part of the stem was only effective in decreasing the rate at which cortical atrophy developed. Less cortical bone loss was observed at six months with proximally coated stems, but at two years there were no differences between partially and fully coated stems.

A similar pattern was seen when comparing uncoated and extensively coated stems. Whether the cementless femoral implant was porous coated or uncoated had no effect on cortical bone loss at a two-year follow-up, although at six months the canines with no porous coating had less proximal cortical loss compared with canines with the coated stems. Therefore, the presence of bone ingrowth fixation may accelerate cortical bone adaptation initially, but in the longer term it does not appear to increase the magnitude of bone loss.

Stem Stiffness

This experimental model, however, showed that stem stiffness may be a design variable that can be used to manipulate bone remodeling behavior. Bone remodeling was compared at six months in titanium alloy stems and composite stems with identical geometries. The composite stem bending stiffness was less than 20% of that of the titanium stem. The composite stem demonstrated more total bone ingrowth and more ingrowth into the proximal and mid aspects of the stem than did the titanium alloy stem. The cancellous bone density increased both proximally and distally for both stem types, although proximal hypertrophy of the cancellous bone was more marked in dogs with composite stems. There was 50% less proximal cortical loss in dogs with composite stems than there was in dogs with titanium alloy stems. The mechanism of proximal cortical resorption also differed, in that no subperiosteal bone resorption was observed. In addition, no evidence of distal cortical hypertrophy was seen in dogs with the composite stems. Because no long-term (two-year) data are yet available regarding composite stems, the long-term efficacy of using more flexible implants to reduce bone loss caused by stress shielding remains hypothetical. Nevertheless, all of these observations seem to reflect drastically different patterns of stress transfer with the use of metallic and composite stems.

In general, our studies have indicated that bone loss and reorganization of the geometry of the femur are responses associated with implantation of cementless porous-coated stems in the experimental animal. The pattern developed is one of proximal cortical bone loss and distal cortical hypertrophy. The most important parameter affecting the phenomenon was the stiffness of the femoral stem, an observation supported by other investigators.[15]

Altering Stem Stiffness

As just described, the stiffness of the stem relative to the stiffness of the femur is an important variable that affects the distribution and extent of bone loss. This relationship depends on the cross-sectional geometry of the stem, the material properties of the stem and the femur, and the location of the stem within the femur. If everything else is constant, an increase in stem stiffness will reduce stress and strain in the proximal femur. As the amount and location of bone tissue alters over time in an attempt to return strain levels to normal, net bone resorption can be expected. With very stiff prostheses, theoretical analysis predicts that the bone might eventually resorb completely.[16]

Clinically, the stem must fill the endosteal area available in the upper femur in order to obtain adequate initial stability and intimate endosteal apposition, both of which are essential requirements for bone ingrowth and successful cementless fixation. Because of their large cross-sections, these large stems are inherently stiff. Several strategies can be used to overcome the problems of stiffness. For example, the implant can be made less rigid by altering its cross-section. Splitting the distal end of the implant, using a hollow implant, or incorporating deep peripheral grooves are three ways of reducing implant stiffness. The use of a hollow implant, demonstrated by Bobyn and associates,[15] appears to be successful, at least in the experimental animal. Several prosthetic devices in clinical use incorporate one of the other two methods, but not enough clinical experience is available with these implants to ascertain their level of success. Unfortunately, all of these strategies can affect the mechanical integrity of a porous coated stem, increasing the risk of fatigue failure of the implant.

Another method of reducing stem stiffness is to use a device manufactured from a low modulus material, such as a composite. In the previous section, we have shown that this approach is successful in reducing bone loss in an experimental model. The clinical experience available with such implants has provided some controversial results.[17,18] One problem with low modulus devices is the possibility of increased relative motion between the more flexible implant and bone, which has the potential for formation of particulate debris and secondary tissue reactions. Thus, to successfully use a low modulus material, it is necessary to achieve biological fixation along the length of the prosthesis.

Clinical Observations

The patterns of bone loss and cortical remodeling described above are also seen in human patients. We recently reviewed our initial experience with the titanium fiber-metal cementless total hip prosthesis.[19] The minimum period of follow-up in this review was 48 months. A total of 126 implants were judged radiologically stable by a series of strict criteria. These stable implants demonstrate a characteristic pattern of remodeling that included proximal cortical resorption and distal cortical hypertrophy. Of the femurs, 91% exhibited a definite loss of proximal cortical density. In addition, longitudinal resorption of the medial femoral cortex, seen in seven patients, ranged from 3 to 11 mm. Distal cortical hypertrophy was noted in more than 30% of the patients and was commonly seen in zones 4, 5, 6, and 7 as described by Gruen and associates.[20] Progression of distal cortical hypertrophy was still seen in 20% of the patients four years after the procedure.

No instances of severe stress shielding were observed. Possible reasons for this include: (1) the use of titanium alloy stems, which have a lower modulus of elasticity than do cobalt chromium alloy stems (see below); (2) the use of proximally coated prostheses with limited areas of porous coating, a variable that can influence the kinetics of cortical resorption; (3) the use of strict patient selection criteria that excluded patients with severe osteopenia or patients who were older than 70 years of age; and (4) the use of an observation time that may have been too short to allow the development of severe cortical atrophy.

Bone remodeling changes, including severe stress shielding, have been reported with porous-coated cobalt chromium alloy stems.[21] Stem diameter, extent of porous coating, the presence of bone ingrowth, age, sex, and the presence of pre-existing osteopenia were factors that influenced the severity of the bone remodeling process. Brown and Ring[1] reported severe bone resorption in the upper portion of the shaft in four patients with cementless porous-coated femoral stems. This resorption was associated with gradual loss of function that necessitated revision in one patient. However, there were factors in this series other than bone remodeling that might have influenced the severity of the resorptive process. In all but one case, a polyethylene femoral head was used, which could contribute large amounts of wear debris to the bone-prosthesis interface.

Thus, bone loss secondary to bone remodeling can lead to failure of the arthroplasty. Although at this time the incidence of clinical problems caused by stress shielding is very low, it is not clear that the process of bone remodeling is self-limited. Consequently, the eventual clinical impact of this phenomenon has yet to be fully determined.

Clinically, stem stiffness is even more significant when the use of cementless devices is considered in bone-deficient femurs, such as are encountered in most revision procedures, often carried out in osteoporotic females or elderly patients. Certainly, the elderly patient with an osteoporotic femur represents a potential problem with this type of fixation. A better understanding of the relationship between stem stiffness and bone remodeling is needed. It is hoped that further research will lead to future improvements in cementless stem designs and applications.

Osteolysis

In contrast to the phenomenon of stress shielding, which has not produced a large scale clinical problem to date, the phenomenon of focal osteolysis has become a clinical problem at relatively short-term follow-up, particularly with cementless fixation.

Clinical Features

Focal osteolysis, also referred to as endosteal erosion, has been well described in the setting of cemented total hip replacement in loose implants. Harris and associates[22] reported on four cases of extensive localized femoral resorption at 33 to 60 months after surgery in patients whose prostheses were described as slightly loose. Carlsson and associates[23] reported 33 cases of localized osteolysis in 70 total hip replacements revised for mechanical loosening. In these studies, infection was ruled out. Histologically, the tissue within the erosive lesions demonstrated sheets of macrophages with few giant cells and multiple small fragments of birefringent material. Radiographically, some studies have found a correlation between a deficiency of the cement mantle and the presence of these lesions.[23,24]

Focal osteolysis in cemented implants has also been reported in the absence of loosening.[25-27] In one study, these lesions developed from 40 to 168 months after surgery, with 70% of the lesions appearing after five years. Of these lesions, 60% were associated with a deficiency in the cement mantle.[26] Furthermore, a communication between the joint cavity and the focal lesion has been demonstrated, which would provide a route whereby debris from the joint could be transported distally.[27] In each case, variable amounts of metal, cement, and polyethylene debris were observed in a tissue infiltrate characterized by macrophages, giant cells, and vascular granulation tissue. One consistent element in these reports was that particles of fragmented bone cement were seen in histiocytes and foreign body granulomata within the femoral osteolytic lesions. Because of this, the term cement disease is used for the clinical description of this phenomenon.[28] One of the driving forces behind the development of cementless technology was concern about this so-called cement disease, endosteal bone loss ascribed to the

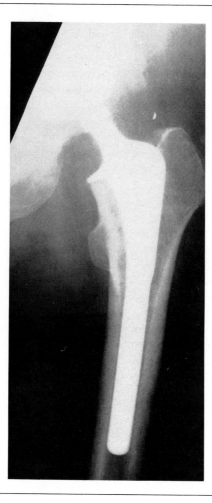 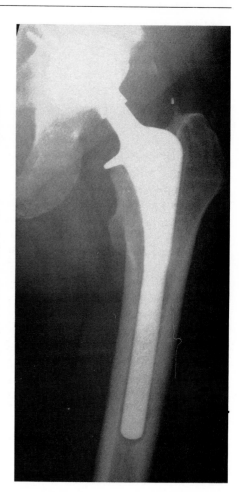

Fig. 2 **Left**, Anteroposterior femoral radiograph at six weeks postoperative following cementless total hip arthroplasty. **Right**, Anteroposterior femoral radiograph at 24 months postoperative. Note the focal endosteal scalloping (endosteal erosion) in the lateral cortex at the tip of the prosthesis (Gruen zones 3 and 4). There is no evidence of femoral component subsidence. (Reproduced with permission from Jacobs JJ, Urban RM, Schajowicz F, et al: Particulate-associated endosteal osteolysis in titanium-base alloy cementless total hip replacement. American Society for the Testing of Materials *Symposium on Biocompatibility of Particulate Implant Materials*, in press.)

presence of fragmented acrylic cement. However, this type of bone loss has been recently recognized in cementless implants as well.

Endosteal bone loss can occur in both stable and unstable cementless implants. In our initial series of 130 titanium fiber-metal cementless total hip prosthesis hips with a minimum 48-month follow-up,[19] there were 12 radiographically unstable implants. In three of these unstable implants, focal endosteal bone loss was seen, for an incidence of osteolysis of 25% in loose implants. Thus, in the unstable implant, the absence of polymethylmethacrylate cement does not preclude bone loss. Implant motion and tissue reaction to abraded particulate metallic and polyethylene debris is the most likely mechanism of bone loss in this setting.

Of more serious concern has been the recognition of endosteal erosions occurring in juxtaposition to stable cementless implants. Maloney and associates[29] reported a 3% incidence of focal femoral osteolysis in patients with well fixed cementless components fabricated from either cobalt-based or titanium-based alloys. All but two of the 16 patients described were active, heavy young men. Of these patients, 14 had excellent clinical results, with Harris hip scores of 90 or greater.

Osteolysis appeared after two years in 15 of the 16 cases. We recently reported on the clinical, radiographic, and histologic features of femoral endosteal osteolysis in cementless titanium alloy total hip prostheses.[30] At a minimum two-year follow-up, the incidence of osteolysis was 4% in patients with stable implants. However, at a minimum of four years after implantation, the incidence increased to 8.2% in stable implants.[19] These lesions appeared at an average of 33 months after implantation (range 12 to 60 months) and generally occurred in the vicinity of the tip of the femoral stem at Gruen zones 3 to 5 (Fig. 2).

While the natural history of focal osteolysis has not been well defined in stable cementless implants, these lesions have been observed earlier than in cemented total hip replacement. In our series, they have resulted in early revision surgery to avoid the risk of progression and subsequent pathological fracture. The apparent increase in incidence with time is particularly disturbing.

Histologic Features

To date, we have performed revision surgery on four cases of focal osteolysis in well-fixed implants. Histologic examination of tissues obtained from these pa-

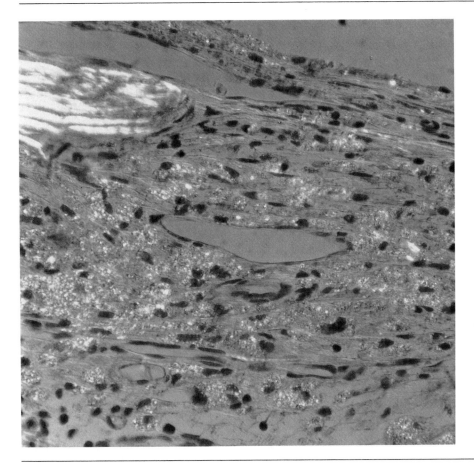

Fig. 3 Representative histologic section obtained from the tissue within the osteolytic lesion seen in Figure 2 at 400X under polarized light. Note the histiocytic infiltrate with abundant intracellular birefringement particles. (Reproduced with permission from Jacobs JJ, Urban RM, Schajowicz F, et al: Particulate-associated endosteal osteolysis in titanium-base alloy cementless total hip replacement. American Society for the Testing of Materials *Symposium on Biocompatibility of Particulate Implant Materials*, in press.)

tients at revision revealed histiocytic proliferation in the capsule, in the membrane surrounding the femoral stem, and at the site of the lytic lesion in the femoral shaft. Under polarized light, abundant strongly birefringent particles were visualized within the cytoplasm of the histiocytes (Fig. 3). That this histiocytic infiltrate has been observed invading adjacent haversian systems documents its aggressive nature. Osteoclasts have been observed but were relatively few in number.

Electron microprobe analysis, analytic electron microscopy, and Fourier transform infrared spectroscopy verified the presence of both polyethylene and titanium alloy particles. In addition, stainless steel particles (presumably contaminants from the surgical tools) and silicate particles have also been observed. Not all of the particles have been positively identified. Specifically, the nature of very fine intracellular particles that appear birefringent on the crossed polars is not clear as yet. Larger birefringent particles have been positively identified as polyethylene by Fourier transform infrared spectroscopy. However, the sensitivity of this technique precludes identification of particles smaller than 5 to 10 μ in size. Although the finer particles are probably submicron polyethylene debris, they could conceivably be very fine metallic particles. Although they are technically not birefringent, submicron me-

tallic particles can appear birefringent under crossed polars because of surface diffraction effects. Sections taken from the area of the porous pads in the four stable implants were examined under back-scattered electron-scanning electron microscopy and demonstrated extensive bone ingrowth, which suggests firm proximal fixation of these prosthetic devices.

Theories of Pathogenesis

Numerous issues with regard to surgical technique, prosthetic design, fabrication, material selection, and method of fixation need to be considered with regard to the pathogenesis of endosteal osteolytic lesions. However, the final common pathway appears to be a histiocytic reaction associated with particulate debris. In attempting to explain this phenomenon, researchers must determine: (1) the origin of the particles and (2) the relative contribution of the various particulates in inciting the osteolytic response.

The polyethylene particles obviously represent wear debris that originates from the joint cavity. Noncircumferential porous coatings allow direct communication between the joint capsule and the femoral canal, which would account for the presence of polyethylene debris near the tip of the stem, even in a well fixed implant. An additional possibility is that debris may be transported through the circulatory system via the perivascular lymphatics, as described by Willert and Semlitsch.[31] In our study, the vast majority of the titanium particles identified were titanium alloy. This suggests that the metal debris originates, not from the porous surface (which is unalloyed titanium), but rather from the uncoated regions of the stem. These particles could be generated by fretting of the stem against the endosteal surface of the bone or from fretting of the cobalt alloy head against the titanium alloy Morse taper. Cobalt chromium debris has also been identified adjacent to the cobalt alloy prostheses (John Callaghan, personal communication) and, in these instances, the origin of the particles may be the uncoated regions of the stem or the porous coating. The silicate particles may represent airborne dust contaminants, but it is probable that they are remnants of the surface processing used to produce the bead blasted surface.

Regarding the relative contribution of the various particles in producing osteolysis, Willert and associates[32] have presented convincing evidence that polyethylene debris is independently capable of producing osteolytic lesions. Other particles may also be implicated. Titanium alloy particles and, to a lesser extent, cobalt alloy particles have been shown to cause a dose-dependent increase in prostaglandin E_2 from monocyte-macrophage cultures.[33] Studies in our laboratory have demonstrated that commercially pure titanium particles 1 to 3 μ in size can cause macrophage-mediated bone resorption.[34] A similar concentration of cobalt-alloy particles results in significant cytotoxicity and cell necrosis in macrophage cultures. These findings preclude the direct comparison of the relative biological activity of cobalt- and titanium-alloy particles.

It is certainly possible that the different particulate substances act synergistically in the activation of histiocytes and the resulting osteolytic response. The determination of the biologic activity of individual particulates is a subject of research at several centers. This work is bound to have important implications with regard to material selection and implant design.

Mechanical factors are important in the generation of particles. A well fixed proximally coated implant may still allow micromotion at the implant tip.[35,36] This has been demonstrated in experimental cadaveric studies with both straight and curved stems.[36] Micromotion and implant/bone fretting would be expected to be more severe in more active individuals or in instances where the component is undersized.

Remedies

To decrease the incidence of endosteal osteolysis, it will be necessary to reduce the particulate burden. It is not quite clear at this time how successfully the magnitude of polyethylene wear can be decreased. Ceramic femoral heads and new ways of manufacturing ultra-high-molecular-weight polyethylene have been introduced, but the effectiveness of these techniques in reducing wear has not been demonstrated in clinical trials.

With regard to the metallic surfaces, a polished surface finish would eliminate the microscopic asperities that predispose the metallic surface to abrasive wear. Polished surface finishes would also eliminate the silica contamination that results from the bead-blasting surface processing. These treatments would be useful for both titanium- and cobalt-base alloy. For titanium alloys, additional surface treatments, such as nitriting or nitrogen ion implantation, would harden the alloy surface and potentially reduce wear debris from the stem and Morse taper. Polishing and nitriting are in use commercially, but it should be noted that the long-term in vivo performance of these surface treatments has not been characterized.

A circumferential porous coating might retard the transport of particulates from the joint cavity to the diaphysis of the femur. More extensive coatings would also minimize micromotion and, thereby, reduce stem-bone fretting. However, more extensive coatings also have disadvantages, including the potential for increased proximal cortical resorption, increased risk of fatigue fracture, increased surface area for metal ion release, and the difficulties inherent in extracting an extensively tissue-ingrown stem.

Surgical technique remains a critical factor. Optimal fit and fill of the implant will minimize implant-bone fretting and provide the most favorable environment for bone ingrowth and, thus, long-term stability.

The role of fretting and corrosion at the Morse taper has yet to be defined. Damage at this location has been observed[37] and may contribute to the local particulate burden. While modularity is a desirable feature and provides the surgeon with considerable flexibility during implantation, it may have a downside that needs to be carefully elucidated in the near future.

Summary

While cementless, porous-coated prosthetic components have shown a high percentage of satisfactory clinical results in short and intermediate term follow-up, there are biologic problems associated with implantation of cementless devices that may predispose to clinical failure at longer term follow-up. Central to the issue of long-term performance is the problem of bone loss secondary either to adaptive bone remodeling processes or to the phenomenon of focal osteolysis. The stiffness of the femoral stem and the relative biologic inertness of the materials used are two properties of critical importance. In the future, continuing developments in the areas of prosthetic design, enhancement of fixation, biocompatibility, and biomaterials research will seek to address and resolve these problems.

References

1. Brown IW, Ring PA: Osteolytic changes in the upper femoral shaft following porous-coated hip replacement. *J Bone Joint Surg* 1985;67B:218–221.

2. Hedley AK, Gruen TA, Borden LS, et al: Two-year follow-up of the PCA noncemented total hip replacement. Proceedings of the Fourteenth Open Scientific Meeting of the Hip Society: *The Hip* 1987;14:225–250.

3. Callaghan JJ, Dysart SH, Savory CG: The uncemented porous-coated anatomic total hip prosthesis: Two-year results of a prospective consecutive series. *J Bone Joint Surg* 1988;70A:337–346.

4. Galante JO: Clinical results with the HGP cementless total hip prosthesis, in Fitzgerald RH (ed): *Non-Cemented Total Hip Arthroplasty*. New York, Raven Press, 1988, pp 427–431.

5. Sumner DR, Galante JO: Determinants of stress shielding: Design vs materials vs interface. *Clin Orthop*, in press.

6. Sumner DR, Turner TM: The effects of femoral component design features on femoral remodeling following cementless total hip arthroplasty, in Fitzgerald RH (ed): *Non-Cemented Total Hip Arthroplasty*. New York, Raven Press, 1988, pp 143–157.

7. Sumner DR, Turner TM, Urban RM, et al: Bone remodeling two years after cementless THA with a proximally porous-coated stem. Presented at the 36th Annual Meeting of the Orthopaedic Research Society, New Orleans, LA, Feb 5–8, 1990.

8. Sumner DR, Turner TM, Urban RM, et al: Long-term femoral remodelling as a function of the presence, type and location of the porous coating in cementless THA. Presented at the 34th Annual Meeting of the Orthopaedic Research Society, Atlanta, GA, Feb 1–4, 1988.

9. Sumner DR, Turner TM, Urban RM, et al: Experimental studies of bone remodeling in total hip replacement. *Clin Orthop*, in press.

10. Sumner DR, Turner TM, Urban RM, et al: Bone remodeling and bone ingrowth at two years in a canine cementless total hip arthroplasty model. *J Bone Joint Surg*, in press.

11. Turner TM, Sumner DR, Urban RM, et al: A comparative study of porous coatings in a weight-bearing total hip-arthroplasty model. *J Bone Joint Surg* 1986;68A:1396–1409.

12. Turner TM, Sumner DR, Urban RM, et al: A comparison of uncoated and porous coated press fit femoral components in a canine total hip arthroplasty (THA) model. *Trans Soc Biomat* 1987;10:2.

13. Turner TM, Sumner DR, Urban RM, et al: Cortical remodeling and bone ingrowth in proximal and full-length porous coated canine femoral stems. *Trans Orthop Res Soc* 1988;13:309.

14. Turner TM, Sumner DR, Urban RM, et al: Effects of stem stiffness and porous coating location on bone ingrowth and bone remodeling in a canine THA model. *Trans Soc Biomat* 1991;14:103.

15. Bobyn JD, Glassman AH, Goto H, et al: The effect of stem stiffness on femoral bone resorption after canine porous-coated total hip arthroplasty. *Clin Orthop* 1990;261:196–213.

16. Huiskes R, Weinans H, Grootenboer HJ, et al: Adaptive bone-remodeling theory applied to prosthetic-design analysis. *J Biomech* 1987;20:1135–1150.

17. Andrew TA, Flanagan JP, Gerundini M, et al: The isoelastic, noncemented total hip arthroplasty: Preliminary experience with 400 cases. *Clin Orthop* 1986;206:127–138.

18. Ritter MA, Keating EM, Faris PM: A porous polyethylene-coated femoral component of a total hip arthroplasty. *J Arthroplasty* 1990;5:83–88.

19. Martel JM, Pierson RH, Jacobs JJ, et al: Primary total hip reconstruction with a cementless titanium fiber coated prosthesis. *J Bone Joint Surg*, in press.

20. Gruen TA, McNeice GM, Amstutz HC: Modes of failure of cemented stem-type femoral components: A radiographic analysis of loosening. *Clin Orthop* 1979;141:17–27.

21. Engh CA, Bobyn JD, Glassman AH: Porous-coated hip replacement: The factors governing bone ingrowth, stress shielding, and clinical results. *J Bone Joint Surg* 1987;69B:45–55.

22. Harris WH, Schiller AL, Scholler JM, et al: Extensive localized bone resorption in the femur following total hip replacement. *J Bone Joint Surg* 1976;58A:612–618.

23. Carlsson AS, Gentz CF, Linder L: Localized bone resorption in the femur in mechanical failure of cemented total hip arthroplasties. *Acta Orthop Scand* 1983;54:396–402.

24. Huddleston HD: Femoral lysis after cemented hip arthroplasty. *J Arthroplasty* 1988;3:285–297.

25. Jasty MJ, Floyd WE III, Schiller AL, et al: Localized osteolysis in stable, non-septic total hip replacement. *J Bone Joint Surg* 1986;68A:912–919.

26. Maloney WJ, Jasty M, Rosenberg A, et al: Bone lysis in well-fixed cemented femoral components. *J Bone Joint Surg* 1990;72B:996–970.

27. Anthony PP, Gie GA, Howie CR, et al: Localised endosteal bone lysis in relation to the femoral components of cemented total hip arthroplasties. *J Bone Joint Surg* 1990;72B:971–979.

28. Jones LC, Hungerford DS: Cement disease. *Clin Orthop* 1987; 225:192–206.

29. Maloney WJ, Jasty M, Harris WH, et al: Endosteal erosion in association with stable uncemented femoral components. *J Bone Joint Surg* 1990;72A:1025–1034.

30. Jacobs JJ, Urban RM, Schajowicz F, et al: Particulate-associated endosteal osteolysis in titanium-base alloy cementless total hip replacement. American Society for the Testing of Materials *Symposium on Biocompatibility of Particulate Implant Materials*, in press.

31. Willert H-G, Semlitsch M: Reactions of the articular capsule to wear products of artificial joints prosthesis. *J Biomed Mater Res* 1977;11:157–164.

32. Willert H-G, Bertram H, Buchhorn GH: Osteolysis in alloarthroplasty of the hip. The role of ultra-high molecular weight polyethylene wear particles. *Clin Orthop* 1990;258:95–107.

33. Goldring SR, Kroop SF, Petrison KK, et al: Metal particles stimulate prostaglandin E_2 (PGE_2) release and collagen synthesis in cultured cells. *Trans Orthop Res Soc* 1990;15:44.

34. Molnar GM, Jacobs JJ, Erhardt P, et al: Particulate titanium induced bone resorption in organ culture. *Trans Orthop Res Soc* 1991;16:553.

35. Vanderby R, Manley PA, Kohles SS, et al: A micromotion comparison of cemented and porous ingrowth total hip replacements in a canine model. *Trans Orthop Res Soc* 1989;14:577.

36. Berzins A, Sumner DR, Rivero D, et al: The influence of functional loads on micromotion at the stem/bone interface in cementless THA. Presented at the Combined Meeting of the Orthopaedic Research Societies of USA, Japan and Canada, Banff, Alberta, Canada, October 21, 1991.

37. Collier JD, Suprenant RE, Jensen RE, et al: Corrosion at the interface of cobalt alloy heads on titanium alloy stems. *Trans Soc Biomater* 1991;14:292.

Advances in Biomaterials and Factors Affecting Implant Fixation

Richard J. Friedman MD, FRCS(C)

Introduction

Thirty years after the advent of total hip arthroplasty by Sir John Charnley, ten- to fifteen-year success rates of around 90% are being reported both for cemented total hip arthroplasty and for total knee arthroplasty. Many earlier problems, such as infection and material failure, have been greatly reduced, and currently these two procedures have gained widespread popularity with consistently reliable results.

Despite improvements in component design, surgical technique, and biomaterials, the long-term mechanical properties of polymethylmethacrylate limit the lifespan of cemented total joint arthroplasty. As a result, methods for cementless fixation have been pursued for many years. The introduction of new biomaterials and innovative design considerations are two promising approaches to improved cementless fixation.

While it is true that the biomaterials in common use today are essentially those that were available when total joint arthroplasty was first performed, a large number of new biomaterials and advances in material technology are the subject of orthopaedic implant research. Calcium phosphate, or bioactive coatings, and carbon fiber-reinforced polymer composites are two newer materials that appear to have some promise for future widespread clinical use.

With the trend towards uncemented fixation for long-term stability, the bone-prosthesis interface is receiving increasing attention. Biologic fixation, achieved with bone ingrowth into a porous coating; press-fit fixation, in which a nonporous coated implant is surrounded by a fibrous tissue layer; and chemical fixation, where a bioactive ceramic chemically bonds to the surrounding bone, are all potential methods to achieve implant fixation with long-term stability.

However, many factors exist that could affect the interface and, therefore, long-term fixation of the prosthesis in a positive or negative way. Therapies used in conjunction with total joint arthroplasty that have the potential to interfere with implant fixation include radiation therapy and various medications. Growth-promoting factors, which act locally to enhance bonding between the prosthesis and bone, have a positive impact.

Bioactive Coatings

The term ceramics has two definitions: (1) the art and technology of making objects treated by fire, also referred to as pottery, and (2) a group of materials made in this way, a group that includes the oldest man-made materials. In the study of biomaterials, ceramics comprise all nonmetallic and inorganic materials. Of the ceramic materials used in the fabrication and fixation of components for total joint arthroplasty, oxide ceramics and calcium phosphate ceramics are most commonly used.

Oxide ceramics have been used primarily as the femoral head component of a total hip prosthesis for articulation with a polyethylene acetabular component. The calcium phosphate ceramics, on the other hand, have only recently seen clinical use as bone substitute materials and as coatings for total joint prostheses. The two most common calcium phosphate ceramics used are tricalcium phosphate and hydroxyapatite.

When placed in hard-tissue sites, hydroxyapatite and tricalcium phosphate provide an osteophilic scaffolding on which bone can proliferate and to which it can bond chemically.[1] The biologic properties of the two materials are very different. Tricalcium phosphate, which has a chemical formula of $Ca_3(PO_4)_2$, has a calcium-to-phosphate ratio of 1.5 to 1. It is bioresorbable, through a combination of physiochemical dissolution and fragmentation, and it has variable in vivo characteristics. Hydroxyapatite, with a chemical formula of $Ca_{10}(PO_4)_6(OH)_2$, has a calcium-to-phosphate ratio of 1.67 to 1 and is relatively insoluble. Its consistent in vivo properties make it a more suitable calcium phosphate coating for total joint prostheses.

The calcium phosphate ceramics, and hydroxyapatite in particular, have been studied for more than 15 years. They are often referred to as bioactive ceramics because of the biological response they generate after implantation. Numerous experimental and in vivo studies have demonstrated their biocompatibility.[2,3] Initial studies and uses of hydroxyapatite were confined to dental and oral surgery applications. More recently, hydroxyapatite has been used to coat metal prostheses, with the aim of providing a chemical bond between the bone and prosthesis.

The developmental process for a hydroxyapatite coating is complex.[4] Neither the coating material nor the mechanical properties of the substrate metal should be adversely altered during the coating process. Ideally, the chemical bond between the coating and the substrate should be permanent, and the expense of the coating process should not significantly increase the cost of the implant.

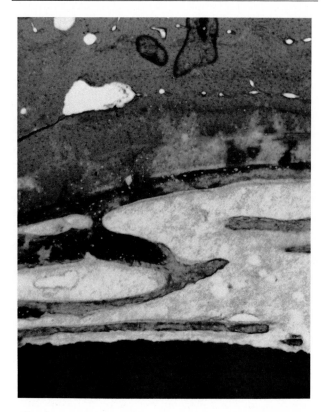

Fig. 1 Photomicrograph of a noncoated titanium rod (black), showing a fibrous membrane separating the smooth rod from the adjacent trabecular bone. (Courtesy of Thomas Bauer, MD, Cleveland, OH).

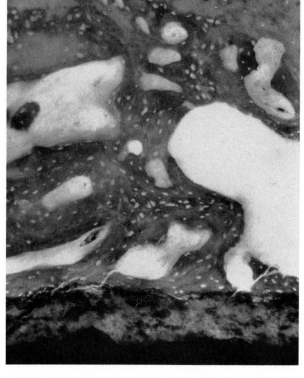

Fig. 2 Photomicrograph of a hydroxyapatite coated (75 μ thick) titanium rod (bottom). Note that the trabecular bone is in intimate contact with the hydroxyapatite coating, with no intervening fibrous membrane. (Courtesy of Thomas Bauer, MD, Cleveland, OH)

Once the coating is made, it must be characterized to ensure that it is in fact hydroxyapatite. The manufacturing and application processes must be consistent, reproducible, and yield reliable results. Also, the coating must behave as predicted, and expected benefits must ensue. Quality control is extremely important to ensure that the coating is really hydroxyapatite.

It should be noted that all hydroxyapatite coatings are not the same, nor are they applied to metallic components in the same way. The coatings can fail if improperly applied, controlled, used, or characterized. They can be characterized by their crystallinity, which measures the degree of atomic organization, by calcium phosphate content, by density, by dissolution properties, and by strength. By itself, hydroxyapatite has poor tensile and shear strength, and is strongest in compression.[5] However, these characteristics change when it is used as a coating.

Although there are many methods of applying the hydroxyapatite powder to a metal surface, the technique of plasma spraying has been used most extensively.[6] Hydroxyapatite powder is introduced into a flame that directs the particles for deposit onto the metal surface. Other coating techniques being investigated include ion sputtering, dip-coating-sintering, and electrolytic and hot isostatic pressing.[4]

Thin coatings, between 30 μ and 90 μ, are recommended, because they do not affect the mechanical properties of the substrate metal.[7] The fatigue strength of the substrate metal is minimally affected by the hydroxyapatite coating. Testing of a hydroxyapatite coating applied to metal has demonstrated that the mechanical properties of the coating are greatly improved in tension and shear, with the shear strength increased three to four times.[8] When applied, a true chemical reaction occurs between the hydroxyapatite and the titanium, which is the most commonly used substrate metal at present, or the chromium cobalt.[7]

Many animal models have been developed to demonstrate the advantages of a hydroxyapatite coating. When hydroxyapatite-coated implants are compared with noncoated devices of the same design, the maximum fixation strength is increased and the time required to achieve adequate fixation strength is shortened.[9,10] In other words, a faster and stronger bond is achieved between the implant and the surrounding bone. Histologic studies have shown that the coating increases the amount of bone-implant contact through preferential deposition of new bone both on the surface of the implant and on the host bed.[11] No fibrous tissue is seen at the interface (Figs. 1 and 2).

Other animal studies have shown that hydroxyapatite coatings increase the amount of bone ingrowth/ongrowth at the interface, and that the histologic response to hydroxyapatite is similar in cortical and cancellous bone.[12,13] The maximum interface strength is achieved at six weeks with hydroxyapatite, compared with 12 to 16 weeks for porous ingrowth. Also, the interface strength is increased more than three times with the hydroxyapatite coating.

Mechanical testing to failure in shear has demonstrated that failure occurs in the bone, but not at the hydroxyapatite-bone interface or between the substrate metal and the hydroxyapatite.[14] Because hydroxyapatite is osteophilic, attachment strength develops more rapidly and the ultimate attachment strength is increased. These characteristics were not affected by the presence of defects in the coating, and they remained true even when there was a gap between the implant and bone.[15] Also, hydroxyapatite enhanced bone implant fixation in a similar manner when it was placed in an allograft host bed.[16]

When comparing hydroxyapatite-coated with porous-coated implants, there are significant differences in the interface. When a femoral stem is press-fit in the femoral canal, only 10% to 20% of it is in direct contact with bone.[17] If a gap of less than 300 μ is present between the pores and bone, bone ingrowth will result. If the gap is greater than 300 μ, then fibrous tissue will ingrow.[18] With a hydroxyapatite coating, the gap between the hydroxyapatite coating and bone can be up to 2,000 μ (2 mm) and bone growth will still result.[7,19] Therefore, hydroxyapatite can fill defects less than 2 mm in size, increasing the contact between the prosthesis and bone, and leading to greater interface stability.

Based on the above results, numerous investigations were carried out to study the effects of a hydroxyapatite-coated total hip prosthesis in a canine model.[20,21] Implants withstood higher compression, shear, and tensile forces than did noncoated controls, and the bonding occurred in a shorter time. There was improved physiologic stress transfer around the implant, and no adverse bone remodeling. Bone scans showed an equilibrium between implant integration and bone metabolism at six months. Histologically, the results were also superior, with no intervening fibrous tissue between the bone and the hydroxyapatite coating. Close apposition between the bone and implant was not required to obtain a stable interface.

Hydroxyapatite-coated titanium and chromium cobalt subperiosteal and endosteal implants have been used clinically by dentists and oral surgeons for approximately seven years.[22] As with other material systems, orthopaedic surgery has borrowed from this experience and applied it to total joint replacement. Clinical trials of a hydroxyapatite-coated total hip prosthesis began in Europe in December 1986, and in this

country four months later with a different prosthetic design and coating. Recently, clinical trials have begun that will evaluate hydroxyapatite-coated total knee prostheses. Overall clinical and radiographic results have been encouraging.

In one series, 100 consecutive hydroxyapatite-coated total hip prostheses were implanted in 88 patients by one surgeon and were followed up for a mean of two years (range 1.5 to 3.3 years).[23] The clinical results, as determined by the Harris hip score, were excellent, with a mean total hip score of over 90 points as early as six months and continuing out to two years. The incidence of thigh pain was low after surgery, and decreased to less than 4% at follow-up examinations. Radiographically, bone apposition and evidence of osteointegration over the coating were seen at six months, and no radiolucent lines were visible around the hydroxyapatite coating. No complications related to the coating occurred. No implants were loose clinically or radiographically, and no revisions for loosening had been performed. It was felt that the early clinical results were comparable to those seen following a cemented total hip replacement.

Another clinical series of hydroxyapatite-coated total hip prostheses was recently reported.[24] A prospective, randomized, controlled multicentered trial was undertaken to compare the clinical and radiographic results of hydroxyapatite-coated total hip prostheses with uncoated press-fit total hip prostheses of the same design (Fig. 3). A total of 361 patients (297 study and 64 control patients) entered into this study, and 163 patients (138 study and 25 control patients) were followed up for a minimum of two years.

At follow-up, the mean total Harris hip score was over 90 points for the study group, which had significantly better scores than did the control patients. Pain relief was also better in the hydroxyapatite group. Radiographically, significantly fewer radiolucent lines were seen around the hydroxyapatite-coated prostheses than around the noncoated implants, and there was good evidence of osteointegration around the hydroxyapatite coating (Fig. 4). One prosthesis in the study group was revised for loosening, compared with two in the control group. No complications occurred related to the hydroxyapatite coating. Again, the clinical course after surgery is similar to that seen with a cemented prosthesis, and superior to that seen with a noncoated prosthesis of the same design. Hydroxyapatite now provides a new means of biologic fixation for an uncemented total hip prosthesis.

Based on numerous laboratory, animal, and, now, human clinical studies, the advantages of hydroxyapatite coatings are now being realized. Calcium and phosphate are naturally occurring biologic substances and are highly biocompatible. Because hydroxyapatite is osteophilic and osteoconductive, it enhances bone ingrowth and ongrowth and promotes interface stability

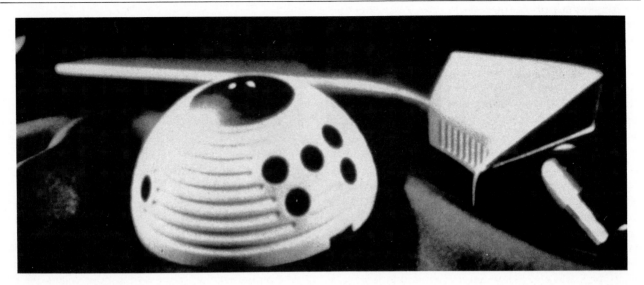

Fig. 3 Photograph of a macrotextured titanium total hip arthroplasty system, with a layer of hydroxyapatite 50 μ thick applied as shown.

through a chemical or biological bond. The coating also acts as a physical barrier to ion release from the substrate metal.

The implications of these results are that, in the future, coated implants will heal more rapidly and be less susceptible to fixation failure. The rapid osteointegration that occurs between hydroxyapatite and bone increases the ultimate stability of the interface. Because there is no intervening fibrous tissue between the bone and prosthesis, more physiologic stress transfer can occur, which gives the implant a potentially longer life span.

Despite these early encouraging results, many questions must still be asked and answered. The exact density, crystallinity, purity, and location of the hydroxyapatite coating remain to be determined. The optimal thickness is unknown, but the trend appears to be toward thinner coatings, as long as mechanical properties are not affected. Hydroxyapatite coatings appear to perform equally well on titanium alloys and on chromium cobalt (R.J. Friedman, K. Garg, R. Draughn, unpublished data). Other substrate materials, such as composites, may be improved by the use of calcium phosphate coatings. The value of applying the coating over a porous surface remains unresolved, but it is being investigated experimentally and clinically (Fig. 5).

Careful follow-up of these implanted coated prostheses is important to determine their long-term behavior and outcome. Will the coatings fracture secondary to fatigue or shear, and, if so, will fractures occur within its substance or along the interface? If the coating resorbs, what will be the status of the interface and the clinical outcome of the arthroplasty?

Newer generations of hydroxyapatite coatings, with improved physiochemical and bonding characteristics, are currently being developed and tested, as the ability to analyze and study surface coatings progresses. The optimal calcium phosphate ceramic for various particular uses must be determined. Not only could different coatings be placed on the different components of an arthroplasty, but various coatings could be used on the same implant to allow a specific biologic response to be directed toward some specific area of the implant. Bioresorbable coatings could stimulate early fixation, and more stable coatings could enhance long-term bone remodeling and interface stability.

The potential exists to influence the biologic response to an implanted prosthesis through coating composition, with the goal of enhancing its long-term stability. Layered coatings could be applied, with a thin inorganically or organically derived surface layer that is osteogenic, but that lacks the ability to provide bone attachment or long-term stability. Underneath, a stable loadbearing coating, which could influence the late bone remodeling response, would provide long-term stability and fixation.

Other ways in which calcium phosphate ceramics can influence implant fixation are being investigated. One technique involves the use of a physiologically active cement. Calcium phosphate cement is biodegradable, and it stabilizes the prosthesis by forming a chemical bond with the surrounding bone after implantation. Preliminary studies in rabbit and canine models have shown favorable results with such a calcium phosphate cement.[25] Continued research in this rapidly developing field promises greater advances in the use of calcium phosphate ceramics for long-term implant fixation.

Composites

Over the last 10 years, the use of porous-coated metal femoral stem components has become more widespread because of the high failure rates of cemented metal stems over time. However, adverse bone remodeling in the proximal femur is of concern because of the relatively high elastic modulus of the metal stem, as compared with the surrounding bone.[26] Reducing the modulus of elasticity of the implant has been shown to cause less stress shielding, osteopenia, and adverse bone remodeling in the surrounding bone in vitro and in vivo.[27]

It is hoped that new materials being developed for use as orthopaedic implants will help overcome these problems, as well as potential problems with metal stems related to metal ion release and biocompatibility. Among these materials are composites, which offer a promising alternative to metal alloys because of their low modulus of elasticity, high bending and fatigue strength properties, and biocompatibility.

Composite materials are formed by combining, either physically or mechanically, two or more substances in such a way that the performance and characteristics of the composite are significantly better than those of either of the materials by themselves. The combination of materials makes it possible to customize the physical, chemical, and material properties of the composite to specific applications. Much work has been done with polymers reinforced with carbon fibers, and, more recently, with carbon fiber-reinforced carbon composites, because of their excellent biocompatibility, high strength, and lower modulus of elasticity, which more closely matches that of bone.

Besides carbon, the other type of fiber being investigated for orthopaedic composites is polyamide. For femoral stem prostheses, various polymers are being tested as the matrix material in which the fiber will be embedded: polysulfone, polyetheretherketone (PEEK) and polyethylene.[28] Many laboratory and animal studies of carbon fiber-reinforced polymers have used polysulfone as the matrix material.

Polysulfone is often used in medical applications because of its high biocompatibility, low toxicity, and favorable mechanical properties.[29,30] Recent investigations of porous polysulfone-coated chromium cobalt femoral stems (a composite by definition) demonstrated excellent biocompatibility with no adverse tissue reactions after having been implanted for longer than four years.[31] Bone ingrowth into the porous surface has also been observed.

However, longer follow-up with this composite femoral stem has revealed unsatisfactory results, with a high rate of loosening and clinical failure.[32,33] Similar results were also observed with chromium cobalt stems coated with a low modulus polymeric porous coating, polytetrafluoroethylene, which had a 36% failure rate at a mean follow-up of 37 months.[34]

Although these two prostheses are composites by definition, their technology is like that of present-day cement technology. Both are high modulus metal alloy

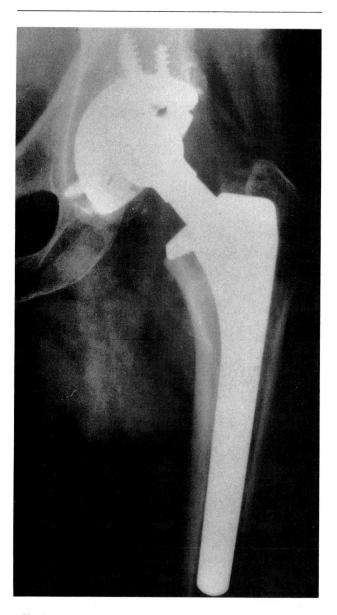

Fig. 4   Radiograph of the hydroxyapatite coated total hip arthroplasty system seen in Figure 3. No radiolucent lines are present, and bone is in intimate apposition to the hydroxyapatite coating.

stems surrounded by a low modulus polymer, either polysulfone or polytetrafluoroethylene, instead of polymethylmethacrylate. Their lack of success, therefore, is not unexpected. As stated, most current composite technology uses carbon fibers in place of metal alloys.

The biocompatibility of various forms of carbon, including carbon fiber-reinforced carbon, has been well documented.[35] However, carbon fiber-reinforced polysulfone has not been extensively studied. Canine studies with carbon fiber-reinforced polysulfone femoral stems implanted for up to eight months showed no carbon fibers or polysulfone in the reticuloendothelial system, and the stems were felt to be biocompatible and biomechanically stable.[36] Other canine trials with a similar

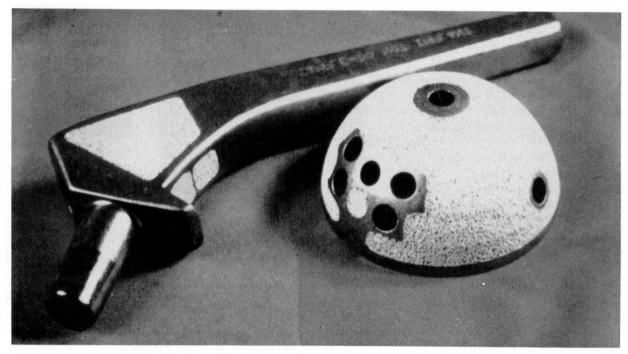

Fig. 5 Photograph of a porous-coated titanium total hip arthroplasty system, with the hydroxyapatite (50 μ thick) applied over the commercially pure titanium porous coating.

composite femoral component followed for up to two years showed a benign host tissue response with few inflammatory cells, no adverse reactions to the material, and no infections.[37] These studies have now been extended to more than four years, and the in vivo performance of this composite femoral stem in the canine model has demonstrated a positive bone remodeling response and excellent clinical success.[38]

A biomechanical advantage of carbon fiber-reinforced polysulfone is that its elastic modulus is close to that of cortical bone, which is many times less than that of chromium cobalt and titanium. The strength and modulus of the material can be altered by varying the fiber content and properties of the composite. The ultimate strength for a polysulfone composite can be made equal to or higher than that of the two metal alloys currently used.[39] The fatigue limit is approximately 40% to 60% of the ultimate load, with no evidence of failure at 10^6 cycles. The elastic modulus can be made 30% lower than that of titanium alloy and 65% lower than that of cast chromium cobalt alloy.

At high loads, the plastic deformation that occurs in the composite matrix prevents delamination and inhibits crack propagation into the fibers. This behavior is very different from that seen in metal implants.[40] Scanning electron microscopy has shown that when failure does occur, the interface between the fibers and matrix is not damaged, because the carbon fibers are still covered with polysulfone. Catastrophic failure of the composite is unlikely. Finite element analyses of composite

stems, implanted both in humans and in canine models, demonstrate transfer of bending loads in the proximal femur, rather than the more distal transfer seen with metal alloys.[41]

The technology required to fabricate composite material is very different from that used with metal alloys.[28] Continuous, rather than chopped, carbon fibers are arranged in thin layers, called plies, and are impregnated with the polymer matrix. A stack of plies is then compressed and molded into plates. The prosthesis is machined into its final shape from the plate. The mechanical properties of the plate depend on the ply orientation and stacking sequence, of which there are many permutations and combinations.

While various properties of the composite materials make them appropriate for use in orthopaedic implants, the interfacial bond formed between the polymer matrix and fiber is the most important. The fibers reinforce the matrix through this bond and the matrix, in turn, supports the fibers and transfers load between them.

Because most analyses have been done in a dry environment, there is concern regarding the effects of moisture on the interfacial bond. Recent characterization of the interfacial bond strength suggests that water and saline ions, in either physiologic saline or acellular inflammatory exudate, can significantly weaken the bond and, therefore, the strength of the composite.[42] Further studies are needed to characterize the interfacial bond in in vivo environments to help predict the long-term performances of these composite materials.

Carbon fiber-reinforced polymer composites have other potential disadvantages. Because they have poor impact resistance, they must be implanted with great care to avoid sharp blows. Because they are radiolucent, radiographic testing for quality control during the manufacturing process is not possible, and postoperative radiographic analysis of device performance is difficult. Other quality control measures and difficulties involved in manufacturing these components may make them more expensive than current metal implants.

Satisfactory short-term clinical results have been reported[35,43] for a carbon fiber-reinforced carbon femoral stem with a ceramic head. No complications related to the composite material were reported, but the follow-up is too short to draw any conclusions.

To date, no information exists on the clinical performance of a carbon fiber-reinforced polysulfone femoral stem, but clinical trials have begun. The composite stem has a low elastic modulus with flexural, torsional, compressive, tensile, fatigue, and shear strengths comparable to currently used metal stems. The composite is completely encapsulated in a textured polysulfone coating to prevent any exposure of the carbon fibers and particulate wear debris and to provide a greater mechanical interlock with the femur.

Another area of research likely to receive increasing attention is the value of coating composite orthopaedic components with substances that will help attach the implant to the surrounding bone. Experimental evidence in rabbits with hydroxyapatite-coated polysulfone implants showed direct bone attachment to both rough- and smooth-surfaced hydroxyapatite-polysulfone implants. Attachment strength was greater for the rough-surfaced implants.[44]

Further studies have been performed with a canine model. Carbon fiber-reinforced triazin resin femoral stems were implanted, both with and without a full hydroxyapatite coating. Clinical (with gait analysis), radiographic and histologic analyses demonstrated that bone bonding, or osteointegration, was enhanced by the presence of a hydroxyapatite-coated stem.[45] Surrounding trabecular and cortical bone structures were not compromised, and no adverse bone remodeling was seen.

Another study involved carbon fiber-reinforced polysulfone acetabular components coated with hydroxyapatite and implanted in dogs. The animals were sacrificed 14 months later.[46] Radiographic and histologic analyses revealed that the composite material remained intact, with no evidence of delamination of the composite or the hydroxyapatite coating. Bone was in direct contact with all areas of the implant, and no intervening fibrous tissue was seen. Large amounts of bone were present at the interface, and no adverse remodeling occurred.

Currently, composite biomaterials are being intensively studied on many fronts. The development of a composite femoral stem appears to be a reasonable goal, but the need for composite technology in other joints is unproven. Their success will depend on obtaining long-term stable fixation to surrounding bone, and osteophilic bioceramic coatings may be of some value in achieving this goal. While biocompatibility has been established, many difficulties remain to be resolved concerning the mechanical properties and the long-term performance of composite biomaterials.

Medications

Indomethacin, a commonly prescribed nonsteroidal anti-inflammatory, is a potent inhibitor of fracture healing and bone remodeling in therapeutic doses.[47,48] It has been used clinically to inhibit heterotopic bone formation after total hip replacement.[49] Clinical studies have suggested that indomethacin may increase acetabular erosion and protrusio in the arthritic patient before total joint arthroplasty.[50]

With the advent of porous-coated implants for biologic fixation of prosthetic components, concern has arisen over the effects of indomethacin and other nonsteroidal anti-inflammatory medications on bone ingrowth.[51] Because, on a histological basis, the process of bone ingrowth is similar to fracture healing, factors or conditions that inhibit one may also inhibit the other.

Using a rabbit model with quantitative histomorphometry, it has been shown that indomethacin, compared with a placebo, causes a significant decrease in the amount of ingrowth into a porous titanium cylinder at eight weeks, independent of the pore size.[52] Subsequent studies with a porous-coated chromium cobalt cylinder in the same animal model showed that therapeutic dosages of indomethacin, aspirin, and ibuprofen all caused a statistically significant decrease in bone ingrowth, as compared with a control group.[53] A dose-response effect was found for the first two nonsteroidal anti-inflammatory medications, with a greater inhibitory effect resulting from higher doses.

In addition to the histologic evidence of indomethacin inhibiting bone ingrowth into a porous-coated implant, studies have shown that the interface strengths are also decreased. Porous-coated chromium cobalt cylinders were implanted into male greyhound dogs, and the effects of indomethacin versus placebo were evaluated with mechanical push-out tests.[54] The maximal load to failure and the interface strengths were significantly decreased in the animals that received indomethacin rather than placebo.

Until the mechanism of inhibition of bone ingrowth by nonsteroidal anti-inflammatory medications is defined and understood, caution should be exercised when using these medications immediately after surgery with patients having a porous-coated total joint replacement. If bone is inhibited from growing into the pores directly after surgery, fibrous tissue will fill the available pores instead. Once this has occurred, it is unlikely that bone can replace the fibrous ingrowth, even if the inhibitory medications are withdrawn. Fibrous ingrowth weakens the interface between the bone and the prosthesis and can lead to early failure.[55]

The clinical implications of this are widespread. Aspirin is widely used for pharmacologic prophylaxis against deep venous thrombosis and pulmonary embolism following total joint arthroplasty of the lower extremity, despite its questionable efficacy and success rate.[56] Indomethacin is used in high risk patients to prevent heterotopic bone formation following total hip replacement, but this may also inhibit bone ingrowth.

Many patients undergoing total joint replacement have similar, but less severe symptoms in other major weightbearing joints, and require these nonsteroidal anti-inflammatory medications after surgery to control their pain and to make physical therapy more comfortable. While definitive guidelines are not yet available, it would be prudent to use other therapies where possible, and either avoid any nonsteroidal anti-inflammatory medications or use the lowest possible dose to minimize their effects on bone ingrowth and fixation.

While the effects of various nonsteroidal anti-inflammatory medications and radiation on the bone-prosthesis interface have been studied both experimentally and clinically, it is likely many other factors exist that we are not yet aware of that can affect the interface either in a positive or negative way. A recent study examining the effects of warfarin on bone ingrowth provides an example.

Osteocalcinin is a noncollagenous bone protein that is synthesized by osteoblasts and regulates the calcification of bone, with vitamin K as a mediator. Warfarin, a vitamin K antagonist, has been shown in a rabbit model to decrease the interface strength and the energy absorbed to failure in porous-coated implants.[57] This suggests that warfarin, an agent commonly used as prophylaxis against thromboembolic disease, may affect bone ingrowth, but the clinical significance is unknown.

Radiation Therapy

An alternate method used to prevent heterotopic bone formation, which is significant in 10% to 15% of patients undergoing an uncemented total hip replacement, is 1,000 rad of cobalt irradiation.[58] Although this treatment has been shown to be effective, recent studies suggest that it may weaken the interface strength of a porous-coated implant. Porous titanium fiber-metal plugs were implanted in dogs and subsequently radiated with 10 Gy given in four daily fractions of 2.5 Gy.[59] At six weeks, the pullout strength of the irradiated implants, compared with controls, was reduced by 19%. Metabolic activity monitored with bone scans was also significantly reduced in the irradiated extremity compared with the nonirradiated side. Histologic evaluations of the bone-prosthesis interface were not performed.

Other investigators have found comparable results.[60] Using similar implants in dogs, dosages of 1,000 rads were found to decrease the fixation strength early on by inhibiting bone ingrowth. This decrease was demonstrated both histologically and mechanically. However, the effects of radiation treatment on bone ingrowth were found to depend both on the dose and on the amount of time that had passed since receiving the radiation. The interface strength was unchanged at two and four weeks when treated with only 500 rads, although the amount of bone formation was slightly decreased.

While lower dosages of postoperative irradiation are being studied, such as 500 or 700 rads in a single dose, the long-term effects of any radiation to the bone-prosthesis interface are unknown. Patients who are felt to require irradiation following total hip replacement should either have a cemented arthroplasty, or should have any porous-coated implants shielded as much as possible to minimize any effects to the interface.

The clinical relevance of this data is unclear without further long-term studies to document the incidence of prosthetic loosening, failure, and bone resorption in patients with irradiated prostheses. In a recent multicenter study, 42 noncemented porous-coated total hip prostheses were shielded and received 1,000 rads after surgery as prophylaxis against heterotopic ossification.[61] With a short follow-up (mean, 30 months), the incidence of heterotopic ossification was significantly lower in the irradiated group (7%) than in the control group (32%). However, there was no difference in the clinical or radiographic results between the two groups, and no evidence of loosening. Further study of these and other patients will clarify the long-term effects of irradiation on the bone-prosthesis interface.

Growth-Promoting Factor

Another example, which demonstrates a positive effect on the bone-prosthesis interface, may have far-reaching clinical implications. Growth-promoting factors, such as platelet-derived growth factor (PDGF), epidermal growth factor (EGF), fibroblast growth factor (FGF), and transforming growth factor beta (TGF-β) are naturally occurring proteins that are mitogenic and chemotactic for mesenchymal cells.[62] They are normally found in wound fluids and potentially could accelerate and/or enhance bone ingrowth into porous implants.[63]

Preliminary studies in a dog model have demonstrated that the percentage of bone ingrowth into a porous titanium implant coated with equal amounts of

PDGF, EGF, and TGF-β is nearly doubled. Although further studies are needed, these preliminary findings have important clinical ramifications for achieving early stabilization with bone ingrowth.

Another study has demonstrated that TGF-β, in combination with PDGF and EGF, appears to have a positive effect on the rate of fracture healing in the rat femur.[64] In rats receiving the growth factors, more bone, cartilage, fibrous tissue, and total callous area were evident as early as one week postoperatively compared to controls, indicating an accelerated rate of fracture repair. Because the biologic process of fracture healing and bone ingrowth are similar, these growth-promoting factors may play a role in the long-term fixation of porous-coated components.

Clearly, many aspects of biologic fixation are not yet well understood, either on a cellular or mechanical level. Several factors that have the potential to affect the fixation, either in a positive or negative manner, are only now being understood. Because so many questions remain unanswered, caution must be exercised when employing the principles of biologic fixation.

References

1. Lemons JE: Hydroxyapatite coatings. *Clin Orthop* 1988;235:220–223.
2. Jarcho M: Calcium phosphate ceramics as hard tissue prosthetics. *Clin Orthop* 1981;157:259–278.
3. Jarcho M, Kay JF, Gumaer KL, et al: Tissue, cellular and subcellular events at a bone-ceramic hydroxyapatite interface. *J Bioeng* 1977;1:79–92.
4. Lacefield WR: Hydroxyapatite coatings. *Ann NY Acad Sci* 1988;523:72–80.
5. de Groot K: Ceramics of calcium phosphates: Preparation and properties, in de Groot K (ed): *Bioceramics of Calcium Phosphate.* Boca Raton, CRC Press, 1982, pp 99–114.
6. de Groot K, Geesink RGT, Klein CPAT, et al: Plasma sprayed coatings of hydroxylapatite. *J Biomed Mater Res* 1987;21:1375–1381.
7. Geesink RG, de Groot K, Klein CP: Chemical implant fixation using hydroxyl-apatite coatings. The development of a human total hip prosthesis for chemical fixation to bone using hydroxylapatite coatings on titanium substrates. *Clin Orthop* 1987;225:147–170.
8. Cook SD, Thomas KA, Kay JF, et al: Hydroxyapatite-coated titanium for othopedic implant applications. *Clin Orthop* 1988;232:225–243.
9. Thomas KA, Kay JF, Cook SD, et al: The effect of surface macrotexture and hydroxyapatite coating on the mechanical strengths and histologic profiles of titanium implant materials. *J Biomed Mater Res* 1987;21:1395–1414.
10. Thomas KA, Cook SD, Kay JF, et al: Attachment strength and histology of hydroxylapatite coated implants. *Biomater Med Devices Artif Organs* 1986;14:73–74.
11. Cook SD, Thomas KA, Kay JF, et al: Hydroxyapatite-coated porous titanium for use as an orthopaedic biologic attachment system. *Clin Orthop* 1988;230:303–312.
12. Richardson DC: The response of cancellous and cortical canine bone to hydroxyapatite coated titanium rods. *Trans Soc Biomater* 1989;12:176.
13. Magee FP, Kay JF, Hedley AK: Interface strength and histology

14. Manley MT, Kay JF, Uratsuji M, et al: Hydroxyapatite coatings applied to implants subjected to functional loads. *Trans Soc Biomater* 1987;10:210.
15. Cook SD, Thomas KA: Coating defects in hydroxyapatite coated implants. *Trans Soc Biomater* 1989;12:172.
16. Soballe K, Hansen ES, Rasmussen HB, et al: Early fixation of allogenic bone graft in titanium and hydroxyapatite coated implants. *Trans Orthop Res Soc* 1989;14:385.
17. Noble PC, Alexander JW, Lindahl LJ, et al: The anatomic basis of femoral component design. *Clin Orthop* 1988;235:148–165.
18. Harris WH, White RE, McCarthy JC, et al: Bony ingrowth fixation of the acetabular component in canine hip joint arthroplasty. *Clin Orthop* 1983;176:7–11.
19. Søballe K, Hansen ES, Rasmussen HB, et al: Enhancement of osteopenic and normal bone ingrowth into porous coated implants by hydroxyapatite coating. *Trans Orthop Res Soc* 1989;14:554.
20. Thomas KA, Cook SD, Haddad RJ, et al: Biologic response to hydroxyapatite-coated titanium hips: A preliminary study in dogs. *J Arthroplasty* 1989;4:43–53.
21. Mahomed N, Maistrelli G, Fornasier V: Interfacial shear strength of hydroxapatite coated hip implants. *Orthop Trans* 1990;14:710–711.
22. Kay JF, Golec TS, Riley RL: Hydroxapatite-coated subperiosteal dental implants: Design rationale and clinical experience. *J Prosth Dent* 1987;58:334–339.
23. Geesink RGT: Hydroxyapatite-coated total hip prosthesis: Two year clinical and roentgenographic results of 100 cases. *Clin Orthop* 1990;261:39–58.
24. Friedman RJ, Dorr LD, Gustke KA, et al: Hydroxyapatite coated total hip arthroplasty. Presented at the 58th Annual Meeting of the American Academy of Orthopaedic Surgeons, Anaheim, CA, Mar 9, 1991.
25. Constantz BR, Young SW, Kienapfel H, et al: Pilot investigations of a calcium phosphate cement in a rabbit femoral canal model and a canine humeral plug mode. Presented at the 17th Annual Meeting of the Society for Biomaterials, Scottsdale, AZ, May 1–5, 1991.
26. Engh CA, Bobyn JD: The influence of stem size and extent of porous coating on femoral bone resorption after primary cementless hip arthroplasty. *Clin Orthop* 1988;231:7–28.
27. Bobyn JD, Glassman AH, Goto H, et al: The effect of stem stiffness on femoral bone resorption after canine porous-coated total hip arthroplasty. *Clin Orthop* 1990;261:196–213.
28. Skinner HB: Composite technology for total hip arthroplasty. *Clin Orthop* 1988;235:224–236.
29. Imai V, Kus YS, Watanabe A, et al: Evaluation of polysulfone as a potential biomedical material. *J Bioeng* 1978;2:103–107.
30. Spector M, Davis RJ, Lunceford EM, et al: Porous polysulfone coatings for fixation of femoral stems by bony ingrowth. *Clin Orthop* 1983;176:34–41.
31. Spector M, Heyligers I, Roberson JR: Porous polymers for biological fixation. *Clin Orthop* 1988;235:207–219.
32. Spector M, Roberson JR, deAndrade JR, et al: Bone growth into porous polysulfone. *J Orthop Surg Tech* 1987;3:21–30.
33. Gaines RK, Bierbaum BE, Roberson JR, et al: Porous polysulfone-coated titanium femoral stems: A prospective multicenter study. Presented at the 58th Annual Meeting of the American Academy of Orthopaedic Surgeons, Anaheim, CA, Mar 9, 1991.
34. Tullos HS, McCaskill BL, Dickey R, et al: Total hip arthroplasty with a low modulus porous coated femoral component. *J Bone Joint Surg* 1984;66A:888–898.
35. Christel PS: The application of carbon fiber reinforced carbon composites in orthopaedic surgery. *CRC Critical Rev Biocomp* 1986;2:189–218.
36. Mendes DG, Roffman M, Soundry M, et al: A composite hip implant. *Orthop Rev* 1988;17:402–407.

37. Magee FP, Weinstein AM, Longo JA, et al: A canine composite femoral stem: An in vivo study. *Clin Orthop* 1988;235:237–252.

38. Longo JA, Magee FP, Koeneman JB: Long-term performance of a canine carbon composite femoral hemiarthroplasty. *Trans Soc Biomater* 1990;13:126.

39. St. John KR: Application of advanced composites in orthopaedic implants, in *Biocompatible Polymers, Metals and Composites.* Lancaster, Technomic Publishing, 1983, pp 861–871.

40. Huettner W, Keuscher G, Nietert M: Carbon fiber-reinforced polysulfone-thermoplastic composites, in Ducheyne P, Van der Perre G, Aubert AE (eds): *Biomaterials and Biomechanics 1983.* Amsterdam, Elsevier Science, 1984, pp 167–172.

41. Weinstein AM, Koenemann JB, Johnson RH, et al: Design and testing of a composite material K9 femoral component. *Trans Orthop Res Soc* 1987;12:486.

42. Latour RA, Black J, Miller B: Interfacial bond degradation of carbon fiber-polysulfone thermoplastic composite in simulated in vivo environments. *Trans Soc Biomater* 1990;13:69.

43. Christel PS, Meunier A, Leclerq S, et al: Development of a carbon-carbon hip prosthesis. *J Biomed Mat Res* 1987;21(A2 suppl): 191–218.

44. Zimmerman MC, Scalzo H, Parsons JR: The attachment of hydroxyapatite coated polysulfone to bone. *J Appl Biomater* 1990; 1:295–305.

45. Maistrelli GL, Garbuz D, Fornasier V, et al: HA and non HA coated carbon composite femoral stems in the canine model: A preliminary report, in Heimke G, Soltesz V, Lee AJC (eds): *Clinical Implant Materials—Advances in Biomaterials.* Amsterdam, Elsevier Science, 1990, vol 9, pp 289–295.

46. Magee FP, Longo JA, Mather SE, et al: One year performance of a HA coated composite acetabular component. *Trans Soc Biomater* 1989;12:206.

47. Sudmann E: Effects of indomethacin on bone remodelling in rabbit ear chambers. *Acta Orthop Scand Suppl* 1975;160:91–115.

48. Allen HL, Wase A, Bear WT: Indomethacin and aspirin: Effect of nonsteroidal anti-inflammatory agents on the rate of fracture repair in the rat. *Acta Orthop Scand* 1980;51:595–600.

49. Ritter MA, Gioe TJ: The effect of indomethacin on para-articular ectopic ossification following total hip arthroplasty. *Clin Orthop* 1982;167:113–117.

50. Newman NM, Ling RSM: Acetabular bone destruction related to non-steroidal anti-inflammatory drugs. *Lancet* 1985;2(8445): 11–14.

51. Longo JA, Hedley AK, Weinstein AM, et al: Comparative effects of EHDP, radiation therapy and indomethicin on bone ingrowth in rabbits. *Trans Soc Biomater* 1985;8:161.

52. Keller, JC, Trancik TM, Young FA, et al: Effects of indomethacin on bone ingrowth. *J Orthop Res* 1989;7:28–34.

53. Trancik T, Mills W, Vinson N: The effect of indomethacin, aspirin, and ibuprofen on bone ingrowth into a porous-coated implant. *Clin Orthop* 1989;249:113–121.

54. Longo JA, Magee FP, Hedley AK, et al: The effect of chronic indomethacin on fixation of porous implants to bone. *Trans Orthop Res Soc* 1989;14:337.

55. Engh CA, Glassman AH, Suthers KE: The case for porous-coated hip implants: The femoral side. *Clin Orthop* 1990;261:63–81.

56. Harris WH, Athanasoulis CA, Waltman AC, et al: Prophylaxis of deep-vein thrombosis after total hip replacement: Dextran and external pneumatic compression compared with 1.2 or 0.3 gram of aspirin daily. *J Bone Joint Surg* 1985;67A:57–62.

57. Lavernia CJ, Yoshida G, Reindel E, et al: Effects of warfarin on the ingrowth kinetics of porous coated devices. *Trans Orthop Res Soc* 1988;13:312.

58. Ayers DC, Pellegrini VD Jr, Evarts CM: Prevention of heterotopic ossification in high-risk patients by radiation therapy. *Clin Orthop* 1991;263:87–93.

59. Wise MW III, Robertson ID, Lachiewicz PF, et al: The effects of radiation therapy on the fixation strength of an experimental porous-coated implant in dogs. *Clin Orthop* 1991;261:276–280.

60. Sumner DR, Turner TM, Pierson RH, et al: Dose and time-dependent effects of radiation treatment on early bone ingrowth in a canine model. *Trans Orthop Res Soc* 1989;14:556.

61. Kennedy WF, Gruen TA, Chessin H, et al: Radiation therapy to prevent heterotopic ossification after cementless total hip arthroplasty. *Clin Orthop* 1991;262:185–191.

62. Canalis E: Effect of growth factors on bone cell replication and differentiation. *Clin Orthop* 1985;193:246–263.

63. Keller J, Grotendorst G, Slayton L, et al: Growth factor enhancement of bone ingrowth. *Trans Soc Biomater* 1987;10:50.

64. Friedman RJ, Acurio MT, Davis R, et al: Effects of growth factors and indomethacin on fracture healing. *Trans Orthop Res Soc* 1992; 17:421.

Current Biomaterial Problems in Implants

Harry B. Skinner, MD, PhD

Introduction

The technology used in orthopaedics has become increasingly complex over the years. Many new types of prosthetic implants have been designed that represent notable advances in the field. However, these innovations also represent the potential for new problems, partly because manufacturers of devices frequently lack the clinical insight to anticipate difficulties that may arise with long-term use. Current issues in joint arthroplasty now relate to such topics as the efficacy of hydroxyapatite and hydroxyapatite coatings, wear problems, fatigue problems, growth factors, and porous coatings. Therefore, any orthopaedist who wishes to avoid the pitfalls of implant surgery must understand the field from an engineering standpoint as well as from a clinical point of view. This discussion presents the current technology of orthopaedic implants and covers the important issues related to their use.

Morse Taper Fittings

A Morse taper is one of several designs of interference joints. It consists of a taper shank and matching socket held together by friction (Fig. 1).[1] This mechanism was first used in machine tools to allow the quick connection and release of a removable part, such as the chuck of a drill press. The American Standard of Morse Tapers includes a range of sizes numbered from 1 to 7, with the addition of No. $4^{1}/_{2}$. Other well-known tapers include the Reed lathe center taper, the Standard Tool Company taper (for twist drill shanks), the Cleveland twist drill taper, the Sellers taper, and the Brown & Sharpe taper. Table 1 compares three of the clinically important Morse tapers and one smaller variety.

Actually, none of the manufactured orthopaedic implants conforms fully to the specifications of a Morse taper (Fig. 2; Table 2). In fact, for some reason, the orthopaedic device industry uses a taper angle that is almost twice that of the Morse.[1] Because of space considerations, shank length and socket depth are shorter than in standard tapers (Fig. 3). The taper, which is approximately 500 μ per centimeter of length, varies from one manufacturer to the next, as does the diameter of the shank and socket at the gauge line. Thus, with one exception, tapers from one manufacturer cannot be used with sockets from another—a restriction that has great clinical importance. Aluminum oxide "ceramic" heads, which are made by the Feldmühle firm in Germany, are available under a license agreement through Smith & Nephew Richards and Depuy, Inc. Zirconia (ZrO_2) heads will become available in the near future.

Use of the wrong shank with any given socket can result in inadvertent separation of the two components. Use of the wrong taper shank with a ceramic head can lead to catastrophic failure of the latter, because routine loads can lead to markedly greater stress than its design allows. Thus, it is critical that the metal taper and ceramic head be compatible. When the dimensions of the various Morse tapers used in orthopaedics are compared, the extent of the differences between manufacturers is apparent (Table 2). The American Society for Testing and Materials has attempted to standardize the Morse taper, but manufacturers have resisted this measure because it would entail expensive retooling.

There may be other consequences to incompatibility. For example, one manufacturer's long-neck femoral head placed on another's prosthesis might result in excessive bending moment in the latter because of a greater head-neck offset than design specifications permit. A larger bending moment results in greater stress on the lateral aspect of the prosthesis and prosthesis neck, increasing the risk of fatigue failure.

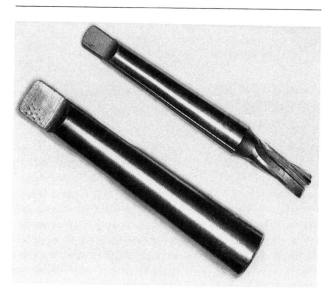

Fig. 1 Typical Morse tapers used in machine tools.

Table 1
Dimensions of Morse tapers*

Number of Taper	Included Angle of Taper (°)	Shank		Socket	
		Length (cm)	Exposed Length (cm)	Depth (cm)	Diameter at Gauge Line (cm)
0.375†	2.40	4.207	0.238	4.127	0.953
1	2.86	5.556	0.125	5.556	1.207
2	2.86	6.827	0.186	6.747	1.778
3	2.88	8.414	0.186	8.414	2.383

*Adapted with permission from Carmichael C (ed): *Kent's Mechanical Engineer's Handbook, Design and Production Volume,* ed 12. New York, Wiley Engineering Handbook Series, 1950.
†Non-standard Morse taper

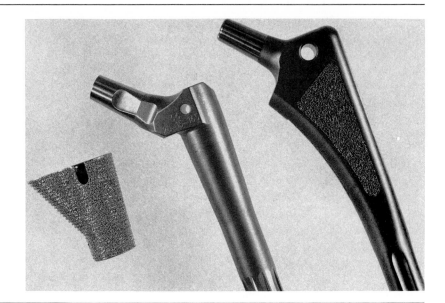

Fig. 2 From **left** to **right**: A porous-coated Morse taper socket for biologic fixation; an S-ROM femoral prosthesis showing the Morse taper stem for fixation to the socket at its left; and a Harris-Galante femoral component with a Morse taper for connection to a femoral head.

Thus, strict adherence to compatibility among Morse tapers and femoral heads is essential. This caveat is particularly important when planning a revision procedure that may require changing the femoral head without revising the femoral shaft component.

Metal-Backed Components

The total joint components usually reinforced by metal backing are the patellar and tibial components of a total knee prosthesis and the acetabular component of a hip prosthesis. The first acetabular components were fabricated from ultra-high-molecular-weight polyethylene. When total knee prostheses were developed later, they, too, were designed with all-polyethylene tibial and patellar components. Eventually, stress analysis, radiographic signs of loosening, and long-term fixation requirements suggested the advisability of backing the acetabular components with metal. Similar considerations prompted the metal backing of tibial components, although the impetus to do the same for patellar components largely derived from the requisites of biologic fixation.

Acetabular Components

High acetabular loosening rates[2] motivated a reassessment of the load stress environment. Using two-dimensional finite element analysis, Carter and associates[3,4] found that metal-backing of the acetabular component significantly reduced stress in the cancellous bone of the pelvis. Crowninshield and associates[5] came to a similar conclusion by studying an axisymmetric model of the acetabular region. When Harris[6] compared an investigation of metal-backed acetabular components in young patients[7] with a similar study involving acetabular components without metal backing,[8] he concluded that the former were associated with lower loosening rates.

These data apparently conflict with a recent report by Ritter and associates,[9] who showed that, after an average of 5.2 years, cemented ultra-high-molecular-weight polyethylene acetabular components produced significantly fewer radiolucent lines, less loosening, and

Table 2
Approximate dimensions of some of the Morse tapers used in orthopaedic implants

Manufacturer	Included Angle of Taper	Shank Length (cm)	Socket Diameter at Gauge Line (cm)
Zimmer	6°	2.00	1.016
Howmedica	5°40′	—	1.138
Joint Medical Products	6°	2.09	1.349
Orthomet			
Perfecta	5°35′	1.60	1.365
Proforma	2°34′40″	1.52	1.365
Smith & Nephew Richards	5°43′30″	1.50	1.430
Feldmühle			
A	5°43′30″ ± 2′	—	1.026
B	5°43′30″ ± 2′	—	1.113
C	5°43′30″ ± 2′	—	1.433
FDA suggested requirements for Al_2O_3 heads	5°35′ to 5°42.5′	Engagement area of stem 50% of length of bore	Bore angle > cone angle

a lower revision rate than metal-backed components. The fact that this study used 28-mm femoral heads may be important in light of the work by Hoeltzel and associates,[10] which suggested that optimal (minimal) surface strain in a ultra-high-molecular-weight polyethylene acetabular component was obtained with a 26-mm head. An observation along the same lines was reported by Morrey and Ilstrup.[11] In their epidemiologic study of total hip arthroplasty cases at the Mayo Clinic, they saw lower acetabular loosening rates for 22-mm heads than for 32-mm heads. Thus, serious consideration should be given to using ultra-high-molecular-weight polyethylene acetabular components, and, if one elects to do so, to use them in conjunction with a 26- or 28-mm head. Cost, if that were the only consideration, would favor all-polyethylene acetabular components, but these types also have other advantages in that they are more easily revised than metal-backed components, and they cause less damage to the bony acetabulum.

If an ultra-high-molecular-weight polyethylene cup without metal backing is selected for cemented use, it is important that it have no stress concentration sites (sharp deep grooves) that would predispose it to catastrophic failure.[12-14] The metal portion of a metal-backed cup can fracture if there is insufficient acetabular bone stock to provide adequate support, regardless of whether or not the cup is cemented (Fig. 4).[15] Finite element studies have suggested that stresses can exceed fatigue endurance limits under certain conditions of use for porous ingrowth cups.[16]

Patellar and Tibial Components

Early total knee prosthesis designs used a polyethylene tibial component and allowed for the option of resurfacing the patella. Patellar resurfacing has essentially become routine. However, a 1982 report by Bartel and associates[17] documented problems with all-polyethylene tibial components, and suggested that

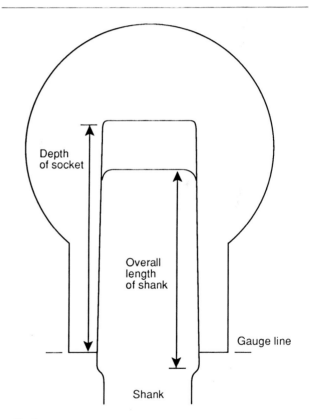

Fig. 3 The Morse taper used in orthopaedics is shown with its standard dimensions.

deformation could predispose them to early failure, especially in the presence of asymmetric loading conditions. Finite element stress analysis has demonstrated excessive bone and cement stresses under such conditions, providing a reason to favor the use of metal-backed tibial components.

Reilly and associates[18] found that a metal-backed stemmed tibial component would tolerate varus/valgus

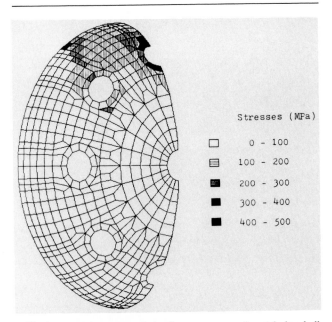

Fig. 4 Finite element analysis of a porous-coated acetabular shell. The stress distribution is shown under the conditions of reduced bony support from a deficient acetabulum. (Reproduced with permission from Burton DT, Skinner HB, Eng M: Stress analysis of a total hip acetabular component: An FEM study. *Biomater Artif Cells Artif Organs* 1989;17:371–383.)

loading better than would an all-plastic stemmed component. In strain-gauge studies, they also showed that, when all possible loading configurations are considered, a metal-backed tibial component deflects the least, which implies that fewer radiolucent lines would result. These investigators pointed out that load bypassing through the stem and higher cost are the trade-offs for possible improved fixation.[19] The early clinical results of a metal-backed tibial component used in total knee replacement seem to verify the superior performance that metal backing provides. In their review of 124 consecutive total condylar knee replacements, Ewald and associates[20] found only insignificant radiolucent lines two to four years after operation. These data suggest that the patellar component would also be improved with metal backing. Indeed, metal backing is necessary if an uncemented ingrowth surface is desired.

On the other hand, when Dorr[21] compared metal-backed tibial components with all-plastic designs, the latter were shown to achieve adequate fixation without radiolucent lines. The study of Ranawat and Boachie-Adjei[22] supports these findings. In their analysis, all-plastic tibial components had a survivorship of 94.1% after 11 years.

It is important to remember that a metal backing takes up some space that would otherwise be occupied by polyethylene. For example, a nominal 8-mm tibial component with metal-backing may have only 5 mm of polyethylene in certain areas of the bearing surface. This is an important concern, because thicknesses of less than approximately 5 mm result in excessively high contact stresses,[23] which in turn can lead to excessive wear of the component and eventual fracture. Finally, as stated earlier, an all-polyethylene component has the advantage of being easier to revise than a metal-backed component with a tibial stem.

Metal backing has introduced unique problems for tibial components. Some of the early designs had inherent flaws that predisposed the metal trays toward fracture.[24] Even appropriate designs can lead to fatigue failure under certain conditions, such as stress shielding of the plateau by a metal stem (Fig. 5).[25–27] More recent designs incorporate supportive fins to reduce the cantilever effect if the plateau is inadvertently left without support. This modification will undoubtedly tend to increase the transfer of stress to the tip of the stem, which could possibly unload the cancellous bone under the metal tibial plateaux and cause radiolucent fibrous membranes.

The problems of metal-backed patellar components are well known.[28–30] There have been cases where the anchoring pegs used for biologic fixation have failed, where the polyethylene has worn through to the metal backing,[29] and where shearing and dissociation of the polyethylene from the metal base have occurred. Obviously, appreciable stress is experienced by the patellar component, which can result in significant shear stresses of the bone-prosthesis interface and cause peg failure. The problem of excessive stress can be exacerbated by malalignment. Indeed, lack of conformity to the femoral component has been suggested as a contributing cause of patellar surface wear.[31]

The Osteolysis Problem

Adverse reaction to foreign materials has been a longstanding concern. Implant materials used today have undergone extensive testing and are considered biocompatible. Following implantation, however, the conditions of use may cause wear or degradation of the prosthesis materials, and the particulate matter that accumulates can stimulate a different and adverse tissue response.[32–34] For example, an early study of localized bone resorption around total hip femoral components implicated birefringent particulate material as the source of the pathology. Although not identified, this material was thought to be either polymethylmethacrylate or polyethylene.[35] Since the time of that investigation, the identity of the causative material and the mechanism by which osteolysis occurs have been subjects of intensive study.

Recently, Howie and associates[36] used a rat knee joint model to show that polyethylene particles of wear-debris size caused resorption around a polymethylmethacrylate plug. This study demonstrated that polyethylene particulate debris can cause lysis of bone, but it

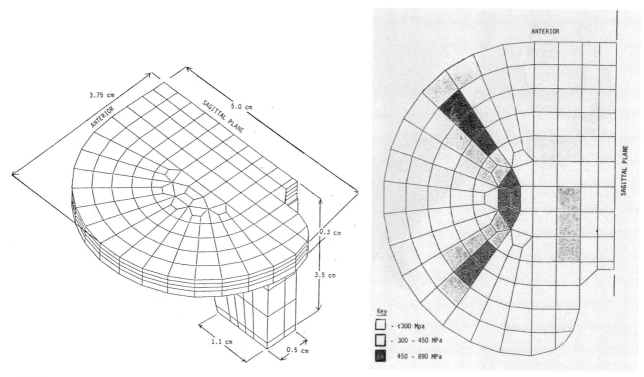

Fig. 5 **Left**, A finite element model of a tibial plateau prosthesis. **Right**, Stress in the plateau under normal loading conditions. (Reproduced with permission from Paganelli JV, Skinner HB, Mote CD Jr: Prediction of fatigue failure of a total-knee replacement tibial plateau using finite element analysis. *Orthopedics* 1988;11:1161–1168.)

did not confirm that polyethylene is the only source of such harmful debris. Reports of lysis adjacent to uncemented prostheses suggest that polyethylene wear may be responsible, but they have also raised suspicion about particulate titanium alloy. A recent American Society for Testing and Materials symposium on particulate materials suggested several possible sources of the wear debris that causes osteolysis, including ultra-high-molecular-weight polyethylene, polymethylmethacrylate bone cement, the barium sulfate from the bone cement, and titanium alloy.

Certainly, wear debris, whether from polyethylene articular surfaces, the fretting of metals,[37] the wearing of metal-bearing surfaces,[38] or the fragmentation of cement, is increasingly recognized as a problem that causes osteolysis and component loosening in total joint arthroplasty. The factors that most influence wear are how well the mating surfaces conform to each other, the contact stress, the hardness of the two articulating surfaces, and surface roughness. Today's prosthetic joints consist of a hard and polished convex surface, made of either metal or ceramic, on which a softer and usually concave surface slides. The prosthetic patella is an exception in that the softer, plastic surface is convex.

The problem encountered when attempting to elucidate the etiology of osteolysis is that experimental duplication of wear conditions in joints is difficult, even for a relatively simple joint like the hip. Two metals, two ceramic materials, and one polymer are involved. Currently, cobalt-chromium alloy is the material of choice for metallic surfaces that articulate with ultra-high-molecular-weight polyethylene. The use of titanium alloy as a bearing surface has been called into question because of recent reports documenting unexplained extreme wear (Fig. 6).[37-39] The polyethylene surface is somewhat in question, too, because manufacturing differences can significantly affect the wear behavior of articulating surfaces.

Solutions to the problem are being pursued along two different paths. The more obvious one is improving the bearing surface of the harder material. For the hip, effort is being devoted to making a ceramic femoral head; aluminum oxide (alumina; Al_2O_3) and zirconium oxide (zirconia; ZrO_2) are the ceramics of choice. Highly polished alumina has been shown to produce low rates of polyethylene wear when it articulates against ultra-high-molecular-weight polyethylene. With their best surface finishes, stainless steel and alumina have produced similar rates of ultra-high-molecular-weight polyethylene wear; at slightly lower-quality surface finishes, alumina has produced less wear, and, because of its greater hardness, is expected to maintain its surface finish even better than the implant alloys.[40]

Efforts to redeem titanium alloy as a bearing surface

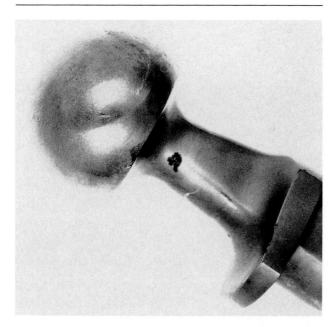

Fig. 6 Wear of the titanium alloy femoral head is shown. This head had been dislocated for several months and was weightbearing against bone and soft tissue.

are devoted to increasing its hardness through ion implantation. This technique involves subjecting the metal to the bombardment of accelerated nitrogen ions, which penetrate the surface to a depth of about 0.5 μ. This process has significantly improved the alloy, even against three-body wear with polymethylmethacrylate.[41] However, three-body wear from bone or cement could remove the thin embedded layer and reopen the surface to wear. For this reason, ion implantation has met with limited enthusiasm.

Changing the properties of polyethylene is another possible way of solving the wear debris problem. The Food and Drug Administration has designated the material properties that define medical grade ultra-high-molecular-weight polyethylene, but the medical grade polyethylene supplied to the orthopaedic device industry has wide ranges of variation: 23% in yield strength, 42% in ultimate strength, 100% in elongation to fracture, and 400% in creep.[42] Only a few manufacturers make medical grade polyethylene, and it constitutes only a small part of their total production of this material.

By carefully controlling manufacturing techniques, the material properties of polyethylene can be significantly improved and still fall within the range of medical grade. Depuy, Inc. has been collaborating with Dupont in developing an ultra-high-molecular-weight polyethylene with lower creep, a higher modulus, and a lower coefficient of friction. Compared with conventional ultra-high-molecular-weight polyethylene, this material is reported to have 17% greater yield strength and a modulus that is 1.7 times greater—changes that are considered to be significant improvements (Table 3). However, these changes must be balanced against the fact that a higher modulus translates into higher contact stress and perhaps greater wear. Also, increases in these parameters may accentuate fatigue crack growth. These new material properties suggest enhancement, but the true indication of improvement will be better performance in the physiologic environment.

Summary

Based on the information presented here, certain recommendations can be made regarding the choice of prosthetic joint components. Morse tapers have the virtue of allowing latitude in the selection of femoral neck length. From the standpoint of wear and loosening, which may be related, a 26- or 28-mm femoral head will cause lower loosening torque for the acetabulum than a large head, and alumina heads in either size should be associated with lower wear rates than those associated with metallic heads. Femoral components for cemented use should probably be made of cobalt-chromium alloy to minimize cement stress; for cementless arthroplasty, a titanium alloy would be expected to cause the least remodeling and pain.[43,44] The acetabular component for cemented use may have a metal backing if a significant polyethylene thickness (>6 mm to 8 mm) is available to reduce contact stress. The metal backing, which is required for porous ingrowth attachment to the acetabulum, can be made of either cobalt-chromium or titanium alloy.

The femoral component of a total knee prosthesis is best made from cobalt-chromium alloy because too many unanswered questions remain about the wear properties of titanium. The more appropriate tibial component design—metal-backed or all-polyethylene—

Table 3
Properties of ultra-high-molecular-weight polyethylene (UHMWPE)

Type of UHMWPE	Tensile Modulus (MPa)	Tensile Yield (MPa)	Elongation at Failure (%)	Creep at 1,000 psi (%)	Shore D Hardness
Enhanced	2,172	28	230	0.7	66
Conventional	1,275	24	260	1.6	62
ASTM F648	—	19.3	>200	<2.0	>60

is yet to be decided. A metal-backed component is probably better if the metal tray allows the plastic to be more than 6 mm to 8 mm thick at the bearing surface. Modularity is a distinct advantage, because it allows selection of a final tibial component of optimal thickness after the other components are in place. Titanium alloy may be preferable to cobalt-chromium as a metal backing, because it permits slightly easier revision, if that becomes necessary. The patellar component should be made of polyethylene.

References

1. Carmichael C (ed): *Kent's Mechanical Engineers' Handbook, Design and Production Volume,* ed 12. New York, Wiley Engineering Handbook Series, 1950.
2. Sutherland CJ, Wilde AH, Borden LS, et al: A ten-year follow-up of one hundred consecutive Müller curved-stem total hip-replacement arthroplasties. *J Bone Joint Surg* 1982;64A:970–982.
3. Carter DR, Vasu R, Harris WH: Stress distribution in the acetabular region: II. Effects of cement thickness and metal backing of the total hip acetabular component. *J Biomech* 1982;15:165–170.
4. Carter DR: Finite element analysis of a metal-backed acetabular component in the hip, in Proceedings of the Eleventh Open Scientific Meeting of the Hip Society: *The Hip.* St. Louis, CV Mosby, 1983, pp 216–228.
5. Crowninshield RD, Pedersen DR, Brand RA, et al: Analytic support for acetabular component metal backing, in Proceedings of the Eleventh Open Scientific Meeting of the Hip Society: *The Hip.* St. Louis, CV Mosby, 1983, pp 207–215.
6. Harris WH: Advances in total hip arthroplasty: The metal-backed acetabular component. *Clin Orthop* 1984;183:4–11.
7. Harris WH, White RE: Socket fixation using a metal-backed acetabular component for total hip replacement. A minimum five-year follow-up. *J Bone Joint Surg* 1982;64A:745–749.
8. Dorr LD, Takei GK, Conaty JP: Total hip arthroplasties in patients less than forty-five years old. *J Bone Joint Surg* 1983;65A:474–479.
9. Ritter MA, Keating EM, Faris PM, et al: Metal-backed acetabular cups in total hip arthroplasty. *J Bone Joint Surg* 1990;72A:672–677.
10. Hoeltzel DA, Walt MJ, Kyle RF, et al: The effects of femoral head size on the deformation of ultra high molecular weight polyethylene acetabular cups. *J Biomech* 1989;22:1163–1173.
11. Morrey BF, Ilstrup D: Size of the femoral head and acetabular revision in total hip-replacement arthroplasty. *J Bone Joint Surg* 1989;71A:50–55.
12. Collins DN, Chetta SG, Nelson CL: Fracture of the acetabular cup: A case report. *J Bone Joint Surg* 1982;64A:939–940.
13. Salvati EA, Wright TM, Burstein AH, et al: Fracture of polyethylene acetabular cups: Report of two cases. *J Bone Joint Surg* 1979;61A:1239–1242.
14. Harley JM, Boston DA: Acetabular cup failure after total hip replacement. *J Bone Joint Surg* 1985;67B:222–224.
15. Cohen MG, Hays MB, Garcia JJ, et al: Fracture of a metal-backed acetabular cup: A case report. *J Arthroplasty* 1988;3:263–265.
16. Burton DT, Skinner HB, Eng M: Stress analysis of a total hip acetabular component: An FEM study. *Biomater Artif Cells Artif Organs* 1989;17:371–383.
17. Bartel DL, Burstein AH, Santavicca EA, et al: Performance of the tibial component in total knee replacement. *J Bone Joint Surg* 1982;64A:1026–1033.
18. Reilly D, Walker PS, Ben-Dov M, et al: Effects of tibial components on load transfer in the upper tibia. *Clin Orthop* 1982;165:273–282.
19. Walker PS, Greene D, Reilly D, et al: Fixation of tibial components of knee prostheses. *J Bone Joint Surg* 1981;63A:258–267.
20. Ewald FC, Jacobs MA, Miegel RE, et al: Kinematic total knee replacement. *J Bone Joint Surg* 1984;66A:1032–1040.
21. Dorr LD: Polyethylene versus metal-backed tibial components. Presented at State-of-the-Art in Total Joint Replacement, Scottsdale, AZ, Nov 21, 1988.
22. Ranawat CS, Boachie-Adjei O: Survivorship analysis and results of total condylar knee arthroplasty: Eight- to 11-year follow-up period. *Clin Orthop* 1988;226:6–13.
23. Wright TM, Bartel DL: The problem of surface damage in polyethylene total knee components. *Clin Orthop* 1986;205:67–74.
24. Skinner HB, Mabey MF, Paganelli JV, et al: Failure analysis of PCA revision total knee replacement tibial component: A preliminary study using the finite element method. *Orthopedics* 1987;10:581–584.
25. Paganelli JV, Skinner HB, Mote CD Jr: Prediction of fatigue failure of a total knee replacement tibial plateau using finite element analysis. *Orthopedics* 1988;11:1161–1168.
26. Scott RD, Ewald FC, Walker PS: Fracture of the metal tibial tray following total knee replacement: A report of two cases. *J Bone Joint Surg* 1984;66A:780–782.
27. Mendes DG, Brandon D, Galor L, et al: Breakage of the metal tray in total knee replacement. *Orthopedics* 1984;7:860–862.
28. Sutherland CJ: Patellar component dissociation in total knee arthroplasty: A report of two cases. *Clin Orthop* 1988;228:178–181.
29. Lombardi AV, Engh GA, Volz RG, et al: Fracture/dissociation of the polyethylene in metal-backed patellar components in total knee arthroplasty. *J Bone Joint Surg* 1988;70A:675–679.
30. Bayley JC, Scott RD, Ewald FC, et al: Failure of the metal-backed patellar component after total hip arthroplasty. *J Bone Joint Surg* 1988;70A:668–674.
31. Stulberg BN, deSwart RJ, Roger S, et al: Factors influencing wear of all-polyethylene patellar components: A retrieval study. Presented at the Meeting of the American Society for the Testing of Materials Symposium on Biocompatibility of Particulate Implant Materials, San Antonio, TX, Oct 31, 1990.
32. Willert H-G, Semlitsch M: Reactions of the articular capsule to wear products of artificial joint prostheses. *J Biomed Mater Res* 1977;11:157–164.
33. Willert H-G, Ludwig J, Semlitsch M: Reaction of bone to methacrylate after hip arthroplasty. A long-term gross, electron microscopic, and scanning electron microscopic study. *J Bone Joint Surg* 1974;56A:1368–1382.
34. Skinner HB, Mabey MF: Soft-tissue response to total hip surface replacement. *J Biomed Mater Res* 1987;21:569–584.
35. Harris WH, Schiller AL, Scholler J-M, et al: Extensive localized bone resorption in the femur following total hip replacement. *J Bone Joint Surg* 1976;58A:612–618.
36. Howie DW, Vernon-Roberts B, Oakeshott R, et al: A rat model of resorption of bone at the cement bone interface in the presence of polyethylene wear particles. *J Bone Joint Surg* 1988;70A:257–263.
37. McKellop HA, Sarmiento A, Schwinn CP, et al: In *vivo* wear of titanium alloy hip prostheses. *J Bone Joint Surg* 1990;72A:512–517.
38. Black J, Sherk H, Bonini J, et al: Metallosis associated with a stable titanium-alloy femoral component in total hip replacement. *J Bone Joint Surg* 1990;72A:126–130.
39. Agins HJ, Alcock NW, Bansal M, et al: Metallic wear in failed titanium-alloy total hip replacements: A histological and quantitative analysis. *J Bone Joint Surg* 1988;70A:347–356.
40. Weightman B, Light D: The effect of the surface finish of alumina and stainless steel on the wear rate of UHMW polyethylene. *Biomaterials* 1986;7:20–24.

41. McKellop AJ, Rostlund TV: The wear behavior of ion implanted Ti-6Al-4V UHWM weight polyethylene. *J Biomed Mater Res* 1990; 24:1413–1425.

42. Collier JP, Mayor MB, Surprenant VA, et al: The biomechanical problems of polyethylene as a bearing surface. *Clin Orthop* 1990; 261:107–113.

43. Skinner HB, Curlin FJ: Decreased pain with lower flexural rigidity of uncemented femoral prostheses. *Orthopedics* 1990;13: 1223–1228.

44. Bobyn JD, Glassman AH, Goto H, et al: The effect of stem stiffness on femoral bone resorption after canine porous-coated total hip arthroplasty. *Clin Orthop* 1990;261:196–213.

Osteotomies of the Hip in the Prevention and Treatment of Osteoarthritis

Michael B. Millis, MD

Robert Poss, MD

Stephen B. Murphy, MD

Introduction

Osteoarthritis of the hip is a common disease in our society. It often affects the young, active patient. Of the more than 100 million adults in the United States aged 20 to 50 years, at least one million have or will develop osteoarthritis of the hip by age 50.[1] While arthroplasty offers a good solution for the painful arthritic hip in the older or inactive patient, the treatment of an active patient in the prime of life with severe osteoarthritis of the hip is problematic. Arthroplasty may fail, and revision arthroplasty is routinely more difficult and shorter lived than the primary operation. Although improving the longevity of primary arthroplasty is desirable, measures to prevent or delay the onset of the osteoarthritis itself seem more appropriate. This chapter focuses on the role of osteotomies of the hip in preventing and treating osteoarthritis.

Etiology

Osteoarthritis (osteoarthrosis) may be considered as primary (idiopathic) or secondary. Idiopathic (primary) osteoarthritis of the hip, representing a biologic failure of articular cartilage in the absence of demonstrable mechanical derangement or deformity, is very rare if it exists at all.[2] Most osteoarthritis of the hip is secondary to pre-existing anatomic deformity. This suggests that many, if not most, cases of osteoarthritis of the hip are theoretically preventable if the predisposing deformity can be prevented or corrected before the osteoarthritis begins. Aronson's careful analysis of large series of patients with end-stage osteoarthritis suggested that as many as 76% had hip dysplasia, Perthes' disease, or slipped capital femoral epiphysis as the etiology of their osteoarthritis (Table 1).[1] Many of these

patients required total hip replacement before age 50. Conversely, long-term follow-up studies of patients with these three developmental hip diseases[3-9] also suggest that such secondary arthritis is a problem of great magnitude. Hip dysplasia historically has led to osteoarthritis by age 50[8,9] in as many as 25% to 50% of patients.[3-5] Perthes' disease has resulted in a 50% incidence of osteoarthritis by age 50.[6,7] Slipped capital femoral epiphysis has led to a 15% to 20% incidence of osteoarthritis by age 50. In these cases, early onset and severity of the secondary osteoarthritis appeared to be related to the degree of deformity present at the end of growth.

There is increasing recognition of the relevance of early intervention in the chain of events that leads to end-stage osteoarthritis. Ideally, primary therapeutic intervention will either prevent or effectively treat the primary disorder that causes the deformity that ultimately leads to the secondary osteoarthritis. Next best is to correct or compensate for, as much as possible, the established deformity from the predisposing developmental hip condition. This is the so-called reconstructive hip osteotomy (Table 2), done at a stage where normal and nearly normal clinical function of the hip can be maintained, and the otherwise poor prognosis of the hip can be restored to normal. Failing this, therapeutic osteotomy can be done after osteoarthritis has developed (salvage osteotomy), to improve present function and to delay the need for arthroplasty.

Table 1
Etiology of endstage osteoarthritis of the hip*

Primary Pathology	(%)
Hip dysplasia	43
Perthes' disease	22
Slipped capital femoral epiphysis	11
Other	12
Idiopathic	12

*Data from Aronson[1]

Table 2
Therapeutic intervention in hip disease: Reconstructive vs salvage osteotomy

Factors	Indications	
	Reconstructive Osteotomy	Salvage Osteotomy
Age	< 20 to 30 (some biologic plasticity remains)	Any
Symptoms	Minimal (but progressive)	Moderate to severe
Motion	Near normal	> 60 degrees flexion
Function	Near normal	Fair to poor
Pathoanatomy	No irreversible changes	Irreversible changes
Radiology	Congruent but malaligned surfaces	Cartilage narrowing and incongruity
Prognosis if untreated	Poor	Poor

The Contemporary Role of Osteotomy in the Prevention of Osteoarthritis of the Hip

It is clear that certain patterns of deformity predispose to the development of osteoarthritis.[2,6,10] In addition, certain developmental hip diseases are often associated with certain of these deformities.[2] The role of reconstructive hip osteotomies as legitimate prophylaxis is increasing.

The poor natural history of acetabular dysplasia, in particular, is now well recognized.[2,4,5,11] More preventive osteotomies are performed for this group of complex deformities than any other. It is problematic that the more severe the symptoms, the easier it is to convince both patient and surgeon that something must be done, and yet the more likely it is that even the best osteotomy may fail to preserve the hip joint for a lifetime. The goal of reconstructive osteotomy is to intervene as early as possible in the disease, before irreversible changes have developed within the joint. The responsibility of the surgeon is clearly great in this relatively asymptomatic group of patients, with good present function and poor prognosis.

Though there is clear evidence of what happens to these hips if corrective surgery is not done, there is not yet the same body of evidence to prove that any osteotomy will significantly improve the natural history. The pioneering work of Wagner,[12] among others, in this most difficult group of patients with severe hip dysplasia, will, over the next decade or two, give us the evidence we require.

The reconstructive osteotomy, whether femoral or pelvic, seeks to normalize joint pressures and unit loads by normalizing pathoanatomy. For the reconstructive hip osteotomy, the assumption usually is that the shape of the articular surfaces is relatively normal and the primary problem is malalignment. The more extreme the malalignment of proximal femur, acetabulum, or both, while congruity and sphericity are preserved, and assuming that normalization of the femoral-acetabular relationship is possible, the more clear the indication is for reconstructive osteotomy.

The theoretical basis of reconstructive osteotomy rests on the following assumptions: (1) Timely correction of the malorientation of the acetabulum and/or proximal femur will restore a normal prognosis to a hip otherwise destined for osteoarthritis; (2) Normal hip anatomy can be adequately characterized to be an achievable goal of surgical treatment; (3) The pathoanatomy (malalignment) of the abnormal hip to be treated can be accurately characterized; and (4) A precise surgical plan can be devised (and carried out) to convert the at-risk hip in the reconstructive stage to a hip with a normal prognosis.

The Contemporary Role of Osteotomy in Treatment of Osteoarthritis[13]

Osteotomy of the hip to treat established osteoarthritis (salvage osteotomy) should be viewed as a complementary rather than a competitive procedure with total hip arthroplasty. As we gain further experience with total hip arthroplasty and are better able to predict the longevity of these procedures (cemented or cementless), the indications for osteotomy and total hip replacement will become clearer. Those patients who are deemed poor candidates for total hip arthroplasty (younger, active patients, with unilateral hip disease) are possibly better candidates for osteotomy. The long-term results of hip replacement suggest increasing longevity with modern prosthetic designs and surgical techniques. As the longevity of hip replacement increases, new problems associated with this longevity emerge: eg, the durability of the bearing surfaces and the preservation of bone stock. Therefore, in the younger, active patient, it is prudent to consider a non-arthroplastic alternative in an attempt to buy time and gain function until arthroplasty is required. The goals of all reconstructive surgery are to relieve pain and improve function, while at the same time preserving bone stock and recognizing that the initial surgery may be the first in a series of operations that the patient will require during a lifetime. When performed in suitable patients, and technically well executed, osteotomy offers an excellent chance of satisfactory long-term results.[14-18] We now treat increasingly well educated patients. They must be advised of the advantages and disadvantages of osteotomy and arthroplasty. The surgeon must be equally comfortable in proposing and executing either procedure. By performing the appropriate procedure in the appropriate patient, the long-term results in both arthroplasty and osteotomy should be optimized and patient satisfaction enhanced.

Principles and Scientific Rationale of Corrective Osteotomy

Bone and cartilage must be loaded to function normally.[19] In comparing the unit load of many joints, both animal and human, a remarkable constancy is observed. The average unit load is approximately 25 kg per cm.[2,20,21] Radiographic features of normal loading in the human hip joint can be seen from the appearance of the subchondral plate in the superior acetabulum, the *sourcil*, as pointed out by Pauwels.[19] Normal load distribution is reflected in a symmetrical subchondral densification on the anteroposterior view. In contrast, in the dysplastic hip, where the unit load is increased because the hip is not well contained, there is an adaptive increase in bone density laterally, and the sourcil becomes eccentric in appearance. Bone and cartilage adapt to increasing loads up to a point, and then they fail. Cartilage degeneration can be arrested, if not reversed, by decreasing excessive unit load, altering the load transmission pattern, and restoring a functional arc of motion. In studies on degenerative arthritis, Mankin and associates[21] have shown that a reparative matrix is secreted by chondrocytes in the early stages of osteoarthritis. Radin and associates[22] demonstrated that repetitive loading of rabbit knees produced deleterious matrix changes, which were reversible with cessation of the repetitive loading. Salter and associates[23] demonstrated a reparative hyaline-like cartilage in rabbits with continuous passive motion.

Degenerative arthritis is accompanied by venous hypertension in the intertrochanteric region. Osteotomy decreases this venous congestion. Investigators have demonstrated that the rest pain of degenerative arthritis is associated with venous hypertension in the intertrochanteric region, and is relieved with decompression.

The beneficial effects of osteotomy in the treatment of osteoarthritis are produced by decreasing unit load (by restoring congruency and decreasing muscle forces) and restoring a functional arc of motion.[10] Remember that osteotomy can also help prevent osteoarthritis by decreasing excessive joint loads before irreversible damage has occurred.

At one time osteotomies were described as either displacement, as popularized by McMurray,[24] or angulation, as popularized by Pauwels.[19] Modern osteotomy combines both angulation and displacement. A varus osteotomy seeks to restore congruency, thus decreasing the unit load, and to decrease muscle forces about the hip by elevating and lateralizing the greater trochanter and by medializing the abductors and psoas. A valgus osteotomy seeks to increase congruency and to transfer the center of hip rotation from the superior aspect of the acetabulum to the medial aspect of the acetabulum, usually to a noninnervated medial osteophyte.[10] When appropriate, a trochanteric osteotomy can be performed in conjunction with the valgus osteotomy to lateralize the greater trochanter.

While it is convenient to think of osteotomies as angulation, displacement, or some combination of both, these distinctions are used more for technical planning than as indications for surgery. It is more useful to recognize that degenerative arthritis is a progressive disease and that intervention at an appropriate time can forestall or reverse the destruction of the joint. Therefore, we recommend that osteotomy be viewed as either a reconstructive or a salvage procedure (Table 2).

A reconstructive osteotomy seeks to restore a normal prognosis to a hip that, although clinically normal or almost normal, is destined for osteoarthritis. A salvage osteotomy is performed in a patient with established arthritis. The goal in salvage osteotomy is to buy time and improve function; ie, to add functional years to

the life of the hip until arthroplasty is required. It is in the salvage group that the difficult decision between arthroplasty and osteotomy must be made. In contrast, the decision in reconstructive osteotomy is whether to undertake preventive or early intervention, or merely to observe the hip. In pelvic osteotomy, reconstructive procedures are those that redirect normally-shaped articular structures to a more physiologic attitude and alignment. Examples of pelvic reconstructive osteotomies are the innominate osteotomies and variants,[25] the periacetabular osteotomy of Ganz and associates,[26] and the acetabular osteotomies of Wagner.[12] Salvage osteotomies include the Chiari[27] and the shelf procedures.

Surgical Planning

In the surgical planning of an osteotomy, a careful clinical evaluation to determine whether the patient is an appropriate candidate is the most important initial task.[28] Technical preparation includes examination under fluoroscopy, tracings, and choice of instrumentation and fixation devices.

Clinical Evaluation of the Patient with Established or Potential Osteoarthritis of the Hip

Patient Selection for Osteotomy

Every patient with potential or established osteoarthritis of the hip requires an assessment of functional demands and functional disability. If osteotomy is to be considered as a treatment, a mechanical etiology must be established for the articular derangement. Next, osteotomy must offer a likelihood of reducing excessive joint pressures. Chronologic and physiologic age, occupation, activity level, habitus, and patient goals are all important secondary factors in deciding for or against an osteotomy. Leg lengths and status of ipsilateral knee and spine are also relevant.

The ideal candidate for reconstructive osteotomy is younger than 25 years of age, with enough biologic plasticity remaining to tolerate major articular alignment.

The ideal candidate for salvage osteotomy is generally younger than 50 years of age, but can be somewhat older if all criteria are met. Ideally, the patient is not obese and is a sedentary worker, rather than one who engages in heavy physical labor.[16] It is essential that a mechanical pathogenesis be demonstrated on radiographs.[10,19] If cartilage and bone demonstrate radiographically a capacity to respond to mechanical overload, then by inference these tissues are capable of a healing process once a proper mechanical environment has been restored. The radiologic criteria demonstrated by an ideal candidate are those of excessive unit load (Fig. 1): A localized increase in radiodensity, localized joint narrowing, and cyst formation. If there is incon-

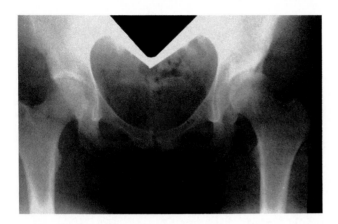

Fig. 1 20-year-old woman with a two-year history of left hip pain. No previous history of hip disease. Left hip demonstrates radiographic signs of excessive unit load associated with acetabular dysplasia, increased subchondral sclerosis, and acetabular cyst formation.

gruity, then improved congruency must be demonstrated on examination under fluoroscopy.

Range of Motion

Range of motion of the involved hip is of crucial importance in the patient with established osteoarthritis for several reasons. First, the discrepancy between functional arcs of motion required in activities of daily living and the limited range of motion present often can lead to the impingement and pain characteristic of advanced osteoarthritis. An important benefit of a successful salvage osteotomy is the restoration of a functional arc of motion, usually achieved by eliminating the flexion-adduction contracture of the hip through the increase in extension and abduction that follows either valgus-extension intertrochanteric osteotomy or Chiari pelvic osteotomy.

Patients who undergo osteotomy usually neither gain nor lose overall hip motion. A minimum of 80 degrees of flexion arc is preferred. Patients with less motion may undergo postoperative spontaneous ankylosis.[10] The magnitude of angular correction in the coronal plane should not significantly exceed the patient's abduction to adduction arc. For example, if a 30-degree valgus osteotomy is performed in a patient who can only adduct 10 degrees, the patient may walk in abduction and experience severe valgus strain in the knee.

Radiographic Evaluation

Radiographic evaluation begins with an anteroposterior pelvis and false profile views.[29] The importance of the false profile view cannot be overemphasized, because some patients with hip dysplasia have nearly normal anteroposterior radiographs, with anterior subluxation seen only on the false profile view (Fig. 2). Functional radiographs in adduction and abduction

and preoperative fluoroscopy are helpful to determine if concentric motion is present or if congruity is improved with certain positions. Arthrography is rarely necessary. Finally, three-dimensional analysis can be used to determine the anatomic deformity as compared with normal anatomy. Preoperative simulation of surgery assists in the selection of the osteotomy that will maximally normalize the patient's hip.[30,31]

Currently, each patient referred to us for surgical evaluation of acetabular dysplasia undergoes three-dimensional imaging study. For younger patients we use magnetic resonance studies, and for patients older than 8 to 10 years of age we use computed tomographic studies. The studies include images through the iliac spines, the hip joint, and the distal femoral condyles.

The image data from the study are transferred to a computing facility, where the images are reformatted and displayed on graphics processors. The bony surfaces of the femurs and pelvis are calculated automatically, based on radiodensity, and are stored as contours. The contours from sequential images are connected using triangular surface tiles to create three-dimensional models of the bone and joint surfaces. The models of the bones can then be displayed in any position or orientation.

Femoral[32] and pelvic[33] reference coordinate systems are used to eliminate the effect of patient positioning on the geometric analysis. The overall orientation of each acetabulum is determined by calculating a plane that best describes all of the points on the acetabular rim. The vector normal to the opening plane of the acetabulum is calculated and resolved to determine the acetabular abduction and anteversion angles.

Analysis of the acetabular and femoral head surfaces is based on the subchondral bone surfaces. Nonarticular portions, such as the fovea and acetabular notch, are specifically excluded. The joint surface points are used to define spheres of specific radius and position that best describe the surfaces of the acetabulum and femoral head. The distance between the centers of the femoral head and acetabulum are measured to quantify the presence or absence of concentric reduction of the joint.

The ability of the acetabulum to contain the femoral head is quantified using two methods: (1) Lateral, anterior, and posterior center-edge (CE) angles are measured to quantify containment relative to the pelvis. (2) Containment of the femoral head by the acetabular rim is measured by modeling the acetabulum as a portion of a globe. This is done by defining the polar axis of the globe as a perpendicular to the opening plane of the rim and then dividing the globe into latitudes and longitudes. The location of the acetabular rim is then calculated in degrees latitude for each longitude. For example, if the acetabulum were a complete hemisphere, each latitude angle would measure 90 degrees. If the acetabulum were one fourth of a sphere, the

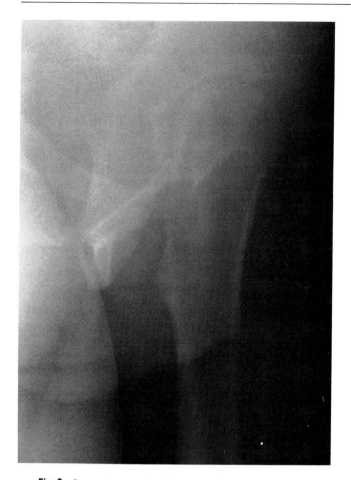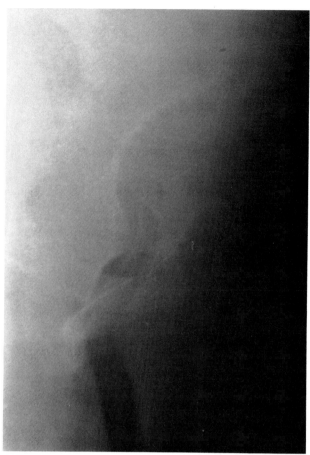

Fig. 2 Same woman as in Figure 1. **Left**, Anteroposterior radiograph showed moderate left acetabular dysplasia. False profile lateral view of right hip shows normal anterior coverage. **Right**, False profile lateral of left hip shows severe anterior dysplasia and proximal subluxation of femoral head.

latitude angles would be 45 degrees. These geometric calculations are made on the patient's hips and then compared with the values of more than 50 normal patients (Murphy SB, Millis MB, Khewski P: Unpublished data). Abnormalities are identified and the goals of surgery are developed.

Using these techniques, various pelvic osteotomy plans can be simulated to determine their normalizing effect. For example, the single innominate osteotomy of Salter[34] is simulated by dividing the pelvis from the sciatic notch to the anterior inferior iliac spine. The distal pelvic fragment, which includes the acetabulum, is then rotated around an axis defined by the pubic symphysis and the sciatic notch. Any degree of rotation can be simulated, but 25 to 30 degrees is about the maximum that can realistically be achieved.

The dial osteotomy is simulated by dividing the acetabulum from the surrounding pelvis using a spherical cut of a defined radius. The free acetabular fragment can then be rotated and translated in any desired position. Following simulation, the geometry of the hip joint can be recalculated and compared with normal

hip geometry to determine the effect of the proposed osteotomy. The osteotomy plan that maximally achieves the surgical goals is then recommended.

Principles: Femoral vs Pelvic Pathology

In general, femoral osteotomy is indicated for primary femoral problems and pelvic osteotomy is indicated for primary acetabular problems. Because osteonecrosis, slipped epiphysis, and Perthes' disease involve the femoral head, femoral osteotomy is usually indicated to correct them.

Conversely, for hip dysplasia, which always involves acetabular deformity, pelvic osteotomy (at least) is usually indicated. If there is a femoral deformity as well (caused either by the disease or by its treatment), then femoral osteotomy may be indicated as well. Hip dysplasia is rarely a primary[15] femoral deformity and, therefore, reconstructive femoral osteotomy alone is very rarely indicated.

Limb Alignment and Limb Length

The planning of the intertrochanteric osteotomy must include an assessment of leg lengths and the effect

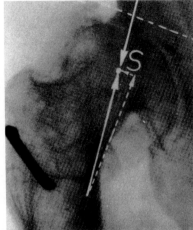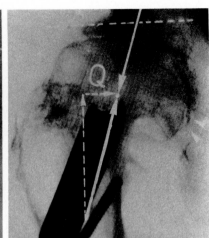

Fig. 3 Valgus osteotomy can stimulate the formation of the roof osteophyte by lateral traction on the superior joint capsule. (Reproduced with permission from Bombelli R: *Osteoarthritis of the Hip.* Springer-Verlag, Berlin, 1983, p 168.)

of osteotomy on the mechanical axis of the limb.[10,28] Of particular importance is the effect of hip realignment on the ipsilateral knee. When varus osteotomy is performed, medial shaft displacement is required so that the mechanical axis of the extremity remains through the center of the knee. Similarly, lateral shaft displacement is required in valgus osteotomy.

Various Intertrochanteric Osteotomies

Varus Osteotomy

The classic radiographic candidate for isolated varus osteotomy is a patient whose hip has a spherical femoral head, little or no acetabular dysplasia (a center-edge angle of at least 15 to 20 degrees), signs of lateral overloading of the sourcil (the acetabular subchondral plate), and a valgus neck-shaft angle of more than 135 degrees. If radiographs in hip abduction demonstrate improved congruity of the hip, the varus osteotomy is indicated. By performing varus osteotomy with medial shaft displacement, the abductors, psoas, and adductors are relatively relaxed, thus unloading the hip joint, and the weightbearing surface is increased. Medial shaft displacement of 10 mm to 15 mm is desirable, not only to decrease the force of the adductors, but also to keep the ipsilateral knee centered under the femoral head, thus maintaining the mechanical axis of the limb.

In various published series, well-selected candidates achieved long-term, good-to-excellent results in more than 90% of cases.[16] Varus osteotomy carries with it, however, the certainty of approximately 1.0 cm of shortening, the presence of a Trendelenburg gait for approximately one year, and a prominent greater trochanter. Patients must be aware of the longer convalescent period intrinsic with this operation.

Valgus Osteotomy (Salvage)

When the femoral head is no longer spherical, the goals of decreasing the unit load and improving con-

gruence often can be achieved by a valgus osteotomy. Osteophytes that form in predictable locations on the femoral head and acetabulum are exploited to achieve the desired result.[10] The capital drop and inferior cervical osteophytes of the femoral head are brought into contact with the floor osteophytes of the acetabulum by adduction of the hip. With these osteophytes now serving as a fulcrum, the superior and lateral joint space is widened. An assessment of the magnitude of correction required can be obtained by examination under fluoroscopy, tracings, or radiographs obtained in various degrees of hip adduction. Sufficient valgus correction should be done so that lateral traction on the superior capsule results in the stimulation of formation of the roof osteophyte (Fig. 3). Pain relief is achieved by: (1) Unloading the hip joint (abductor and psoas relaxation); (2) Changing the bone contact from the painful innervated superior femoral head and acetabulum to noninnervated medial osteophytes; (3) Decreasing the lever arm of body weight by shifting it medially to the new center of rotation of the femoral head, the osteophytes; and (4) Improving the congruity of the joint and thus increasing the weightbearing surface. Further long-term improvement may come with formation of the roof osteophyte, which further increases the weightbearing surface, and cartilage healing.

Extension

In addition to angular correction in the coronal plane, correction in the sagittal plane can increase the effectiveness of osteotomy. Biplane correction is desirable for two reasons: (1) In acetabular dysplasia, the femoral head is uncovered not only laterally (the frontal plane) but anteriorly (the sagittal plane). Better coverage is achieved by correction in both planes; (2) Fixed flexion contractures can be eliminated by extension correction to a degree at least equal to the magnitude of the flexion contracture. By so doing, the functional

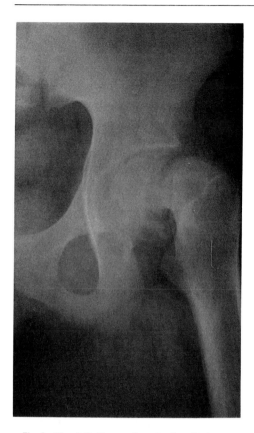

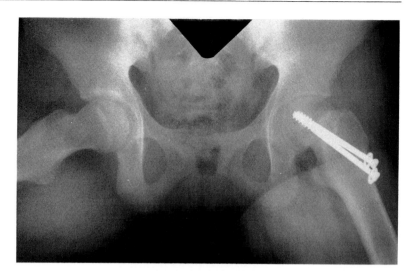

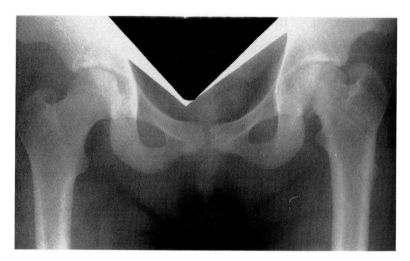

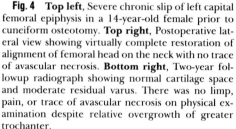

Fig. 4 **Top left**, Severe chronic slip of left capital femoral epiphysis in a 14-year-old female prior to cuneiform osteotomy. **Top right**, Postoperative lateral view showing virtually complete restoration of alignment of femoral head on the neck with no trace of avascular necrosis. **Bottom right**, Two-year followup radiograph showing normal cartilage space and moderate residual varus. There was no limp, pain, or trace of avascular necrosis on physical examination despite relative overgrowth of greater trochanter.

arc of motion is returned to within the anatomic arc, and an important source of pain and impingement is removed.[10] The use of the term extension is often confusing. Extension refers to the angular correction of the femur in the sagittal plane after osteotomy. Thus, with extension, the apex of the angle is directed anteriorly. To achieve this correction, the femur is flexed to the desired degree, the osteotomy is performed, and the distal femoral fragment brought parallel to the floor. Thus, the proximal fragment is flexed, but the final angular correction of the femur is said to be extended.

Rotation

Patients with dysplastic hips have a constellation of anatomic variations in the pelvic and femoral sides of the hip joint. The acetabulum is usually deficient both laterally and anteriorly, the femoral neck may be in excess valgus (greater than 135 degrees), and antever-

sion may be increased. The true degree of femoral anteversion (and hence the true neck shaft valgus) can be determined by fluoroscopic or other methods. It is likely that a neck shaft angle of 150 degrees seen on the anteroposterior radiograph is in reality a combination of a 140- to 145-degree neck shaft angle and a 25-degree femoral anteversion. Preoperative planning for a varus-extension osteotomy should allow for 10 to 15 degrees of derotation (leave 15 degrees of residual internal rotation to allow for a normal gait) and varus correction of 10 to 20 degrees.

Intertrochanteric Osteotomy for Severe Slipped Capital Femoral Epiphysis

The major deformity in chronic severe slipped capital femoral epiphysis is an extension deformity through the upper femoral neck and physis, with an associated severe retroversion and a secondary apparent varus deformity (Fig. 4, *top left*). Most efficient correction of the deformity follows an osteotomy through the open physis, although the hazards of avascular necrosis following surgery at this level are well known. A less hazardous therapeutic option in those cases with deformity severe enough to require correction is a flexion intertrochanteric osteotomy by the method of Imhauser. This osteotomy involves a transverse intertrochanteric osteotomy cut just above the level of the lesser trochanter, with anterior translocation and flexion of the distal fragment, to align the femoral shaft perpendicular to the plane of the physis. A wedge from the distal end of the proximal fragment is not routinely removed (Fig. 4).

An extensive anterior capsulotomy is done for several reasons. First, it facilitates accurate placement of the blade portion of the blade plate routinely used for the internal fixation. Secondly, it facilitates preliminary placement of a cancellous epiphyseal screw before making the osteotomy cut if the physis remains open. Thirdly, the anterior capsulotomy allows the head and neck fragment to extend enough after the intertrochanteric flexion osteotomy so that an unacceptable flexion contracture does not result.

Along with the flexion aspect of the osteotomy, which is the major correction, any necessary derotation can be accomplished easily by simple rotation of the distal fragment (usually internally) before final fixation of the plate portion of the implant to the femoral shaft.

Little correction is necessary in the usual case of severe chronic slipped capital femoral epiphysis in which most of the varus deformity is only apparent. In these cases, major corrective flexion will restore the greater trochanteric tip to an appropriate height with relation to the center of the femoral head.

If a flexion correction of more than 55 or 60 degrees is carried out, some authors prefer to modify the Imhauser osteotomy by making it a three-part osteotomy. A separate trochanteric osteotomy is done to avoid excessive flexion forward of the greater trochanter, which theoretically could impair abductor function.

Intertrochanteric Osteotomy for Osteonecrosis

In selected cases of osteonecrosis, intertrochanteric redirectional osteotomy can greatly improve hip function and can maintain it at a high level for many years. For redirectional intertrochanteric osteotomy to have a good chance of success in this condition, there must be a reasonable range of motion remaining and a reasonable cartilage space. The sum of the arcs of the involved head segments on the anteroposterior and lateral views should be less than 220 degrees. The osteotomy must be able to deliver normal bone into at least 50% of the weightbearing area, but the entire necrotic segment need not be delivered from the weightbearing area. In addition, a functional arc of motion must remain following osteotomy.

In the commonest variety of segmental osteonecrosis

amenable to redirectional intertrochanteric osteotomy, the involved segment is anterolateral. In this situation, a valgus flexion intertrochanteric osteotomy is most likely to yield clinical success.

Varus intertrochanteric osteotomy is occasionally used to treat segmental osteonecrosis if the healthy subchondral bone is central and lateral and the involved segment is more medial than lateral.

Reconstructive Pelvic Osteotomies

Reconstructive osteotomies involve redirecting the existing acetabulum into a more appropriate position. These procedures include the single innominate osteotomy,[34] the double innominate osteotomy,[35] the triple innominate osteotomy,[24,35] and the periacetabular osteotomies.[12,26,37,38] The single innominate osteotomy extends and retroverts the acetabulum around a fixed axis. This osteotomy also tends to lateralize the joint. Because the dysplastic hip joint is usually already excessively lateral, lateralization should be avoided. Also, since the degree of correction by this osteotomy decreases with age, the indication for this operation also decreases with age. The double and triple osteotomies were developed in an attempt to avoid lateralization of the joint and to improve correction. The ischial cut of the Steel osteotomy is quite far from the joint. As a result, significant angular corrections create a large secondary deformity of the ischium and the potential for ischial nonunion. The triple osteotomies described by Tonnis[25] and Jakob (personal communication, 1991) include an ischial osteotomy that is much closer to the acetabulum. The ischial osteotomy of the Tonnis triple osteotomy is performed through a posterior approach with the patient in the prone position. The Jakob triple osteotomy includes an ischial osteotomy via a medial approach, which allows all three osteotomies to be performed with the patient in the supine position. Even so, Jakob reserves the triple osteotomy for the patients with an open triradiate cartilage and recommends a periacetabular osteotomy for the skeletally mature patient.

The periacetabular osteotomies include those described by Eppright,[37] Ganz and associates,[26] and Wagner.[12] The osteotomy described by Eppright is a barrel-shaped osteotomy with an anterior-posterior axis. This osteotomy allows for excellent lateral coverage but is limited in the amount of anterior coverage that can be achieved. Because anterior instability is a major, if not primary component of dysplasia, the osteotomies described by Ganz and Wagner have the greatest versatility. The periacetabular osteotomy described by Ganz and associates involves a series of straight cuts combined with a controlled fracture to separate the acetabulum from the surrounding pelvis. Because there is no medial buttress, the joint can be medialized as needed. In addition, the acetabulum can be extended as necessary to improve anterior stability. Because the external portion of the ischium is left undissected, it is believed that branches of the inferior gluteal artery supply the acetabular fragment in addition to the capsular vessels. The advantage of this osteotomy is that a capsulotomy can be performed, when indicated, to remove labral tears. The disadvantage of the osteotomy lies with the asphericity of the osteotomies. Because the osteotomy is not spherical, extension of the acetabulum causes anterior displacement of the hip joint. Prevention of anterior displacement requires trimming the corners of the acetabular fragment.

The spherical osteotomy of Wagner[38] has the advantage of excellent osteotomy congruity, rapid healing, and intrinsic stability with minimal internal fixation. The disadvantage of type I spherical osteotomy is that the medial buttress of the quadrilateral plate prevents medialization of the joint. Therefore, if medialization is a goal, a type III spherical osteotomy, which includes two osteotomies (the second is an additional Chiari-like cut proximally) must be performed. This osteotomy relies on the capsular blood supply to support the acetabular fragment. Therefore, a capsulotomy for the treatment of intra-articular pathology is relatively contraindicated. Although the complication of avascular necrosis of the acetabulum is often discussed, this has not occurred in our series of over 50 spherical osteotomies.

Salvage Pelvic Osteotomies: Chiari and Shelf Procedures

Pelvic procedures are broadly divided into reconstructive and salvage procedures. The salvage procedures, which include the shelf and Chiari osteotomies, are generally reserved for severely incongruous and unstable hip joints. Care should be taken to avoid condemning a hip to a salvage procedure on the basis of the anteroposterior radiograph. The posterior/inferior portion of the acetabulum is often spared from the disease. If this portion of the acetabulum can be rotated superiorly, the congruity of the joint can be dramatically improved by reconstructive osteotomy.[26] In the rare case where no portion of the acetabulum is spared from the incongruity, a salvage procedure is indicated. The Chiari osteotomy is performed by abducting the acetabulum into a more vertical and medial position and replacing it with joint capsule supported by the bony buttress of the iliac wing.[27]

There are three pitfalls to be avoided when performing Chiari's osteotomy. First, it is necessary to medialize and abduct the distal (acetabular) fragment and to avoid lateralizing the proximal fragment without abducting the distal fragment. Second, if the iliac osteotomy is not angled from distal lateral/anterior to proximal medial/posterior, the iliac buttress will be too horizontal, resulting in a persistently unstable joint laterally. Third, because this osteotomy creates a triangular bony defect anteriorly, this defect must be grafted with a curved plate of bone graft from the iliac wing. Failure to create

an adequate anterior buttress will result in a persistently unstable joint anteriorly, which does not show on the anteroposterior radiograph. Even if this operation is performed correctly, many patients will limp for a prolonged period of time, if not indefinitely.

A torn acetabular labrum can lead to a poor result after Chiari osteotomy. If a Chiari is being done, an arthrogram should rule out a tear. If a torn labrum is found, it should be repaired.

After Chiari osteotomy, two crutches should be used for at least three months to allow the capsule under the iliac buttress to transform into cartilage.

Summary

Osteoarthritis of the hip is common in our society, even in the relatively young patient. Most of this osteoarthritis is mechanical in etiology and is secondary to residual deformity from developmental hip disease. This type of osteoarthritis can often be predicted and prevented if the causative excessive joint pressures are reduced in a timely fashion by corrective osteotomy. Realigning pelvic or intertrochanteric osteotomy of this preventive type is termed reconstructive; those osteotomies performed after osteoarthritis is established are termed salvage.

Corrective osteotomy will be clinically successful only if the mechanical etiology for the potential or established osteoarthritis is clear and if the osteotomy succeeds in reducing the pathologically excessive joint loads. The clinical success of osteotomy also requires precise technical planning preoperatively and careful operative technique.

References

1. Aronson J: Osteoarthritis of the young adult hip: etiology and treatment, in Anderson LD (ed): *Instructional Course Lectures, XXXV.* St. Louis, CV Mosby, 1986, chap 35, 119–128.
2. Harris WH: Etiology of osteoarthritis of the hip. *Clin Orthop* 1986;213:20–33.
3. Wiberg G: Studies on dysplasic acetabula and congenital subluxation of the hip joint with special reference to the complications of osteoarthritis. *Acta Chir Scand Suppl* 1939;83(suppl 58):5–135.
4. Cooperman DR, Wallensten R, Stulberg SD: Post-reduction avascular necrosis in congenital dislocation of the hip: Long-term follow-up study of twenty five patients. *J Bone Joint Surg* 1980;62A:247–258.
5. Cooperman DR, Wallensten R, Stulberg SD: Acetabular dysplasia in the adult. *Clin Orthop* 1983;175:79–85.
6. Stulberg SD, Cooperman DR, Wallensten R: The natural history of Legg-Calvé-Perthes Disease. *J Bone Joint Surg* 1981;63A:1095–1108.
7. McAndrew MM, Weinstein SL: A long term follow-up of Legg-Calvé-Perthes Disease. *J Bone Joint Surg* 1984;66A:860–869.
8. Boyer DW, Mickelson M, Ponseti IV: Slipped capital femoral epiphysis: Long-term follow-up study of one hundred and twenty-one patients. *J Bone Joint Surg* 1981;63A:85–95.
9. Ordeberg G, Hansson LI, Sandstrom S: Slipped capital femoral epiphysis in Southern Sweden: Long term result or symptomatic treatment. *Clin Orthop* 1984;191:95–104.

10. Bombelli R: *Osteoarthritis of the Hip*, ed 2. Berlin, Springer-Verlag, 1983.

11. Weinstein SL: Natural history of congenital hip dislocation (CDH) and hip dysplasia. *Clin Orthop* 1987;225:62–76.

12. Wagner H: Experiences with spherical acetabular osteotomy for the correction of the dysplastic acetabulum. *Prog Orthop Surg* 1978;2:131.

13. Poss R: The role of osteotomy in the treatment of osteoarthritis of the hip: Current concepts review. *J Bone Joint Surg* 1984;66A:144–151.

14. Harris NH, Kirwan E: The results of osteotomy for early primary osteoarthritis of the hip. *J Bone Joint Surg* 1964;46B:477–487.

15. Langlais F, Roure J-L, Maquet P: Valgus osteotomy in severe osteoarthritis of the hip. *J Bone Joint Surg* 1979;61B:424–431.

16. Morscher EW: Intertrochanteric osteotomy in osteoarthritis of the hip, in *The Hip: Proceedings of the Eighth Open Scientific Meeting of the Hip Society*. St. Louis, CV Mosby, 1980.

17. Schneider R: Results of intertrochanteric osteotomies in patients with coxarthrosis 12–15 years after surgery, in Weil UH (ed): *Joint Preserving Procedures of the Lower Extremities*. Berlin, Springer-Verlag, 1980, vol 4, pp 39–43.

18. Miegel RE, Harris WH: Medial-displacement intertrochanteric osteotomy in the treatment of osteoarthritis of the hip. *J Bone Joint Surg* 1984;66A:878–887.

19. Pauwels F: *Biomechanics of the Normal and Diseased Hip: Theoretical Foundation, Technique, and Results of Treatment*. Berlin, Springer-Verlag, 1976.

20. Ewald FC, Poss R, Pugh J, et al: Hip cartilage supported by methacrylate in canine arthroplasty. *Clin Orthop* 1982;171:273–279.

21. Mankin HJ, Dorfman H, Lippiello L, et al: Biochemical and metabolic abnormalities in articular cartilage from osteo-arthritic human hips: II. Correlation of morphology with biochemical and metabolic data. *J Bone Joint Surg* 1971;53A:523–537.

22. Radin EL, Ehrlich MG, Chernack R, et al: Effect of repetitive impulsive loading on the knee joints of rabbits. *Clin Orthop* 1978;131:288–293.

23. Salter RB, Simmonds DF, Malcolm BW, et al: The biological effect of continuous passive motion on the healing of full-thickness defects in articular cartilage: An experimental investigation in the rabbit. *J Bone Joint Surg* 1980;62A:1232–1251.

24. McMurray TP: Osteo-arthritis of the hip joint. *J Bone Joint Surg* 1939;21:1–11.

25. Tonnis D: *Congenital Dysplasia and Dislocation of the Hip in Children and Adults*. Berlin, Springer-Verlag, 1987.

26. Ganz R, Klaue K, Vinh TS, et al: A new periacetabular osteotomy for the treatment of hip dysplasias: Technique and preliminary results. *Clin Orthop* 1988;232:26–36.

27. Chiari K: Medial displacement osteotomy of the pelvis. *Clin Orthop* 1974;98:55–71.

28. Schatzker J: *The Intertrochanteric Osteotomy*. Berlin, Springer-Verlag, 1984.

29. Lequesne M, de Seze S: Le faux profile du bassin: Nouvell incidence radiographique par l'étude de la hanch: Son utilité dans les dysplasies et les differentes coxopathies. *Rev Rhum Mal Osteoartic* 1961;28:643.

30. Klaue K, Wallin A, Ganz R: CT evaluation of coverage and congruency of the hip prior to osteotomy. *Clin Orthop* 1988;232:15–25.

31. Murphy SB, Kijewski PK, Millis MB, et al: The planning of orthopaedic reconstructive surgery using computer-aided simulation and design. *Comput Med Imaging Graph* 1988;12:33–45.

32. Murphy SB, Kijewski PK, Millis MB, et al: Acetabular dysplasia in the adolescent and young adult. *Clin Orthop* 1990;261:213–222.

33. McKibbin B: Anatomical factors in the stability of the hip joint in the newborn. *J Bone Joint Surg* 1970;52B:148–159.

34. Salter RB: Innominate osteotomy in the treatment of congenital dislocation and subluxation of the hip. *J Bone Joint Surg* 1961;43B:518–539.

35. Sutherland DH, Greenfield R: Double innominate osteotomy. *J Bone Joint Surg* 1977;59A:1082–1091.

36. Steel HH: Triple osteotomy of the innominate bone. *J Bone Joint Surg* 1973;55A:343–350.

37. Eppright RH: Dial osteotomy of the acetabulum in the treatment of dysplasia of the hip. *J Bone Joint Surg* 1976;58A:726.

38. Wagner H: Osteotomies for congenital hip dislocation, in *The Hip: Proceedings of the Fourth Open Scientific Meeting of the Hip Society*. St. Louis, CV Mosby, 1976, pp 45–66.

Spine

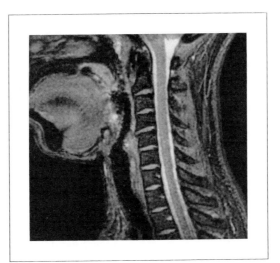

Posterior Screw Plate Fixation in Thoracolumbar Injuries

R. Roy-Camille, MD

Introduction

I have been using plate-and-screw fixation for posterior spine stabilization since 1963. During this time, the instrumentation used has evolved progressively in design in order to face new problems that have arisen from the pathology of the lesions to be treated, or to deal with the different anatomic levels of the spine.[1-18]

Instrumentation

The plates used at the thoracic and thoracolumbar levels (Fig. 1, *left*) are 1 cm wide, and the holes are spaced 13 mm apart. This spacing of the holes has been selected because the mean distance between two ver-tebral pedicles is approximately 26 mm. In order to prevent plate breakage, we have developed plates with reinforced holes. The plates are precontoured to allow them to adapt to or to reconstitute the normal curvature of the posterior aspect of the spine. The concept of precontouring is very important because as the plates are implanted and the screws are tightened into the pedicles, the spine is drawn back towards the plates, restoring its normal curvature.

At the lumbar level, I often use a special short lumbar plate (Fig. 1, *center*), which fits the height of three lumbar vertebrae. The holes in these plates are in a different position. At each end of the plate there are three holes with a distance of 9 mm between them. Another hole is located at the midpoint of the plate. The three holes at either end are used to implant two screws into

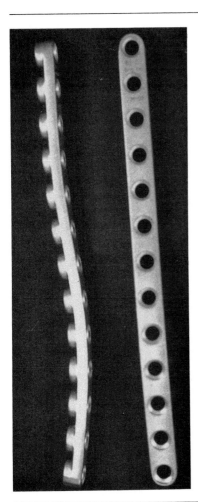
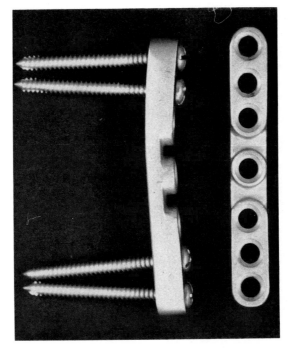
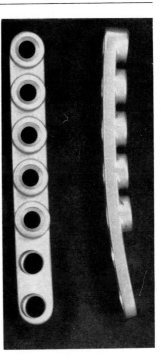

Fig. 1 Left, The plates for thoracic and thoracolumbar levels (they are available in different lengths, from 5 to 21 holes); **Center,** Short special lumbar plate; **Right,** For lumbosacral junction.

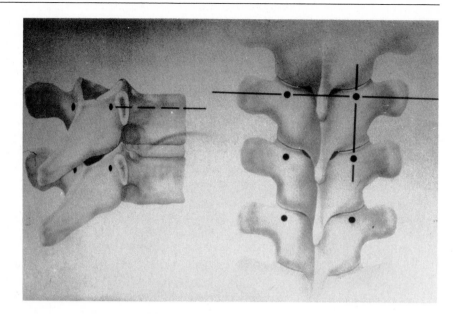

Fig. 2   Point of entry of the screw on the thoracic spine.

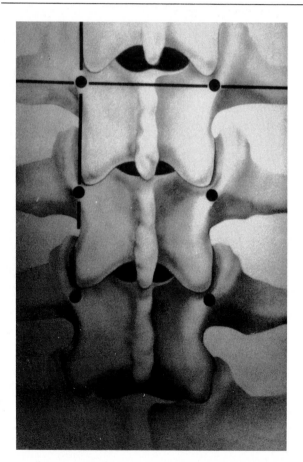

Fig. 3   Point of entry of the screw on the lumbar spine.

one pedicle through two adjacent holes. In the lumbar spine, the vertebral pedicles are broad enough to allow placement of two screws into one pedicle.

Plates used at the lumbosacral junction are flat at the inferior part and have three holes that face obliquely in a lateral direction (Fig. 1, *right*), which means that there must be right- and left-hand plates. Screws are implanted through the inferior holes into the bony lateral part of the sacrum, giving stronger fixation.

The screw-plate interface at the reinforced hole is not rigidly constrained but has a slight clearance, which allows a small amount of motion and helps to avoid screw breakage.

Two types of screws are available with the system. The first type is a standard bone screw, available in diameters of 3.5, 4.0, and 4.5 mm. The second type of screw is specifically designed for implantation into the pedicles. This screw is composed of two sections. The first section, which is implanted into the vertebral body, has a large thread. It comes in diameters of 3.5, 4.0, 4.5, or 5.5 mm and lengths of 30 to 45 mm. The posterior section of the screw, which goes through the plate, has a standard diameter of 5.0 mm and has a fine thread to receive a locknut. This type of screw also has a clearance between screws and plates to decrease screw breakage. This design feature is a basic element of my philosophy of spinal plating.

In working at the thoracic and thoracolumbar levels, the surgeon must be extremely familiar with the anatomic features of the pedicles in order to implant the screws accurately. In my institution the rules are simple and always constant. The screws are implanted perpendicular to the vertebra and straight forward from

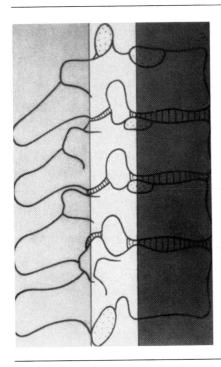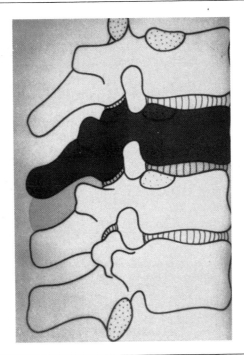

Fig. 4 Left, The three vertical segments of the spine. **Right,** The two horizontal segments of the spine.

the point of entry. The pedicle is at the junction of the transverse process and the lamina. It connects to the superior articular facet just below its inferior edge. Once the facet joint line is exposed, the point of entry is just 1 mm below this facet joint. The facet joint is in a frontal plane, and the point of entry must be exactly in the midline of the joint. This point is at the base of the transverse process on a small crest of bone that usually slopes down medially. The point of entry can also be located at the junction of two crosslines (Fig. 2). One of these is a vertical line in the midpart of the facet joint; the other is a horizontal line that goes through the upper part of the base of the two transverse processes.

In the thoracic spine, the diameter of the pedicles is small. The smallest, T5, is only about 3.5 mm in diameter. The small screws required can be used without the risk of breakage because in this system, too, the screw-plate interface is not rigid and the slight motion allowed limits the stresses imparted to the screws. In the thoracic spine, the screws used are usually between 30 and 35 mm long.

At thoracolumbar junction, the anatomic configuration of the pedicles is the same as in the thoracic spine. At T12-L1 and in the lumbar spine, however, the orientation of the facet joints is more sagittal than coronal. The point of entry is still 1 mm below the inferior edge of the facet joint and on the line of the facet joint. Here, the point of entry of the pedicle can still be located, as in the thoracic spine, at the junction of the same two crosslines (Fig. 3). Another very good landmark at the lumbar level is a crest going up from

the lower facet, lateral to the isthmus. This crest ascends to the level of the point of entry, and it is often necessary to flatten it with a rongeur before drilling into it with the drill bit. The screws used at the thoracolumbar junction are 4 mm in diameter and are usually 40 mm long.

For the lumbosacral spine, S1 is considered to have a normal pedicle. Here, too, the point of penetration is 1 mm below the middle of the facet joint, which is oblique both inferiorly and medially. The screw is directed either perpendicular to the posterior aspect of S1 and straight anteriorly or, better, slightly superiorly so that it can gain purchase in the dense bone below the S1 superior endplate. Lower in the sacrum, the screws are oriented in a lateral direction through the oblique holes of the plates in the thicker bone of the sacral ala. The lower sacral screws are 4 mm in diameter and 40 mm long and have a small, 6-mm head in order to prevent prominence and skin scar. Screws used in the lumbar spine are 4.5 mm in diameter and are usually 45 mm long. Screws 5.5 mm in diameter can also be used, mainly in revision surgery.

Indications for Posterior Spinal Plating in Traumatic Cases

The first indication is a neurologic involvement with cord damage. The best decompression is achieved by the reduction of the displacement with or without a laminectomy. After the decompression, the fixation that is performed with spinal plates is very important,

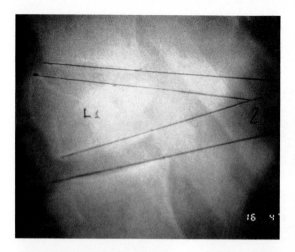
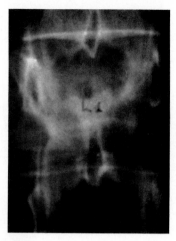
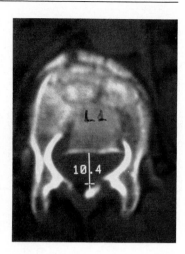
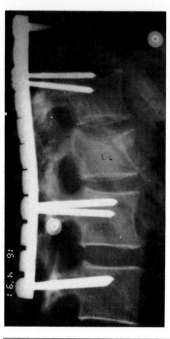
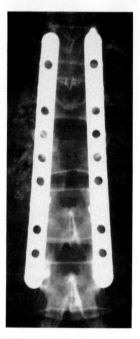

Fig. 5 Reduction and fixation of a fracture of L1, two vertebrae above and two below. **Top left,** Preoperative lateral view; **Top center,** Anteroposterior view; **Top right,** Computed tomography scan; **Bottom left,** Postoperative lateral view, **Bottom center,** Anteroposterior view.

because it must prevent secondary displacement and reestablish the stability of the spine.

The second indication for spinal plating is unstable lesions of the spine even in the absence of neurologic involvement. Here, too, plating is important because of the risk of a secondary displacement, which can induce a late neurologic deterioration. My analysis of the spine usually includes three vertical and two horizontal segments (Fig. 4). The middle vertical segment (posterior wall, pedicles, articular facets) and the mobile horizontal segment (soft tissue between two vertebrae) are the main elements providing stability of the spine. Their damage will induce instability.

The third indication is significant displacement with deformity of the spine. This condition can require treatment even in the absence of a cord syndrome because such a deformity tends to increase progressively, and

because magnetic resonance imaging has demonstrated evidence in some cases of a secondary post-traumatic cyst of the cord at the level of a marked kyphosis. To prevent the development of such a chronic definitive cord syndrome it may be necessary to correct the initial deformity of the spine.

The indications are as follows: (1) kyphosis of more than 20 degrees on the vertebrae immediately above and below, (2) bayonet displacement that narrows the surface area of the spinal canal by more than 50%, or (3) a posterior fragment protruding in the spinal canal with the same decrease in canal area. It is obvious that if the deformity can be corrected by conservative treatment, as for instance Boehler's technique for a thoracolumbar fracture in kyphosis, surgery is not indicated.

In the thoracolumbar spine, posterior plating is well

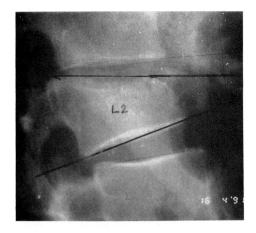
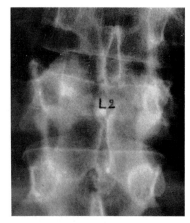
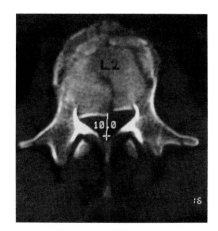
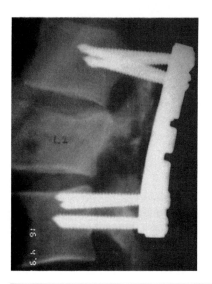
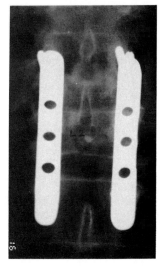

Fig. 6 Reduction and fixation of a fracture of L2, one vertebrae above and one below with two screws in each pedicle. **Top left,** Preoperative lateral view; **Top center,** Anteroposterior view; **Top right,** Computed tomography scan; **Bottom left,** Postoperative lateral view; **Bottom center,** Anteroposterior view.

adapted to the treatment of spinal trauma. The vertebral body can usually be restored to its normal height and shape. In order to achieve adequate stability and leverage for reduction, posterior plating usually requires inclusion of two vertebra above and two vertebra below the lesion (Fig. 5). With this long fixation we usually do a short posterolateral fusion, bridging just one disk above the fractured vertebra, or two disks (one above and one below the fractured vertebra).

In the lumbar spine, posterior plating must be kept as short as possible in order to prevent a significant decrease in the mobility of the lumbar spine. Posterior plating should include, as frequently as possible, only one vertebra above and one vertebra below the injury level (Fig. 6), and the fusion should be of the same length. If the reduction is mainly in the disk instead of in the vertebral body it may be an indication for complementary anterior fixation and grafting (Fig. 7).

It is important to give some practical technical details. The reduction is achieved on a Judet's orthopaedic table by pulling on the lower limbs to reduce the axial compression and by lifting the lower limbs to

reduce the kyphotic deformity. The full reduction is completed surgically. If necessary, a decompression of the dural sac is performed through a laminectomy, which may be enlarged laterally. This approach allows reduction or removal of a posterior protruding fragment of the vertebral body, which is then controlled with ultrasound intraoperatively.

The plates are implanted afterwards. The pedicles are drilled, a Kirschner wire (K-wire) is put into each pedicle, and the K-wires are placed through the appropriate holes in a plate of suitable length. The K-wires are then removed in sequence, and the screws implanted in their place. The progressive tightening of the screws achieves a few more degrees of reduction by pulling the spine back towards the plates, which are shaped to match the normal sagittal configuration.

When special screws for spinal pedicles are used, the technique is simpler. It is not necessary to drill holes. The point of entry of the screw is determined and then the hole in the pedicle is prepared with a thin awl to a depth of only 3 or 4 mm. The spinal screw is then inserted directly, as it is self tapping. The screw will

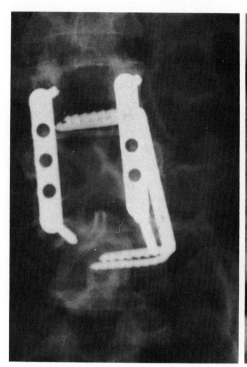
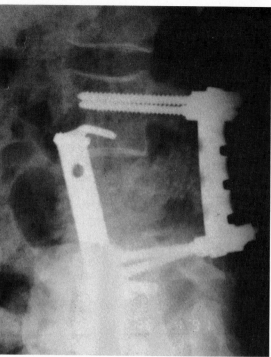

Fig. 7 Reduction and short fixation with a double approach (preoperative neurologic deficit). Posterior plating is done first (**left**), followed by anterior grafting plus staple (**right**).

find its own way into the center of the pedicle. Reduction of the fracture is facilitated by special forceps that apply distraction or contraction on the posterior part of the screws.

In postoperative care for patients without medullary syndrome, the spinal stabilization is strong enough to allow early ambulation. The mechanical results of posterior spinal plating are stable.

At thoracic and lumbar spine levels, in a series of 123 consecutive cases, there was a mean loss in kyphosis of 4 degrees, 4 minutes when the plates were still in place and of 6 degrees, 3 minutes after the plates were removed. Plates are usually removed after one year of follow-up. More precisely, the secondary kyphosis was none in 39% of the cases, 5 degrees in 19%, 5 to 10 degrees in 36%, and 10 to 20 degrees in 6% of the cases.

Conclusion

I want to emphasize the difference between treating the cervical spine, where the screws are implanted into the articular masses because it is anatomically too dangerous to drill a cervical pedicle (except C2 and C7), and the thoracic and lumbar spine where the screws are implanted into the pedicles. Although the technique of implantation is now well known, it remains difficult and requires great precision. For this reason, most surgeons use pedicular screws only on the lumbar spine, where the pedicles are broad.

My personal philosophy of spinal plate fixation leads me to maintain a nonrigidly constrained screw-plate interface with slight clearance. This technique avoids many instances of screw breakage and allows the surgeon to use 3.5-mm screws in the thin thoracic pedicles.

References

1. Bradford DS, Akbarnia BA, Winter RB, et al: Surgical stabilization of fracture and fracture dislocations of the thoracic spine. *Spine* 1977;2:185–196.
2. Cotler JM, Vernace JV, Michalski JA: The use of Harrington rods in thoracolumbar fractures. *Orthop Clin North Am* 1986;17:87–103.
3. Cotrel Y, Dubousset J, Guillaumat M: New universal instrumentation in spinal surgery. *Clin Orthop* 1988;227:10–23.
4. Denis F: The three column spine and its significance in the classification of acute thoracolumbar spinal injuries. *Spine* 1983;8:817–831.
5. Dick W: "The fixateur ixterne" as a versatile implant for spine surgery. *Spine* 1987;12:882–900.
6. Edwards CC, Levine AM: Early rod-sleeve stabilization of the injured thoracic and lumbar spine. *Orthop Clin North Am* 1986;17:121–145.
7. Keene JS, Wackwitz DL, Drummond DS, et al: Compression-distraction instrumentation of unstable thoracolumbar fractures: Anatomic results obtained with each type of injury and method of instrumentation. *Spine* 1986;11:895–902.
8. McAfee PC, Farey ID, Sutterlin CE, et al: Device-related osteo-

porosis with spinal instrumentation: 1989 Volvo award in basic science. *Spine* 1989;14:919–926.

9. McAfee PC, Werner FW, Glisson RR: A biomechanical analysis of spinal instrumentation systems in thoracolumbar fractures: Comparison of traditional Harrington distraction instrumentation with segmental spinal instrumentation. *Spine* 1985;10:204–217.

10. Olerud S, Karlstrom G, Sjostrom L: Transpedicular fixation of thoracolumbar fractures. *Contemp Orthop* 1990;20:285–300.

11. Roy-Camille R, Roy-Camille M, Demeulenaere C: Osteosynthèse du rachis dorsal, lombaire et lombo-sacrè par plaques métalliques vissées dans les pedicules vertébraux et les apophyses articulaires. *Presse Med* 1970;78:1447–1448.

12. Roy-Camille R, Saillant G, Mazel C: Plating of thoracic, thoracolumbar and lumbar injuries with pedicle screw plates. *Orthop Clin North Am* 1986;17(1):147–159.

13. Roy-Camille R, Saillant G, Mazel C: Internal fixation of the lumbar spine with pedicle screw plating. *Clin Orthop* 1986;203:7–17.

14. Roy-Camille R, Saillant G, Mazel CH: Internal fixation of the unstable cervical spine by a posterior osteosynthesis with plates, in *Cervical Spine*. New York, Springer-Verlag, 1989, pp 390–403.

15. Roy-Camille R, Mazel CH, Saillant G, et al: Rationale and techniques of internal fixation in trauma of the cervical spine, in Errico TJ (ed): *Treatment of Surgical Spine Disease*. Philadelphia, JB Lippincott, 1990, pp 163–191.

16. Roy-Camille R, Mazel CH, Saillant G, et al: Treatment of malignant tumors of the spine with posterior instrumentation, in Sundaresan N (ed): *Tumors of the Spine: Diagnosis and Clinical Management*. Philadelphia, WB Saunders, 1990, pp 473–487.

17. Steffee AD, Biscup RS, Sitkowski DJ: Segmental spine plates with pedicle screw fixation: A new internal fixation device for disorders of the lumbar and thoracolumbar spine. *Clin Orthop* 1986; 203:45–53.

18. White AA III, Panjabi MM: The problem of clinical instability in the human spine: A systematic approach, in White AA III, Panjabi MM (eds): *Clinical Biomechanics of the Spine*. Philadelphia, JB Lippincott, 1978, pp 191–192.

Pathophysiology of Spinal Stenosis

Srdjan Mirkovic, MD

Steven R. Garfin, MD

Bjorn Rydevik, MD, PhD

Steven J. Lipson, MD

Definitions

Stenosis is defined as an occlusion (narrowing or stricture) of ducts or canals, caused, among other things, by narrowing of their walls. Pathology is the study of the structural and functional manifestations of a disease process, and physiology deals with physical and chemical processes. The present discussion focuses on spinal degenerative processes that are associated with aging and that lead to anatomic structural changes. These changes narrow the space available for the cauda equina and the spinal nerve roots and can cause abnormal motion. Narrowing of the spinal canal, or spinal stenosis, may lead to physical and chemical alterations that can subsequently produce symptoms including pain, weakness, reflex alterations, and paresthesia.

Anatomy

Anatomically, spinal canal narrowing can be considered either as central narrowing, which compresses the cauda equina, or as lateral (neuroforaminal) narrowing, which compresses the nerve roots.

The central canal is bounded anteriorly by the disk, the posterior longitudinal ligament, and the vertebral body; posteriorly by the ligamentum flavum and lamina; and laterally by the pedicles. Because of anatomic variability, the canal may have a number of configurations (Fig. 1). The round or nearly round canal, which is the most capacious centrally and laterally,[1-4] has an average anteroposterior diameter of 12 mm. Its minimal cross sectional area, the area that accommodates the neural elements, is at least 77 ± 13 mm.[2,5,6] Alternatively, trefoil canals, commonly seen with congenital stenosis, have an unfavorable configuration, particularly in the lateral recess (Fig. 2).

The spinal nerve canals are bounded posteriorly by the facet joints, superiorly and inferiorly by the pedicles, and anteriorly by the vertebral body and disk (Fig. 3). Degeneration or insult to any of these structures can compromise the space available for the spinal nerve root. Additionally, in the lower lumbar spine[7] the pedicles are larger and their caudal borders are more transversely oriented than those of the more superior lumbar pedicles, which are concave inferiorly (Fig. 4). With disk space narrowing and posterior bulging, there is less room in the neuroforamen for the spinal nerve roots. This is particularly important in the lower lumbar

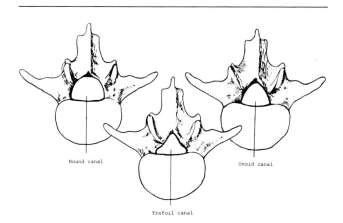

Round canal

Ovoid canal

Trefoil canal

Fig. 1 Generalized shapes for the spinal canal. The round canal (*left*) and ovoid canal (*right*) have relatively capacious central areas and lateral recesses for the cauda equina and the spinal nerve roots, respectively. The trefoil canal shape (center) has less room in the neuroforamen to accommodate changes that occur as a result of aging or degenerative alterations. (Reproduced with permission from DePalma AF, Rothman RH: *The Intervertebral Disc*. Philadelphia, WB Saunders, 1970, p 62.)

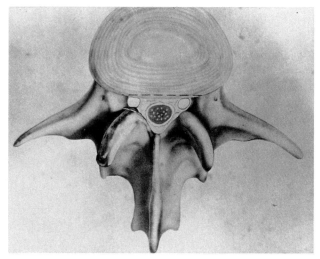

Fig. 2 With facet hypertrophy and a bulging disk, even relatively minor changes can compromise the spinal nerve in the neuroforamen in this trefoil canal as can be seen on the left. (Reproduced with permission from Rothman RH, Simeone FA: *The Spine*. Philadelphia, WB Saunders, 1991.)

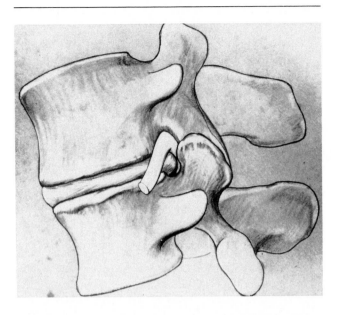

Fig. 3 Lateral view of the spinal nerve root exiting the neuroforamen showing its compromise by the facet joint posteriorly, the pedicle superiorly, and a bulging disk anteriorly and inferiorly. (Reproduced with permission from Rothman RH, Simeone FA: *The Spine.* Philadelphia, WB Saunders, 1991.)

spine, where the pedicles encompass a relatively larger area and have a broader inferior surface.

Classification

Spinal stenosis can be classified as either congenital or acquired.[8] Congenital, or developmental, stenosis is subdivided into chondrodystrophic[9-20] and idiopathic.[21-26] Acquired spinal stenosis can be degenerative, degenerative and congenital, spondylolytic, iatrogenic, or post-traumatic. This chapter focuses on the pathophysiologic changes associated with degenerative spinal stenosis.

Disk Biochemistry

The intervertebral disk consists of the connective tissues between the hyaline cartilage endplates of the vertebral bodies. The three primary biomechanical components of the intervertebral disk are collagen, proteoglycans, and water. These substances constitute 90% to 95% of the normal disk volume. The arrangement of the collagen laminae allows for disk extensibility and provides intervertebral attachment. Proteoglycan hydrodynamic and electrostatic properties control tissue turgor by regulating fluid exchanges within the disk matrix. Proteoglycan content and disk hydration are thus closely interrelated throughout life.

Water

Mechanically, although the water content of a disk depends on the disk load, it normally comprises up to 80% of the nucleus pulposus and 78% of the annulus fibrosis. With the normal aging process, the proteoglycan content of both the nucleus and the annulus decreases five fold between adolescence and the eighth decade, resulting in disk dehydration.[27-31] The content of water in both the annulus and the nucleus falls to about 70% with degeneration. These changes, which are more pronounced in the nucleus pulposus,[32,33] vary with the spinal level involved. As the nucleus pulposus dehydrates, its ability to distribute stresses declines,[34,35] leading to fissuring of the annular tissue.

Collagen

Both type I collagen (collagen of skin, tendon, and bone) and type II collagen (collagen of cartilage) are found in the intervertebral disk and provide it with properties of tensile strength. The nucleus consists almost exclusively of type II collagen fibrils,[36,37] in which the intermolecular spacing is greater than in type I. This feature is associated with increased water content, implying higher levels of hydration and, thus, better performance under compressive and deforming loads.

The annulus fibrosis consists of approximately 60% type II and 40% type I collagen. The distribution of type I collagen increases progressively from the inner to the outer annulus, and it is the predominant component of the outer annulus.[38,39] In both humans[40] and animals (pigs), the proportion of type I to type II collagen changes with aging, with an increase in type I in disks of older individuals.[39,40] In the younger spine, total collagen content varies little.

Irreducible cross-linking in the collagen accumulates with age. The major irreducible cross-link of adult collagen is hydroxypyridinium,[37,41] which increases with aging and decreases with disk herniation, indicating new collagen synthesis.[42] Reducible cross-links, on the other hand, are commonly absent by age 25.

With aging, immunofluorescent studies demonstrate the appearance of type III collagen. Disk degeneration is thus accompanied by alterations in collagen subtypes, with type I replacing type II collagen, the appearance of type III collagen, and the overall accumulation of irreducible crosslinks. Regional appearance of new collagen synthesis may represent a cellular response to tensile loads.[39]

Proteoglycans

Intervertebral disk proteoglycans are similar to those found in articular cartilage,[43] but they are smaller in

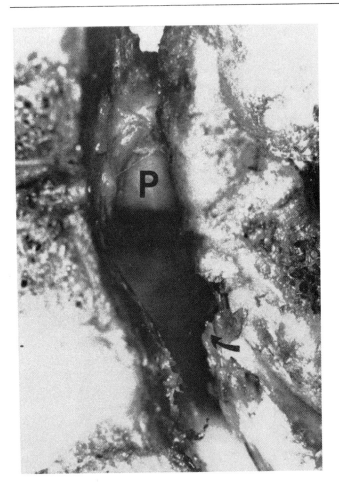 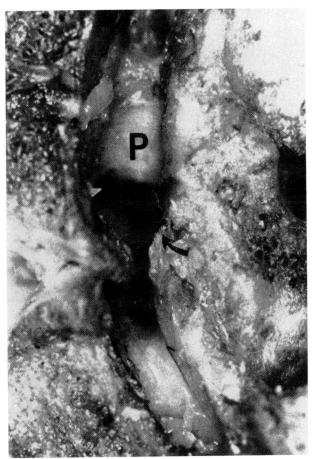

Fig. 4 **Left**, The L4-5 facet joints have been debrided of capsular tissue and the L4 pedicle (P) is visible. The arrow points to a small osteophyte off the L4-5 facet joint. The view is into the L4-5 neuroforamen. **Right**, The L4-5 disk has been removed and there is compression across the motion segment. As shown, the neuroforamen becomes smaller. The osteophyte at L4-5 moves significantly closer to the L4 pedicle and potentially could entrap, or impale, the exiting nerve root. (Reproduced with permission from Lancourt JE, Glenn WV, Wiltse LL: Multiplanar computerized tomography in the normal spine and in the diagnosis of spinal stenosis. *Spine* 1979;4:379–390.)

size,[44] have a shorter core protein, and include keratin sulfate and chondroitin sulfate chains.

Compressibility is governed by proteoglycans, which are present in higher concentration in the nucleus than in the annulus.[29,38,45,46] With age and degeneration, as demonstrated by Pearce and associates,[47] total proteoglycan content decreases.[29,33,35,48-50] Decreased protein aggregation,[51] associated with a decrease in core protein size,[32] is also observed.

With aging, general slowing in the rate of proteoglycan synthesis is noted, probably accompanied by degradation in the hyaluronic acid binding region. The ratio of keratin sulfate to chondroitin sulfate increases with age.[28,48,51-53]

Intervertebral disks elaborate collagenolytic, gelatinolytic, and elastinolytic enzymes,[54] as well as serum proteinases.[55] It is thought that activation of proteolytic activity in the disk may play a role in degenerative

changes, and that some proteoglycan degeneration is caused by proteolysis.

Link proteins stabilize the noncovalent bonding of aggregating proteoglycans to hyaluronic acid. Of the link proteins isolated, the largest occur in the young.[56] With aging, the smaller link proteins, along with their fragmentation products,[56,57] accumulate. The concentration of smaller link proteins is particularly high within the annulus.

Further insights into the biochemical changes associated with aging have been gained from animal models. A rabbit model of surgically induced ventral herniation[58,59] demonstrated progressive fibrocartilaginous metaplasia with tissue proliferation, as well as alteration in disk architecture, which is similar to an end-stage degenerative disk. In this model, after an acute loss, water content was regained by the fourth day after the injury and then gradually diminished with

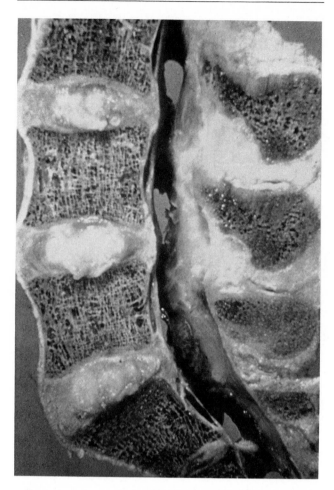

Fig. 5 In this young specimen the gelatinous nucleus bulges significantly. The annulus is well seen, particularly in the disk in the center. (Reproduced with permission from Kirkaldy-Willis WH, Wedge JH, Yong-Hing K, et al: Pathology and pathogenesis of lumbar spondylosis and stenosis. *Spine* 1978;3:319–328.)

tracellular matrix, often in association with collagen fibrils. The proteoglycan granules exhibit regional differences in both chemical structure and aggregate formation, allowing variations in the hydrodynamic and mechanical properties of the tissue. Their main role, as in other cartilaginous tissue, is to offer resistance to compression.

Disk Pathoanatomic Changes

In the majority of cases, disk degeneration has been shown to be the first stage in the degenerative process of the spine[60-64] that leads to spinal stenosis. Videman and associates,[65] however, have demonstrated that, in 20% of cases, facet arthritis precedes disk degeneration.

The originally gelatinous nucleus pulposus (Fig. 5) undergoes fibrocartilaginous metaplasia with appearance of chondrocytes within the inner lamellae. The original sharp borders between the nucleus and annulus gradually become indistinct after the second decade (Fig. 6, *top left*).[66-71] In addition to gradual cavitation, desiccation, and fibroblastic proliferation, deposition of calcium salt occurs, and the nuclear area eventually is replaced by fibrocartilage (Fig. 6, *top right* and *bottom left*).[66]

The annular contour and the intact disk in youth are smooth, and the lamellar structures are clearly distinct from the gelatinous nucleus pulposus (Fig. 5). With aging, the annular lamellae become coarser, with progressive fissuring and hyalinization. Disk degeneration continues and, by the fourth decade, nests of chondrocytes can be noted that are associated with annular conversion to more disorganized fibrocartilage. The appearance of random periodic acid-schiff-reactive fibrous material implies an alteration in the collagen-proteoglycan relationship and subsequent irreversible changes in the mechanical properties of the annulus fibrosis.[71]

Based on these observations, Nachemson,[72] as summarized by Miller and associates,[73] classified disk degeneration into four grades. In grade I, the nucleus is shiny and gelatinous, is well delineated from the annulus, and is free of macroscopic fissures or discolorations. In grade II, the nucleus remains clearly distinct from the intact annulus but has grown more fibrous. In grade III, the nucleus is even more fibrous but is still soft, the annulus boundary has become indistinct, and annular fissures have appeared. In grade IV, macroscopic differences in annulus and nucleus are seen, with fissures and cavities present in both and with the appearance of marginal osteophytes. The first evidence of disk degeneration usually presents itself in the second decade in males and the third in females.[73] The greatest increase in degeneration has been found between 25 and 35 years of age. By the age of 40, 80% of male and 65% of female disks are moderately de-

time. Proteoglycans follow a similar course, in which an initial loss is followed by rapid proteoglycan synthesis. The aggregating population of proteoglycans reaccumulates by the third week after injury and then diminishes at weeks six and seven. This model raises the possibility of repair attempts by the tissue.

Histologic studies (at an electron microscopic level) demonstrate that the biochemical constituents of the intervertebral disk display an architectural array that reflects their biomechanical properties. The annulus fibrosis is composed of collagen fibrils organized in lamellar layers of fibers that cross at angles of 40 to 70 degrees and that provide tensile strength. The tightly packed annular fibers become less dense and less organized at the nucleus annulus border and form a loose network within the nucleus pulposus. With age, fibril diameters increase and become more variable and dense throughout the intervertebral disk, including the nucleus. Proteoglycans form small granules in the ex-

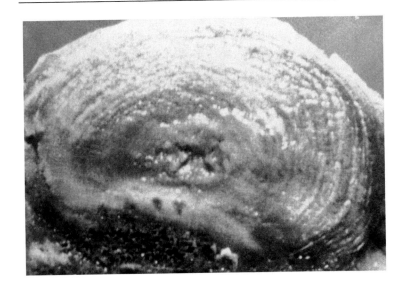

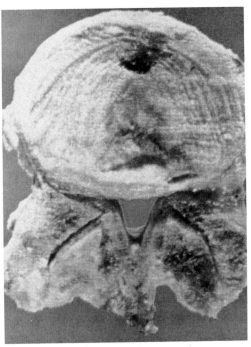

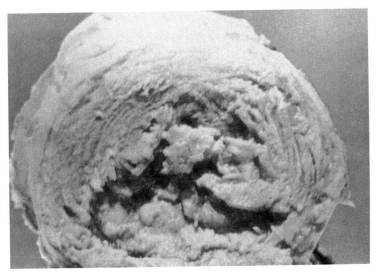

Fig. 6 Top left, An example of a relatively healthy disk. The nucleus, although it is drying, remains distinct from the annulus with its concentric lamellae. **Top right,** Aging and/or degeneration lead to some dehydration of the annulus and nucleus. Small tears may develop in the annulus as can be seen in the posterior aspect of this specimen. Additionally, degenerative changes can occur concurrently in the facets, resulting in thickened facets, narrowed interlaminar space, and stenosis of the central canal. As the degenerative process progresses, the tears coalesce and develop into large radial tears. This example shows significant disruption of the disk from the degenerative process. **Bottom left,** The end point of this degenerative process is significant degenerative change, secondary to dehydration and chemical alterations. The dried, disrupted, nucleus becomes nearly indistinguishable from the annular lamellae. (Reproduced with permission from Kirkaldy-Willis WH, Wedge JH, Yong-Hing K, et al: Pathology and pathogenesis of lumbar spondylosis and stenosis. *Spine* 1978;3:319–328.)

generated. The L5-S1, L4-5, and L3-4 levels are the most commonly involved.

The biomechanical and biochemical changes discussed thus far lead to a decrease in disk height, narrowing the intervertebral disk space. Disk fissuring, collapse, and subsequent narrowing of the intervertebral disk space bring about annular bulging along the posterior longitudinal ligament, as well as frank disk herniation and osteophyte formation. These pathologic alterations, as well as those associated with facet degeneration and instability (described below), cause progressive central and lateral foraminal stenosis. These age-related changes usually occur first in the lower, more mobile disk segments of L5-S1 and L4-5 and then proceed cephalad, eventually involving most disks.

Facet Degeneration

Radiographs of normal facet joints show some evidence of sclerosis, particularly in the concavity of the superior facet. With aging, the porosity of bone in the facets increases, with concurrent loss of the joint space (Fig. 7). With time, sclerosis decreases, suggesting alterations in the stress distribution across the facet joint secondary to the degenerative process. Further facet degeneration is characterized by hypertrophy and the presence of osteophytes.

Kirkaldy-Willis and Farfan,[61] in their depiction of spine motion segments, visualized a large tripod with a disk as one joint and the facets completing the two posterior supports of a three-joint complex (Fig. 2). In a well preserved facet joint, the cartilage is intact with

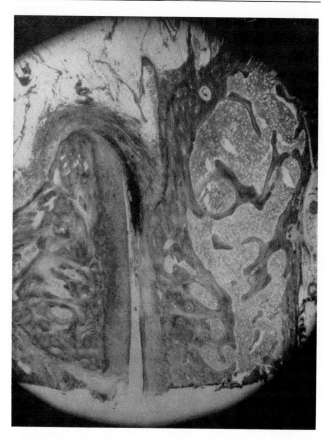

Fig. 7 This longitudinal section through a facet joint shows early, typical alterations, including loss of cartilage, fissuring of the cartilage, and narrowing of the joint space. Additionally, osteoporotic changes, reflected as porosis radiographically, can be seen in the center of the facet joints with increased bone density subchondrally. (Reproduced with permission from Sutro CJ: Lumbar facets—spinal stenosis and intermittent claudication: A mini review. *Bull Hosp Jt Dis* 1979;40:13–36.)

a well contoured gliding surface.[74,75] The central portion of the facet is cancellous and the synovial joint is covered with a capsule. Involvement of any of the three joints of the tripod (usually the disk as a primary dysfunctional unit) causes abnormal biomechanical stresses on the facet joints. These increased facet joint stresses[49,76,77] induce arthritic changes, which follow the predictable course seen in most other joints.[49,78–82] As the cartilage surface begins to erode (Fig. 7) and the bone loses its mass and normal function, articular surfaces become irregular and override. Settling and erosion of the facet joints follows.[83,84] In the early stages, subtle retrolisthesis of the superior vertebral body on the inferior one, coupled with overriding facets and bulging disk spaces, is observed (Fig. 8).

Compression of the emerging nerve roots may be subarticular, as they pass underneath the medial border of the superior articular facet before they swing around the pedicle to emerge through the foramen between the hypertrophied superior articular facet and the dor-

sal aspect of the vertebral body (Fig. 9). Radicular kinking may occur as the disk height decreases, causing the upper vertebral body to descend and its pedicle to compress or deform the emerging nerve root. Most commonly, however, compression occurs in the gutter formed by the diffuse lateral bulge of the disk and the pedicle above, commonly seen with L5-S1 spondylolisthesis. Foraminal stenosis can result from compression between the superior facet and the pedicle above. Finally, in the late stages, with osteophyte development, additional narrowing may occur between the superior articular facet and the posterior aspect of the vertebral body (Fig. 8).[85] Degenerative changes in the facet joints, degenerative spondylolisthesis, and osteophyte formation contribute markedly to this stenotic pattern, both dynamically and statically.[86]

Ligaments

A gradual increase in lordosis is another sequel of degenerative disk disease. Breig[87] noted that with progressive spine extension the ligamentum flavum becomes broader and wider. This, coupled with a posterior bulging of the disks and the already compromised neural canal, results in a relative increase in spinal stenosis.

Segmental Instability

The tripod configuration of the spine with normal disks, facet joints, and ligaments allows smooth and symmetrical accommodation of rotational motion, as well as flexion and extension, by the spinal motion segment (vertebral body-disk-vertebral body) and the neuroforamen, without significantly altering the space available. With time, however, the central canal and the neuroforamen become less accommodating in rotation (Fig. 10) because of narrowing and altered torsional stresses.[63,88] These changes, which are secondary to the advanced disk degeneration associated with ligament buckling[89] and facet hypertrophy, can cause motion segment instability[90–93] and produce irritation or inflammation of the spinal nerves and cauda equina.

Common occurrences seen with segmental instability are anterior and posterior subluxation.[94–98] Retrolisthesis usually occurs when disk collapse exceeds facet arthritic changes with posterior overriding of the facet joints. With anterolisthesis, as seen in the anterior and posterior column, degeneration occurs concurrently with erosion, hypertrophy, and gradual realignment and redistribution of forces across the facet joints. The frequent presence of anterolisthesis at the L4-5 level is thought to be the result of the restraining effect of iliolumbar ligaments on the L5 vertebral body and transverse processes, which allows subluxation and increased motion at L4-5.[99]

The abnormal biomechanical stresses across the motion segment are seen radiographically as a collapsed disk space with endplate sclerosis (Fig. 8). Radiographically, this can resemble infection; however, the sclerosis is confined to the motion segment areas adjacent to the disk space. Instability is frequently suspected in the presence of large osteophytes. This end-stage clinical and radiographic picture has been called benign idiopathic vertebral sclerosis.

Mechanical Compression

The foregoing conclusion, thus far, is that some degree of mechanical compression is an inevitable sequel of the degenerative processes associated with aging. Mechanical compression can lead to chronic and, at times, acute impairment of neurologic function and compromise of cauda equina blood supply (Fig. 11).[100,101] These changes can be accompanied by chronic inflammation, which, when combined with metabolic alterations and intraneural tissue reactions, can lead to demyelinization,[102] subsequent lowering of the pain threshold,[89] and neurologic alterations.[103–108]

Physiology of Spinal Stenosis

The effect of compression on neurologic elements has been studied experimentally using cadaver spines and circumferential clamps to narrow the cauda equina. Schönström and associates[5,6,109] were able to demonstrate that the minimal cross sectional area necessary to accommodate the neural elements, including the dural sac, was 77 ± 13 mm² at L3. This represents 45% of the normal cross sectional area of the dural sac at this level.[110,111] To generate 50 mm of Hg pressure in the neural elements, the cross sectional area had to be narrowed to 63 ± 13 mm², which represents 37% of the normal noncompressed dural sac area. At pressures of 100 mm Hg, neural tissues had been narrowed to 33% of their normal size. It appears that symptoms rarely occur at pressures less than 100 mm Hg. A number of researchers have demonstrated that pressures greater than 50 mm Hg cause capillary constriction and electrophysiologic alteration in spinal nerve roots.[112–116] Others have used animal models to show that even low pressures, on the order of 5 to 10 mm Hg, can lead to venous congestion.[103–108,114] Complete ischemia of the compressed nerve root segments occurred in a porcine model with compression in excess of 130 mm Hg, which exceeded the mean arterial pressure in this animal model. Studies involving solute transport (HC-labeled methyl-glucose) showed a 45% reduction of flow across nerve root segments compressed at as little as 10 mm Hg.[112] Intraneural edema was observed after a 2-minute compression at 50 mm Hg.[117]

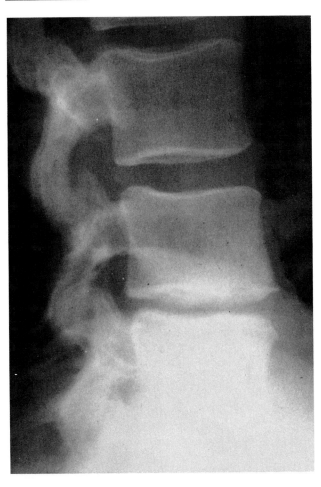

Fig. 8   Radiograph showing marked narrowing of a disk space, endplate sclerosis, traction spurs anteriorly, and slight retrolisthesis of the superior vertebrae. (Reproduced with permission from Rothman RH, Simeone FA (eds): *The Spine*. Philadelphia, WB Saunders, 1991.)

Afferent and efferent electrophysiologic conduction impairment was consistently elicited in the porcine cauda equina compressed at 100 mm Hg for two hours (Fig. 12). Following pressure relief, motor nerves recovered faster and to a greater degree than sensory nerve roots, which might explain the continued subjective complaints of pain and discomfort observed clinically with spinal nerve root compression.

Delamarter and associates[118] studied the effect of cauda equina constriction on neurologic deficits in a beagle dog model. They found that motor and sensory deficits were elicited by 50% or greater constriction of the cross sectional area of the cauda equina. These findings are consistent with those of Schönström and associates.[5,6,109]

Pain and Spinal Stenosis

Spinal stenosis would be of little consequence if pain were not a major symptom, because grave neurologic

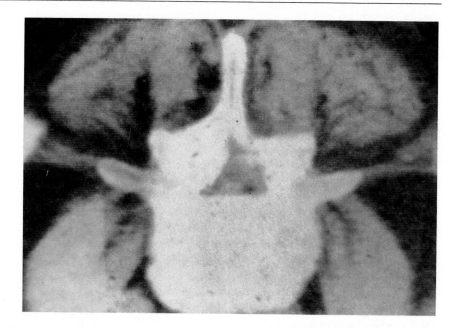

Fig. 9 Computed tomographic scan shows significant unilateral facet hypertrophy, which leads to marked narrowing of the neuroforamen and entrapment of the underlying nerve, coupled with deformation caused by the bony overgrowth. (Reproduced with permission from Rothman RH, Simeone FA (eds): *The Spine*. Philadelphia, WB Saunders, 1991.)

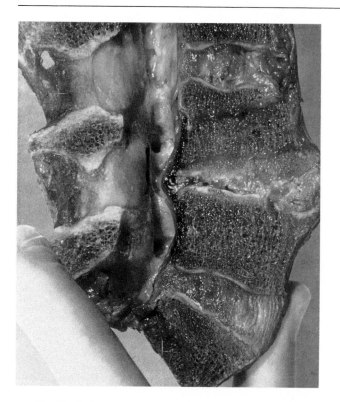
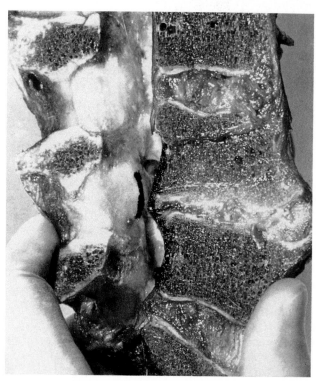

Fig. 10   Left, This specimen has a clockwise force applied to it. The neuroforamen and central canal can be seen. A black dye line is placed between the ligamentum flavum posteriorly and the posterior bulging of the disk with osteophytes on the anterior portion of the canal/neuroforamen. **Right,** With a counterclockwise force there is significant narrowing in the neuroforamen, as shown by the near apposition of the dye lines. This graphically depicts the effects of rotation on a degenerative, compromised nerve canal. (Reproduced with permission from Kirkaldy-Willis WH, Wedge JH, Yong-Hing K, et al: Pathology and pathogenesis of lumbar spondylosis and stenosis. *Spine* 1978;3:319–328.)

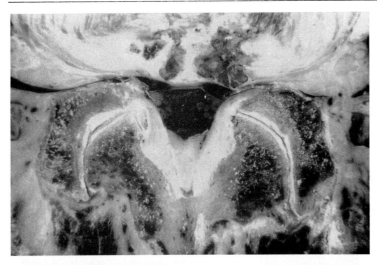

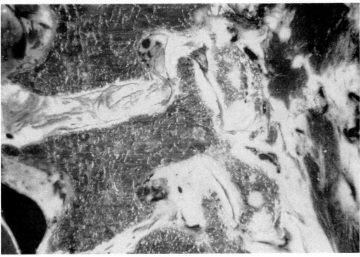

Fig. 11 Top, This cadaveric specimen shows marked narrowing of the neuroforamen caused by hypertrophied facets and a bulging disk. Additionally, this elegant preparation demonstrates vascular intrusion, or perhaps evidence of inflammation, in the posterior aspect of the prominent posterior disk. Central narrowing can be seen, as can facet joint and cartilage alterations. **Bottom**, Sagittal section laterally through the neuroforamen. The spinal nerve root and vessels can be seen centrally. The neuroforamen is narrowed by the facet, facet capsule, and ligaments posteriorly, and by the bulging disk inferiorly and anteriorly. (Reproduced with permission from Rauschning W: Normal and pathologic anatomy of the lumbar root canals. *Spine* 1987;12:1008–1019.)

changes are extremely rare. If spinal stenosis is a normal function of aging, why then do some people have pain and what is its etiology? The changes observed with spinal stenosis related to aging can be found in a large number of asymptomatic individuals. Unfortunately, mechanical instability or isolated nerve root compression cannot explain why patients' symptoms tend to be intermittent and why only a limited number of older individuals develop symptoms.

A likely source of pain in spinal stenosis and degenerative disk disease could be mechanical irritation or inflammation of the sinovertebral nerve or the posterior ramus[4,74,119,120] secondary to instability (Fig. 13). However, these nerves are extremely small and, although they are present in all humans, they are difficult to isolate and implicate with any certainty as a source of pain.

Although Arnoldi and associates[8] demonstrated increased venous pressures in patients with spinal stenosis, this finding does not explain why symptoms are intermittent and worsen with extension and improve with flexion. A generous arteriovenous anastomosis surrounds the spine, which should not decompress rapidly just with postural changes. If the symptoms are related to congestion and hypertension, relief of pain with decreased activity should be slow. Rapid relief, however, is achieved by simply changing posture. Furthermore, if congestion and hypertension were causative factors in the pain complaints, a narrow laminectomy would be sufficient to decompress the veins. However, unless the nerve roots are individually decompressed, symptoms frequently persist or recur shortly after surgery, which suggests that the venous system is not the primary component in the generation of pain.

Presently, a more acceptable explanation of pain in the patient with spinal stenosis relates to the arterial and nutritional support systems of the cauda equina.[2,13,75,110,121] Parke and associates[122,123] have shown that cauda equina nerve roots are supplied with blood by arteries that emerge from the central spinal artery, as well as by radicular arteries and their segmental

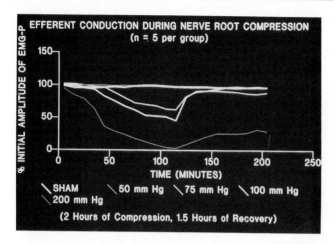

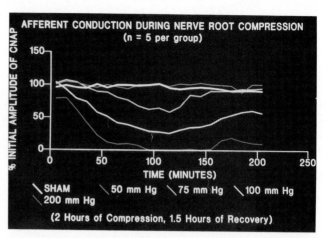

Fig. 12 **Left,** This graph demonstrates efferent conduction during experimental nerve root compression in a pig model of cauda equina compression. After a compression time of two hours, the compression was removed, and the recovery period was followed for the next one hour and a half. As the magnitude of compression (50 mm Hg - 75 mm Hg - 100 mm Hg - 200 mm Hg) increases, the loss of amplitude becomes more apparent. Similarly, during the recovery period there is a differential in the amount of efferent conduction that returns. **Right,** The same model. This graph, however, shows the monitoring of the afferent conduction (related to sensory roots). Again, the differential in conduction, which relates to magnitude of compression, is seen. This effect is demonstrated both during the compression and recovery phase. (Reproduced with permission from Rothman RH, Simeone FA (eds): *The Spine.* Philadelphia, WB Saunders, 1991.)

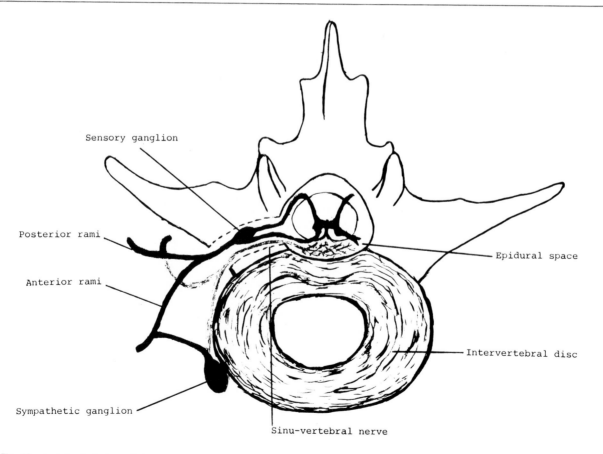

Fig. 13 Artist's depiction of the sinuvertebral nerve and posterior primary ramus. These structures, which innervate middle and posterior column structures, may contribute to the symptoms of low back pain. (Reproduced with permission from Rothman RH, Simeone FA (eds): *The Spine.* Philadelphia, WB Saunders, 1991.)

branches. Arterial dilatation occurs with exercise, and oxygen use increases with stimulation of the nerve.[124,125] Along the spinal nerve roots and cauda equina, an area of relative hypovascularity is noted where the central and radicular systems approach each other. Further studies of the human cauda equina and peripheral nerves show a decreased number of microvessels per cross sectional area in the cauda equina.[121,123] Spinal stenosis, with constriction of both blood vessels and neural elements, can thus diminish oxygen supply, especially during exercise, and can cause ischemia.[121,123] This situation is distinct from the dorsal root ganglia, where a rich and extensive microvascular web is present,[110] and the vessels are more permeable than intraneural vessels at other levels.[110,126] The increased vascularity, coupled with microvascular permeability in the dorsal root ganglia, suggests increased metabolic demand. The dorsal root ganglion also appears to be the site where synthesis of several essential pain-mediating substances, such as substance P, occurs.[110] Any compromise in the blood supply secondary to chronic compression, inflammation, fibrosis, or ischemia can alter the diffusion processes, and can further contribute to symptoms and signs of spinal stenosis.

Conclusion

Despite some knowledge of the biochemical foundation underlying the disk's functional and biomechanical construct, the onset of events leading to disk degeneration and spinal stenosis are incompletely understood. Because of anatomic variation, the degree of compression varies between individuals and with time in the same individual. Although several theories attempt to elucidate the etiology of such symptoms as pain and neurologic dysfunction, the most plausible explanation appears to be ischemia and metabolic nutritional deficiencies.

References

1. Dupuis PR, Yong-Hing K, Cassidy JD, et al: Radiologic diagnosis of degenerative lumbar spinal instability. *Spine* 1985;10:262–276.
2. Dommisse GF: Morphological aspects of the lumbar spine and lumbosacral region. *Orthop Clin North Am* 1975;6:163–175.
3. Postacchini F, Ripani M, Carpano S: Morphometry of the lumbar vertebrae. An anatomic study in two caucasoid ethnic groups. *Clin Orthop* 1983;172:296–303.
4. Sinclair DC, Feindel WH, Weddell G, et al: The intervertebral ligament as a source of segmental pain. *J Bone Joint Surg* 1948;30B:515–521.
5. Schönström N, Hansson T: Pressure changes following constriction of the cauda equina: An experimental study in situ. *Spine* 1988;13:385–388.
6. Schönström N, Lindahl S, Willér J, et al: Dynamic changes in the dimensions of the lumbar spinal canal: An experimental study in vitro. *J Orthop Res* 1989;7:115–121.
7. Sutro CJ: Lumbar facets—spinal stenosis and intermittent claudication: A mini review. *Bull Hosp Joint Dis* 1979;40:13–37.
8. Arnoldi CC, Brodsky AE, Cauchoix J, et al: Lumbar spinal stenosis and nerve root entrapment syndromes: Definition and classification. *Clin Orthop* 1976;115:4–5.
9. Alexander E Jr: Significance of the small lumbar spinal canal: Cauda equina compression syndromes due to spondylosis. Part 5: Achondroplasia. *J Neurosurg* 1969;31:513–519.
10. Bailey JA II: Orthopaedic aspects of achondroplasia. *J Bone Joint Surg* 1970;52A:1285–1301.
11. Bergström K, Laurent U, Lundberg PO: Neurological symptoms in achondroplasia. *Acta Neurol Scand* 1971;47:59–70.
12. Caffey J: Achondroplasia of pelvis and lumbo-sacral spine. Some roentgenographic features. *AJR* 1958;80:449–457.
13. Duvoisin RC, Yahr MD: Compressive spinal cord and root syndromes in achondroplastic dwarfs. *Neurology* 1962;12:202–207.
14. Epstein JA, Malis LI: Compression of spinal cord and cauda equina in achondroplastic dwarfs. *Neurology* 1955;5:875–881.
15. Freund E: Spastic paraplegia in achondroplasia. *Arch Surg* 1933;27:859–867.
16. Hancock DO, Phillips DG: Spinal compression in achondroplasia. *Paraplegia* 1965;3:23–33.
17. Lutter LD, Langer LO: Neurological symptoms in achondroplastic dwarfs: Surgical treatment. *J Bone Joint Surg* 1977;59A:87–92.
18. Schreiber F, Rosenthal H: Paraplegia from ruptured discs in achondroplastic dwarfs. *J Neurosurg* 1952;9:648–651.
19. Spillane JD: Three cases of achondroplasia with neurological complications. *J Neurosurg* 1952;15:246–252.
20. Yamada H, Nakamura D, Tajima M, et al: Neurological manifestations of pediatric achondroplasia. *J Neurosurg* 1981;54:49–57.
21. Edwards WC, LaRocca SH: The developmental segmental sagittal diameter in combined cervical and lumbar spondylosis. *Spine* 1985;10:42–49.
22. Eisenstein S: Measurements of the lumbar spinal canal in 2 racial groups. *Clin Orthop* 1976;115:42–46.
23. Porter RW, Wicks M, Ottewell D: Measurement of the spinal canal by diagnostic ultrasound. *J Bone Joint Surg* 1978;60B:481–484.
24. Hibbert CS, Porter RW: Relationship between the spinal canal and other skeletal measurements in a Romano-British population. *Ann R Coll Surg Engl* 1981;63:437.
25. Sarpyener MA: Congenital stricture of the spinal canal. *J Bone Joint Surg* 1945;27A:70–79.
26. Sarpyener MA: Spina bifida aperta and congenital stricture of the spinal canal. *J Bone Joint Surg* 1947;29A:817–821.
27. Eyring EJ: The biochemistry and physiology of the intervertebral disk. *Clin Orthop* 1969;67:16–28.
28. Gower WE, Pedrini V: Age-related variations in proteinpolysaccharides from human nucleus pulposus, annulus fibrosus, and costal cartilage. *J Bone Joint Surg* 1969;51A:1154–1162.
29. Hirsch C, Paulson S, Sylven B, et al: Biophysical and physiological investigations of cartilage and other mesenchymal tissues. *Acta Orthop Scand* 1952;22:175–181.
30. Naylor A, Horton WG: The hydrophilic properties of the nucleus pulposus of the intervertebral disc: VI. Characteristics of human pulposi during aging. *Rheumatism* 1955;11:32–35.
31. Roberts S, Beard HK, O'Brien JP: Biochemical changes of intervertebral discs in patients with spondylolisthesis or with tears of the posterior annulus fibrosus. *Ann Rheum Dis* 1982;41:78–85.
32. Lyons G, Eisenstein SM, Sweet MBE: Biochemical changes in intervertebral disc degeneration. *Biochem Biophys Acta* 1981;673:443–453.
33. Mitchell PEG, Hendry NGC, Billewicz WZ: The chemical background of intervertebral disc prolapse. *J Bone Joint Surg* 1961;43B:141–151.

34. DePalma A, Rothman R: *The Intervertebral Disc*. Philadelphia, WB Saunders, 1970.
35. Naylor A: The biophysical and biochemical aspects of intervertebral disc herniations and degeneration. *Ann R Coll Surg Engl* 1962;31:91–114.
36. Eyre DR, Muir H: Types I and II collagens in intervertebral disc. Interchanging radial distributions in annulus fibrosus. *Biochem J* 1976;157:267–270.
37. Herbert CM, Lindberg KA, Jayson MIV, et al: Changes in the collagen of human intervertebral discs during aging and degenerative disc disease. *J Mol Med* 1975;1:79–81.
38. Adams P, Eyre DR, Muir H: Biochemical aspects of development and aging of human lumbar intervertebral discs. *Rheumatol Rehabil* 1977;16:22–29.
39. Brickley-Parsons D, Glimcher MJ: Is the chemistry of collagen in intervertebral discs an expression of Wolff's Law? A study of the human lumbar spine. *Spine* 1984;9:148–163.
40. Eyre DR: Biochemistry of the intervertebral disc. *Int Rev Connect Tissue Res* 1979;8:227–291.
41. Eyre DR, Koob TJ, Van Ness KP: Quantitation of hydroxypyridinium crosslinks in collagen by high-performance liquid chromatography. *Anal Biochem* 1984;137:380–388.
42. Lipson SJ: Metaplastic proliferative fibrocartilage as an alternative concept to herniated intervertebral disc. *Spine* 1988;13:1055–1060.
43. Stevens RL, Erwins RJF, Revell PA, et al: Proteoglycans of the intervertebral disc. *Biochem J* 1979;179:561–572.
44. Stevens RL, Dondi PG, Muir H: Proteoglycans of intervertebral disc. Absence of degradation during isolation of proteoglycans from the intervertebral disc. *Biochem J* 1979;179:573–578.
45. Melrose J, Ghosh P, Taylor TKF: Neutral proteinases of the human intervertebral disc. *Biochim Biophys Acta* 1987;923:483–495.
46. Sylvén B: On the biology of the nucleus pulposus. *Acta Orthop Scand* 1951;20:275–279.
47. Pearce RH, Grimmer BJ, Adams ME: Degeneration and the chemical composition of the human lumbar intervertebral disc. *J Orthop Res* 1987;5:198–205.
48. Hallén A: Hexosamine and ester sulphate content of the human *nucleus pulposus* in different ages. *Acta Chem Scand* 1958;12:1862–1869.
49. Lewin T: Osteoarthritis of the lumbar synovial joints: A morphologic study. *Acta Orthop Scand Suppl* 1964;73:1–112.
50. Urban JP, McMullin JF: Swelling pressure of the lumbar intervertebral discs. Influence of age, spinal level, composition, and degeneration. *Spine* 1988;13:179–187.
51. Adams P, Muir H: Qualitative changes with age of proteoglycans of human lumbar discs. *Ann Rheum Dis* 1976;35:289–296.
52. Lyons H, Jones E, Quinn FE, et al: Protein-polysaccharide complexes of normal and herniated intervertebral discs. *Proc Soc Exp Biol* 1964;115:610–614.
53. Lyons H, Jones E, Quinn FE, et al: Changes in the protein-polysaccharide fractions of nucleus pulposus from human intervetral disc with age and disc herniation. *J Lab Clin Med* 1966;68:930–939.
54. Sedowofia KA, Tomlinson IW, Weiss JB, et al: Collagenolytic enzyme systems in human intervertebral disc. Their control, mechanism, and their possible role in the initiation of biomechanical failure. *Spine* 1982;7:213–222.
55. Malinsky J: Histochemical demonstration of carbohydrates in human intervertebral discs during postnatal development: Histology of intervertebral discs, 5th communication. *Acta Histochem* 1958;5:120–128.
56. Pearce RH, Mathieson JM, Mort JS, et al: Effect of age on the abundance and fragmentation of link protein of the human intervertebral disc. *J Orthop Res* 1989;7:861–867.
57. Donohue PJ, Jahnke MR, Blaha JD, et al: Characterization of link protein(s) from human intervertebral-disc tissues. *Biochem J* 1988;251:739–747.
58. Lipson SJ, Muir H: Experimental intervertebral disc degeneration. Morphologic and proteoglycan changes over time. *Arthritis Rheum* 1981;24:12–21.
59. Lipson SJ, Muir H: 1980 Volvo award in basic science. Proteoglycans in experimental intervertebral disc degeneration. *Spine* 1981;6:194–210.
60. Kirkaldy-Willis WH: The relationship of structural pathology to the nerve root. *Spine* 1984;9:49–52.
61. Kirkaldy-Willis WH, Farfan HF: Instability of the lumbar spine. *Clin Orthop* 1982;165:110–123.
62. Kirkaldy-Willis WH, Paine KW, Cauchoix J, et al: Lumbar spinal stenosis. *Clin Orthop* 1974;99:30–50.
63. Kirkaldy-Willis WH, Wedge JH, Yong-Hing K, et al: Pathology and pathogenesis of lumbar spondylosis and stenosis. *Spine* 1978;3:319–328.
64. Knutsson S: The instability associated with disc degeneration in the lumbar spine. *Acta Radiol* 1944;25:593–609.
65. Videman T, Malmivaara A, Mooney V: The value of the axial view in assessing discograms: An experimental study with cadavers. *Spine* 1987;12:299–304.
66. Coventry MB, Ghormely RK, Kernohan JW: The intervertebral disc: Its microscopic anatomy and pathology. Part II. Changes in the intervertebral disc concomitant with age. *J Bone Joint Surg* 1945;27A:233–247.
67. Coventry MB, Ghormley RK, Kernohan JW: The intervertebral disc: Its microscopic anatomy and Pathology. Part III. Pathological changes in the intervertebral disc. *J Bone Joint Surg* 1945;27A:460–474.
68. Eckert C, Decker A: Pathological studies of intervertebral discs. *J Bone Joint Surg* 1947;29A:447–454.
69. Friberg S, Hirsch C: Anatomical and clinical studies on lumbar disc degeneration. *Acta Orthop Scand* 1949;19:222–242.
70. Harris RI, Macnab I: Structural changes in the lumbar intervertebral discs: Their relationship to low back pain and sciatica. *J Bone Joint Surg* 1954;36B:304–322.
71. Van Den Hooff A: Histological age changes in the annulus fibrosus of the human intervertebral disc with a discussion of the problem of disc herniation. *Gerontologia* 1964;9:136–149.
72. Nachemson A: Lumbar intradiscal pressure: Exerimental studies on post mortem materials. *Acta Orthop Scand Suppl* 1960;43:43–44.
73. Miller JA, Schmatz C, Schultz AB: Lumbar disc degeneration: Correlation with age, sex, and spine level in 600 autopsy specimens. *Spine* 1988;13:173–178.
74. Edgar MA, Ghadially JA: Innervation of the lumbar spine. *Clin Orthop* 1976;115:35–41.
75. Crock HV, Yoshizawa H: *The Blood Supply of the Vertebral Column and Spinal Cord in Man*. New York, Springer-Verlag, 1977.
76. Badgley CE: The articular facets in relationship to low-back pain and sciatic radiation. *J Bone Joint Surg* 1941;23A:481–496.
77. Lorenz M, Patwardhan A, Vanderby R Jr: Load-bearing characteristics of lumbar facets in normal and surgically altered spinal segments. *Spine* 1983;8:122–130.
78. Eisenstein SM, Parry CR: The lumbar facet arthrosis syndrome. Clinical presentation and articular surface changes. *J Bone Joint Surg* 1987;69B:3–7.
79. Engel R, Bogduk N: The menisci of the lumbar zygapophysial joints. *J Anat* 1982;135:795–809.
80. Epstein JA, Epstein BS, Lavine LS, et al: Lumbar nerve root compression at the intervertebral foramina caused by arthritis of the posterior facets. *J Neurosurg* 1973;39:362–369.
81. Lewinnek GE, Warfield CA: Facet joint degeneration as a cause of low back pain. *Clin Orthop* 1986;213:216–222.
82. Taylor JR, Twomey LT: Age changes in lumbar zygapophyseal joints. On structure and function. *Spine* 1986;11:739–745.
83. Gotfried Y, Bradford DS, Oegema TR Jr: Facet joint changes after chemonucleolysis-induced disc space narrowing. *Spine* 1986;11:944–950.

84. Yang KH, King AI: Mechanism of facet load transmission as a hypothesis for low-back pain. *Spine* 1984;9:557–565.

85. Lancourt JE, Glenn WV Jr, Wiltse LL: Multiplanar computerized tomography in the normal spine and in the diagnosis of spinal stenosis: A gross anatomic-computerized tomographic correlation. *Spine* 1979;4:379–390.

86. Macnab I: The traction spur: An indicator of segmental instability. *J Bone Joint Surg* 1971;53A:663–670.

87. Breig A: *Adverse Mechanical Tension in the Central Nervous System.* New York, John Wiley, 1978.

88. Troup JDG: Biomechanics of the lumbar spinal canal. *Clin Biomech* 1986;1:31–43.

89. Towne EB, Reichert FL: Compression of the lumbosacral roots of the spinal cord by thickened ligamenta flava. *Ann Surg* 1931; 94:327–336.

90. Farfan HF, Gracovetsky S: The nature of instability. *Spine* 1989; 9:714–719.

91. Frymoyer JW, Selby DK: Segmental instability. Rationale for treatment. *Spine* 1985;10:280–286.

92. Gertzbein SD, Seligman J, Holtby R, et al: Centrode patterns and segmental instability in degenerative disc disease. *Spine* 1985;10:257–261.

93. Stokes IA, Frymoyer JW: Segmental motion and instability. *Spine* 1987;12:688–691.

94. Epstein JA, Epstein BS, Lavine LS, et al: Degenerative lumbar spondylolisthesis with an intact neural arch (pseudospondylolisthesis). *J Neurosurg* 1976;44:139–147.

95. Farfan HF: The pathological anatomy of degenerative spondylolisthesis: A cadaver study. *Spine* 1980;5:412–418.

96. Johnsson KE, Willner S, Johnsson K: Postoperative instability after decompression for lumbar spinal stenosis. *Spine* 1986;11: 107–110.

97. Newman PH: Stenosis of the lumbar spine in spondylolisthesis. *Clin Orthop* 1976;115:116–121.

98. Rosenberg NJ: Degenerative spondylolisthesis. Predisposing factors. *J Bone Joint Surg* 1975;57A:467–474.

99. Leong JC, Luk KD, Chow DH, et al: The biomechanical functions of the iliolumbar ligament in maintaining stability of the lumbosacral junction. *Spine* 1987;12:669–674.

100. Rydevik B, Lundborg G, Bagge U: Effects of graded compression on intraneural blood flow: An in vivo study on rabbit tibial nerve. *J Hand Surg* 1981;6:3–12.

101. Rydevik B, Nordborg C: Changes in nerve function and nerve fibre structure induced by acute, graded compression. *J Neurol Neurosurg Psychiatry* 1981;43:1070–1082.

102. Weinstein JN, La Motte R, Rydevik B, et al: Nerve, in Frymoyer JW, Gordon SL, (eds): *New Perspectives on Low Back Pain.* Park Ridge, IL, American Academy of Orthopaedic Surgeons, 1989, pp 35–130.

103. Dahlin LB, Rydevik B, McLean WG, et al: Changes in fast axonal transport during experimental nerve compression at low pressures. *Exp Neurol* 1984;84:29–36.

104. Hasue M, Kikuchi S, Sakuyama Y, et al: Anatomic study of the interrelation between lumbosacral nerve roots and their surrounding tissues. *Spine* 1983;8:50–58.

105. Lundborg G: *Nerve Injury and Repair.* Edinburgh, Churchill Livingstone, 1988.

106. Rydevik B, Brown MD, Lundborg G: Pathoanatomy and pathophysiology of nerve root compression. *Spine* 1984;9:7–15.

107. Rydevik B, Garfin S: Spinal nerve root compression, in Szabe RM (ed): *Nerve Compression Syndromes—Diagnosis and Treatment.* Thorofare, NJ, Slack, 1989, pp 247–262.

108. Sunderland S: *Nerves and Nerve Injuries,* ed 2. Edinburgh, Churchill Livingstone, 1978.

109. Schönström N, Bolender NF, Spengler DM, et al: Pressure changes within the cauda equina following constriction of the dural sac: An in vitro experimental study. *Spine* 1984;9:604–607.

110. Arvidson B: Distribution of intravenously injected protein tracers in peripheral ganglia of adult mice. *Exp Neurol* 1979; 63:388–410.

111. Schonstrom NS, Bolender NF, Spengler DM: The pathomorphology of spinal stenosis as seen on CT-scans of the lumbar spine. *Spine* 1985;10:806–811.

112. Olmarker K, Rydevik B, Hansson T, et al: Compression-induced changes of the nutritional supply to the porcine cauda equina. *J Spinal Dis* 1990;3:25–29.

113. Olmarker K, Rydevik B, Holm S: Intraneural edema formation in spinal nerve roots of the porcine cauda equina induced by experimental, graded compression. *Trans Orthop Res Soc* 1988; 13:136.

114. Olmarker K, Rydevik B, Holm S, et al: Effects of experimental graded compression on blood flow in spinal nerve roots: A vital microscopic study on the porcine cauda equina. *J Orthop Res* 1989;7:817–823.

115. Pedowitz RA, Garfin SR, Massie JB, et al: Effects of magnitude and duration of compression on spinal nerve root conduction. *Spine* 1990, (in press).

116. Rydevik BL, Pedowitz RA, Hargens AR, et al: Effects of acute, graded compression on spinal nerve root function and structure: An experimental study of the pig cauda equina. *Spine,* in press.

117. Olmarker K, Rydevik B, Holm S: Edema formation in spinal nerve roots induced by experimental, graded compression: An experimental study on the pig cauda equina with special reference to differences in effects between rapid and slow onset of compression. *Spine* 1989;14:569–573.

118. Delamarter RB, Bohlman HH, Dodge LD, et al: Experimental lumbar spinal stenosis: Analysis of the cortical evoked potentials, microvasculature, and histopathology. *J Bone Joint Surg* 1990;72A:110–120.

119. Inman VT, Saunders JB deCM: Referred pain from skeletal structures. *J Nerv Ment Dis* 1944;99:660–667.

120. Stillwell DL: Nerve supply of vertebral column. *Anat Rec* 1956; 125:139–142.

121. Watanabe R, Parke WW: Vascular and neural pathology of lumbosacral spinal stenosis. *J Neurosurg* 1986;64:64–70.

122. Parke WW, Gammell K, Rothman RH: Arterial vascularization of the cauda equina. *J Bone Joint Surg* 1981;63A:53–62.

123. Parke WW, Watanabe R: The intrinsic vasculature of the lumbosacral spinal nerve roots. *Spine* 1985;10:508–515.

124. Blau JN, Logue V: Intermittent claudication of the cauda equina: An unusual syndrome resulting from central protrusion of a lumbar intervertebral disc. *Lancet* 1961;1:1081–1086.

125. Blau JN, Rushworth G: Observations on the blood vessels of the spinal cord and their responses to motor activity. *Brain* 1958;81:354–363.

126. Olsson Y: The involvement of vasa nervorum in the diseases of peripheral nerves, in Vinken PJ, Bruyn GW (eds): *Handbook of Clinical Neurology. Vascular Diseases of the Nervous System, Part II.* New York, American Elsevier, 1972, vol 12, pp 644–664.

Epidemiology of Spinal Stenosis

Thomas A. Martinelli, MD

Sam W. Wiesel, MD

Introduction

The concept of spinal stenosis dates back to at least 1803, when Portal[1] proposed that stenotic vertebral canals could cause low back pain. The exact definition of spinal stenosis has varied among authors,[2–5] and objective criteria have varied with advances in imaging technology. These variations have made historical comparisons and prevalence studies difficult to interpret.

We use the definition of Postacchini,[6] which considers lumbar spinal stenosis as an "abnormal narrowing of the osteoligamentous vertebral canal and/or the intervertebral foramina, which is responsible for compression of the dural sac and/or the caudal nerve roots." His definition specifically excludes disk herniation as a causative agent. This distinction is important, because the two conditions have vastly different prognoses and pathophysiologies.

Incidence

Given the varied definitions of spinal stenosis, it is not surprising that the incidence varies widely from one report to another. Roberson and associates[7] noted 33 cases of lumbar spinal stenosis in a series of 2,000 lumbar myelograms. De Villiers and Booysen[8] noted a 6% incidence of "stenosis of the thecal sac" in a series of 850 myelograms, but they made no mention of why the myelograms were done. Other reports[4,9,10] simply indicate relative incidences of stenosis (developmental, congenital, degenerative, and so forth) in a cohort of stenotics, but the absolute incidence in the general population remains to be quantified.

Age

Again, the age at onset of symptoms has varied with the criteria used to define stenosis. In a study by Paine,[11] which included conditions with or without disk herniation, provided that a narrow canal preexisted, the mean age was 30. Most of the other studies,[12–14] and our own experience, place the average age of onset of symptoms in the fifth to sixth decades. Exceptions to this include achondroplasia, where the average age is in the fourth decade,[15] and the congenital/developmental stenoses, where the average age at onset is between the third and fifth decades.[6] Degenerative spondylolisthesis is infrequent in patients younger than 50.[16,17]

Sex

Both the developmental and combined forms of lumbar spinal stenosis show a male preponderance in most studies.[4,6,9] Getty,[17] however, reports equal distribution of stenosis between men and women. There are several cohorts of unusual morphology with cervical and/or lumbar stenoses in the Japanese literature in which men appear to predominate.[18] The one noteworthy exception is in degenerative spondylolisthesis with spinal stenosis, which has been reported to occur four to six times as frequently in women as in men.[10,19]

Somatotype

Several reviews have attempted to correlate phenotype with canal diameter. McRae[20] noted that "thickset individuals" tended to develop spinal stenosis. Babin[21] states that the anteroposterior diameter of the canal varies with biotype, race, and muscular strains in sports and professions. Nightingale[22] correlated increasing canal diameter in the cervical spine with increasing length of the humerus and shorter trunk length, but there were large standard errors, and values for the arm and trunk were not predictive for cervical spine stenosis.

Porter,[5] however, stated, "the clinically important mid-sagittal diameter of the vertebral canal is independent of other anthropometric measurements—it cannot be predicted, and must be measured directly." Postacchini[6] also states that there is no significant relationship between phenotype and stenosis, with the exception of achondroplasia.

Occupation

Postacchini[6] states that degenerative stenosis occurs more frequently in workers who do heavy manual labor. He also noted a higher incidence of degenerative changes in the lumbar spine in this group and postulated that this in part explains the increased incidence in males. He does qualify this, however, by noting this relationship to be "somewhat generic." In contradistinction, Porter[5] and Getty[17] note canal size to be unrelated to occupation, even among heavy laborers.

Outline 1
Conditions associated with the development of spinal stenosis.

Achondroplasia
Acromegaly
Ankylosing spondylitis
Autosomal dominant osteosclerosis
Calcium pyrophosphate deposition disease
Cheirolumbar dysostosis
Chondrodysplasia punctata
Diffuse idiopathic skeletal hyperostosis
Down's syndrome
Epidural lipomatosis
Fluorosis
Hypoparathyroidism
Hypophosphatemic vitamin D resistant rickets
Kneist's disease
Léri's pleonosteosis
Malnutrition
Metatrophic dwarfism
Morquio's syndrome
Multiple epiphyseal dysplasia
Osteopoikilosis
Oxalosis
Paget's disease
Renal osteodystrophy
Rheumatoid arthritis
Schuermann's disease
Scoliosis: Idiopathic or degenerative
Spina bifida
Spondyloepiphyseal dysplasia

Race

Eisenstein,[23] in his extensive review, established average canal diameters for South African Negroes and Caucasians, and found the average canal diameter to be smaller in Negroes than in Caucasians. He noted, however, that in his personal experience and in verbal reports from his colleagues, clinically significant stenosis is rare in the black population.

Syndromes

Many disease states and syndromes have been implicated in the development of spinal stenosis both in the lumbar and cervical spine.[4,6,12,15,17,24–39] Outline 1 lists all these states. The majority of these are discrete syndromes that have only occasionally been implicated as causative agents in spinal stenosis. For the most part, they still depend on the presence of degenerative changes to produce symptoms, but they do so at an earlier age than would otherwise be expected. Verbiest,[40] Varughese and Quartey,[41] and Postacchini and associates[42] have all reported familial developmental stenosis in the absence of other disease stigmata.

An interesting theory was expounded by Clark and associates,[43] who implicated prenatal and infantile malnutrition in the etiology of adult spinal stenosis. They studied the Dickson Mounds archaeologic site, where a shift from a protein-rich to a protein-poor environment occurred with a change from hunter-gatherer to agricultural society. They noted smaller canal diameters, particularly anteroposterior diameters, in the protein-deficient population. This finding was confirmed experimentally by Platt and Stewart,[44] who noted a 20% smaller canal size in malnourished versus normal littermates. A catch-up phenomenon may occur, but the clinically important midsagittal diameter approaches adult size by age 10, and diet would have to change early in growth and development to accomplish this. The corresponding study in a modern populace remains to be undertaken.

Summary

Although spinal stenosis has been recognized for nearly 190 years, no exact definition has yet been agreed on, a fact that has made incidence and prevalence studies all but impossible to interpret. The age at onset clearly correlates with the underlying pathomechanics. The disease appears to affect more men than women, except for degenerative spondylolisthesis, which affects more women. Occupation and somatotype do not appear to correlate with the development of symptomatic spinal stenosis. Although they are statistically more likely to have a smaller canal diameter, the black population does not seem to have a high incidence of symptomatic stenosis. Finally, although many syndromes have been reported to be associated with the development of spinal stenosis, the concomitant presence of degenerative changes appears to be a prerequisite to the development of symptomatic spinal stenosis.

References

1. Portal A: Cours d'anatomie medicale on elemens de l'anatomie del'homme. Paris, Baudovin, 1803, pp 293–319.
2. Eisenstein S: Measurements of the lumbar spinal canal in two racial groups. *Clin Orthop* 1976;115:42–46.
3. Kirkaldy-Willis WH, Paine KW, Cauchoix J, et al: Lumbar spinal stenosis. *Clin Orthop* 1974;99:30–50.
4. Verbiest H: Pathomorphologic aspects of developmental lumbar stenosis. *Orthop Clin North Am* 1975;6:177–196.
5. Porter RW: Spinal stenosis in the central and root canal, in Jayson M (ed): *The Lumbar Spine and Back Pain*, ed 3. New York, Churchill-Livingstone, 1987, pp 383–400.
6. Postacchini F: *Lumbar Spine Stenosis.* New York, Springer-Verlag Wien, 1989, pp 49–74.
7. Roberson GH, Llewellyn HJ, Taveras JM: The narrow lumbar spinal canal syndrome. *Radiology* 1973;107:89–97.
8. De Villiers PD, Booysen EL: Fibrous spinal stenosis: A report on 850 myelograms with a water-soluble contrast medium. *Clin Orthop* 1976;115:140–144.
9. Paine KW: Clinical features of lumbar spinal stenosis. *Clin Orthop* 1976;115:77–82.
10. Rosenberg NJ: Degenerative spondylolisthesis. Predisposing factors. *J Bone Joint Surg* 1975;57A:467–474.

11. Paine KW: Results of decompression for lumbar spinal stenosis. *Clin Orthop* 1976;115:96–100.
12. Moreland LW, López-Mendez A, Alarcón GS: Spinal stenosis: A comprehensive review of the literature. *Semin Arthritis Rheum* 1989;19:127–149.
13. Epstein JA, Epstein BS, Lavine LS, et al: Degenerative lumbar spondylolisthesis with an intact neural arch (pseudospondylolisthesis). *J Neurosurg* 1976;44:139–147.
14. Surin V, Hedelin E, Smith L: Degenerative lumbar spinal stenosis: Results of operative treatment. *Acta Orthop Scand* 1982; 53:79–85.
15. Wynne-Davies R, Walsh WK, Gormley J: Achondroplasia and hypochondroplasia. Clinical variation and spinal stenosis. *J Bone Joint Surg* 1981;63B:508–515.
16. Newman PH: Stenosis of the lumbar spine in spondylolisthesis. *Clin Orthop* 1976;115:116–121.
17. Getty CJ: Lumbar spinal stenosis: The clinical spectrum and the results of operation. *J Bone Joint Surg* 1980;62B:481–485.
18. Cauchoix J, Benoist M, Chassaing V: Degenerative spondylolisthesis. *Clin Orthop* 1976;115:122–129.
19. Iida H, Shikata J, Yamamuro T, et al: A pedigree of cervical stenosis, brachydactyly, syndactyly, and hyperopia. *Clin Orthop* 1989;247:80–86.
20. McRae DL: Radiology of the lumbar spinal canal, in Weinstein PR, Ehni G, Wilson CB (eds): *Lumbar Spondylosis; Diagnosis, Management and Surgical Treatment.* London, Year Book Medical, 1977, pp 92–114.
21. Babin E: Radiology of the narrow lumbar canal, in Wackenheim A, Babin E (eds): *The Narrow Lumbar Canal. Radiologic Signs and Surgery.* New York, Springer-Verlag, 1980, pp 1–10, 147–155.
22. Nightingale S: Development spinal canal stenosis and somatotype. *J Neurol Neurosurg Psychiatry* 1989;52:887–890.
23. Eisenstein S: The morphometry and pathological anatomy of the lumbar spine in South African negroes and caucasoids with specific reference to spinal stenosis. *J Bone Joint Surg* 1977;59B:173–180.
24. Yasuda Y, Dokoh S, Seko K, et al: Autosomal dominant osteosclerosis associated with familial spinal canal stenosis. *Neurology* 1986;36:687–692.
25. Weisz GM: Lumbar spinal canal stenosis in Paget's disease. *Spine* 1983;8:192–198.
26. Metcalfe RA, Butler P: Spinal cord compression in Léri's pleonosteosis. *Br J Radiol* 1985;58:1117–1119.
27. Weisz GM: Stenosis of the lumbar spinal canal in Forestier's disease. *Int Orthop* 1983;7:61–64.
28. Weisz GM: Lumbar spinal canal stenosis in osteopoikilosis. *Clin Orthop* 1982;166:89–92.
29. Epstein N, Whelan M, Benjamin V: Acromegaly and spinal stenosis: Case report. *J Neurosurg* 1982;56:145–147.
30. Lipson SJ, Naheedy MH, Kaplan MM, et al: Spinal stenosis caused by epidural lipomatosis in Cushing's syndrome. *N Engl J Med* 1980;302:36.
31. Epstein BS, Epstein JA, Jones MD: Cervical spine stenosis. *Radiol Clin North Am* 1977;15:215–226.
32. Yoshikawa S, Shiba M, Suzuki A: Spinal cord compression in untreated adult cases of vitamin-D resistant rickets. *J Bone Joint Surg* 1968;50A:743–752.
33. Epstein JA, Epstein BS, Jones MD: Symptomatic lumbar scoliosis with degenerative changes in the elderly. *Spine* 1979;4:542–547.
34. Bethem D, Winter RB, Lutter L, et al: Spinal disorders of dwarfism: Review of the literature and report of eighty cases. *J Bone Joint Surg* 1981;63A:1412–1425.
35. Singh A, Dass R, Hayreh SS, et al: Skeletal changes in endemic fluorosis. *J Bone Joint Surg* 1962;44B:806–815.
36. Friedman H: Intraspinal rheumatoid nodule causing nerve root compression: A case report. *J Neurosurg* 1970;32:689–691.
37. Becker DH, Conely FK, Anderson ME: Quadriplegia associated with narrow cervical canal, ligamentous calcification and ankylosing hyperostosis. *Surg Neurol* 1979;11:17–19.
38. Blaw ME, Langer LO: Spinal cord compression in Morquio-Brailsford's disease. *J Pediatr* 1969;74:593–600.
39. Sarpyener MA: Spina bifida aperta and congenital stricture of the spinal canal. *J Bone Joint Surg* 1947;29A:817–821.
40. Verbiest H: Neurogenic intermittent claudication. Lesions of the spinal cord and cauda equina, stenosis of the vertebral canal, narrowing of intervertebral foramina and entrapment of peripheral nerves, in Vinken PJ, Bruyn GW (eds): *Handbook of Clinical Neurology.* New York, Elsevier, 1976, pp 678–679.
41. Varughese G, Quartey GR: Familial lumbar spinal stenosis with acute disc herniations: Case reports of four brothers. *J Neurosurg* 1979;51:234–236.
42. Postacchini F, Massobrio M, Ferro L: Familial lumbar stenosis: Case report of three siblings *J Bone Joint Surg* 1985;67A:321–323.
43. Clark GA, Panjabi MM, Wetzel FT: Can infant malnutrition cause adult vertebral stenosis? *Spine* 1985;10:165–170.
44. Platt BS, Stewart RJC: Transverse trabeculae and osteoporosis in bones in experimental protein-calorie count. *Br J Nutr* 1962;16:483–494.

Spinal Stenosis: Clinical Evaluation

Harry N. Herkowitz, MD

Since its initial description by Verbiest[1] in 1954, spinal stenosis has become a well recognized clinical entity. The symptoms and signs of spinal stenosis have been confused with those of vascular claudication, and, in fact, peripheral vascular disease remains the primary clinical disorder in the differential diagnosis. The purpose of this chapter is to outline the natural history and clinical evaluation of a patient with suspected spinal stenosis. In addition, factors differentiating spinal stenosis from lumbar disc herniations, peripheral vascular disease, and peripheral neuropathy will be highlighted.

Natural History

Little information is available on the natural history of spinal stenosis. Johnsson and associates (unpublished data) studied three groups of patients with myelographically proven spinal stenosis. Group I consisted of 19 patients who received nonsurgical treatment. Group II consisted of 30 surgical patients without a complete myelographic extradural block. Group III was composed of 14 surgical patients with total myelographic occlusion of the dural sac. The mean duration of follow-up for the three groups was 29, 41, and 43 months, respectively. In group I, 11 patients (58%) showed improvement, in seven patients (37%) there was no change, and symptoms worsened in the last patient. In group II, improvement was noted in 19 patients (63%), and there was no change in 11 (36%). No patient in this group deteriorated as a result of the surgery. Of the 14 patients with complete block, nine (64%) improved, four (29%) were unchanged, and one was more debilitated than before the surgery.

Because diminished walking capacity is a common indication for surgery, walking capacity was evaluated in the three groups. In patients treated without surgery (group I), improved walking capacity was noted in eight (42%), six (32%) were unchanged, and five patients (26%) were worse. In group II, 15 (50%) showed improved walking capacity, eight (27%) were unchanged, and seven (23%) were worse. In the group with complete myelographic blockage (group III), 11 (79%) were improved, and three (32%) had reduced walking capacity. These results are less favorable than in most series, in which surgical success rates of 85% to 90% are reported.[2-8]

The authors also compared the postoperative results with the duration of symptoms in the different groups. Although better results were noted in those patients with a shorter duration of symptoms, this was not statistically significant.

In our experience, intermittent episodes of pain occur in 85% of patients with documented spinal stenosis, while only 15% demonstrate progressive deterioration. In those patients with episodic symptoms, it is impossible to predict the longevity or severity of each attack.

History

The age of onset of symptoms is related, in part, to the type of spinal stenosis.[6,9-11] Patients with congenital or developmental stenosis often note symptoms beginning in their early thirties. Both in a patient of normal stature, who has a congenitally narrow canal, and in a patient with achondroplastic dwarfism, symptom onset coincides with the development of osteoarthritis in a spinal canal with no reserve space.

Onset of degenerative stenosis, the most common form of spinal stenosis, occurs in the patient's mid to late fifties or early sixties.[12,13] Several early series reported significantly more males than females (3 to 1). However, with the increased recognition of this disorder, the ratio appears to favor females over males (5 to 1).[6,14] Degenerative spondylolisthesis also affects females significantly more often than males, perhaps because of hormonal factors leading to ligamentous laxity of the motion segment.[15,16]

Although low back pain is commonly associated with spinal stenosis, this symptom usually is not the reason for referral to the orthopaedic surgeon.[13] The quality of back pain is that seen in osteoarthritis—ache and stiffness, which is often worse in inclement weather. In addition, the back pain is usually insidious in onset rather than acute.[17] Patients rarely have a "sciatic list" or significant back spasm, as is seen in an individual with a herniated disk. The back pain is mechanical—activity aggravates it, and rest relieves the discomfort. Radiation of pain to the coccyx or buttocks is typical.[18] A clue that the low back pain may be associated with a narrow spinal canal is the development of progressive buttock discomfort, tightness, or burning brought about by walking or standing.[19] The patient may also walk with a forward list, because pain in the buttock or low back is lessened by this maneuver. Complaints of limited spine movement, although common, occur much less frequently than in patients with a lumbar disk herniation. In most patients, extension of the spine, such as in reaching up to get something out of a cabinet, is limited, but forward bending is not. Often extension leads to jolts of pain that move down the buttocks or legs. Patients with degenerative spondylolisthesis associated with spinal stenosis tend to have quantitatively and qualitatively more back pain than those with stenosis secondary to osteoarthritis alone.[20,21]

Complaints of leg pain, which prompt the referral to the orthopaedic surgeon, can be grouped into two types.[3,6,13,14,22] One type, typical sciatica, usually involves one extremity, in which aching or sharp pain follows a specific dermatomal distribution. Reflex changes and/or motor weakness may occur. The fifth lumbar nerve root is the most commonly involved, producing extensor hallucis longus or tibialis anterior weakness. Weakness occurs when the nerve root is entrapped in the lateral recess(es) or when a disk herniation is associated with the underlying spinal stenosis.

The second type, neurogenic claudication or pseudoclaudication, is the more common form of leg pain associated with spinal stenosis. Patients complain of pain, numbness, tingling, weakness, or cramping in one or, more commonly, both lower extremities. Neurogenic claudication is caused by central canal compression, which typically has an "hourglass" or "washboard" appearance on a myelogram. Classically, the pain begins in the low back or buttocks and radiates into the legs without following a specific dermatomal distribution. The symptoms may stop at the knee, but, as activity increases or the condition progresses, it will radiate to the lower leg and foot. Typically, walking or standing precipitates symptoms, and sitting and leaning forward or lying alleviates the extremity discomfort. A sudden worsening of symptoms or progression of neurologic findings may indicate a disk herniation associated with the spinal stenosis.

Claudication caused by vascular disease can be confused with claudication related to spinal stenosis.[23,24] Patients with peripheral vascular disease usually complain of cramping or tightness in the calves, with symptoms that begin distally and progress proximally. Extremity symptoms in patients with spinal stenosis begin proximally and progress distally. In addition, patients with vascular claudication obtain relief by standing, and those with neuroclaudication have persistent pain while standing, which is improved by sitting forward.[25] The claudication of vascular disease usually occurs after walking a constant distance, while patients with spinal stenosis walk a variable distance before symptoms occur (Table 1).

Peripheral neuropathy is another condition that can be confused with neuroclaudication.[26] In an elderly population, diabetes or other conditions that can cause neuropathy are often present in patients with suspected spinal stenosis. Burning or paresthesias that begins in the feet and progresses proximally is a typical neuropathic symptom. Usually the pain is worse at night and has no relation to activity. Patients may also complain of an inability to feel their feet, caused by posterior column involvement. In severe cases, weakness may occur in one or both lower extremities. A burning stocking distribution of discomfort below the knees, which is not related to activity, is the hallmark of neuropathy. This diagnosis can be confirmed by prolonged nerve conduction velocities on electrodiagnostic testing.

Urinary dysfunction is uncommon in patients with stenosis, occurring in only 3% to 4% of cases.[6] Because of the advanced age of many of these individuals, it is not uncommon for them to have bladder abnormalities unrelated to stenosis. Bladder complaints that are related to spinal stenosis usually involve incontinence.

Physical Examination

Palpation of the lower back usually does not elicit severe pain. Patients usually complain of discomfort deep within the muscles. Occasionally point tenderness may be elicited over the sacroiliac joint(s) and in the sciatic notch region. In performing range-of-motion maneuvers patients often can forward flex without difficulty, but extension is significantly limited. Brieg[27] has shown in cadaver studies that when the spine moves from flexion to extension, the following occurs: (1) spinal canal is shortened by 2.2 mm; (2) nervous tissue shortens and becomes broader; (3) ligamentum flavum shortens and broadens; (4) posterior protrusion of the disk occurs; and (5) there is interference with microcirculation of the nerve roots and cauda equina. All of these factors can contribute to the precipitation of buttock and/or leg pain when an individual with a compromised spinal canal attempts extension of the spine.

A straight leg raising test usually does not cause pain in spinal stenosis. It is more likely to produce pain in cases with an associated disk herniation.

Strength testing more often than not reveals little or no loss of function. Because the L4-L5 level is the most common vertebral level involved, the usual neurologic findings are mild extensor hallucis longus or tibialis anterior weakness. At the time of examination, the neurologic evaluation may be normal. The pathogenesis and pathophysiology of spinal stenosis are such that exercise can induce muscular weakness or a loss of a

Table 1
Comparison of vascular to neurogenic claudication.

Evaluation	Vascular	Neurogenic
Claudication distance	Fixed	Variable
Relief of pain	Standing	Sitting-flexed
Walk up hill	Pain	No pain
Bicycle ride	Pain	No pain
Type of pain	Cramp, tightness	Numbness, ache, sharp
Pulses	Absent	Present
Bruit	Present	Absent
Skin	Loss of hair, shiny	Normal
Atrophy	Rarely	Occasional
Weakness	Rarely	Occasional
Back pain	Uncommon	Common
Limitations of spinal movement	Uncommon	Common

reflex. In the office setting, patients are asked to walk up and down the hall several times or climb stairs, after which they are re-examined. At that time, objective neurological findings may be present. Atrophy may be seen in the thighs or calves in patients with longstanding neural compression. Patients with lateral recess stenosis tend to have weakness or atrophy more often than patients with central stenosis only.[28] The fifth lumbar nerve root is also the most common spinal level involved in lateral recess stenosis.

Reflex testing is often unreliable, because reflex loss is common in elderly patients.[3] Sensory deficits are also uncommon but, when present, are seen most often in the L4 or L5 dermatome. Diffuse sensory loss is more indicative of peripheral neuropathy.

By history, spinal stenosis presents a recognizable clinical picture. The paucity of physical findings may confuse the clinician initially as to the etiology of the patient's complaints. As the condition progresses and becomes more obvious, imaging studies will confirm the presence of a narrow spinal canal.

References

1. Verbiest H: A radicular syndrome from developmental narrowing of the lumbar vertebral canal. *J Bone Joint Surg* 1954;36B:230–237.
2. Bolesta MJ, Bohlman HH: Degenerative spondylolisthesis, in Barr JS Jr (ed): American Academy of Orthopaedic Surgeons *Instructional Course Lectures, XXXVIII.* Park Ridge, IL, American Academy of Orthopaedic Surgeons, 1989, chap 10, pp 157–165.
3. Grabias S: Current concepts review: The treatment of spinal stenosis. *J Bone Joint Surg* 1980;62A:308–313.
4. Herkowitz HN, Garfin SR: Decompressive surgery for spinal stenosis. *Semin Spine Surg* 1989;1:163–167.
5. Paine KWE: Results of decompression for lumbar spinal stenosis. *Clin Orthop* 1976;115:96–100.
6. Spengler DM: Current concepts review: Degenerative stenosis of the lumbar spine. *J Bone Joint Surg* 1987;69A:305–308.
7. Tile M, McNeil SR, Zarins RK, et al: Spinal stenosis: Results of treatment. *Clin Orthop* 1976;115:104–108.
8. Wiltse LL, Kirkaldy-Willis WH, McIvor GWD: The treatment of spinal stenosis. *Clin Orthop* 1976;115:83–91.
9. Blau JN, Logue L: Intermittent claudication of the cauda equina: An unusual syndrome resulting from central protrusion of a lumbar intervertebral disc. *Lancet* 1961;1:1081–1086.
10. Lipson S: Clinical diagnosis of spinal stenosis. *Semin Spine Surg* 1989;1:143–144.
11. Nelson MA: Lumbar spinal stenosis. *J Bone Joint Surg* 1973;55B:506–512.
12. Jones RAC, Thomson JLG: The narrow lumbar canal: A clinical and radiological review. *J Bone Joint Surg* 1968;50B:595–605.
13. Kirkaldy-Willis WH, Paine KWE, Cauchoix J, et al: Lumbar spinal stenosis. *Clin Orthop* 1974;99:30–50.
14. Hall S, Bartleson JD, Onfrio BM, et al: Lumbar spinal stenosis: Clinical features, diagnostic procedures and results of surgical treatment in 68 patients. *Ann Intern Med* 1985;103:271–275.
15. Cauchoix J, Benoist M, Chassaing V: Degenerative spondylolisthesis. *Clin Orthop* 1976;115:122–129.
16. Fitzgerald JAW, Newman PH: Degenerative spondylolisthesis. *J Bone Joint Surg* 1976;58B:184–192.
17. Evans JG: Neurogenic intermittent claudication. *Br Med J* 1964;2:985–987.
18. Wilson CB: Significance of the small lumbar spinal canal: Cauda equina compression syndromes due to spondylosis. Part 3: Intermittent claudication. *J Neurosurg* 1969;31:499–506.
19. Joffe R, Appleby A, Arjona V: Intermittent ischaemia of the cauda equina due to stenosis of the lumbar canal. *J Neurol Neurosurg Psychiatr* 1966;29:315–318.
20. Macnab I: Spondylolisthesis with an intact neural arch - the so-called pseudo-spondylolisthesis. *J Bone Joint Surg* 1950;32B:325.
21. Newman PH: Stenosis of the lumbar spine in spondylolisthesis. *Clin Orthop* 1976;115:116–121.
22. Schatzker J, Pennal GF: Spinal stenosis: A cause of cauda equina compression. *J Bone Joint Surg* 1968;50B:606–618.
23. Dodge LD, Bohlman HH, Rhodes RS: Concurrent lumbar spinal stenosis and peripheral vascular disease. *Clin Orthop* 1988;230:141–148.
24. Hawkes CH, Roberts GM: Neurogenic and vascular claudication. *J Neurosurg Sci* 1978;38:337–345.
25. Dyke P, Doyle JB: "Bicycle test" of Van Gelderen in diagnosis of intermittent cauda equina compression syndrome.. *J Neurosurg* 1977;46:667–670.
26. Thomas PK: Clinical features and differential diagnosis, in Dyck P, Thomas P, Lambert E, et al (eds): *Peripheral Neuropathy,* ed 2. Philadelphia, WB Saunders, 1984, pp 1169–1190.
27. Brieg A: *Biomechanics of the Central Nervous System.* Stockholm, Almquist & Wiksell, 1960.
28. Ciric I, Mikhael MA, Tarkington JA, et al: The lateral recess syndrome: A variant of spinal stenosis. *J Neurosurg* 1980;53:433–443.

Biomechanics of Lumbar Disk Disease

Malcolm H. Pope, DMSc, PhD

Daniel S. Pflaster, MS

Martin H. Krag, MD

Disparate Functions of the Spine

The lumbar spine has many challenging, and in some ways conflicting, demands placed upon it.[1] The spine must be mobile enough to permit the activities of daily living. In the lumbar spine, the mobility is mostly in flexion and extension. At the same time, the spine must be able to support loads, both those produced by the mass of the body segments and any external loads applied to the body. In addition, the spine must also be able to protect the neural structures—the spinal cord and the exiting nerve roots. Finally, the spine must be able to control precisely each portion of its individual motion segments in three-dimensional space. The structures that provide these functions may be thought of as passive elements (disks, ligaments, facet joints) and active elements (muscles and tendons).

The intervertebral disk plays a vital role in each of these functions. The disk, which is flexible and conforms to the vertebrae as they move, provides some shock absorption and mechanical protection of the vertebrae. Anatomically, because the disk represents one margin of the vertebral canal and intervertebral foramina, it can compromise the neural structures if it is injured. Finally, the disk provides some stability to the system. If a disk is diseased, degenerated, or injured,

some of these roles are compromised and loads are shifted to other structures.

Disk Structure

The functional unit of the lumbar spine includes the two adjacent vertebrae, the ligaments, and the intervertebral disk. Schmorl and Junghanns[2] termed this unit the motion segment. It can be thought of as a three-joint complex made up of the intervertebral disk and the two facet joints. The mechanical behavior of the motion segment is complex. For example, motion typically occurs as complex, coupled motions (the one or more motions that regularly occur with the main motion).

The disk itself forms the primary articulation and has a major role in weightbearing. The outer part of the disk (Fig. 1), the annulus fibrosus, is made up of as many as 90 collagen sheets loosely bonded together. The fibers in one sheet run obliquely to those in the adjacent sheet. The structure (Fig. 2) can be thought of as an inflated tire with the nucleus as a pressurized

Nucleus Pulposus   Posterior

Laminae

Annulus Fibrosus

Fiber

Anterior   Disk Axis

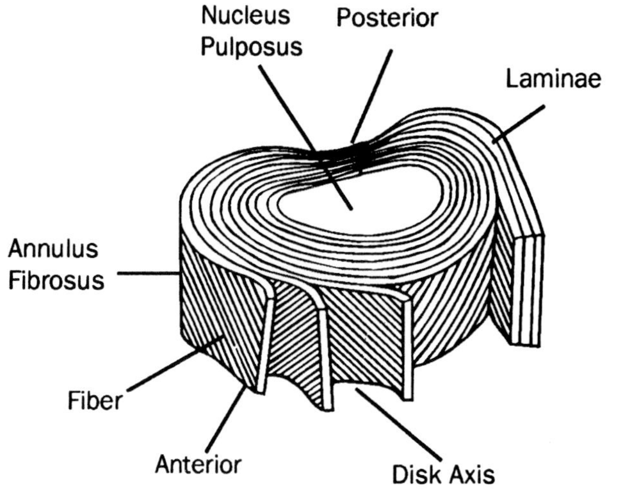

Fig. 1 The outer part of the disk, the annulus fibrosus, is made up of as many as 90 collagen sheets loosely bonded together.

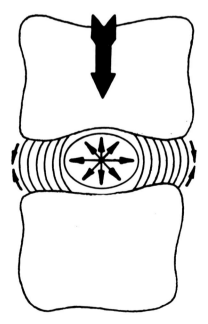

Fig. 2 The structure can be thought of as an inflated tire with the nucleus as a pressurized cavity that causes primarily tensile stresses in the annulus.

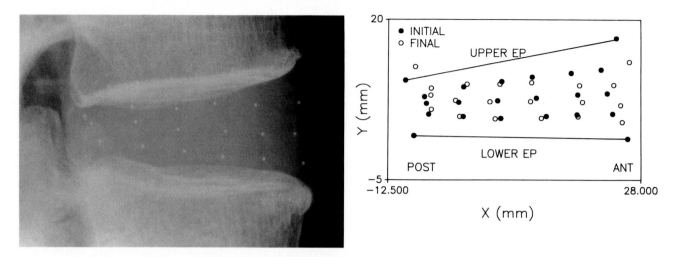

Fig. 3 Under flexion the nucleus moves posteriorly, under extension it moves anteriorly. These directions are opposite to those of the endplate. (Reproduced with permission from Seroussi RE, Krag MH, Muller DL, et al: Internal deformations of intact and denucleated human lumbar discs subjected to compression, flexion, and extension loads. *J Orthop Res* 1989;7:122–131.)

cavity that causes primarily tensile stresses in the annulus. White and Panjabi[3] have shown that, in the absence of a nuclear pressure, the stresses in the annulus become primarily compressive and larger in magnitude. This is closely related to the inward bulging of the annulus that we have shown to occur after denucleation.[4] Thus, we can envision how chemonucleolysis, degeneration, or nuclectomy could change the stress distribution and perhaps increase the rate of degeneration.

The nucleus pulposus is a well hydrated tissue. Kolditz and associates[5] have shown that the water content of the disk nucleus decreases from approximately 90% in the first year of life to 74% in the eighth decade. This water content is largely controlled by macromolecules (mucopolysaccharides) in the nucleus, which bind water and, as a result, cause fluid to flow into (or out of) the nucleus until the applied pressure and the osmotic pressure are in equilibrium. This interplay between mechanical and osmotic forces is vital both for the mechanical functioning of the disk and disk nutrition.[6] Thus, the intervertebral disk should be thought of as an osmotic system in which the outer periphery of the segment (the cartilaginous endplates and annulus fibrosus) behaves like a semipermeable membrane. Solute diffusion depends on the permeability of the particular pathway and also on the ionic nature of the solute in question. Glucose diffuses mainly through the endplates; sulfate ions are excluded from the highly charged nucleus and diffuse mainly through the annulus.[7] Nutrition is affected by aging, probably through changes in the relative amounts of proteoglycans and collagen, loss of nutritional pathways through the endplate,[8] immobilization,[9] and exposure to smoking.[10] Holm and Nachemson[11] and Holm and Rosenquist[12] showed in animal studies that whole-body vibrations

can disturb the nutrition of the intervertebral disks, leading to an intradiskal accumulation of metabolites. This has, as we shall see, possible relevance to the etiology of disk herniation in industrial workers exposed to sustained heavy mechanical loads.

Biomechanical Behavior

The intervertebral disk adapts well to the loads that are placed upon it. In axial compression, the increased intradiskal pressure is counteracted by annular fiber tension, disk space narrowing, and disk bulge.[1] We have developed a technique for the placement of radioopaque spheres in a matrix throughout the sagittal plane of the disk.[4,13] These experiments show that under flexion or extension, the nucleus moves posteriorly or anteriorly, respectively, in a direction opposite to that of the endplate (Fig. 3). This probably substantially reduces the high endplate stresses that would result without this shift mechanism.[13] In the denucleated disk, there is the appearance of inward bulging of the inner margin of the disk annulus that suggests delamination of the annulus.[4] Modic (personal communication, 1991) noted such delamination on magnetic resonance imaging and believes it to be a reliable sign of disk degeneration. Disk injury has also been shown[14] to produce changes in viscoelastic behavior of the motion segment. These mechanical events—altered stress distribution, inward bulging, and altered viscoelasticity— are probably closely related to the process of disk degeneration.

In axial rotation, the annulus fibers of one orientation are stretched significantly while those on the opposite side are shortened or crimped.[15] During torsion,

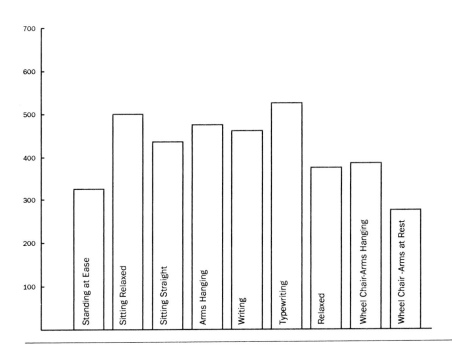

Fig. 4   The pressure increases in the standing posture as compared with the recumbent and is even greater in unsupported seating.

there is a tendency for the disk bulge to be reduced, the disk height to be increased, and the disk pressure to be increased. The mathematical models of Kraus[16] as well as those of Spilker[17] suggest that under torsion, there will be a significant stress concentration in the posterolateral margin of the annulus, a frequent site of disk herniation. Adams and Hutton,[18] in some unique in vitro tests, demonstrated that disks do not rupture under compression loading but that an endplate fracture can occur. Asymmetric loading, such as lateral bending or axial rotation, accompanied by compression, was necessary to cause a herniation. Wilder and associates[19] showed that cyclic loading can also herniate the disk.

Arguably, the greatest impact upon our knowledge of the disk has come from the work of Nachemson[20] and Nachemson and Elfström.[21] Nachemson reasoned that the disk nucleus behaves hydrostatically and, thus, the pressure measured there is indicative of the load on the disk. The pressure is approximately 1.5 times the mean applied pressure over the area of the endplate. Nachemson and Elfström[21] introduced a needle into the nucleus of normal human volunteers and found that the pressure varied substantially with posture and load. As shown in Figure 4, the pressure increases in the standing posture as compared with the recumbent and is even greater in unsupported seating.

The mechanical properties of the disk are influenced by the magnitude, the duration, and the frequency of the applied load, which suggests that the disk behaves in a viscoelastic manner.[22–28] The creep rate for a constant load decreases with time but is dependent on the load applied. The creep rate is faster in the degenerated

state.[25,26] As creep occurs, the stiffness of the motion segment unit increases. The mechanism that causes creep has been discussed earlier. When loaded, the disk loses fluid and decreases in height, and when unloaded the disk height recovers, absorbs fluid, and increases in height.[29]

Creep has also been estimated in vivo by the measurement of overall height changes. De Puky[30] first demonstrated this phenomena and also showed changes in diurnal height loss with age. Other workers[31,32] have improved the technique by more careful control of posture and by more closely spaced measurements to clarify the rate of height loss and recovery.[32] In a recent paper, an adaptation of the Eklund and Corlett[31] device was used to measure height loss in female subjects in three different age groups during static sitting. The load exposure time was five minutes, and repeated measurements were performed with 10 minutes intermission for rest.[33] The average height loss for subjects was 4.53 mm during exposure to static sitting. The height loss in the group aged 60 to 65 years was significantly larger than in the 40- to 45-year-old group, 6.28 mm and 3.46 mm respectively (Fig. 5).

More recently, we have developed a technique to measure creep in vivo[34] using the intersegmental motion device shown in Figure 6. This device was used to measure sagittal plane compression, rotation, and anteroposterior shear between two vertebrae by means of three strain-gauge extensometers mounted on pins rigidly fixed to the spinous processes. Posture was carefully controlled by means of rods. Segmental motion was measured continuously in three women during five

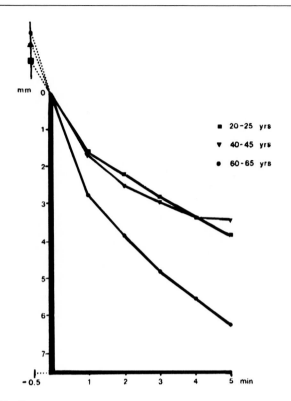

Fig. 5 Height loss in individuals 60 to 65 years of age is significantly greater than it is in those between 40 and 45 years of age, 6.28 mm and 3.46 mm, respectively. (Reproduced with permission from Magnusson M, Hult E, Lindstrom I, et al: Measurement of time-dependent height loss during sitting. *Clin Biomech* 1990;5:132–142.)

posterior elements. Further research is needed in this area.

Ergonomic Issues

Sitting is related to a higher incidence of low back pain.[34-38] Kelsey[38] found that sedentary workers were more likely to have a herniated disk and that the relative incidence increased in those over 35 years of age.

The classic work of Nachemson and Elfström[21] showed that there is a 40% increase in intradiskal pressure in sitting as compared with standing. In sitting, the lumbar spine flattens and the effective lever arm decreases for certain muscles, which results in higher levels of muscle activity and higher resultant forces through the disk. Andersson and associates[39-42] examined the effects of a backrest and a lumbar support. They showed that both myoelectric activity and disk pressure decreased when the back was supported by a backrest. This effect was optimal when the backrest was tilted 20 degrees backwards from vertical and was equipped with a lumbar support that protruded 4 cm from the backrest. This effect occurs because when a person leans against a backrest, part of the body weight is transferred to the backrest, which reduces the load on the lower back.

Many studies have shown that an increase in seated whole body vibration is associated with an increased incidence of low back pain.[43-48] Fewer studies have shown a relationship between whole body vibration and herniated nucleus pulposus, although Kelsey[38] and Kelsey and Hardy[49] found that male truck drivers are up to four times more likely to suffer a herniated disk. Early degenerative changes of the intervertebral disk in drivers of heavy vehicles have been found in the studies of Christ and Dupuis,[50] Rosegger and Rosegger,[51] and Gruber.[52] Several workers[45,48,53] have hypothesized that these findings may be explained by the results of their work, which shows that certain vehicles vibrate the spine at the first natural frequency and lead

minutes of quiet and erect sitting. The segmental motion is shown in Table 1.

It is clear from these reports that there is a loss of disk height during the day, and that there are additional losses when the disk is exposed to external loads. Some individuals may be more susceptible to disk symptoms in the morning (well hydrated disk); others may be more susceptible after loading or at the end of the day, when loads are transferred to other structures, such as the

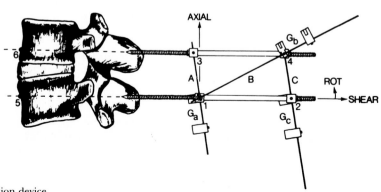

Fig. 6   Intersegmental motion device.

Table 1
Quasistatic segmental motion during quiet sitting*

Subject	Measured Response		
	Rotation (degree)	Axial (mm)	Shear (mm)
1	0.07	−0.22	0.00
2	0.07	−1.08	0.05
3	0.07	−0.88	0.05

* Duration = 300 seconds

to higher spinal loading. The first natural frequency is the frequency at which the excitation of the spine exceeds the input to it.

The National Institute for Occupational Safety and Health guidelines[54] summarize studies relating higher low back injury rates and severity rates to jobs in which: (1) heavy objects are lifted; (2) bulky objects are lifted (load-moment increases); (3) lifting starts at the floor; and (4) lifting is frequent. Although many sophisticated and complex mathematical models exist, relatively simple calculations can be used to show the magnitude of forces acting on the motion segment and thus on the disk. The model relies on the equilibrium of forces and moments. In practice, forces up equal forces down and clockwise moments equal counterclockwise moments. As shown in Figure 7, forces across the motion segment can be extremely high.

Effect of Surgery

In 1974, Markolf and Morris[55] proposed that disk injuries do not have lasting mechanical effects. In contrast, Panjabi and associates,[56] in 1981, showed that a partial excision of the annulus had substantial effects, with the greatest effect being on instability in axial rotation. Furthermore, when coupled with nucleotomy, such excision had major effects on instability in flexion, lateral bending, and axial rotation. Thus, such surgery should not be considered benign in terms of the biomechanics of the disk.

Conclusions

The intervertebral disk is an integral part of the functional spinal unit. Its composition is conducive to its role as a flexible, loadbearing structure. The constituents of the disk lend to it being an osmotic system that increases hydration with decreasing loads. The disk is susceptible to injury under asymmetric loads. The disk is subjected to large compressive forces, but compressive loads do not lead to disk failure. Surgery to the disk has profound mechanical consequences, particularly if the nucleus is removed.

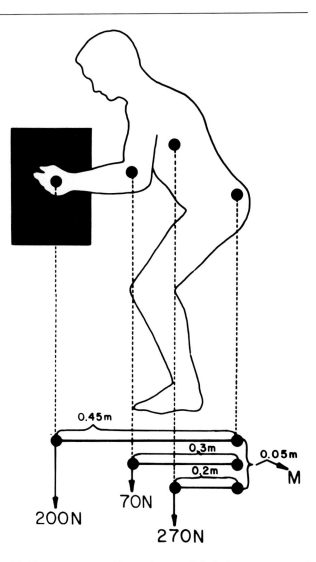

Fig. 7 Forces up equal forces down, and clockwise moments equal counterclockwise moments.

References

1. Pope MH, Andersson GBJ, Chaffin DB, et al: *Occupational Low Back Pain*. St. Louis, CV Mosby, 1990.
2. Schmorl G, Junghanns H: *Die gesunde und die kranke WirbeRsaule in Rontgenbild und Klinik 5*. Stuttgart, Aufl Thieme, 1968.
3. White AA, Panjabi MH: *Clinical Biomechanics of the Spine*. Philadelphia, JB Lippincott, 1990.
4. Seroussi RE, Krag MH, Muller DL, et al: Internal deformations of intact and denucleated human lumbar discs subjected to compression, flexion, and extension loads. *J Orthop Res* 1989;7:122–131.
5. Kolditz D, Kramer J, Gowin R: Wasser und elektrolytyehalt der bandscherben des menschen und wechselnder belastung. *Z Orthop* 1985;123:235–241.
6. Maroudas A, Stockwell RA, Nachemson A, et al: Factors involved in the nutrition of the human lumbar intervertebral disc: Cellularity and diffusion of glucose *in vitro*. *J Anat* 1975;120:113–130.
7. Urban JPG, Holms S, Maroudes A, et al: Nutrition of the intervertebral disc. *Clin Orthop* 1977;129:101–114.

8. Krämer J: Pressure dependent fluid shifts in the intervertebral disc. *Orthop Clin North Am* 1977;8:211–216.

9. Holm S, Nachemson A: Nutritional changes in the canine intervertebral disc after spinal fusion. *Clin Orthop* 1982;169:243–258.

10. Holm S, Nachemson A: Nutrition of the intervertebral disc: Acute effects of cigarette smoking: An experimental animal study. *Ups J Med Sci* 1988;93:91–99.

11. Holm S, Nachemson A: Nutrition of the intervetebral disc: Effects induced by vibrations. Presented at the International Society for the Study of the Lumbar Spine, Sydney, Australia, May 1985.

12. Holm S, Rosenquist AL: Morphological and nutritional change in the intervertebral disc after spinal motion. Presented at the European Society of Osteoarthrology, Kuopio, Finland, May 1986.

13. Krag MH, Seroussi RE, Wilder DG, et al: Internal displacement distribution from *in vivo* loading of human thoracic and lumbar spinal motion segments: Experimental results and theoretical prediction. *Spine* 1987;12:1001–1007.

14. Panjabi MM, Krag MH, Chung TQ: Effects of disc injury on mechanical behavior of the human spine. *Spine* 1984;9:707–713.

15. Stokes IAF: Surface strain on human intervertebral discs. *J Orthop Res* 1987;5:348–355.

16. Kraus H: Stress analysis, in Farfan HF (ed): *Mechanical Disorders of the Low Back*. Philadelphia, Lea & Febiger, 1973, p 112–133.

17. Spilker RL: Mechanical behavior of a simple model of an intervertebral disk under compressive loading. *J Biomech* 1980;13:895–901.

18. Adams MA, Hutton WC: Prolapsed intervertebral disk: A hyperflexion injury. *Spine* 1982;7:184–191.

19. Wilder DG, Pope MH, Frymoyer JW: The biomechanics of lumbar disk herniation and effect of overload and instability: Annual award of the American Back Society. *J Spinal Disorders* 1988;1:16–32.

20. Nachemson A: Disc pressure measurements. *Spine* 1981;6:93–97.

21. Nachemson AL, Elfström G: Intravital dynamic pressure measurements in lumbar discs: A study of common movements, maneuvers and exercises. *Scand J Rehabil Med Suppl* 1970;2:1–40.

22. Hirsch C, Nachemson A: New observations on the mechanical behavior of lumbar discs. *Acta Orthop Scand* 1954;23:254–283.

23. Hirsch C: The reaction of intervertebral discs to compression forces. *J Bone Joint Surg* 1955;37A:1188–1196.

24. Brown T, Hansen RJ, Yorra AJ: Some mechanical tests on the lumbosacral spine with particular reference to the intervertebral discs. *J Bone Joint Surg* 1957;39A:1135–1164.

25. Kazarian LE: Dynamic response characteristics of the human vertebral column: An experimental study on human autopsy victims. *Acta Orthop Scand* 1972;146(suppl):pp 1–186.

26. Kazarian LE: Symposium on the lumbar spine: Creep characteristics of the human spinal column. *Orthop Clin North Am* 1975;6:3–18.

27. Panjabi MM, Krag MH, White AA III, et al: Effects of preload on load displacement curves of the lumbar spine. *Orthop Clin North Am* 1977;8:181–192.

28. Keller TS, Hansson TH, Holm SH, et al: In vivo creep behavior of the normal and degenerated porcine intervertebral disc: A preliminary report. *J Spinal Dis* 1989;1:267–278.

29. Krämer J: *Biomekanische Veranderungen im Lumbalen Bewegungssegment*. Stuttgart, Hippokrates-Verlag, 1973.

30. De Puky P: The physiological oscillation of the length of the body. *Acta Orthop Scand* 1935;6:338–347.

31. Eklund JAE, Corlett EN: Shrinkage as a measure of the effect of load in the spine. *Spine* 1984;9:189–194.

32. Krag MH, Cohen MC, Haugh LD, et al: Body height change during upright and recumbent posture. *Spine* 1990;15:202–207.

33. Magnusson M, Hult E, Lindström I, et al: Measurement of time-dependent height loss during sitting. *Clin Biomech* 1990;5:137–142.

34. Kaigle AM, Pope MH, Fleming BC, et al: A method for the intravital measurement of interspinous kinematics, technical note. *J Biomech*, in press.

35. Hult L: The Munkfors investigation: A study of the frequency and causes of the stiff neck-brachialgia and lumbago-sciatica syndrome as well as observations on certain signs and symptoms from the dorsal spine and the joints of the extremities in industrial and forest workers. *Acta Orthop Scand* 1954;16(suppl):1–76.

36. Magora A: Investigation of the relation between low back pain and occupation. 3. Physical requirements: Sitting, standing and weight lifting. *Ind Med Surg* 1972;41:5–9.

37. Lawrence J: *Rheumatism in Populations*. London, William Heinemann Medical Books, 1977.

38. Kelsey JL: An epidemiological study of acute herniated lumbar intervertebral discs. *Rheum and Rehabil* 1975;14:144–159.

39. Andersson BGJ, Jonsson B, Örtengren R: Myoelectric activity in individual lumbar erector spinae muscles in sitting: A study with surface and wire electrodes. *Scand J Rehab Med* 1974;(suppl 3):91–108.

40. Andersson BGJ, Örtengren R: Lumbar disc pressure and myoelectric back muscle activity during sitting: I. Studies on an experimental chair. *Scand J Rehabil Med* 1974;6:104–114.

41. Andersson GBJ, Örtengren R: Lumbar disc pressure and myoelectric back muscle activity during sitting: II. Studies on an office chair. *Scand J Rehabil Med* 1974;6:115–121.

42. Andersson GBJ, Örtengren R, Nachemson A, et al: Lumbar disc pressure and myoelectric back muscle activity during sitting: IV. Studies on a car driver's seat. *Scand J Rehabil Med* 1974;6:128–133.

43. Vihko V, Hasan J: Biomedical aspects of low frequency vibration: A bibliography of reference. *Work Environ Health* 1970;7:91–107.

44. Wickström G: Effect of work on degenerative back disease: A review. *Scand J Work Environ Health* 1978;4(suppl 1):1–12.

45. Pope MH, Wilder DG, Frymoyer JW: Vibration as an etiologic factor in low back pain. *Orthop Trans* 1980;4:344–345.

46. Backman A-L: Health survey of professional drivers. *Scand J Work Environ Health* 1983;9:36–41.

47. Frymoyer JW, Pope MH, Clements JH, et al: Risk factors in low-back pain: An epidemiological survey. *J Bone Joint Surg* 1983;65A:213–218.

48. Wilder DG, Frymoyer JW, Pope MH: The effect of vibration on the spine of the seated individual. *Automedica* 1985;6:5–35.

49. Kelsey JL, Hardy RJ: Driving of motor vehicles as a risk factor for acute herniated lumbar intervertebral disc. *Am J Epidemiol* 1975;102:63–73.

50. Christ W, Dupuis H: Über die beanspruchung der wirbelsaüle unter dem einfluss sinusförmiger und stochastischer schwingungen. *Int Z Angew Physiol Arbeitsphysiol* 1966;22:258–278.

51. Rosegger R, Rosegger S: Health effects of tractor driving. *J Agric Eng Res* 1960;5:241–276.

52. Gruber GL: Relationships between whole body vibration and morbidity patterns among interstate truck drivers. Cincinnati, National Institute for Occupational Health and Safety, 1977.

53. Wilder DG, Woodworth BB, Frymoyer JW, et al: Vibration and the human spine. *Spine* 1987;12:243–254.

54. NIOSH (National Institute for Occupational Health and Safety): A Work Practices Guide for Manual Lifting. Cincinnati, Technical Report No. 81–122, 1981.

55. Markolf KL, Morris JM: The structural components of the intervertebral disc: A study of their contributions to the ability of the disc to withstand compressive forces. *J Bone Joint Surg* 1974;56A:675–687.

56. Panjabi MM, Hausfeld JN, White AA III: A biomechanical study of the ligamentous stability of the thoracic spine in man. *Acta Orthop Scand* 1981;52:315.

CHAPTER 21

The Radiologic Evaluation of Lumbar Degenerative Disk Disease and Spinal Stenosis in Patients With Back or Radicular Symptoms

Richard J. Herzog, MD

Introduction

Patients with back or leg pain have always been a challenge to the treating physician. Up to the early 1900's, given the limited understanding of most physicians of the anatomy and pathophysiology of the spine, patients with spine symptoms were usually diagnosed as having some type of rheumatologic condition and were treated empirically. The approach to patients with neural dysfunction changed radically after Mixter and Barr[1] reported that a herniated lumbar disk could cause back or leg pain. For the first time, it was possible to define precisely the cause of the patient's symptoms, a fact that altered not only the physician's decision-making process in patient evaluation, but also the expectation of the patient undergoing treatment. As patients became aware that a definitive surgical procedure had the potential of eliminating their pain, surgery quickly became the gold standard against which other therapeutic regimens were measured. The description of a herniated disk as a "ruptured disk" also implied an association between the occasion that marked the onset of symptoms, for example, an injury incurred at work or as a result of an accident, and a specific acute traumatic event.

More than 50 years have passed since the initial description of disk herniation. It is now evident that herniations are only one of a myriad causes of back and leg pain, and that disk herniation is just one manifestation of the degenerative process affecting the spinal motion segment. Approximately 50% of patients with a disk herniation can remember a precise traumatic episode that antedated the onset of their pain, but even these patients, when questioned further, are often able to remember short episodes of nondebilitating back pain that preceded the event that they feel precipitated their herniated disk.

Kirkaldy-Willis[2] was one of the first investigators to stress the importance of the dynamic nature of disk degeneration and herniation. Many stages of disk degeneration may be subclinical or cause mild intermittent discomfort. Even when a degenerating disk causes few symptoms, the biomechanics of the spinal motion segment are affected by the disk's altered viscoelastic properties. The abnormal biomechanics may result in segmental spinal instability, facet arthrosis, and, eventually, spinal stenosis. Any component of this degenerative cascade may be the cause of the patient's initial episode of back or radicular pain.

With the development and implementation of such advanced radiologic imaging studies as computed tomography with multiplanar reformations (CT/MPR) and magnetic resonance imaging (MRI), it is now possible to delineate accurately any pathomorphologic changes at an abnormal spinal motion segment in a patient with acute or chronic back or radicular pain. Frequently, disk disease is associated with degenerative osseous changes that must be defined precisely to allow a rational choice between alternative therapeutic regiments. The following section discusses MRI and CT evaluation of disk disease and spinal stenosis in patients with either acute or chronic back or leg pain.

Degenerative Disk Disease

Both CT/MPR and MRI provide excellent delineation of morphologic changes of disk degeneration. The major difference between the imaging modalities resides in the ability of MRI to delineate pathoanatomic and physiochemical changes in a degenerating disk before the disk contour has altered. Both the nucleus pulposus and annulus fibrosus consist of water, collagen, and proteoglycans, with the major differences between the two being the relative amount of these components, level of hydration, and the particular type of collagen that predominates.[3] MRI precisely delineates the different parts of disk architecture. On T_2-weighted images, the high signal intensity in the central portion of the disk originates from both the nucleus pulposus and the inner annular fibers.[4] The outer annular fibers demonstrate very low signal intensity, as do the adjacent anterior and posterior longitudinal ligaments[5] (Fig. 1). The signal intensity in the disk is related to its state of hydration and the physiochemical state of the diskal tissue.[6,7] With aging, there is gradual breakdown of proteoglycans in the nucleus, gradual desiccation of the mucoid nuclear material, and loss of anatomic delineation between the nucleus and inner annular fibers.[8] In individuals older than 30, an intranuclear cleft, which represents ingrowth of fibrous tissue,[9] can be identified in normal disks on T_2-weighted MR images.

Both experimentally and clinically, the occurrence of a radial annular tear may be the necessary step in the development of disk degeneration or herniation.[10,11] It is now possible with MRI to delineate small tears in the outer annulus with T_2-weighted[11] or gadolinium-diethylenetriamine penta-acetic acid (Gd-DTPA) enhanced T_1-weighted images[12] (Fig. 2). When the radial tear communicates with the nucleus, the disk begins to degen-

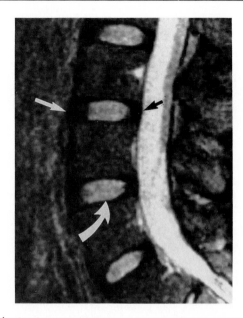

Fig. 1 On the sagittal MR T$_2$-weighted image, there is high signal intensity within the nucleus pulposus and inner annular fibers (curved white arrow). In the anterior outer annular fiber/anterior longitudinal ligament complex (straight white arrow) and posterior outer annular fiber/posterior longitudinal ligament complex (straight black arrow), there is absence of an MR signal.

erate and demonstrates decreased signal intensity on T$_2$-weighted images. Disk herniations result from the possible displacement of nuclear material through these communicating radial tears. Displacement of the nuclear material into the region of the outer annular-posterior longitudinal ligament complex will alter the morphology of the peripheral contour of the disk, resulting in a focal protrusion of the disk beyond the margin of the vertebral body endplates. A contained disk herniation is displaced nuclear material that is still bound by the outer annular fibers and/or the posterior longitudinal ligaments. Both CT/MPR and MRI delineate these contour changes clearly (Fig. 3).[13,14]

In some patients, the development of annular fissures may lead to internal disk disruption[15] or intervertebral disk resorption[16] without the displacement of nuclear material. MRI is helpful in evaluating these situations, because it demonstrates altered signal intensity in the abnormal disk. Unfortunately, it is relatively common to detect disk levels that have decreased signal intensity, but that are totally asymptomatic.[17] For this reason, some patients with persistent back pain who have had an MR study delineating decreased signal intensity at one or more disk levels are further evaluated with diskography and CT diskography. In addition to the information these tests provide on abnormal morphology

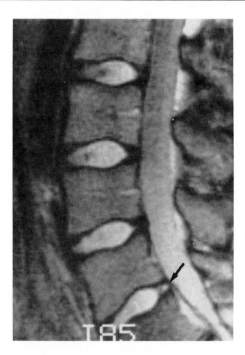

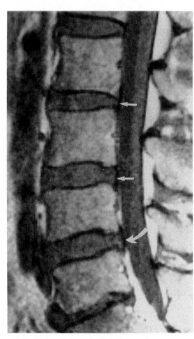

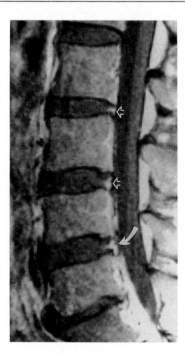

Fig. 2 On the sagittal MR T$_2$-weighted image (**left**) at the L5-S1 level, there is a posterior annular fissure (black arrow). The fissure has increased signal intensity when compared with the normal posterior outer annular fibers at the superjacent normal disk level. In another patient, on the MR T$_1$-weighted sagittal image (**center**), at the L2-3 and L3-4 levels, the posterior annular fibers (straight white arrows) have normal morphology and signal intensity. At the L4-5 disk level, there is a small posterior disk protrusion (curved white arrow). After the intravenous injection of Gd-DTPA on a repeat sagittal T$_1$-weighted sequence (**right**), posterior annular fissures demonstrating increased signal intensity are identified at the L2-3 and L3-4 disk levels (open white arrows) and increased signal intensity is present in the small posterior disk protrusion at the L4-5 disk level (curved white arrow). There is no increased signal intensity in the normal L1-2 disk.

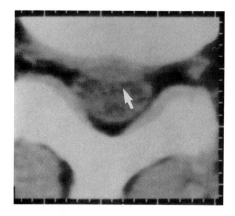

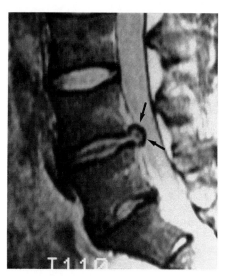

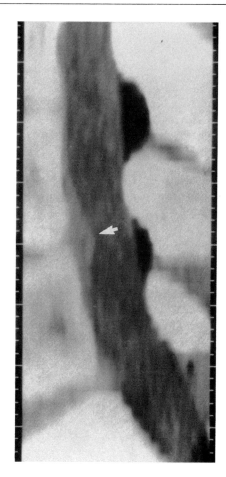

Fig. 3 On the axial CT/MPR image (**top left**) and the sagittal reconstructed image (**right**), there is a posterior midline contained disk herniation (white arrow). The herniation has smooth contours and is elevating the posterior longitudinal ligament. On the sagittal MR T_2-weighted image (**bottom left**), there is a posterior contained disk herniation at the L4-5 disk level. An intact posterior longitudinal ligament (black arrows) is delineated surrounding the disk herniation.

of the disk, the diskogram is a provocative test to demonstrate the patient's pain response when the disk is injected (Fig. 4). When performing lumbar diskography, the suspected abnormal disk level and the contiguous disk levels are routinely injected, even when these disks appear normal on the MR evaluation. There have been several reports documenting disks that had normal signal intensity on MRI, but that proved to be abnormal morphologically on diskography.[18,19]

With the superb soft-tissue resolution of MRI, it is frequently possible to determine whether the disk herniation is contained by the outer annular-posterior longitudinal ligament complex or whether it has extruded through this complex to become an extruded, noncontained herniation (Fig. 5).[20] This information is needed for the successful application of percutaneous diskectomy[21] and chemonucleolysis. It is also important as an indicator of surgical outcome for lumbar disk herniation.[22] The diagnosis of disk extrusion from CT studies depends on the configuration of the herniated disk.[23,24] Axial images are always needed on either the MR study or the CT/MPR study to evaluate neural displacement or impingement and to detect posterolateral or lateral disk herniations.

Herniated disk material may separate from the disk of origin and become a sequestered fragment. MRI is useful in differentiating between a disk extrusion and sequestration. Compared with the degenerated disk of origin, sequestered disk fragments usually generate increased signal intensity on T_2-weighted images. In one prospective study, the accuracy of MRI in differentiating sequestered disk fragments from other forms of lumbar disk herniation was 85%, compared with a 65% accuracy for CT myelography.[25] The differential diagnosis of a sequestered disk fragment includes epidural abscess,[26] extradural tumor,[27] conjoined nerve root,[28] nerve root sheath tumor or cyst,[29] and epidural hematoma.[30]

After herniation, the disk continues to degenerate, and on an MR study, the degenerated disk demonstrates decreased signal intensity on the T_2-weighted sequence. To date, there has been no prospective study to determine the length of time necessary for a normally hydrated disk to become desiccated after it her-

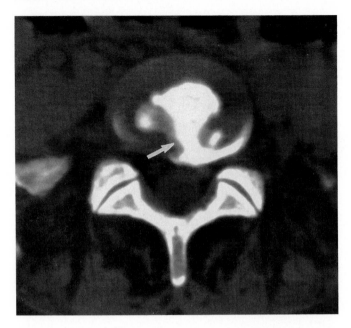

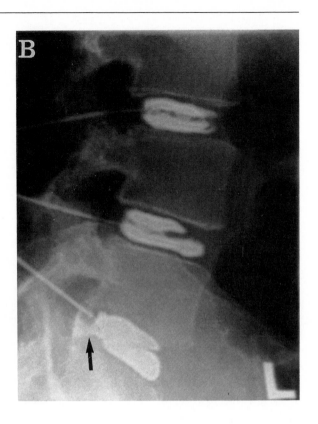

Fig. 4 On an axial CT image (**left**) from a CT diskogram, a posterior annular fissure is identified (white arrow). Contrast extends posteriorly into the outer annular fibers and is contained by the posterior annular/posterior longitudinal ligament complex. At the time of diskography (**right**), the patient experienced severe concordant back pain when the L5-S1 disk level was injected and the posterior annular fissure filled with contrast (black arrow). There was no pain when the normal L3-4 and L4-5 disk levels were injected.

Fig. 5 On the sagittal MR proton density-weighted image (**left**) at the L5-S1 disk level, there is a posterior disk extrusion (open black arrow) that has penetrated through the posterior annular/posterior longitudinal ligament complex (curved black arrow). On the T$_2$-weighted image (**right**) the interrupted posterior annular/posterior longitudinal ligament complex (curved black arrow) is delineated. In addition, the posterior displacement of the right S1 nerve root (black arrow head) by the disk extrusion is delineated.

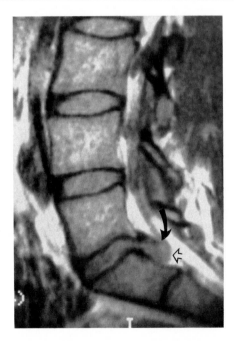

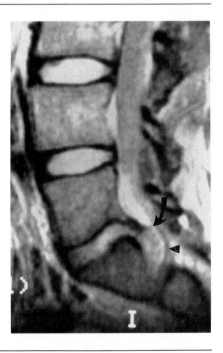

niates. Therefore, it is not possible to date the exact occurrence of a disk herniation if a prior study is not available for comparison. Even when secondary degenerative changes, such as endplate osteophytes, are identified, a disk herniation still can represent an acute process superimposed on a chronic degenerative state. In

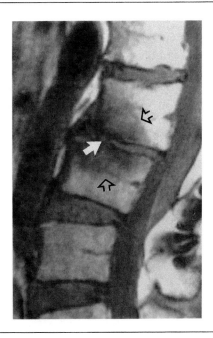 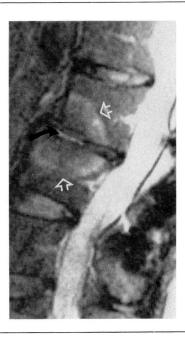

Fig. 6 On the sagittal MR T_1-weighted image (**left**) at the L2-3 disk level, moderately severe decreased disk height (white arrow) is present along with a minimal retrolisthesis. There is a hemispheric region of decreased signal intensity (open black arrows) in the cancellous bone adjacent to the degenerative diskovertebral joint. On the T_2-weighted image (**right**), there is increased signal intensity (open white arrows) in the cancellous bone compatible with grade I endplate degenerative changes. Increased signal intensity present in the anterior portion of the disk space (curved black arrow) most likely represents fluid in degenerative fissures.

cases of long-standing disk degeneration, fluid-containing fissures may be present in the degenerative disk along with ingrowth of granulation tissue.[31] These pathologic changes may result in increased signal intensity in the disk on T_2-weighted images, and this should not be confused with an inflammatory process (Fig. 6).[32] Calcification or gas in a degenerated disk may be difficult to detect on T_2-weighted images because of the decreased signal intensity in the disk and the absence of a MR signal from the calcium or gas. T_1-weighted or gradient echo images are more useful when a vacuum phenomenon or disk calcification is to be delineated.[33]

The excellent characterization of normal and abnormal disks by MRI and CT/MPR has made possible the noninvasive study of the natural history of disk degeneration and herniation. Multiple studies have reported the excellent sensitivity, specificity, and accuracy of MRI[34,35] and CT[23,36,37] in the diagnosis of disk disease. For this reason, invasive studies, such as myelography and CT myelography, are rarely indicated for the evaluation of disk abnormalities. Even when there is evidence of disk degeneration or herniation, it is important to remember that asymptomatic lumbar disk herniation is relatively common.[38–40] The increased use of MRI has made it clear that disk degeneration and herniation afflict adolescents[41,42] and young adults,[43] as well as patients over the age of 30.

Disk degeneration and herniation alter the biomechanics of the diskovertebral joint. Endplate degenerative changes are frequently associated with degenerative disk disease. MRI is extremely sensitive to degenerative changes in the adjacent vertebral body endplates, and Modic and associates[44] have described the pathologic alterations in the vertebral body marrow adjacent to disks undergoing degeneration. Compared with normal marrow, type I endplate degeneration shows a decrease in signal intensity in the subchondral cancellous bone on a T_1-weighted image and an increase on a T_2-weighted image. This region of altered signal intensity pathologically represents prominent fibrovascular tissue in the marrow adjacent to the vertebral body endplate. Type II endplate degenerative changes, which pathologically represent increased fat in the subchondral bone marrow, display signal hyperintensity on T_1-weighted images and slight hyperintensity or isointensity on T_2-weighted images, when compared with normal marrow. Type III endplate degenerative changes represent coarsening and thickening of the subchondral trabeculae, which is depicted on T_1- and T_2-weighted images as decreased signal intensity. Gradient echo sequences are frequently part of the routine MR evaluation of the lumbar spine. These sequences are less sensitive to signal intensity changes within the disk or the adjacent vertebral body marrow associated with disk degeneration [33] than are standard spin echo T_1- and T_2-weighted sequences (Fig. 7). On CT/MPR evaluation, only endplate sclerosis can be delineated, and this is not necessarily correlated to type III changes identified by MRI. On the T_1-weighted image, the MR signal intensity of the vertebral body is predominantly determined by the amount of fat present in the marrow. It is, therefore, possible to maintain normal signal intensity in a vertebra with thickened trabeculae if there is still a critical amount of residual fat present in the marrow.

Endplate osteophytosis is frequently associated with disk degeneration. The excellent delineation of osseous

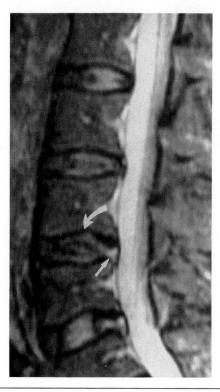

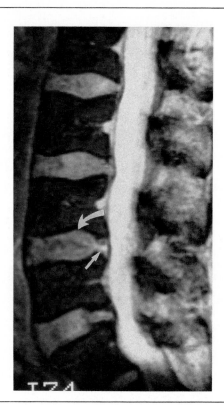

Fig. 7 On the sagittal MR T$_2$-weighted (**left**), there is moderate disk desiccation identified at the L4-5 disk level (curved white arrow) and a posterior annular fissure (straight white arrow). On the same patient on a sagittal gradient echo image (**right**), the signal intensity within the L4-5 disk (curved white arrow) is almost identical to the normal superjacent L3-4 disk. It is difficult to detect that disk desiccation is present. The posterior annular fissure (straight white arrow) is also difficult to delineate because of the increased signal intensity within the degenerated disk.

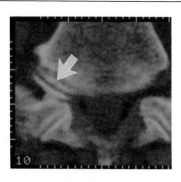

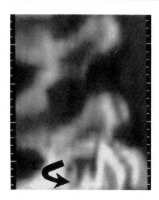

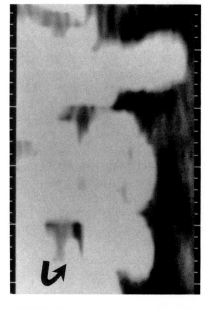

Fig. 8 On the axial CT/MPR image (**left**), at the L5-S1 disk level, there are spondylotic ridges (white arrow) projecting into the right intervertebral canal. The sagittal reconstructed images (**center** and **right**) optimally delineate the degree of stenosis secondary to the degenerative ridges (curved black arrow). Impingement of the exiting L5 nerve root is identified on image (**right**).

structures and superior spatial resolution possible with CT make it more accurate than MRI in the evaluation of the location and size of endplate ridges. CT permits accurate delineation of the position of endplate proliferative changes in relation to neural structures and differentiation of ridges from disk material (Fig. 8). With MRI, it may be difficult to distinguish an osseous ridge from herniated disk material because of the hypointensity of both structures on T$_1$- and T$_2$-weighted sequences. This problem is not uncommon in the inter-

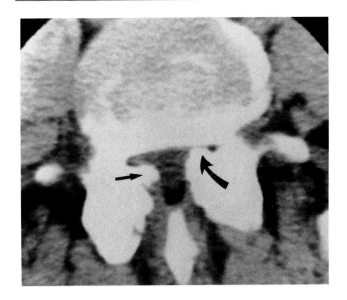

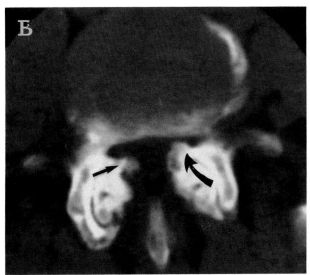

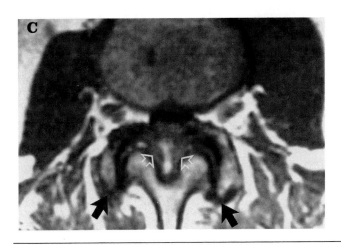

Fig. 9   On the axial CT images (**top left** and **top right**) severe facet degenerative changes are delineated, with hyperostotic ridges projecting off the anteromedial margin of the right facet joint (straight black arrow) and left facet joint (curved black arrow) causing severe central canal stenosis. In addition, the degenerative changes of the left facet joint are causing severe stenosis of the subarticular lateral recess. On the axial MR image (**bottom**), the hypertrophic degenerative changes of the facet joints (straight black arrows) and the hypertrophied ligamenta flava (white arrows) are causing narrowing of the central spinal canal.

vertebral canal, where posterolateral disk herniations are frequently associated with osseous ridges that project from the vertebral body endplates.

Spinal Stenosis

Spinal stenosis, defined as a local, segmental, or generalized narrowing of the central or intervertebral canals by bony or soft-tissue elements, can eventually encroach on neural structures. The narrowing may involve the bony canal alone, the dural sac, or both.[45] The degenerative changes most often associated with stenosis include hyperostotic ridging of the vertebral body endplates, hypertrophy and degenerative ridging of the facet joints, and hypertrophy of the ligamenta flava and anterior facet capsules.[46,47] The role of MRI and CT/MPR in the evaluation of patients with back pain, radiculopathy, or intermittent claudication is not just to demonstrate that stenosis is present, but to define the relative contributions of each component of the stenotic process (Fig. 9).

In the lumbar spine, it has become clear that patients of any age can have disk degeneration superimposed on a stenotic process, or they can have isolated stenosis as a cause of leg or back pain.[48,49] In order to determine the true diameter of the central spinal canal, axial images orthogonal to the long axis of the spinal canal or midline sagittal images must be performed. With the excellent spatial resolution of osseous structures, CT/MPR provides the optimal technique to ascertain precise osseous spinal measurements.

The classification of spinal stenosis as congenital, developmental, and acquired is extremely helpful when evaluating a small spinal canal.[50,51] Congenital stenosis results from disturbed fetal development and can occur as one element of a congenital malformation of the lumbar spine. Developmental stenosis is a growth disturbance of the posterior elements, involving the pedicles, lamina, or articular processes, resulting in decreased volume of the spinal canal.[52] A true midline osseous sagittal diameter measuring less than 12 mm is considered relative stenosis, and a diameter of less than 10 mm is considered absolute stenosis.[53] This diameter is measured from the middle of the posterior surface of the vertebral body to the point of junction of its spinous process and laminae. With relative stenosis, the reserve capacity of the spinal canal is reduced, thus predisposing the neural elements to impingement or compression by a small disk herniation or mild degenerative changes. Acquired stenosis is the narrowing of the central or intervertebral canals by degenerative changes of the diskovertebral joints, facet joints, and ligamenta flava.[47,50,54]

In a prospective study, the spines of 60 patients with suspected lumbar disk herniations and/or central stenosis were studied with surface coil MRI, CT, and/or myelography, and the results were compared with the findings at surgery. The surgical diagnosis of stenosis agreed with MRI in 77% of the cases, with CT in 79%, and with myelography in 54%.[55] This study did not differentiate between central and intervertebral canal stenosis, and the CT study did not include multiplanar reformations, which are extremely helpful in the evaluation of central and intervertebral canal stenosis.[56,57] With MRI, the cross-sectional area of the thecal sac can also be evaluated. In one study using CT myelography, this measurement was found to be useful in the evaluation of patients with central stenosis and neurogenic claudication.[58]

In addition to osseous degenerative changes that can lead to stenosis of the spinal canal, other osseous abnormalities that can narrow the central spinal canal include post-traumatic deformity, overgrowth of a spinal fusion,[59] Paget's disease,[60] fluorosis, vertebral hemangiomas,[61] diffuse idiopathic skeletal hyperostosis,[62] and hypertrophy and ossification of the posterior longitudinal ligament and ligamenta flava.[63] Intraspinal masses can also cause neurogenic claudication. Disease processes to consider in patients with spinal claudication include intraspinal synovial cysts,[2,64–67] intra and extradural tumors,[68–70] multiple myeloma, metastatic disease, and hypertrophy of the extradural fat.[71,72]

The importance of intervertebral canal stenosis as a cause of radicular symptoms[73] and its significance in failed back surgery has been well-documented.[48] Considering that all intervertebral canals in the spinal column have a vertical and horizontal dimension, as well as a length (up to 12 mm at the L5-S1 disk level), the canals are truly a three-dimensional structure and should not be designated as foramen. Pathologic changes of any component of the intervertebral canal may impinge or compress the exiting nerve root. The intervertebral canal at the L5-S1 disk level is unique in its morphometry and, because of its length, it can be stenotic at its entrance, mid, or exit zone. The most common etiology of stenosis at this level is osteophytic ridges that project from the inferior endplate of L5 or, less commonly, the superior endplate of S1.[46,74] De-

generative changes of the facet joint or the anterior facet capsule can decrease the volume of the posterior and superior compartment of the intervertebral canal and can cause neural compression. Extracanalicular (far out) stenosis[75] can also occur at the L5-S1 disk level in young patients with spondylolisthesis or in elderly patients with disk degeneration and scoliosis.[76] The stenosis is secondary to the apposition of the base of the junction of the transverse process and pedicle of L5 to the adjacent sacral ala. In addition, osseous ridges can project from the lateral margin of the vertebral body endplates of L5 and S1 and impinge the L5 nerve root in the paravertebral gutter (far-far out stenosis). The pathoanatomy of this region is optimally delineated by CT and the three-dimensional images created from the CT data (Fig. 10).

Degenerative spondylolisthesis is an important cause of central canal stenosis and most frequently involves the L4-5 disk level.[77] Disk degeneration, along with degenerative changes of sagittally oriented facet joints,[78] predisposes the motion segment to an anterolisthesis that, because of the intact neural arch, rarely progresses beyond a grade I slip. The combination of hyperstotic ridges projecting from the anteromedial margin of the facet joints, hypertrophy of the ligamenta flava, annular redundancy, and an anterolisthesis can result in severe central canal and subarticular lateral recess stenosis. There is usually at least mild narrowing of the intervertebral canals in the cephalocaudal direction secondary to the decreased disk height and the anterolisthesis.

Both disk degeneration and spinal stenosis are frequently detected in patients with isthmic spondylolisthesis. The occurrence of disk herniation has been reported both at the spondylolytic level[79] and at the superjacent motion segment.[80,81] Intervertebral canal stenosis at the L5-S1 disk level is also relatively common because of the decreased cephalocaudal dimension of the canal secondary to the anterolisthesis. This predisposes the L5 nerve root to dynamic impingement and entrapment by osseous ridges that encroach on the canal.

Conclusion

Both CT/MPR and MRI are excellent noninvasive imaging studies used to delineate pathomorphologic changes of the spinal motion segment. The transformation of the data from these exams into useful clinical information requires precise correlation of exam results with the patient's clinical condition and any additional diagnostic tests, such as electromyographs, that have been performed. It is now evident that proliferative osseous degenerative changes occur concurrently with disk degeneration and herniation. For this reason, it is necessary that all components of the spinal motion

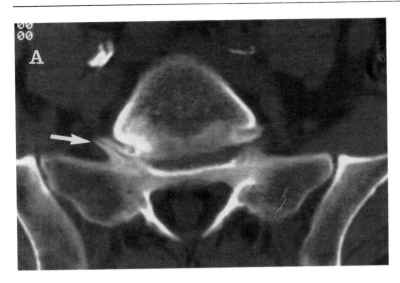
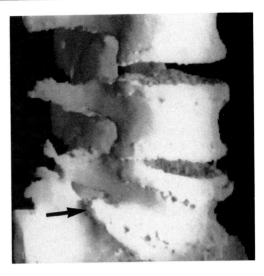

Fig. 10   On the axial CT image (**left**) at the L5-S1 disk level, spondylotic ridges (white arrow) are projecting off the vertebral body endplates at the exit zone of the right intervertebral canal. The size and position of the spondylotic ridges (black arrow) are easier to appreciate on the three-dimensional image (**right**) constructed from the CT data.

segment be completely evaluated in each patient who has back or leg pain in order to determine the pathoetiology of their symptom complex.

References

1. Mixter WJ, Barr JS: Rupture of the intervertebral disc with involvement of the spinal canal. *N Engl J Med* 1934;211:210–214.
2. Kirkaldy-Willis WH: The pathology and pathogenesis of low back pain, in Kirkaldy-Willis WH (ed): *Managing Low Back Pain*. New York, Churchill Livingstone, 1988, p 49–75.
3. Ghosh P (ed): *The Biology of the Intervertebral Disc*. Boca Raton, CRC Press, 1988, vol 1, p 245.
4. Yu SW, Haughton VM, Ho PS, et al: Progressive and regressive changes in the nucleus pulposus: Part II. The adult. *Radiology* 1988;169:93–97.
5. Pech P, Haughton VM: Lumbar intervertebral disk: Correlative MR and anatomic study. *Radiology* 1985;156:699–701.
6. Ghosh P (ed): *The Biology of the Intervertebral Disc*. Boca Raton, CRC Press, 1988, vol 2, p 207.
7. Hickey DS, Aspden RM, Hukins DW, et al: Analysis of magnetic resonance images from normal and degenerate lumbar intervertebral discs. *Spine* 1986;11:702–708.
8. Miller JA, Schmatz C, Schultz AB: Lumbar disc degeneration: Correlation with age, sex, and spine level in 600 autopsy specimens. *Spine* 1988;13:173–178.
9. Aguila LA, Piraino DW, Modic MT, et al: The intranuclear cleft of the intervertebral disk: Magnetic resonance imaging. *Radiology* 1985;155:155–158.
10. Lipson SJ, Muir H: Proteoglycans in experimental intervertebral disc degeneration. *Spine* 1981;6:194–210.
11. Yu S, Haughton VM, Sether LA, et al: Criteria for classifying normal and degenerated lumbar intervertebral disks. *Radiology* 1989;170:523–526.
12. Ross JS, Modic MT, Masaryk TJ: Tears of the anulus fibrosus: Assessment with Gd-DTPA-enhanced MR imaging. *AJR* 1990; 154:159–162.
13. Kambin P, Nixon JE, Chait A, et al: Annular protrusion: Path-

ophysiology and roentgenographic appearance. *Spine* 1988;13: 671–675.
14. Williams AL, Haughton VM, Meyer GA, et al: Computed tomographic appearance of the bulging annulus. *Radiology* 1982; 142:403–408.
15. Blumenthal SL, Baker J, Dossett A, et al: The role of anterior lumbar fusion for internal disc disruption. *Spine* 1988;13:566–569.
16. Jaffray D, O'Brien JP: Isolated intervertebral disc resorption: A source of mechanical and inflammatory back pain? *Spine* 1986; 11:397–401.
17. Boden SD, Davis DO, Dina TS, et al: Abnormal magnetic-resonance scans of the lumbar spine in asymptomatic subjects. *J Bone Joint Surg* 1990;72A:403–408.
18. Zucherman J, Derby R, Hsu K, et al: Normal magnetic resonance imaging with abnormal discography. *Spine* 1988;13:1355–1359.
19. Bernard TN Jr: Lumbar discography followed by computed tomography: Refining the diagnosis of low-back pain. *Spine* 1990; 15:690–707.
20. Grenier N, Greselle J-F, Vital J-M, et al: Normal and disrupted lumbar longitudinal ligaments: Correlative MR and anatomic study. *Radiology* 1989;171:197–205.
21. Mink JH: Imaging evaluation of the candidate for percutaneous lumbar discectomy. *Clin Orthop* 1989;238:83–103.
22. Hurme M, Alaranta H: Factors predicting the result of surgery for lumbar intervertebral disc herniation. *Spine* 1987;12:933–938.
23. Fries JW, Abodeely DA, Vijungco JG, et al: Computed tomography of herniated and extruded nucleus pulposus. *J Comp Assist Tomogr* 1982;6:874–887.
24. Glenn WV Jr, Rhodes ML, Altschuler EM, et al: Multiplanar display computerized body tomography applications in the lumbar spine. *Spine* 1979;4:282–352.
25. Masaryk TJ, Ross JS, Modic MT, et al: High-resolution MR imaging of sequestered lumbar intervertebral disks. *AJR* 1988;150: 1155–1162.
26. Post MJD, Quencer RM, Montalvo BM, et al: Spinal infection: Evaluation with MR imaging and intraoperative US. *Radiology* 1988;169:765–771.
27. Sze G, Krol G, Zimmerman RD, et al: Malignant extradural spinal

tumors: MR imaging with Gd-DTPA. *Radiology* 1988;167:217–223.

28. Peyster RG, Teplick JG, Haskin ME: Computed tomography of lumbosacral conjoined nerve root anomalies: Potential cause of false-positive reading for herniated nucleus-pulposus. *Spine* 1985;10:331–337.

29. Goyal RN, Russell NA, Benoit BG, et al: Intraspinal cysts: A classification and literature review. *Spine* 1987;12:209–213.

30. Levitan LH, Wiens CW: Chronic lumbar extradural hematoma: CT findings. *Radiology* 1983;148:707–708.

31. Coventry MB, Ghormley RK, Kernohan JW: The intervertebral disc: Its microscopic anatomy and pathology. Part II. Changes in the intervertebral disc concomitant with age. *J Bone Joint Surg* 1945;27A:233–247.

32. Modic MT, Feiglin DH, Piraino DW, et al: Vertebral osteomyelitis: Assessment using MR. *Radiology* 1985;157:157–166.

33. Modic MT, Masaryk TJ, Ross JS. et al: Imaging of degenerative disk disease. *Radiology* 1988;168:177–186.

34. Edelman RR, Shoukimas GM, Stark DD, et al: High-resolution surface-coil imaging of lumbar disk disease. *AJR* 1985;144:1123–1129.

35. Forristall RM, Marsh HO, Pay NT: Magnetic resonance imaging and contrast CT of the lumbar spine: Comparison of diagnostic methods and correlation with surgical findings. *Spine* 1988;13:1049–1054.

36. Firooznia H, Benjamin V, Kricheff II, et al: CT of lumbar spine disk herniation: Correlation with surgical findings. *AJR* 1984;142:587–592.

37. Haughton VM, Eldevik OP, Magnaes B, et al: A prospective comparison of computed tomography and myelography in the diagnosis of herniated lumbar disks. *Radiology* 1982;142:103–110.

38. Powell MC, Wilson M, Szyprt P, et al: Prevalence of lumbar disc degeneration observed by magnetic resonance in symptomless women. *Lancet* 1986;2(8520):1366–1367.

39. Weinreb JC, Walbarsht LB, Cohen JM: Prevalence of lumbosacral intervertebral disk abnormalities on MR images in pregnant and asymptomatic nonpregnant women. *Radiology* 1989;170:125–128.

40. Wiesel SW, Tsourmas N, Feffer HL, et al: A study of computer-assisted tomography: I. The incidence of positive CAT scans in an asymptomatic group of patients. *Spine* 1984;9:549–551.

41. Epstein JA, Epstein NE, Marc J, et al: Lumbar intervertebral disk herniation in teenage children: Recognition and management of associated anomalies. *Spine* 1984;9:427–432.

42. Erkintalo M, Salminen JJ, Paajanen H, et al: Disk degeneration in 14-year-old children: MR imaging study on low back pain and asymptomatic groups in radiology. Presented at the 75th Anniversary Scientific Assembly and Annual Meeting of the Radiological Society of North America, Chicago, IL, Nov 26-Dec 1, 1989.

43. Paajanen H, Erkintalo M, Kuusela T, et al: Magnetic resonance study of disc degeneration in young low-back pain patients. *Spine* 1989;14:982–985.

44. Modic MT, Steinberg PM, Ross JS, et al: Degenerative disk disease: Assessment of changes in vertebral body marrow with MR imaging. *Radiology* 1988;166:193–199.

45. Arnoldi CC, Brodsky AE, Cauchoix J, et al: Lumbar spinal stenosis and nerve root entrapment syndromes: Definition and classification. *Clin Orthop* 1976;115:4–5.

46. Rauschning W: Normal and pathologic anatomy of the lumbar root canals. *Spine* 1987;12:1008–1019.

47. Schneck CD: The anatomy of lumbar spondylosis. *Clin Orthop* 1985;193:20–37.

48. Burton CV, Kirkaldy-Willis WH, Yong-Hing K, et al: Causes of failure of surgery on the lumbar spine. *Clin Orthop* 1981;157:191–199.

49. Hasso AN, McKinney JM, Kileen J, et al: Computed tomography

50. Verbiest H: Fallacies of the present definition, nomenclature, and classification of the stenoses of the lumbar vertebral canal. *Spine* 1976;1:217–225.

51. Verbiest H: Words, images, knowledge, and reality: Some reflections from the neurosurgical perspective. *Acta Neurochir (Wein)* 1983;69:163–193.

52. Roberson GH, Llewellyn HJ, Taveras JM: The narrow lumbar spinal canal syndrome. *Radiology* 1973;107:89–97.

53. Verbiest H: Results of surgical treatment of idiopathic developmental stenosis of the lumbar vertebral canal: A review of twenty-seven years experience. *J Bone Joint Surg* 1977;59B:181–188.

54. Schnebel B, Kingston S, Watkins R, et al: Comparison of MRI to contrast CT in the diagnosis of spinal stenosis. *Spine* 1989;14:332–337.

55. Modic MT, Masaryk T, Boumphrey F, et al: Lumbar herniated disk disease and canal stenosis: Prospective evaluation by surface coil MR, CT and myelography. *AJR* 1986;147:757–765.

56. Lancourt JE, Glenn WV Jr, Wiltse LL: Multiplanar computerized tomography in the normal spine and in the diagnosis of spinal stenosis: A gross anatomic-computerized tomographic correlation. *Spine* 1979;4:379–390.

57. McAfee PC, Ullrich CG, Yuan HA, et al: Computed tomography in degenerative spinal stenosis. *Clin Orthop* 1981;161:221–234.

58. Bolender NF, Schönström NS, Spengler DM: Role of computed tomography and myelography in the diagnosis of central spinal stenosis. *J Bone Joint Surg* 1985;67A:240–246.

59. Kirkaldy-Willis WH, Wedge JH, Yong-Hing K, et al: Pathology and pathogenesis of lumbar spondylosis and stenosis. *Spine* 1978;3:319–328.

60. Weisz GM: Lumbar spinal canal stenosis in Paget's disease. *Spine* 1983;8:192–198.

61. Ross JS, Masaryk TJ, Modic MT, et al: Vertebral hemangiomas: MR imaging. *Radiology* 1987;165:165–169.

62. Karpman RR, Weinstein PR, Gau EP, et al: Lumbar spinal stenosis in a patient with diffuse idiopathic skeletal hypertrophy syndrome. *Spine* 1982;7:598–603.

63. Kurihara A, Tanaka Y, Tsumura N, et al: Hyperostotic lumbar spinal stenosis: A review of 12 surgically treated cases with roentgenographic survey of ossification of the yellow ligament at the lumbar spine. *Spine* 1988;13:1308–1316.

64. Jackson DE Jr, Atlas SW, Mani JR: Intraspinal cynovial cysts: MR imaging. *Radiology* 1989;170:527–530.

65. Kurz LT, Garfin SR, Unger AS, et al: Intraspinal synovial cyst causing sciatica. *J Bone Joint Surg* 1985;67A:865–871.

66. Liu SS, Williams KD, Drayer BP: Synovial cysts of the lumbosacral spine: Diagnosis by MR imaging. *AJR* 1990;154:163–166.

67. Maupin WB, Naul LG, Kanter SL: A case report: Synovial cyst presenting as a neural foraminal lesion: MR and CT appearance. *AJR* 1989;153:1231–1232.

68. Gennuso R, Zappulla RA, Strenger SW: A localized lumbar spinal root arteriovenous malformation presenting with radicular signs and symptoms. *Spine* 1989;14:543–546.

69. McGuire RA, Brown MD, Green BA: Intradural spinal tumors and spinal stenosis. *Spine* 1987;12:1062–1066.

70. Yang WC, Zappulla R, Malis L: Case report: Neurolemmoma in lumbar intervertebral foramen. *J Comput Assist Tomogr* 1981;5:904–906.

71. Badami JP, Hinck VC: Symptomatic deposition of epidural fat in a morbidly obese woman. *AJNR* 1982;3:664–665.

72. Stambough JL, Cheeks ML, Keiper GL: Nonglucocorticoid-induced lumbar epidural lipomatosis: A case report and review of literature. *J Spinal Disorders* 1989;2:201–207.

73. Porter RW, Hibbert C, Evans C: The natural history of root entrapment syndrome. *Spine* 1984;9:418–421.

of children and adolescents with suspected spinal stenosis. *J Comput Assist Tomogr* 1987;11:609–611.

74. Bohatirchuk F: The aging vertebral column (macro- and histo-radiographical study). *Br J Radiol* 1955;28:389–404.

75. Wiltse L: Far-out syndrome, in Rothman LG, Glenn WV Jr (eds): *Multiplanar CT of the Spine*. Baltimore, University Park Press, 1985, pp 384–393.

76. Grubb SA, Lipscomb HJ, Coonrad RW: Degenerative adult onset scoliosis. *Spine* 1988;13:241–245.

77. Macnab I: Spondylolisthesis with an intact neural arch—the so-called pseudo-spondylolistheses. *J Bone Joint Surg* 1950;32B: 325–333.

78. Sato K, Wakamatsu E, Yoshizumi A, et al: The configuration of the laminas and facet joints in degenerative spondylolisthesis: A clinicocardiologic study. *Spine* 1989;14:1265–1271.

79. Szypryt EP, Twining P, Mulholland RG: The prevalence of disc degeneration associated with neural arch defects of the lumbar spine assessed by magnetic resonance imaging. *Spine* 1989;14: 977–981.

80. Grenier N, Kressel HY, Scheibler ML, et al: Isthmic spondylolysis of the lumbar spine: MR imaging at 1.5T. *Radiology* 1989;170: 489–493.

81. Rothman SL, Glenn WV Jr: CT multiplanar reconstruction in 253 cases of lumbar spondylolysis. *ANJR* 1984;5:81–90.

CHAPTER 22

The Pathophysiology and Diagnosis of Low Back Pain and Sciatica

Mark D. Brown, MD, PhD

Introduction

There have been many recent advances in the clinical and basic sciences concerning the cause and cure of back pain and sciatica. This chapter interprets these new findings in light of my 20 years of experience in the management of patients who suffer from back and leg pain.

The increased understanding of the natural history of disk degeneration and disk herniation is of help to the diagnostician. Evidence indicates that the consequences of disk degeneration account for most back and leg pain syndromes. A study demonstrating the tissue origin of pain that results from disk failure has been of help to me in diagnosis and is also included, as is a simple and helpful categorization of all causes of back and leg pain syndromes.

Familiarity with the pathophysiology of various painful conditions affecting the spine is essential to obtain an accurate patient history of present illness, understand physical examination findings, and interpret the significance of confirmatory tests. Pain drawings and magnetic resonance imaging (MRI) have improved our diagnostic acumen, and current knowledge in these areas is also presented.

Diagnostic Groups for Low Back Pain and Leg Pain

One helpful strategy in diagnosing the cause of back and leg pain syndromes is to assign patients to one of five diagnostic groups. These are (1) benign etiologies, (2) radiculopathy from a herniated disk, (3) radiculopathy secondary to spinal stenosis, (4) serious underlying disorders, and (5) behavioral disorders.[1]

Benign Disorders

Benign etiologies for low back pain include many causes, which have in common a poorly localized source of pain, a self-limiting clinical course, and spontaneous resolution of symptoms despite treatment. Low back sprain, facet syndrome, osteoarthritis, acute annular tear, bulging disk, and degenerative disk disease are among the many diagnostic terms included in the benign low back pain group.

Radiculopathy

Herniated Disk I place the nerve root pain from a herniated disk and that caused by spinal stenosis into sep-

arate categories because the symptoms and signs that accompany these two disorders differ. Radiculopathy secondary to a herniated disk occurs when tension and compression on a lumbar nerve root result in irritation and ectopic stimulus of the root.[2] The pain pattern can be presented by the patient on a pain drawing in a typical dermatomal distribution. Patients complain of pain that radiates from proximal to distal in the sciatic or femoral nerve distribution. On physical examination, their ability to carry out straight leg raising or the femoral stretch test is limited and produces pain along the course of the sciatic or femoral nerve, respectively, associated with one or more reflex, sensory, or motor deficits.

Spinal Stenosis Radiculopathy secondary to spinal stenosis is caused by a slow circumferential constriction of the lumbar nerve root(s). It usually does not lead to irritation of the spinal nerve roots, and ectopic stimulus resulting in the radicular pain seen with an acute herniated disk is absent. Spinal stenosis may lead to venous congestion,[3] loss of nutrition through the spinal fluid to the roots,[4] and ischemia of the roots.[5] Any or all three of these mechanisms can cause neurogenic claudication, which is characterized by pain in the back and lower extremities with activity, relieved by rest. On physical examination, these patients exhibit a normal range of motion of the spine, normal straight leg raising without pain, and no neurologic deficits. The pain drawing by the patient typically shows a bilateral multiradicular distribution.

Serious Underlying Disorders

Serious underlying disorders encompass a variety of other causes of back and/or leg pain.[6] Hematogenous disk space infection, impending posterior rupture of an aortic aneurysm, pathologic fractures, and intrathecal neurofibromas are among the diagnoses included in this category.

Behavioral Disorders

Psychogenic regional pain disturbance[7] or behavioral disorders form a diagnostic and prognostic category for low back and leg pain. Patients who suffer from litigation neurosis with pending liability claims for injuries commonly come under this category. The very common condition of medication-induced depression with pain enhancement also fits into this category.

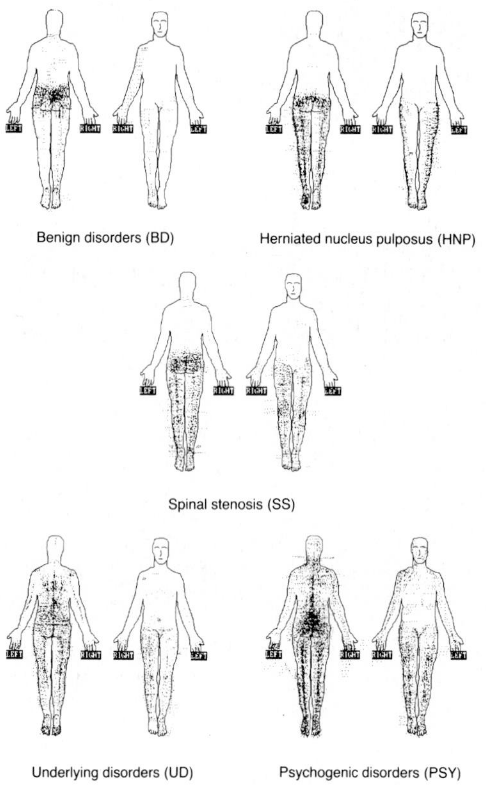

Benign disorders (BD)   Herniated nucleus pulposus (HNP)

Spinal stenosis (SS)

Underlying disorders (UD)   Psychogenic disorders (PSY)

Fig. 1 Computer generated superimposition of 50 patients' pain drawings in each of five diagnostic categories of low back pain and sciatica. (Reproduced with permission from Mann NH III, Brown MD: Artificial intelligence in the diagnosis of low back pain. *Orthop Clin North Am* 1991;22:303–314.)

Chief Complaints

The patient's chief complaint is easily depicted on a pain drawing. In the case of a unilateral first sacral radiculopathy secondary to a displaced lumbosacral disk, the pain drawing may show a highly specific dermatomal distribution. Conversely, the patient suffering from psychogenic regional pain disturbance with a strong hysterical and hypochondriacal component may place pain symbols over the entire anterior and posterior silhouette of the pain drawing, with qualifying remarks and symbols outside the silhouette.[8] In such cases, one picture speaks a thousand words. Because their pain does not arise from a specific organic source, it is difficult for these patients to provide a verbal chief complaint. There is a direct correlation between the degree of hysteria and hypochondriasis and certain bizarre features of the pain drawing. Because, in my experience, the pain drawing is an accurate and effective method of determining the patient's chief complaint, I have attempted to determine its usefulness as a diagnostic tool.

Certain characteristic pain patterns depicted by the patient on an anterior and posterior silhouette can be recognized easily by the clinician. Pain drawings not only give a qualitative diagnostic representation of the patient's pain, but also provide a quantitative estimate of the severity of the pain. When we superimposed pain marks from fifty patients in each of the five diagnostic categories on a single anteroposterior silhouette (Fig. 1), we saw that patients within the benign disorders group placed their pain markings on the area corresponding to the low back.[9] Patients with a herniated lumbar disk placed markings in the mid aspect of posterior leg and lateral aspect of the thigh and calf. The markings were more common on the left side than the right side, corresponding to the more common incidence of herniated disks on the left side.

Our finding, that patients with spinal stenosis had a more frequent distribution of pain markings on the anterior thigh and lower leg than those with herniated disks, probably reflects the fact that spinal stenosis is more common at the L3-L4 and L4-L5 level, whereas disk herniation is more common at L4-L5 and L5-S1.

Patients with underlying disorders place pain markings over the lower thoracic and upper lumbar spine area in the midline. Patients with behavioral disorders placed pain markings over the entire anterior and posterior silhouette and outside the silhouettes.

A computerized artificial intelligence neural network was programmed to recognize characteristic pain drawings in five different categories of diagnosis. The computer's ability to recognize the correct diagnostic group from 50 patients' pain drawings was compared with that of seven low back pain medical experts. The computer's ability to detect the correct diagnosis from the pain drawing alone was equal to that of the seven spine experts. Fifty percent of the time both the computer and the experts picked the correct group, a rate significantly better than could be expected by chance alone (20%).

We found that the pain drawing should be completed by the patient. An attendant shows the patient how it is done, but should not fill it out for the patient. Certain characteristic pain drawings are easily recognized by the computer or the experts. For example, patients with radiculopathy (Fig. 2) and patients with behavioral disorders (Fig. 3) frequently make easily recognizable pain drawings. We found that patients who suffer from benign disorders and serious underlying disorders (Fig. 4) are less likely to depict a characteristic pain drawing. The pain drawing also may be a clue to other causes of leg pain such as osteoarthritis of the hip (Fig. 5).

Anatomic Sources of Low Back and Leg Pain

In a classic study,[10] pain responses to tissue stimulation were recorded during operations on the lumbar

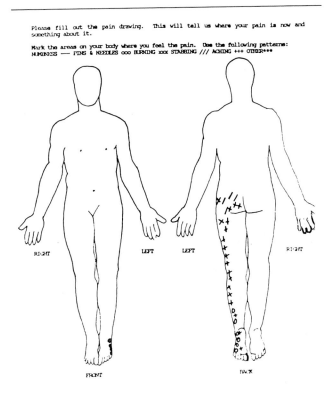

Fig. 2 Patient-generated pain drawing typical of a first sacral nerve root radiculopathy. A fifth lumbar disk displacement involving the nerve root was confirmed by MRI scan.

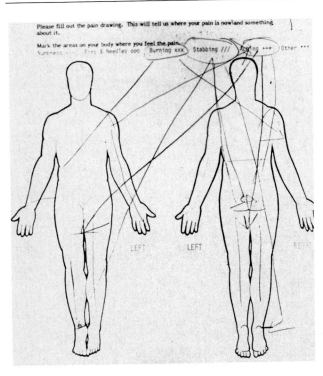

Fig. 3 Typical patient-generated pain drawing by patient suffering from a psychogenic regional pain disturbance.

spine using local anesthesia. The results of this study have helped me understand the source of low back pain and sciatica.

When stimulated at the time of surgery, the skin and a compressed nerve root are always painful. When a compressed or irritated nerve root was stimulated, the patient experienced back and/or leg pain 99% of the time, whereas stimulating a normal nerve root caused pain in only 11% of patients being operated on under local anesthesia. The pain was severe in less than 9% of cases where a normal nerve root was stimulated but was severe in 90% of irritated and compressed nerve roots. In the latter cases patients felt pain as far as the foot, but when normal nerve roots were stimulated, pain was never felt below the knee.

In this study, the peripheral annulus fibrosus and posterior longitudinal ligament were a frequent source of pain production when stimulated, but all the other structures of the motion segment unit rarely produced pain. No pain was produced by stimulation of the ligamentum flavum, the spinous processes, or noncompressed nerve roots, and there was rarely any pain when the supraspinous and intraspinous ligament, facet capsules, and muscle attachments to the spinous processes and lamina were stimulated.

These observations are very pertinent to the diagnostician. One may assume from them that the majority

of attacks of low back pain occur when disk displacement stimulates the free nerve endings in the posterior longitudinal ligament and annulus fibrosus. Sciatic pain, however, results from irritation of a nerve root by a disk herniation.

In one frequent chronology, patients experience recurring attacks of low back pain presumably caused by a radial tear in the inner annulus fibrosus with partial herniation of the nucleus pulposus, which creates tension on the peripheral annulus fibrosus and posterior longitudinal ligament. Subsequently, when the annulus fibrosus ruptures completely and the nucleus pulposus is displaced in the spinal canal, leg pain develops because of compression of the nerve root. When this happens, the back pain may be relieved because there is no longer tension on the free nerve endings in the peripheral annulus fibrosus and posterior longitudinal ligament. When a patient gives a history of this sequence of pain experience, it is fairly certain that the patient is suffering from an extruded disk.[11]

Cauda Equina Syndrome

Cauda equina syndrome from massive disk prolapse in the lumbar spine is uncommon.[12] However, the diagnostician must be aware that it can occur. These patients have acute severe back pain and bilateral leg pain, are unable to stand or void, and have various degrees of neurologic deficits in both lower extremities. They may have decreased rectal tone and perianal anesthesia.

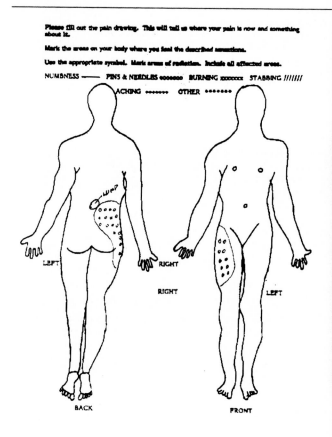

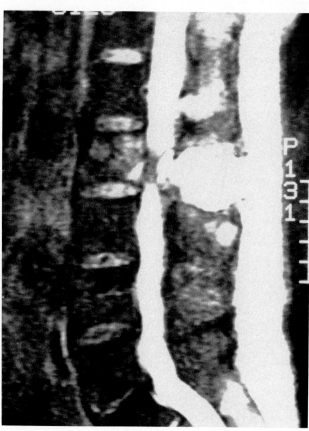

Fig. 4 **Left,** Patient-generated pain drawing which was specific for a serious underlying disorder. Note the patients descriptive "lump" with an arrow to a circle. The pain referral pattern to the upper lateral flank is typical of a serious disorder. **Right,** The diagnosis of a malignant neoplasm was confirmed by MRI scan and biopsy. Note the lesion in the second lumbar vertebral body and spinous process. (Reproduced with permission from Brown MD: Low back pain and sciatica: An easy approach to diagnosis and prognosis. *Consultant* 1991;31:23–25.)

The problem with cauda equina syndrome is that, despite immediate recognition, confirmation of diagnosis by MRI or myelogram, and decompression of the cauda equina, it may be too late for restoration of function.

The levels of pressure occurring during compression of the cauda equina that will produce irreversible changes in physiologic function have recently been determined.[13] It is known that the normal cauda equina in animals can sustain compression of as much as 200 mm Hg for less than two hours and still recover to some degree following release of compression. However, this amount of compression for a period longer than two hours will irreversibly damage the cauda equina. A displaced nucleus pulposus within the spinal canal can generate swelling pressures in excess of 200 mm Hg and, therefore, can account for the paralysis, infrequently seen, but certainly possible, from massive disk prolapse.[14]

The diagnostician must always be alert to the possibility of the occasional patient with a cauda equina syndrome. For most patients who come to the emergency room because of acute back pain, the cause is an an-

nular tear into the region of the posterior longitudinal ligament and posterior annulus fibrosus. Other patients with acute low back pain are chemically dependent on narcotic analgesics and are suffering from an acute psychogenic regional pain disturbance.

It is not infrequent for a patient with an acute severe back pain who is seen in the emergency room to be given an injection of narcotics and then develop urinary retention. These patients are difficult to differentiate from those with early cauda equina syndrome caused by massive disk prolapse. A careful history, physical examination, and emergency confirmatory test such as a magnetic resonance imaging scan, along with an awareness of the possibility of these various causes of acute back and leg pain, will allow a rapid and accurate differential diagnosis.

Pain-Related Sleep Disturbance

Patterns of pain-related sleep disturbances can provide important clues to the differential diagnosis of

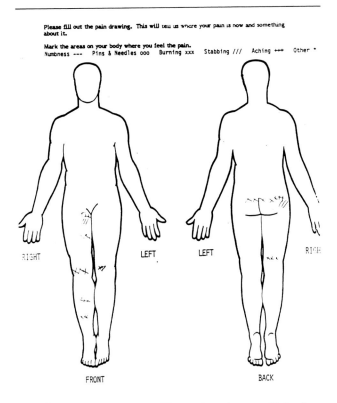

Please fill out the pain drawing. This will tell us where your pain is now and something about it.

Mark the areas on your body where you feel the pain.
Numbness --- Pins & Needles ooo Burning xxx Stabbing /// Aching +++ Other *

RIGHT   LEFT   LEFT   RIGHT

FRONT   BACK

Fig. 5 Pain drawing generated by a patient who was suffering from L4 radiculopathy secondary to a lumbar disk displacement and symptomatic osteoarthritis of the hip on the same side.

Table 1

Typical patient history elicited for various pain related sleep disturbances

Complaint	Differential Diagnosis
Difficulty getting to sleep, once asleep, no disturbance	Benign
Unable to sleep on side or prone	Herniated nucleus pulposus and/or stenosis
Turning awakens patient	
Able to get back to sleep	
Sleep disturbance every night	Tumor
Progressive and relentless	
Distal extremity pain severe	
Must walk around for relief	
Requires sleeping pills	Psychogenic regional pain disturbance
Awakens 4:00 a.m. every night and takes pain pills	

back pain (Table 1).[15] Lateral recess stenosis in an unstable degenerated motion segment unit can cause painful sleep disturbance when the patient turns while sleeping. An uncontrolled twisting maneuver leads to nerve root entrapment in the lateral recess, stimulus of an ectopic impulse from the nerve root, the experience of radicular pain, awakening, repositioning, and usually the ability to get back to sleep within a very short period of time. These patients state that they are able to sleep in some positions, such as the lateral decubitus or fetal positions, but not others, for example, the prone position.

The patient who is suffering from a slow-growing intrathecal neurofibroma will have a different pattern of sleep disturbance (Fig. 6).[16] These patients are usually men over the age of 60 with a classic history of progressive severe night pain that awakens them and does not allow them to get back to sleep. The pain, which is relentless and progressive, occurs every night. The patient gives a history of getting up and walking around for pain relief and having difficulty getting back to sleep. These patients, who are usually exhausted and anxious and require pain medication, can be easily confused with patients suffering from a behavioral disorder.

Sleep disturbance from behavioral disorders is usually secondary to a dependency upon some chemical, such as nicotine, narcotic analgesics, sleeping pills, muscle relaxants, or some combination of these. Such patients have a sleep disturbance pattern characterized by awakening at 4:00 a.m. They then are unable to get back to sleep. Careful questioning will disclose that a physiologic dependency on a chemical substance, not pain, is the primary reason for the sleep disturbance.[17]

Differentiating these three patterns of sleep disturbance and correlating this history with the pain drawing, subsequent physical examination, and diagnostic tests are of great importance in arriving at a correct diagnosis.

Smoking and Low Back Pain and Sciatica

Peripheral vascular disease and spinal stenosis can occur together in a patient over 60 years of age who has a long history of smoking. The association of smoking and peripheral vascular disease has been established clearly in the past. More recently, there has also been established a clear association between long-term smoking and chronic low back pain,[18,19] which is probably related to premature and progressive disk degeneration as the result of starving the disk of needed oxygen. Smokers have a lower average Po_2 and mean O_2 saturation than do nonsmokers. They also have a 15% carboxyhemoglobin, resulting in a 25% reduction in available tissue oxygen supply.[20]

There may also be an association between smoking and ischemia-induced sciatic leg pain.[21] I have encountered patients suffering from acute severe radiculopathy who have obtained relief of pain within a 72-hour period by not smoking. I attribute the relief of pain to restoration of the normal O_2 saturation and ridding the body of carboxyhemoglobin. With an addition of 25% oxygen supply at the tissue level, this may be enough to remove the ischemic stimulus of ectopic impulses in a compressive radiculopathy.

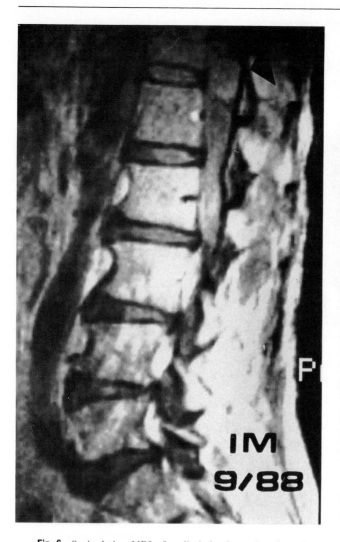 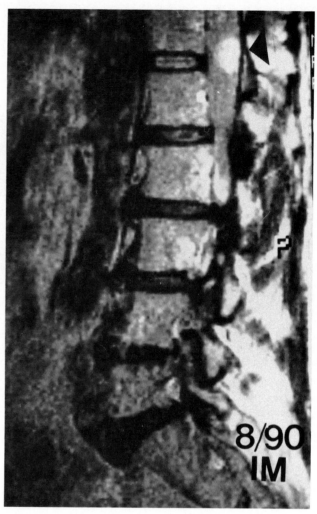

Fig. 6 Sagittal view MRI of scoliotic lumbar spine, from September 1988 (**left**) and August 1990 (**right**) of same patient. Note the high signal intensity lesion posterior to the twelfth thoracic disk displacing the conus medularis anteriorly. This biopsy-proven meningioma was finally recognized on both MRI scans after correlation of the patient's history of pain-related sleep disturbance with MRI findings.

Activity-Related Pain

An accurate history of activity-related leg pain can help in differentiating between neurogenic and vascular claudication.[22] Patients with vascular insufficiency complain of a cramping sensation in the calves with walking a specific distance. Once the pain begins, they prefer to stand for relief, because this position maintains arterial perfusion to the lower extremities. They are unable to perform other forms of exercise, such as bicycling and swimming, without suffering pain secondary to muscular ischemia.

Patients with spinal stenosis complain of more proximal pain, which radiates from the buttocks down to the posterior thigh and leg with walking or standing in an upright posture. They may be able to ride a bicycle, to walk leaning on a shopping cart, or to dance leaning on a partner but they cannot walk upright. They usually

have good days and bad days. On a good day they can walk more than a mile without pain. On bad days they can walk less than a hundred yards. They sit or lean against a wall to flex the spine for relief of the pain. Flexion of the spine stretches the buckled ligamenta flavum and posterior annulus fibrosus. By opening up the spinal canal, this relieves pressure on the cauda equina.[23]

It is not uncommon for leg pain caused by spinal stenosis and by peripheral vascular insufficiency to occur simultaneously in the older patient with a long history of smoking (Fig. 7). On close questioning, the patient is usually able to distinguish the pain of neurogenic claudication from that caused by vascular claudication. I have operated on patients with severe spinal stenosis who have subsequently had relief of their neurogenic claudication. Even though their vascular claudication persisted, these patients have been satis-

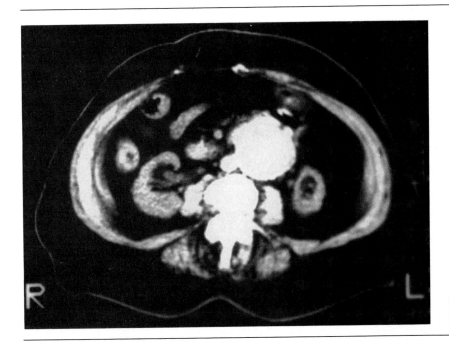

Fig. 7 Transverse view, computed tomographic scan, showing enlarged aorta with impending posterior rupture in an elderly male smoker who presented with low back pain.

fied with the results. This lead me to believe that patients tolerate neurogenic claudication less well than they do vascular claudication.

Inherited Predisposition to Low Back Pain

A recent study has shown that there is an inherited predisposition to the development of symptoms of low back pain, sciatica, and disk herniation.[24] The familial predisposition to these symptoms is prevalent in the entire human population.

The chemical manifestations of this inherited predisposition result in the production of abnormal proteoglycans in the nucleus pulposus, leading to disk instability in the early stages of disk degeneration.[25,26] With slight disk narrowing, within physiologic ranges of torsion, radial tears in the annulus occur towards the posterior lateral corner of the disk.[27] When these tears disrupt the free nerve endings in the region of the peripheral annulus fibrosus and posterior longitudinal ligament, the initial manifestations of low back pain are felt.[28] Usually occurring within the second and third decade of life, this phenomenon probably accounts for the majority of patients suffering from self-limiting, poorly localized benign back pain syndromes.

Stimulus of the free nerve endings in the peripheral annulus fibrosus and posterior longitudinal ligament stimulates secretion of substance P from the sensory root ganglia down the sensory nerves to the local tissues.[29] A series of events stemming from degranulation of tissue-bound mast cells by the substance P takes place. Mast cell granules contain histamine vasodilators, proteases, and collagenase. Release of these substances

into the tissue results in pain, edema, and lysis of local connective tissue and probably represents a normal defense mechanism. For example, when disk displacement occurs beyond the annulus fibrosus, the stimulus to secrete substance P, with its effect on mast cells, may be one way for autochemonucleolysis to occur.

We know now that in the majority of patients who have lumbar disk herniations, the condition spontaneously improves over time.[30] This improvement seems to correlate with a reduction in the size and displacement of the herniation as seen on serial MRI scans (Fig. 8).[31]

Biopsies in the region of herniated disks have not revealed round-cell inflammatory infiltrates.[32] The inflammation seen in this condition probably results from the action of neuromediators, such as substance P, on the tissue-bound mast cells. I know from numerous observations in the clinical setting that the acute pain from a disk herniation can be relieved by injecting steroids into the epidural space. The mechanism of action of locally injected steroids may be related to stabilization of the tissue-bound mast cells.

Mechanical Low Back Pain

In the early stages of disk degeneration, the motion segment unit becomes destabilized.[26] In the middle stages of disk degeneration, where we see failure of the annulus fibrosus and disk displacement, the motion segment unit is the most unstable as compared with normal disks. In the late stages of disk degeneration, with narrowing of the disk and complete loss of signal intensity of the nucleus on MRI, the motion segment unit be-

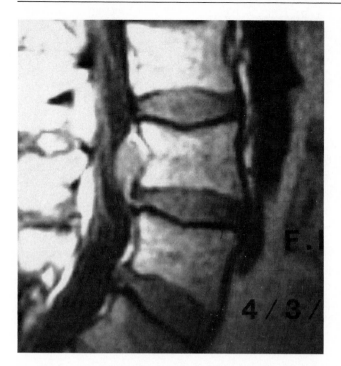 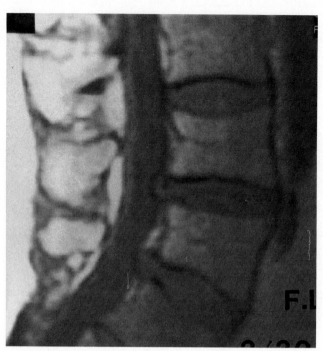

Fig. 8 Mid-sagittal MRI of lumbar spine (**left**). A large extruded, almost sequestrated, disk displacement is apparent behind the fourth lumbar vertebral body. Patient suffered from symptoms of cauda equina syndrome for one week following onset of pain. At the time of MRI scan his symptoms had resolved spontaneously. Because of the high signal intensity on MRI of the displaced fragment it was felt the disk would be resorbed spontaneously and no treatment was prescribed. (Reproduced with permission from Brown MD: Low back pain and sciatica: An easy approach to diagnosis and prognosis. *Consultant* 1991;31:23–25.) One year later, the patient was asymptomatic with no evidence of disk displacement on MRI (**right**).

comes stiffer than normal. This stiffness probably results from reactive changes at the point of attachment of the annulus fibrosus to the vertebral bodies. With abnormal stress at this junction, osteophytes form and new collagen is produced. In the absence of repeated trauma with subsequent disk narrowing and osteophyte formation, the motion segment unit becomes stiffer than normal, with subsequent resolution of the mechanical low back pain.[33]

In some cases, chronic mechanical back pain recurs because the normal restiffening process does not take place. Because the pathophysiology and the pathologic changes described here occur over months and years, the patient's history of present illness must also span months and years and must include an account of the patient's activities.

In my experience, the history of recurring attacks of low back pain brought on by mechanical stress, a spinal list, several severe traumatic episodes in the past, and evidence of abnormal degenerative changes in one or more disks on MRI scan are diagnostic of mechanical insufficiency of the motion segment unit. I have *not* found a painful response during diskography,[34] standing flexion and extension lateral stress films,[35] or traction and compression radiography[36] to be of help in confirming the diagnosis of mechanical insufficiency of

the motion segment unit from degenerative disk disease.

Diagnostic Studies

The plain roentgenograms of the low back should include standing anteroposterior, lateral, and oblique films. An anteroposterior roentgenogram of the pelvis, including both hips, should also be performed in those patients in whom a clear view of the sacroiliac joints and/or hips is required to rule out arthritic conditions. Plain roentgenograms provide a presumptive confirmation of mechanical insufficiency of the spine when spondylolysis or spondylolisthesis is detected, and of spinal stenosis when one notes a narrow degenerated disk with facet hypertrophy.[37] Also, destructive lesions of the spine or erosion secondary to tumor and/or infections can be detected with plain films. Because plain films are superior to other imaging techniques in determining variations in spinal segmentation as well as spinal deformity, such as scoliosis, they are a necessary prerequisite to planning surgery of the spine.

In my experience, the most cost effective and safest diagnostic technique for low back pain and sciatica is MRI.[38] Because MRI scans clearly differentiate soft-

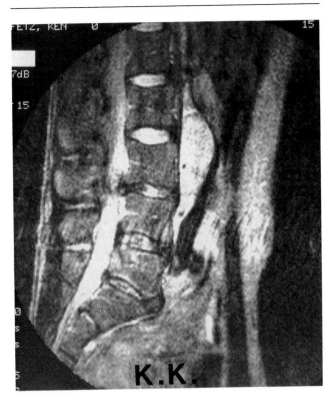

Fig. 9 Mid-sagittal MRI spine in a patient who had spinal stenosis L3-L4 (symptomatic) and a large retro-aortic lymphoma (asymptomatic). (Reproduced with permission from Brown MD: Low back pain and sciatica: An easy approach to diagnosis and prognosis. *Consultant* 1991;31:23–25.)

tissue lesions as well as physiologic changes, they offer the best way of demonstrating the various degrees of disk displacement (bulging, herniated, extruded, or sequestrated disks)[39] into the spinal canal and/or foramen.

In addition to showing the degree of disk degeneration, MRI also makes it possible to see how edematous or fibrous the displaced disk is. From this information one can determine the prognosis for spontaneous resorption. A correlation of the patient's history with the morphology of the disk herniation and size and shape of the spinal canal as seen on MRI allows some prediction concerning prognosis. An extruded and/or sequestrated disk with a high signal intensity (T_2 image), indicating a high water content, in the normal size and shaped spinal canal is more likely to resorb spontaneously than is a fibrotic disk protrusion (low signal intensity on T_2 MRI) into a small spinal canal (Fig. 8).

Magnetic resonance scans are the method of choice for demonstrating epidural hematoma, infectious lesions, and tumors in and around the spinal canal (Fig. 9). With the ability to enhance the vasculature by the use of intravenously injected gadolinium, lesions such as neurofibromas of the conus medullaris are more easily detected by MRI than by myelogram.[40]

MRI replaces the myelogram as a global picture of the lumbar spine, and it is better than the myelogram with computed tomography scan for picking up disk herniations in the foramen.[41] It is more subtle than the bone scan for picking up inflammatory processes and tumors.

Problems with availability, quality, and cost of MRI scanning, which existed when the technique was first introduced in the late 1980's, have for the most part been resolved even in rural communities of North America. In my opinion, magnetic resonance imaging is unquestionably the most accurate, humane, and cost effective diagnostic technique for confirmation of the cause of back pain and sciatica.

The few disadvantages of MRI are length of exam time, artifacts from motion, and limited spinal resolution.[42] An occasional patient with severe radiculopathy has difficulty lying flat due to leg pain. I have performed an epidural local anesthetic block in these patients to allow for the successful completion of the study. I will sedate the patient who is known to be claustrophobic to allow for completion of the scan without motion artifacts.

Our current indications for myelography are: when MRI scanning is contraindicated because of ferromagnetic implants that would distort the image, when the patient has a pacemaker, and when treating the occasional rare individual who is so claustrophobic that a MRI scan cannot be tolerated. The non-ionic, iodine, water contrast myelographic media are safe, but a spinal tap is required to inject them. Spinal fluid analysis can be obtained, which is helpful in diagnosing myelopathy secondary to demyelinating conditions. However, in my opinion, the MRI scan is safer and more accurate than myelography for the detection of demyelinating diseases.

In sensitivity, specificity, and predictive value, MRI is superior in every category to all other methods of diagnosis.[43] It is necessary to remember, however, that the value of a diagnostic study ultimately depends on the physician's history, physical examination, differential diagnosis, and judgment. The MRI scan result must be correlated with the history and physical examination before decisions are made confirming the diagnosis and planning conservative or surgical care. One must always remember to treat the patient and not the MRI scan.

An MRI study in asymptomatic women showed that only 46% of the disks were normal, and of the 54% that were abnormal, 44% were bulging and 10% were herniated.[44] These women had no history of back or leg pain. In another study, MRI was performed on asymptomatic individuals of different age groups.[45] Under the age of 60, 20% of the subjects had a herniated lumbar disk, and 55% of those individuals over the age of 60 had abnormal scans. There was evidence of a herniated nucleus pulposus in 35% and spinal stenosis in 20% of asymptomatic individuals over the age of sixty.

Conclusions

A careful, thorough history and physical examination remains the key to accurate diagnosis of the cause of low back pain and/or leg pain. Pain drawings and MRI scans are very useful adjuncts to diagnosis and, in the case of leg pain, may be definitive.

An understanding of the pathophysiology of degenerative disk disease and the neuropathology of nerve root injury helps in the understanding of common sources of low back pain and sciatica and enables one to distinguish the source of pain from etiologies other than degenerative diseases of the motion segment unit.

References

1. Mathew B, Norris D, Hendry D, et al: Artificial intelligence in the diagnosis of low-back pain and sciatica. *Spine* 1988;13:168–172.
2. Rydevik B, Brown MD, Lundborg G: Pathoanatomy and pathophysiology of nerve root compression. *Spine* 1984;9:7–15.
3. Parke WW: The significance of venous return impairment in ischemic radiculopathy and myelopathy. *Orthop Clin North Am* 1991;22:213–222.
4. Rydevik B, Holm S, Brown MD, et al: Diffusion from the cerebrospinal fluid as a nutritional pathway for spinal nerve roots. *Acta Physiol Scand* 1990;138:247–248.
5. Parke WW, Watanabe R: The intrinsic vasculature of the lumbosacral nerve roots. *Spine* 1985;10:508–515.
6. McCowin PB, Borenstein D, Wiesel SW: The current approach to the medical diagnosis of low back pain. *Orthop Clin North Am* 1991;22:315–325.
7. Engel GL: "Psychogenic" pain and pain-prone patient. *Am J Med* 1959;26:899–918.
8. Ransford AO, Cairns D, Mooney V: The Pain Drawing as an aid to the psychologic evaluation of patients with low-back pain. *Spine* 1976;1:127–134.
9. Mann NH III, Brown MD: Artificial intelligence in the diagnosis of low back pain. *Orthop Clin North Am* 1991;22:303–314.
10. Kuslich SD, Ulstrom CL, Michael CJ: The tissue origin of low back pain and sciatica. *Orthop Clin North Am* 1991;22:181–188.
11. Murphey F: Sources and patterns of pain in disc disease. *Clin Neurosurg* 1968;15:343–351.
12. Choudury AR, Taylor JC: Cauda equina syndrome in lumbar disc disease. *Acta Orthop Scand* 1980;51:493–499.
13. Olmarker K, Rydevik B: Pathophysiology of sciatica. *Orthop Clin North Am* 1991;22:223–234.
14. Glover MG, Hargens AR, Mahmood MM, et al: A new technique for the in vitro measurement of nucleus pulposus swelling pressure. *J Orthop Res* 1991;9:61–67.
15. Brown MD: The diagnosis of pain syndromes of the spine. *Orthop Clin North Am* 1975;6:233–248.
16. McGuire RA, Brown MD, Green BA: Intradural spinal tumors and spinal stenosis: Report of two cases. *Spine* 1987;12:1062–1066.
17. Pilowsky I, Crettenden I, Townley M: Sleep disturbance in pain clinic patients. *Pain* 1985;23:27–33.
18. Frymoyer JW: Back pain and sciatica. *New Engl J Med* 1988;318:291–300.
19. Hanley EN Jr, Shapiro DE: The development of low back pain after excision of a lumbar disc. *J Bone Joint Surg* 1989;71A:719–721.
20. Brown CW, Orme TJ, Richardson HD: The rate of pseudoarthrosis (surgical nonunion) in patients who are smokers and patients who are nonsmokers: A comparison study. *Spine* 1986;11:942–943.
21. Kelsey JL, Githens PB, O'Conner T, et al: Acute prolapsed lumbar intervertebral disc: An epidemiologic study with special references to driving automobiles and cigarette smoking. *Spine* 1984;9:608–613.
22. Hawkes CH, Roberts GM: Neurogenic and vascular claudication. *J Neurol Sci* 1978;38:337–345.
23. Magnaes B: Clinical recording of pressure on the spinal cord and cauda equina: Part 1: The Spinal Block infusion test methods and clinical studies. Part 2: Position changes in pressure on the cauda equina in central lumbar stenosis. *J Neurosurg* 1982;57:48–63.
24. Varlotta GP, Brown MD, Kelsey JL, et al: Familial predisposition for herniation of a lumbar disc in patients who are less than twenty-one years old. *J Bone Joint Surg* 1991;73A:124–128.
25. Brown MD: The pathophysiology of the intervertebral disc. *Orthop Clin North Am* 1971;2:359–370.
26. Brown MD, Holmes DC, Eckstein EC, et al: In vitro and in vivo measurement of lumbar spine motion segment unit stiffness. *Orthop Trans* 1990;14:110.
27. Hickey DS, Hukins DWL: Relation between the structure of the annulus fibrosus and the function and failure of the intervertebral disc. *Spine* 1980;5:106–116.
28. Brown MD: The sources of low back pain and sciatica. *Semin Arthritis Rheum* 1989;18(suppl 2):67–72.
29. Weinstein J: Neurogenic and nonneurogenic pain and inflammatory mediators. *Orthop Clin North Am* 1991;22:235–246.
30. Weber H: Lumbar disc herniation: A controlled, prospective study with ten years of observation. *Spine* 1983;8:131–140.
31. Saal JA, Saal JS, Herzog RJ: The natural history of lumbar intervertebral disc extrusions treated nonoperatively. *Spine* 1990;15:683–686.
32. Yoshizawa H, O'Brien JP, Smith WT, et al: The neuropathology of intervertebral discs removed for low-back pain. *J Pathol* 1980;132:95–104.
33. Kirkaldy-Willis WH, Farfan HF: Instability of the lumbar spine. *Clin Orthop* 1982;165:110–123.
34. Bernard TN Jr: Lumbar discography followed by computed tomography: Refining the diagnosis of lowback pain. *Spine* 1990;15:690–707.
35. Knuttsson F: The instability associated with disc degeneration in the lumbar spine. *Acta Radiol* 1944;25:593–609.
36. Friberg O: Lumbar instability: A dynamic approach by traction-compression radiography. *Spine* 1987;12:119–128.
37. Frymoyer JW, Newberg A, Pope MH, et al: Spine radiographs in patients with low-back pain. *J Bone Joint Surg* 1984;66A:1048–1055.
38. Modic MT, Ross JS: Magnetic resonance imaging in the evaluation of low back pain. *Orthop Clin North Am* 1991;22:283–302.
39. Masaryk TJ, Ross JS, Modic MT, et al: High-resolution MR imaging of sequestered lumbar intervertebral disks. *AJR* 1988;150:1155–1162.
40. Valk J: Gd-DTPA in MR of spinal lesions. *AJR* 1988;150:1163–1168.
41. Osborn AG, Hood RS, Sherry RG, et al: CT/MR spectrum of far lateral and anterior lumbosacral disk herniations. *Am J Neuroradiol* 1988;9:775–778.
42. Miller GM, Forbes GS, Onofrio BM: Magnetic resonance imaging of the spine. *Mayo Clin Proc* 1989;64:986–1004.

43. Modic MT, Masaryk TJ, Boumphrey F, et al: Lumbar herniated disc disease and canal stenosis: Prospective evaluation by surface coil MR, CT, and myelography. *AJR* 1986;147:757–765.

44. Weinreb JC, Wolbarsht LB, Cohen JM, et al: Prevalence of lumbosacral intervertebral disk abnormalities on MR images in pregnant and asymptomatic nonpregnant women. *Radiology* 1989;170:125–128.

45. Boden SD, Davis DO, Dina TS, et al: Abnormal magnetic-resonance scans of the lumbar spine in asymptomatic subjects. *J Bone Joint Surg* 1990;72A:403–408.

CHAPTER 23

Lumbar Disk Disease: Epidemiology

John W. Frymoyer, MD

Introduction and Definitions

An Italian anatomist, Domenico Cotunio,[1] distinguished sciatica from the more general aching discomfort usually associated with low back pain. Over the next 200 years, it became recognized that this condition is caused by compression of the anterior primary rami of the L5 or S1 nerve roots. The less discreet leg pain associated with back disorders arises from posterior primary ramus innervated structures.[2]

Following Mixter and Barr's[3] classic article, lumbar disk herniation was identified as the most common cause of sciatica. Today we recognize the etiology to be such diseases as lateral recess stenosis, epidural hemorrhage and abscesses, tumors and facet ganglia, tumors, and, perhaps, local compression of the sciatic nerve in the buttocks.[4] Furthermore, we recognize that lumbar disk herniation is not always associated with back pain or sciatica. Surveys using myelography,[5] computed tomography scan (CT),[6] and magnetic resonance image (MRI)[7] have revealed that as many as 30% of the adult population have bulging or herniated lumbar disks but have never experienced back or sciatic pain.

In analyzing the epidemiology of sciatica, these points must be kept in mind: (1) sciatica is a symptom, not a pathologic diagnosis; (2) leg pain associated with back pain is not necessarily sciatica; (3) not all sciatic pain is caused by lumbar disk herniation; and (4) lumbar disk herniation does not necessarily cause sciatic pain.

In this chapter, the epidemiology of sciatica and lumbar disk herniation will be analyzed from the perspectives of prevalence, incidence, natural history, risk factors, and surgical intervention.

Prevalence and Incidence

Lifetime Incidence

The lifetime incidence of low back pain ranges from 50% to 70%,[8-14] as determined by epidemiologic studies, whereas the incidence of sciatica is only 13% to 40%.[15] Heliovaara[16] surveyed 8,000 adult Finnish citizens from 20 to 60 years of age. Of the total, 3,637 were men and 4,363 were women. Data collected included medical histories, physical examinations, and anteroposterior and lateral radiographs. The subjects were divided into three groups: Those with herniated lumbar disks, confirmed by surgery or myelography; those with sciatica, based on symptoms and physical findings; and those with other low back syndromes. Asymptomatic subjects were used as controls. Forty percent of the test group reported having had sciatica sometime during their life; 20% had experienced that symptom during the past month; and 20% had experienced recurrent symptoms. Despite the high prevalence of these complaints, only 3% had required bedrest during the past five years, and fewer than 3% reported the symptom as continuous.

The association of sciatica with back pain becomes more apparent when the severity of the low back pain is quantified. In one study,[11] 22% of a male cohort aged 18 to 55 reported they had experienced severe low back pain at sometime during their adult life. The severity of the subjective complaint correlated significantly with the frequency with which health professionals were consulted and with time lost from work. Of this 22%, half (11% of the entire cohort) reported sciatica, often associated with numbness, tingling, or weakness. Table 1 shows the significant correlations between these subjective complaints. In another study,[17] adult males and females representative of the United States population were analyzed. Although back pain was a common complaint, only 14% reported pain lasting longer than two weeks. In the entire sample, only 2% of the subjects reported sciatica. Of individuals who reported two weeks of back pain, 15% had experienced that symptom.

Annual Incidence

The annual incidence of low back pain is 5% to 20%. These variations seem to be related to the individual's occupation.[18] The corresponding annual incidence of sciatica ranges from 1% to 5%.

Table 1
Men reporting symptoms in the lower limbs associated with low back pain

Symptoms*	Men (%)	
	Moderate (n = 565)	Severe (n = 288)
Pain	28.9	54.5†
Numbness	14.0	37.4†
Weakness	17.9	44.0†

*A subject may have reported one or more of these symptoms.
† < 0.001, chi-square analysis.
(Reproduced with permission from Frymoyer JW, Pope MH, Clements JH, et al: Risk factors in low-back pain. An epidemiological survey. *J Bone Joint Surg* 1983;65A:213–218.)

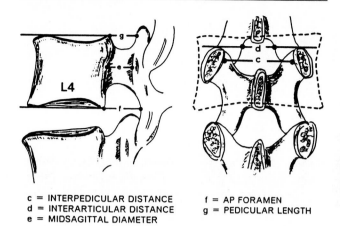

c = INTERPEDICULAR DISTANCE
d = INTERARTICULAR DISTANCE
e = MIDSAGITTAL DIAMETER

f = AP FORAMEN
g = PEDICULAR LENGTH

Fig. 1 A schematic drawing presenting the landmarks for radiographic measurements. (Reproduced with permission from Vanharanta H, Korpi J, Heliovaara M, et al: Radiographic measurements of lumbar spinal canal and their relation to back mobility. *Spine* 1985; 10:461–466.)

Radiographic Surveys

Few attempts have been made to define sciatica more strictly on the basis of physical examination or imaging studies. In the cohort study of men aged from 15 to 55 years,[19] a representative sample of 360 individuals had spine radiographs and were evaluated for nerve root tension signs and neurologic abnormalities. Few subjects had objective findings. None of the radiographic measurements correlated with low back pain or sciatica, except L4-L5 disk space narrowing. In similar studies reported by Lawrence in 1969[20] and 1977,[21] physical examinations were not included specific to neurologic dysfunction. At the time of his earlier evaluation, 3.1% of women and 1.3% of men had sciatica. Again, many radiographic abnormalities were recorded, most of which were age-related. Perhaps these

negative results should not be surprising. Hakelius and Hindmarsh[22] extensively analyzed the predictive value of spinal radiography in patients with myelographically proven lumbar disk herniation. Disk space narrowing was found to be a poor, if not negative, predictor.

Another approach has been to correlate radiographic indices of spinal stenosis with subjective complaints of sciatica. The measurements made from plain spinal radiographs are shown in Figure 1. In subjects with proven lumbar disk herniation or definite sciatica, the interarticular distance was found to be narrower than it was in a control group or in another group who reported only low back pain.

Natural History

The natural history of recovery from acute low back pain has been reported to be favorable in most surveys, one of which is depicted in Figure 2. Hakelius and Hindmarsh[23] retrospectively studied patients with sciatica caused by disk herniations proven by myelogram. Some were treated surgically and others were treated conservatively. Figure 2 also shows the natural recovery for sciatica in patients who did and did not undergo surgery.

Weber[24] prospectively analyzed patients with unequivocal sciatica and who had myelographic confirmation of lumbar disk herniation. His patients were randomly allocated to surgical and nonsurgical treatment. Although this study shows a favorable likelihood of recovery without surgical treatment, his data require more detailed analysis.

First, he eliminated from the randomization patients with cauda equina dysfunction, "functionally significant or progressive muscle weakness," as well as patients with "unrelenting pain" despite conservative treatment. Twenty percent of the cohort fulfilled those

Fig. 2 The natural history of recovery of surgically and nonsurgically treated patients with sciatica. Note that in this retrospective study the two treatments had similar outcomes. (Reproduced with permission from Hakelius A: Prognosis in sciatica: A clinical follow-up of surgical and non-surgical treatment. *Acta Orthop Scand* 1970;129(suppl): 1–76.)

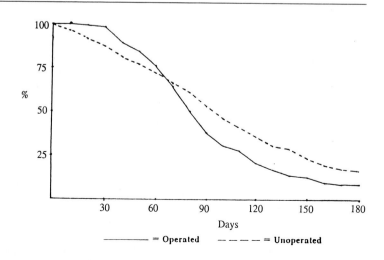

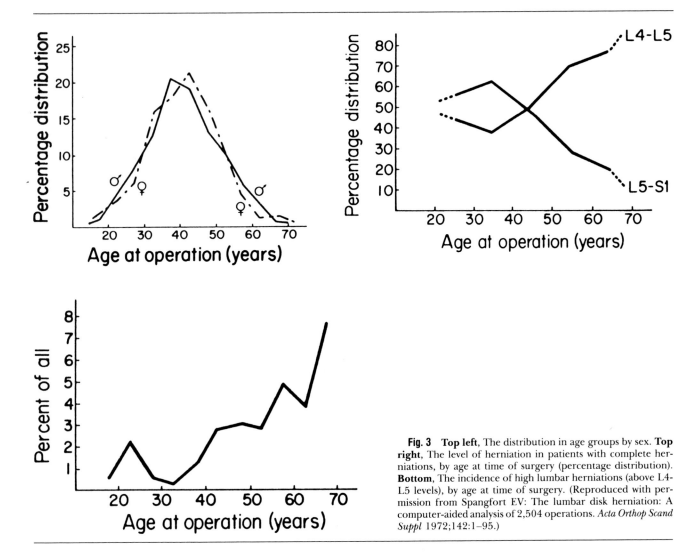

Fig. 3 **Top left**, The distribution in age groups by sex. **Top right**, The level of herniation in patients with complete herniations, by age at time of surgery (percentage distribution). **Bottom**, The incidence of high lumbar herniations (above L4-L5 levels), by age at time of surgery. (Reproduced with permission from Spangfort EV: The lumbar disk herniation: A computer-aided analysis of 2,504 operations. *Acta Orthop Scand Suppl* 1972;142:1–95.)

criteria. Until the fourth year the surgically treated group fared better with respect to symptoms and function. In the ensuing six and 10-year surveillance, the operated patients and controls have fared equivalently.

Saal and Saal[25] used MRI to monitor patients who had unequivocal lumbar disk herniations and sciatica and were treated conservatively. Serial MRI appeared to confirm the hypothesis that over time the protruded portion of the disk undergoes dehydration and resorption, although clinical and functional recovery often precedes morphologic change.

Risk Factors

The risk factors for sciatica have been analyzed in two general cohort types—patients with the symptom but no confirmation of the causation, and patients with symptoms caused by lumbar disk herniation.

Gender

Most studies have reported men to be affected more often than women, although the differences are fairly small in absolute terms. In Heliovaara's cohort, 5.3% of men and 3.7% of women reported sciatica.[16] The risk factor for low back pain and sciatica has been reported as equal for men and women,[26–29] and sex-linked variation has generally been weak or minimal for lumbar disk herniation. However, an increase in back symptoms, with associated pain in the buttocks and sacroiliac joints, has been reported[30] and these symptoms may have been confused with sciatica.

Age

Sciatica, like lumbar disk herniation, rarely starts before the age of 20, reaches its peak in the fifth decade of life, and then declines. This age distribution is also typical of those who require surgical treatment of lumbar disk herniation. Spangfort[31] analyzed both his own large series of patients and accumulated series reported in the literature. Figure 3, *top left*, shows the ages at which surgery was performed in these groups. Herniation occurred at an earlier age at the L5-S1 level than at L4-L5 (Fig. 3, *top right*). Herniations at higher levels, as L3-4, L2-3, occurred in older age groups (Fig. 3,

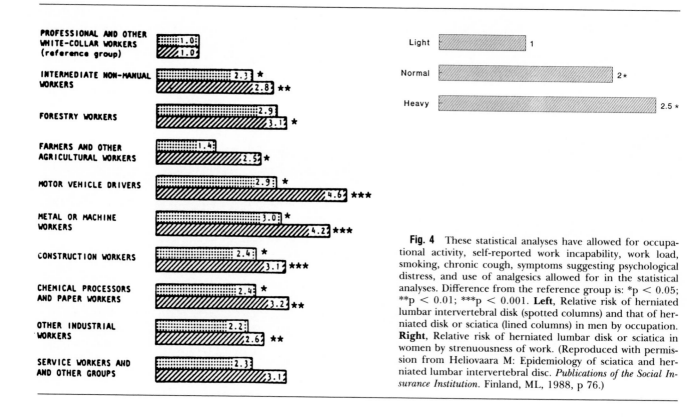

Fig. 4 These statistical analyses have allowed for occupational activity, self-reported work incapability, work load, smoking, chronic cough, symptoms suggesting psychological distress, and use of analgesics allowed for in the statistical analyses. Difference from the reference group is: *p < 0.05; **p < 0.01; ***p < 0.001. **Left**, Relative risk of herniated lumbar intervertebral disk (spotted columns) and that of herniated disk or sciatica (lined columns) in men by occupation. **Right**, Relative risk of herniated lumbar disk or sciatica in women by strenuousness of work. (Reproduced with permission from Heliovaara M: Epidemiology of sciatica and herniated lumbar intervertebral disc. *Publications of the Social Insurance Institution.* Finland, ML, 1988, p 76.)

bottom). This observation is consistent with imaging studies that demonstrate that lumbar disk degeneration proceeds from caudal to cephalad.[32]

Anthropometrics

Height, weight, and body mass have been analyzed as risk factors for back pain and sciatica with varying results. Most studies suggest minimal increased risk, with the possible exception of individuals who are in the highest quintile for weight and height. For example, Heliovaara[16] found a cutoff for height was 170 cm in women and 180 cm in males. Subjects taller than those heights had an increased risk in men of 2.3% and in women of 3.7%. In his study, weight and body mass were not predictive.

Genetic and Social Factors

A genetic causation for lumbar degeneration and possibly for disk herniation has been suggested by Wynn-Davies and Scott.[33] However, the associations were not striking. A more convincing genetic antecedent has been reported by Varlotta and associates,[34] who studied adolescents with unequivocal lumbar disk herniation. A significant increase in lumbar disk herniations in first degree relatives of these patients suggests a genetic determinant, possibly autosomal. The degree to which spinal canal dimensions are genetically determined is also conjectural, with the exception of rarer diseases, such as achondroplasia. The association between spinal canal dimensions and sciatica described

earlier in this review does not prove or disprove a genetic determinant.

Regional variations are also identified between countries and even within different areas of the same country in the reported prevalence of back pain, sciatica, and lumbar disk herniation. For example, comparisons of nonindustrialized and industrialized countries show low back pain and sciatica to be more prevalent in the nonindustrialized populations.[21] Although in Heliovaara's study, sciatica and disk herniation were found to be more prevalent in the urban than in the rural residents of Finland, he concluded that too many confounding variables were present to give the observation significance.[16]

Exposures

Three separate exposures have been analyzed—smoking, vibration, and occupation. In most studies, cigarette smoking has been identified as a risk factor for low back pain, sciatica, and lumbar disk herniation.[11,16,35–40] Gyntelberg[37] found the association to be mediated by the presence or absence of cough, thus implicating a mechanical causation. Others[11] have thought a direct chemical effect of one or more constituents of tobacco might be operative. This hypothesis is consistent with laboratory experiments,[41] which show reduced lumbar disk nutrition in animals exposed to smoke.

A second exposure is vibration, which again has been identified as a risk factor for low back pain, sciatica,

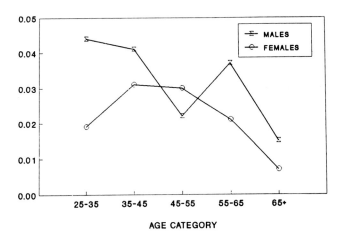

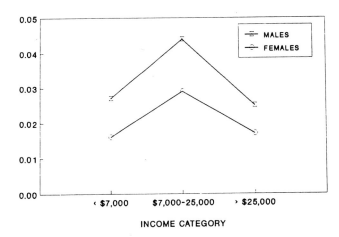

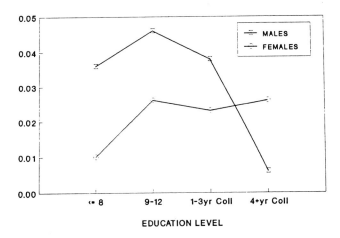

Fig. 5 Top, The vertical gives the lifetime incidence of a lumbar spinal operation. For example, .02 (2%) of women age 25–35 reported they had surgery. **Center,** Note the effects of total family income on the probability of a subject undergoing lumbar surgery. **Bottom,** The effects of education on surgical rates are calculated. Note the least and most educated are less likely to have undergone surgery.

and lumbar disk herniation.[16,19,36,38] The association is most evident in those patients with myelographically proven disk herniations who were exposed to extensive automobile driving. It seems likely that vibration in the range of 4 to 5 Hertz, which coincides with a resonating frequency of the seated human spine, is common in vehicular driving.[42,43] The resultant large energy transfers appear to have a direct mechanical effect, both on the lumbar disk and on its nutritional pathways.

The last and most important of the exposures are the multiple factors associated with occupation. Since the earliest epidemiologic studies, occupational exposures to heavy lifting have been recognized as a risk factor for low back pain and leg pain.[44,45] In fact, the annual incidence of back symptoms is reported to vary between 1% and 20% as a function of occupation.[18] Figure 4, *left*, demonstrates these variations in men as reported by Heliovaara.[16] Note in this graph that the relative risks are quantified for lumbar disk herniation and sciatica. Figure 4, *right*, demonstrates similar results for women, broken down only by the classification of light, normal, and heavy occupational requirements. However, it is known that nurses, in particular, are at unusual risk for low back symptoms and sciatica. There is probably greater complexity to these data than simple lifting.

A more detailed analysis of lifting postures and lumbar disk herniation[46] showed little risk for lifting in the sagittal plane and significant risks for lifting in a twisted and asymmetric posture. Also, the self-reports of back symptoms in the industrial setting are heavily influenced by other factors, such as job satisfaction, the requirements for repetitive and monotonous tasks, and the general job atmosphere.[47,48] Few data are available to show how these factors relate to psychological distress, except when resultant disability becomes a major consideration. For example, Heliovaara found a weak association between sciatica and lumbar disk herniation and complaints of nervousness, fatigue, excessive sweating, heart pounding, etc., but concluded there were too many confounding factors to reach any conclusions.[16] Many of these same complaints have been found to occur more frequently in chronically disabled low back pain patients.[49]

Epidemiology of Lumbar Surgery

The epidemiology of lumbar surgery is quite different from the epidemiology of either sciatica or lumbar disk herniation. This difference probably exists because most surgical interventions are done to relieve pain rather than to correct major neurologic dysfunction. Most studies[24,31,50] report the only absolute indication for lumbar disk excision, cauda equina syndrome, occurs in 1% to 3% of patients who have an established lumbar herniation. Major, functionally significant mus-

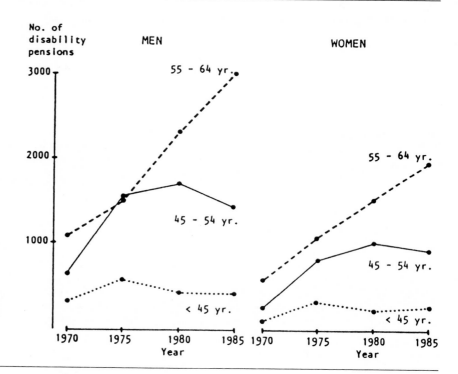

Fig. 6 Number of current disability pensions having been granted by the Social Insurance Institution on the basis of sciatica or intervertebral disk displacement (ICD codes 353.99, 725.00–.99) by sex, age, and calendar year. (Reproduced with permission from Heliovaara M: Epidemiology of sciatica and herniated lumbar intervertebral disc. *Publications of the Social Insurance Institution.* Finland, ML, 1988, p 76.)

cle weakness, which is a strong relative indication, seems to occur in no more than 20% of the patients who undergo surgery. Thus, the major indication is pain.

The lifetime incidence of lumbar disk excision varies between 1% and 3%, consistent with the self-reports of severe sciatica in a relatively small percent of the population.[11,51] However, annual surgical rates vary widely between countries and even within countries. The highest rates (0.1% per year) are recorded in the United States,[52] and the lowest (0.01% per year) are recorded in England and Sweden.[53] Significant regional variations (as great as ten fold) are reported within the United States (R. Deyo, personal communication, 1991). Even more impressive, significant variations can occur within a region simply as a function of surgeon's preference for surgical versus nonsurgical treatment.[54]

A summation of the available information suggests the following are additional important determining factors: (1) Age: The age relationships have been discussed in the prior section. (2) Gender: Although there are modest differences between males and females for the prevalence and incidence of lumbar disk herniation and sciatica, males have a three times greater probability of surgical intervention. The reason for these differences is uncertain. (3) Occupation: Just as occupation is a determinant of back pain and sciatica, it also plays a significant role in the likelihood of surgery, the highest rates being in heavy occupations. Unfortunately, the success rates are significantly lower in the blue collar worker, particularly when compensation is involved.[55]

(4) Social Factors: Figure 5 demonstrates the significant variations in the lifetime prevalence of disk surgery, as calculated from national probability cohorts.[56] Note that income and education are factors.

Social Consequences of Sciatica

The major consequence of sciatica, particularly when it results from lumbar disk herniation, is disability. It has been observed that disability caused by low back pain has increased at a rate disproportionate to population growth or any other health condition during the past 20 years.[57] How much of this problem is attributable specifically to sciatica is uncertain. A number of studies suggest it is a significant proportion.[53,58,59] Heliovaara's study also confirms an increase in disability pension awards for sciatica for the age group 55 to 64 (Fig. 6).

Another unanswered question is the degree to which surgical intervention based on uncertain criteria contributes to disability. A number of studies suggest that it is significant. For example, Norton[60] found poor results and extraordinary costs following lumbar disk excision or chymopapain injection in patients with compensation and "lumbar disk hernia." (The quotations reflect the fact that for a high proportion of patients the diagnosis did not fulfill the basic criteria as published by the American Academy of Orthopaedic Surgeons.)[61] Similarly, a disproportionately high number of patients entering chronic pain and rehabilitation programs have undergone one or more unsuccessful surgical interventions.[62]

Summary

Sciatica is a common symptom that affects as many as 40% of the adult population at some time. However, clinically significant sciatica is much less common and occurs in only 4% to 6% of the population. Exactly how often the symptom is caused by lumbar disk herniation is uncertain; it is known that herniation can occur independent of symptoms. Among the factors associated with its occurrence are age, gender, occupation, cigarette smoking, and exposure to vehicular vibration. The contribution of other factors such as height, weight, and genetics is less certain. The majority of patients with sciatica appear to recover. Approximately 20% of patients with sciatica caused by lumbar herniation have a strong indication for surgical intervention. In the remainder, indications are based primarily on pain rather than functionally significant neurologic deficits. Because pain is the principle indication, there are wide variations in the rates of surgical intervention between countries, and, even within countries, there are significant regional variations. These variations appear to be driven less by specific medical factors and more by gender, occupation, income, education, and the surgeon's preference. Although the contribution of sciatica to low back pain disability remains uncertain, disability caused by low back pain and sciatica appears to be increasing at a rate disproportionate to population growth. To what degree surgery now contributes to that disability is uncertain, but limited information suggests that it may be substantial.

References

1. Cotunio D: *De Ischiade Nervos Canmentarius.* Naples, Simoncos Brothers, 1764.
2. Weinstein JN, LaMotte R, Rydevik B: Nerve: Future directions, in Frymoyer JW, Gordon SL (eds): *New Perspectives on Low Back Pain.* Park Ridge, IL, American Academy of Orthopaedic Surgeons, 1989, pp 125–130.
3. Mixter WJ, Barr JS: Rupture of the intervertebral disc with involvement of the spinal canal. *N Engl J Med* 1934;211:210–215.
4. Frymoyer JW: Back pain and sciatica. *N Engl J Med* 1988;318: 291–300.
5. Hitselberger WE, Witten RM: Abnormal myelograms in asymptomatic patients. *J Neurosurg* 1968;28:204–206.
6. Wiesel SW, Tsourmas N, Feffer HL, et al: A study of computer-assisted tomography. I. The incidence of positive CAT scans in an asymptomatic group of patients. *Spine* 1984;9:549–551.
7. Boden SD, Davis DO, Dina TS, et al: Abnormal magnetic-resonance scans of the lumbar spine in asymptomatic subjects: A prospective investigation. *J Bone Joint Surg* 1990;72A:403–408.
8. Biering-Sørensen F: Low back trouble in a general population of 30–40-, 50-, and 60-year-old men and women. Study designs, representativeness, and basic results. *Dan Med Bull* 1982;29:289.
9. Hirsch C, Jonsson B, Lewin T: Low-back symptoms in a Swedish female population. *Clin Orthop* 1969;63:171–176.
10. Hult L: Cervical, dorsal, and lumbar spinal syndromes: A field investigation of a non-selected material of 1200 workers in different occupations with special reference to disc degeneration and so-called muscular rheumatism. *Acta Orthop Scand Suppl* 1954;17:1–102.
11. Frymoyer JW, Pope MH, Clements JH, et al: Risk factors in low-back pain: An epidemiological survey. *J Bone Joint Surg* 1983; 65A:213–218.
12. Nagi SZ, Riley LE, Newby LG: A social epidemiology of back pain in a general population. *J Chron Dis* 1973;26:769–779.
13. Svensson HO, Andersson GB, Johansson S, et al: A retrospective study of low-back pain in 38- to 64-year-old women. Frequency of occurrence and impact on medical services. *Spine* 1988;13: 548–552.
14. Valkenburg HA, Haanen HCM: The epidemiology of low back pain, in White AA III, Gordon SL (eds): *Symposium on Idiopathic Low Back Pain.* St. Louis, CV Mosby, 1982, pp 9–22.
15. Andersson GBJ, Pope MH, Frymoyer JW, et al: Epidemiology and cost, in Pope MH, Andersson GBJ, Frymoyer JW, et al (eds): *Occupational Low Back Pain: Assessment, Treatment and Prevention.* Chicago, Mosby-Year Book, 1991, pp 95–113.
16. Heliovaara M: Epidemiology of sciatica and herniated lumbar intervertebral disc. *Publications of the Social Insurance Institution,* Finland, ML, 1988, p 76.
17. Deyo RA, Tsui-Wu YJ: Descriptive epidemiology of low-back pain and its related medical care in the United States. *Spine* 1987;12: 264–268.
18. Snook SH: Low back pain in industry, in White AA III, Gordon SL (eds): American Academy of Orthopaedic Surgeons *Symposium on Idiopathic Low Back Pain.* St. Louis, CV Mosby, 1982, pp 23–38.
19. Frymoyer JW, Newberg A, Pope MH, et al: Spine radiographs in patients with low back pain: An epidemiological study in men. *J Bone Joint Surg* 1984;66A:1048–1055.
20. Lawrence JS: Disc degeneration: Its frequency and relationship to symptoms. *Ann Rheum Dis* 1969;28:121–138.
21. Lawrence J: *Rheumatism in Populations.* London, Heinemann, 1977.
22. Hakelius A, Hindmarsh J: The comparative reliability of preoperative diagnostic methods in lumbar disc surgery. *Acta Orthop Scand* 1972;43:234–238.
23. Hakelius A, Hindmarsh J: The significance of neurological signs and myelographic findings in the diagnosis of lumbar root compression. *Acta Orthop Scand* 1972;43:239–246.
24. Weber H: Lumbar disc herniation: A controlled prospective study with ten years of observation. *Spine* 1983;8:131–140.
25. Saal JA, Saal JS: Non-operative treatment of herniated lumbar intervertebral disc with radiculopathy: An outcome study. *Spine* 1989;14:431–437.
26. Frymoyer JW, Pope MH, Costanza MC, et al: Epidemiologic studies of low-back pain. *Spine* 1980;5:419–423.
27. Biering-Sørensen F: A prospective study of low back pain in a general population: II. Location, character, aggravating and relieving factors. *Scand J Rehabil Med* 1983;15:81–88.
28. O'Connell JEA: Lumbar disc protrusions in pregnancy. *J Neurol Neurosurg Psychiatry* 1960;23:138–141.
29. Videman T, Nurminen T, Tola S, et al: Low-back pain in nurses and some loading factors of work. *Spine* 1984;9:400–404.
30. Andersson GBJ: Low back pain in pregnancy, in Weinstein JN, Wiesel SW (eds): *The Lumbar Spine.* Philadelphia, WB Saunders, 1990, pp 840–845.
31. Spangfort EV: The lumbar disc herniation: A computer-aided analysis of 2,504 operations. *Acta Orthop Scand Suppl* 1972;142: 1–95.
32. Andersson GBJ, Pope MH: The patient, in Pope MH, Andersson GBJ, Frymoyer JW, et al (eds): *Occupational Low Back Pain: As-*

sessment, Treatment and Prevention. Chicago, Mosby-Year Book, 1990, pp 132–147.

33. Wynn-Davies R, Scott JH: Inheritance and spondylolisthesis: A radiographic family survey. *J Bone Joint Surg* 1979;61B:301–305.

34. Varlotta GP, Brown MD, Kelsey J, et al: Familial predisposition for herniation of a lumbar disc in patients who are less than twenty-one years old. *J Bone Joint Surg* 1991;73A:123–128.

35. Kelsey JL: An epidemiological study of acute herniated lumbar intervertebral discs. *Rheum Rehab* 1975;14:144–159.

36. Kelsey JL, Githens PB, O'Conner T, et al: Acute prolapsed lumbar intervertebral disc: An epidemiologic study with special reference to driving automobiles and cigarette smoking. *Spine* 1984; 9:608–613.

37. Gyntelberg F: One year incidence of low back pain among male residents of Copenhagen aged 40–59. *Dan Med Bull* 1974;21: 30–36.

38. Frymoyer JW, Pope MH, Costanza MC, et al: Epidemiologic studies of low-back pain. *Spine* 1980;5:419–423.

39. Svensson HO, Vedin A, Wilhelmsson C, et al: Low-back pain in relation to other diseases and cardiovascular risk factors. *Spine* 1983;8:277–285.

40. Biering-Sørensen F, Thomsen C: Medical, social and occupational history as risk indicators for low-back trouble in a general population. *Spine* 1986;11:720–725.

41. Holm S, Nachemson A: Immediate effects of cigarette smoke on the nutrition of the intervertebral disc of the pig. *Orthop Trans* 1984;8:380.

42. Wilder DG, Woodworth BB, Frymoyer JW, et al: Vibration and the human spine. *Spine* 1982;7:243–254.

43. Wilder DG, Frymoyer JW, Pope MH: The effect of vibration on the spine of the seated individual. *Automedica* 1985;6:5–35.

44. Hult L: The Munkfors investigation: A study of the frequency and causes of the stiff neck-brachialgia and lumbago-sciatica syndromes, as well as observations on certain signs and symptoms from the dorsal spine and the joints of the extremities in industrial and forest workers. *Acta Orthop Scand Suppl* 1954;16:1–76.

45. Horal J: The clinical appearance of low back disorders in the City of Gothenburg, Sweden. *Acta Orthop Scand Suppl* 1969;18: 1–109.

46. Kelsey JL, Githens PB, White AA III, et al: An epidemiologic study of lifting and twisting on the job and risk for acute prolapsed lumbar intervertebral disc. *J Orthop Res* 1984;2:61–66.

47. Svennson HO, Andersson GB: Low-back pain in 40- to 47-year-old men: Work history and work environment factors. *Spine* 1983;8:272–276.

48. Vallfors B: Acute, subacute and chronic low back pain: Clinical symptoms, absenteeism and working environment. *Scand J Rehabil Med* 1985;11(suppl 11):1–98.

49. Frymoyer JW, Rosen JC, Clements J, et al: Psychologic factors in low-back-pain disability. *Clin Orthop* 1985;195:178–184.

50. Kostuik JP, Harrington I, Alexander D, et al: Cauda equina syndrome and lumbar disc herniation. *J Bone Joint Surg* 1986;68A: 386–391.

51. Andersson GBJ, Pope MH, Frymoyer JW: Epidemiology, in Pope MH, Frymoyer JW, Andersson G (eds): *Occupational Low Back Pain.* New York, Praeger, 1984.

52. Pokras R, Graves EJ, Dennison CF: Surgical operations in short-stay hospitals: United States, 1978. *Vita Health Stat* 1982;13:61.

53. Benn RT, Wood PHN: Pain in the back: An attempt to estimate the size of the problem. *Rheum Rehab* 1975;14:121–128.

54. Keller RB, Soule DN, Wennberg JE, et al: Dealing with geographic variations in the use of hospitals: The experience of the Maine Medical Assessment Foundation orthopaedic study group. *J Bone Joint Surg* 1990;72A:1286–1293.

55. Kahanovitz N, Viola K, Watkins R, et al: A multicenter comparative analysis of workmen's compensation and private patients undergoing surgical diskectomy. Presented at the Meeting of the International Society for Study of the Lumbar Spine, Miami, FL, 1988.

56. Frymoyer JW, Nachemson A: Natural history of low back disorders, in Frymoyer JW, (ed): *The Adult Spine: Principles and Practice.* New York, Raven Press, 1991.

57. National Center for Health Statistics: Prevalence of selected impairments. United States-1977, series 120, No 132, DHHS Publication (PHS) 81–1562, Hyattsville, MD, 1981.

58. Anderson JAD: Back pain and occupation, in Jayson MIV (ed): *The Lumbar Spine and Back Pain,* ed 2. Tunbridge Wells, Pitman Medical, 1980, pp 57–82.

59. Anderson JA: Epidemiological aspects of back pain. *J Soc Occup Med* 1986;36:90–94.

60. Norton WL: Chemonucleolysis versus surgical discectomy: Comparison of costs and results in workers' compensation claimants. *Spine* 1986;11:440–443.

61. Task Force on Clinical Policies: *Orthopaedic Clinical Policies.* Park Ridge, IL, American Academy of Orthopaedic Surgeons, 1989.

62. Long DM, Filtzer DL, BenDebba M, et al: Clinical features of the failed-back syndrome. *J Neurosurg* 1988;69:61–71.

Low Back Pain: Fusion

James N. Weinstein, DO

Background and History: Lumbar Spinal Fusion

The historic role of fusion has been to treat painful joints and to augment the correction of deformity. Pain of musculoskeletal origin, as we currently understand it, arises from many components of the functional spinal unit, although the precise mechanisms involved in spinal pain have yet to be clearly elucidated.[1] Motion (stretch), particularly when it is abnormal in character or degree, often is thought to be a potent stimulus for peripheral nociceptors. Deformity and/or loss of structural integrity may also contribute to abnormal motion and mechanical stresses, further activating nociceptors and resulting in pain.

Pain: Anatomy and Function

Late 19th century anatomists and psychologists recognized that nerve fibers have anatomically distinct endings. Max Von Fry, a German physician, proposed that each anatomically distinct nerve ending responds to a different type of stimulus: touch, temperature, and pain. Pain was considered a specific sensation transmitted along a unique class of nerve fibers. Well before this, however, a 17th century French philosopher, Rene Descartes, wrote of the existence of the specific pathways that transmit pain information from an injured part of the body through the spinal cord to a pain center in the brain (Fig. 1). This "telephone cable view" of the transmission of pain messages has been accepted for many years. The fact that transecting the cable that carries pain messages does not consistently alleviate the pain reveals a very important concept about the generation of pain itself. Pain is, therefore, a complex perception and depends not only on the intensity of stimulus but also on the situation experienced and, more importantly, on the component parts of the individual experiencing the stimulus. Thus pain can be, and often is, very subjective. In some cultures, young men are asked to cross rivers with grappling hooks imbedded in their stomachs to prove their manhood. In viewing pictures of these men, it is certainly not obvious that they are in pain. However, the expression of pain and the severity of pain differs from one individual to another.

It is the subjective nature of pain that makes its study so difficult. In fact, little is known regarding the cortical mechanisms involved in the perception of back pain. To date, investigators of pain have been unable to communicate a good understanding of their patients' back pain. In fact, several investigators, studying pain, have themselves submitted to having their own nerves crushed, cut, or resutured in order to observe and describe their sensory experiences. None of these investigators have ever agreed with each other.[2]

Definition

The taxonomy committee of the International Association for the Study of Pain (1979) defined pain as "an unpleasant sensory and emotional experience associated with actual or potential tissue damage, or described in terms of such damage."[1] The nature of back pain and its impact on industrialized countries have imposed a sense of urgency for a better understanding of the various pain pathways in neuromechanisms. Treatment modalities are so varied that an appropriate analysis of efficacy has been, at best, difficult. Today, if one method of treatment fails, another method is tried. If it fails, a further method is tried. Therefore, it is hard to study the natural history of any one condition or the result of any one specific treatment. It is only through a better understanding of pain and its neurophysiology that responsible decisions can be made regarding treatment.

Neuroanatomy of the Functional Spinal Unit

Dorsal primary rami provide nerve fibers that innervate each functional spinal unit of the lumbar spine. The medial branches from each dorsal ramus of the spinal nerves send fibers to the vertebral periosteum, facet joint capsules, and ligamentous connections of the neural arches. The sinovertebral nerve provides innervation to structures within the spinal canal (Fig. 2). There is general agreement that the dorsal primary ramus is a branch off the spinal nerve just distal to the dorsal root ganglion. Direct stimulation of the posterior longitudinal ligament is known to elicit back pain in humans. Pederson and associates[3] showed that stimulation of these tissues in cats resulted in changes in blood pressure and respiration similar to those elicited by painful stimuli in other areas of the body. Thresholds of these pain fibers can be altered by various pathologic conditions. On the other hand, in a patient who has

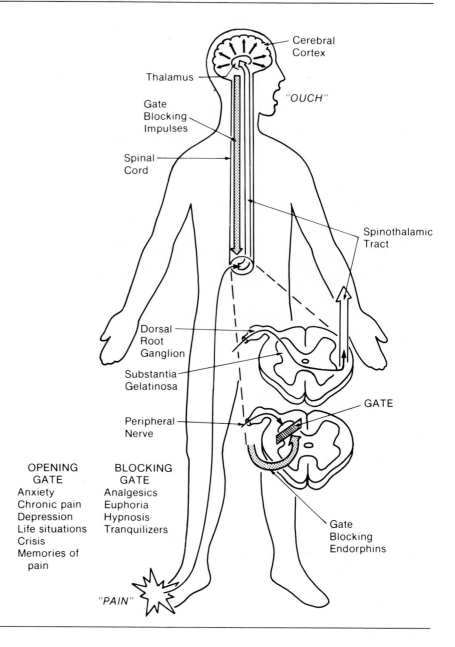

Fig. 1 A diagrammatic sketch of the gate control theory of pain. Descartes first described such a pathway in 1664. (1) First toe is injured; this causes a release of various pain modulators, such as substance P, and other chemicals are released. This starts the pain signal on its way as an electrical impulse. (2) The message reaches the dorsal horn of the spinal cord (substantia gelatinosa). (3) It is relayed via the spinothalamic tract to the thalamus, the area of the brain where the painful stimulus first becomes conscious. (4) The message then reaches the cerebral cortex, where the location of pain and its intensity are perceived. (5) Gate blocking impulses are transmitted from the brain via the spinal cord to provide pain relief. (6) In the dorsal horn, chemicals like endorphins are released to diminish the pain message from the injured toe. (Reproduced with permission from Weinstein JN: The perceptions of pain, in Kirkaldy-Willis W (ed): *Managing Low Back Pain*, ed 2. New York, Churchill-Livingstone, 1988, p 88.)

never had a history of back pain and no history of injury to the back and/or the surrounding structures, C-fiber thresholds may be normal. In such an individual, therefore, walking or sitting may not cause pain, while those who have had an injury and an altered thermostatic setting or threshold for pain often experience severe pain even with the slightest of motions.[4]

There may be several potential causes of localized pain in the lower back in an individual with proven pathology. Pain originating in the lumbar spine typically arises from mechanical and/or chemical irritation of primary sensory neurons. Abnormal mechanical stresses may be accompanied by a changing chemical environment, which may induce changes in several tissue components in the functional spinal unit. Resultant static and dynamic changes in tissue morphology and function can lead to pain.[2,4,5]

The nerve root and/or its branches may be involved. Chronic nerve root irritation may result in edema, fibrosis, and development of segmental demyelination. There is evidence that nerve root tissue that has been altered in this manner can become mechanically sensitive in terms of reacting with a pain response, even with minor mechanical deformation. Chronic abnormal motion in association with, for example, degenerative spondylolisthesis or isthmic spondylolisthesis, may produce repeated micro stretching injuries and friction to the nerve roots. These factors may be a significant mechanism behind the occurrence of radicular pain in such situations.[4]

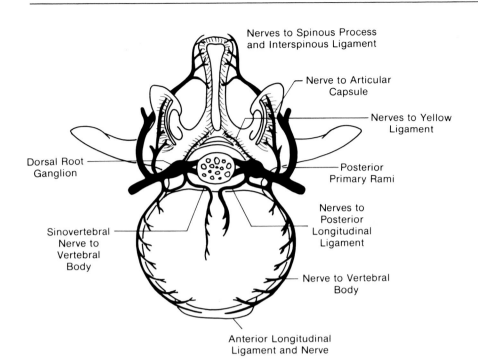

Nerves to Spinous Process
and Interspinous Ligament

Nerve to Articular
Capsule

Nerves to Yellow
Ligament

Dorsal Root
Ganglion

Posterior
Primary Rami

Nerves to
Posterior
Longitudinal
Ligament

Sinovertebral
Nerve to
Vertebral
Body

Nerve to Vertebral
Body

Anterior Longitudinal
Ligament and Nerve

Fig. 2 The three-joint complex receives pleurisegmental innervation by a combination of nerves (sinuvertebral). (Reproduced with permission from Weinstein JN: The perceptions of pain, in Kirkaldy-Willis W (ed): *Managing Low Back Pain*, ed 2. New York, Churchill-Livingstone, 1988, p 86.)

Fusion Versus Arthroplasty

A major component of orthopaedic surgery has been to eliminate pain originating from joints.[6] Two major approaches to achieving this goal in orthopaedics have been the obliteration of motion by arthrodesis or by arthroplastic joint replacement. In the spine, efforts at developing clinically useful arthroplasty have either been unsuccessful or are still experimental. Thus, fusion remains the method of choice for surgical relief of spinal pain. Bone grafting alone has a number of drawbacks. First, most grafting techniques have little or no capacity to correct spinal deformity. Second, most posterior grafting techniques do not provide early control of motion, because control cannot occur until after graft consolidation. Third, pseudarthrosis occurs with an unacceptable frequency, particularly when multiple levels are incorporated in the fusion. For these reasons, orthopaedists have searched for adjuncts to bone grafting, such as electrical stimulation or internal fixation devices, which will alleviate or eliminate these three problems.

Hypothesis

"When pathologic motion is eliminated by immobilization or arthrodesis, pain relief may follow."[5] When deformity is corrected, fusion maintains skeletal alignment and prevents recurrence. Based on these general premises, spinal arthrodesis has been employed to control pain attributed to unstable motion or to mechanical

insufficiency produced by traumatic, degenerative, inflammatory, neoplastic, and infectious processes. Likewise, spinal fusion has been used to maintain the correction of spinal deformities associated with these pathologic processes as well as progressive deformities secondary to various developmental conditions.

The first clinical report of spinal fusion using internal fixation was in 1887 by Captain B. F. Wilkins of Ottawa, Kansas, who wired a T12-L1 fracture dislocation in a baby.[6] In 1911 Albee[7] and Hibbs[8] used a different technique for Pott's disease. Hibbs observed natural ankylosis in the infected spine and reasoned that the surgical acceleration of this process might result in a more rapid and certain healing. Albee implanted a tibial graft in the spinous processes with the thought that it might provide an internal splint and hasten stabilization of the spine. In 1917, DeQuervain and Hoessly and others made use of the scapular spine as an internal splint and source and bone graft. In the same year Hibbs reported on spinal fusion to prevent the increasing deformity of scoliosis. No internal fixation was used even though Hadra[9] in 1891 had reported a technique for wiring the spine, and Lange[10] in 1902 had developed a system that used steel rods with a celluloid cylinder.

Modified and expanded applications of the more popular Hibbs technique advanced over the next 30 years. In addition to infection this technique was used to manage fractures and various developmental deformities (scoliosis). In 1943 Howorth broadened the indications for fusion as an adjunctive method for treatment of the ruptured nucleus pulposus, following the lead of Mixter and Barr.[11] He concluded that fusion—

the quickest and most economical method of pain relief—offered a financial advantage to patient, hospital, and community. In more recent times, indications for spinal fusion have broadened, except for the dwindling enthusiasm for its use in conjunction with excision of primary lumbar disk herniations in adults. Techniques for spinal fusion have now evolved to include a wide variety of internal fixation devices. These devices attempt to provide greater correction of deformities and to increase the rates of spine fusion.

In the past decade, posterior fixation devices have achieved increasing popularity because of their capacity to correct spinal deformity and provide early stabilization. There is substantial evidence, if not extensive proof, that they also increase the rate of solid arthrodesis, particularly when multiple functional spinal units are included in the fusion area. The elimination of pain and improvements in function that result from solid arthrodesis require further investigation.

More recently, a variety of bone-grafting methods and substitutes have been tried, including vascularized grafts, allografts, decalcified bone, and periosteal strippings. However, despite the best attempts, posterolateral spinal fusion continues to have a significant rate of clinical and biological failure.

Fusion and Pain

There are numerous reasons why a solid fusion may not achieve pain relief. This information has grown out of studies that compared grafting with nongrafting after partial diskectomy either retrospectively or prospectively. The reasons for failure may include incorrect diagnosis or inadequate length of fusion to bridge all the pain sources. A more subtle cause is a presence of excessive springiness or deflection despite the presence of contiguous arthrodesis.[12-14] This movement tends to occur to a greater extent when the bone graft is placed more posteriorly. Conversely, intertransverse process or interbody grafts are less subject to this problem, because the lever arm between the grafts and loading axis is less. Others have suggested that nonosseous spinal structures are the source of residual pain. Proposed structures include the supraspinous and interspinous ligaments, the posterior primary rami that supplies the dorsal muscles, facet joints of the neural arch, and the facet joint capsules. Likewise, muscle damage intraoperatively secondary to a retractor-induced ischemia may be a cause. Graft impingement on adjacent facets, nerve roots, laminar hypertrophy, or the continued presence of a degenerative painful disk itself must also be considered.

The onset of pain following fusion may result from accelerated degeneration of the adjacent functional spinal unit. Biomechanical events that promote the accelerated breakdown have been studied both in vitro and in vivo.[14,15] Biochemical aspects of this problem also need to be studied.

Implant Evolution

The development of internal fixation devices was directly stimulated by the problem of pseudarthrosis, particularly in patients with mechanical insufficiencies.[16-18] Deformities are a multilevel problem. Recently, external fixation devices have been used as a diagnostic tool to determine before surgery whether temporary spinal stabilization will eliminate or reduce pain. The variety of devices available are usually described based on where they attach to the vertebra; facet joint screws, spinous process plates, laminar hooks and rods, segmental wires, smooth rods, transpedicular screws, and external fixation devices.

A variety of issues remain to be resolved regarding transpedicular screws. These include the optimal thread design, the optimal position for screw placement, the optimal method for monitoring screw placement, the optimal depth of insertion, the proper preparation of the screw hole, the length of spine segment to be instrumented, the use of crosslinking, and the optimal mechanical characteristics of various pedicle fixation devices. A final issue to be resolved is the current clinical experience with such devices.

Although these issues have yet to be resolved, we do know that pedicular fixation has opened new vistas for the experienced spine surgeon. Unfortunately, the less experienced surgeon should not consider such techniques without proper training. The care and treatment of surgically treated spine fractures, tumors, and osteotomies have clear and distinct advantages when treated with pedicular devices. In spine fractures, double or even single level fusions may be in the best interest of both surgeon and patient. In the treatment of spine tumors, primary or secondary, reconstructive procedures never before possible can now be achieved with pedicular fixation. In experienced hands, this technique should lead to better tumor surgery, reduced morbidity, and improved survival. Patients indicated for spinal osteotomies for posttraumatic kyphosis or ankylosing spondylitis have also benefitted directly as a result of pedicular devices now available to experienced spine surgeons.

Technique: Pedicle Screws

Using a traditional midline approach, the paravertebral muscles are stripped laterally, with care taken not to injure the facet joint capsules. The surgeon must also take extreme care to avoid disrupting the facet joint capsules while releasing the deep muscles. Using electrocautery, lateral to the facet joint capsules, one can clearly identify and expose the transverse processes, initiating the exposure for performing a posterolateral fusion. Under C-arm (radiograph) control, with a No. 4 Penfield, the center of the pedicle is identified. This is done by having the C-arm perpendicular to the long axis of the pedicle. Now, a high speed burr or fine curette is used to remove the outer cortex of the pedicle, rechecking once again with the No. 4 Penfield on the anteroposterior image. The entrance point for lumbar screws is the lateral cortex of the superior facet where it meets the transverse process. A probe (straight or slightly curved) is used to help insure screw placement into the cancellous bone of the pedicle. I suggest tapping the pedicle. The tap should be allowed to find its own way into the pedicle, and should not be forced.[19] Some surgeons use a drilling technique, but this may have extra inherent risks. Some suggest that predrilling can weaken pullout strength, but others discount this.

The direction and depth of pedicle screw placement varies depending on the desired goals of the surgeon for the particular case. In treating a trauma patient, it may be desirable to have deep penetration, 80% to 90%, whereas in degenerative disease 50% penetration of pedicle may be adequate. Directing the screw medially and superiorly is recommended by some authors. This appears to reduce the risk of shearing at the screw-bone interface.

Complications

Spinal pedicle fixation has tremendously advanced the care and treatment of various spinal problems. There is, however, a learning curve and the surgeon should be well aware of this.[19] Likewise, spinal surgeons should also be aware that radiographs are very unreliable in determining whether they are in or out of the pedicle. This, however, must be weighed against the consequences of not using radiograph at all. If screws placed through the pedicle of L3, L4, or L5 breech the anterior vertebral cortex, neurovascular structures can be injured. These include the aorta, inferior vena cava, obturator nerve, and others. Although this is not a likely complication, the mortality of such complications is probably in the 60% to 80% range. What is acceptable? Extrinsic placement of pedicle screw is not desirable, although Weinstein and associates[19] suggest that pedicle penetration or breach occurs in as many as 20% of screw placements.

What about hardware failure? Hardware failure, or screw breakage, does not necessarily mean that the system is bad or the surgeon has not achieved the other objectives. Screw breakage need not necessarily be interpreted as a complication, because the dynamics of fusion and the biology of bone fusion may require such breakage to occur to allow appropriate fusion to take place. Screw breakage does not necessarily represent failure. On the contrary, it may have allowed fusion to occur.

Methylmethacrylate can be used as an adjunct to pedicle fixation in severely osteoporotic bone. Mechanical studies by Zindrick and associates[20] demonstrate significantly improved pullout strengths, but this technique is not without risks.

In the final analysis, a spinal surgeon must approach each motion segment individually, realizing the biology of the problem being treated and assessing objectively each level and each facet joint within each level. Some functional spinal units may require rigid fixation; others may require less rigid fixation or none at all. Today's surgeon must be open to many options and not use one particular device or one particular operation for all problems. Over the last century we have gone to great lengths to achieve successful spinal fusion. In the next century we must learn how to use this knowledge to provide our patients with the best clinical outcomes.

References

1. Wall PD, Melzack R: *Textbook of Pain.* New York, Churchill-Livingstone, 1984.
2. Weinstein JN: Anatomy: Neurophysiologic mechanisms of pain, in Frymoyer JW, Weinstein JN, Kostuik JP, et al (eds): *The Adult Spine: Principles and Practice.* New York, Raven Press, 1991, p 593.
3. Pederson HE, Blunck CF, Gardner E: Anatomy of lumbosacral posterior rami and meningeal branches of spinal nerves (sinuvertebral nerves) with experimental study of their functions. *J Bone Joint Surg* 1956:38A:377–391.
4. Weinstein JN: Nerve, in Frymoyer JW, Gordon SL (eds): *New Perspectives on Low Back Pain.* Park Ridge, IL, American Academy of Orthopaedic Surgons, 1989, pp 35–130.
5. Weinstein J, Rydevik B: The pain of spondylolisthesis. *Semin Spine Surg* 1989:1:100–105.
6. Wiltse L: The history of spinal disease, in Frymoyer JW, Weinstein JN, Kostuik JP, et al (eds): *The Adult Spine: Principles and Practice.* New York, Raven Press, 1991, p 30.
7. Albee FH: Transplantation of a portion of the tibia into the spine for Pott's disease: A preliminary report. *JAMA* 1911;57:885–886.
8. Hibbs RA: An operation for progressive spinal deformities: A preliminary report of three cases from the service of the orthopaedic hospital. *NY Med J* 1911;93:1013–1016.
9. Hadra B: Wiring of the vertebrae as a means of immobilization in fracture and Pott's disease. *Am Orthop Assn Trans* 1891;4:206.
10. Lange F: Support for the spondylitic spine by means of buried steel bars attached to the vertebrae. *Am J Orthop Surg* 1910:8:344–361.
11. Mixter WJ, Barr JS: Rupture of the intervertebral disc with involvement of the spinal canal. *N Engl J Med* 1934;211:210–215.
12. Bosworth DM: Technique of spinal fusion: Pseudoarthrosis and method of repair, in Blount WP (ed): American Academy of Orthopaedic Surgeons *Instructional Course Lectures, V.* Ann Arbor, JW Edwards, 1948, pp 295–313.
13. DePalma AF, Rothman RH: The nature of pseudarthrosis. *Clin Orthop* 1968;59:113–118.
14. Rolander SD: Motion of the lumbar spine with special reference to the stabilizing effect of posterior fusion: An experimental study on autopsy specimens. *Acta Orthop Scand* 1966;90(suppl):1–44.

15. Lehmann TR, Spratt KF, Tozzi JE, et al: Long-term follow-up of lower lumbar fusion patients. *Spine* 1987:12:97–104.
16. Frymoyer JW, Hanley E, Howe J, et al: Disc excision and spine fusion in the management of lumbar disc disease: A minimum ten-year follow-up. *Spine* 1978;3:1–6.
17. Frymoyer JW, Selby DK: Segmental instability: Rationale for treatment. *Spine* 1985;10:280–286.
18. Hanley EN Jr, Shapiro DE: The development of low-back pain after excision of a lumbar disc. *J Bone Joint Surg* 1989;71A:719–721.
19. Weinstein JN, Spratt KF, Spengler D, et al: Spinal pedicle fixation: Reliability and validity of roentgenogram-based assessment and surgical factors on successful screw placement. *Spine* 1988; 13:1012–1018.
20. Zindrick MR, Patwardhan A, Lorenz M: Effect of methylmethacrylate augmentation upon pedicle screw fixation in the spine. Proceedings of the International Society for the Study of the Lumbar Spine, Dallas, TX, May 1986.

Osteoporosis and Fusion

Neil Kahanovitz, MD

Introduction

The direct relationship between osteoporotic bone and the probability of obtaining a solid lumbar fusion is poorly understood. The actual question of whether an osteoporotic spine is more prone to pseudoarthrosis formation following spinal fusion has not been conclusively answered in either a clinical setting or a basic science model. Because this question has not been addressed, it is extremely difficult to determine whether an osteoporotic spine fuses as well without internal fixation or whether the internal fixation is worth the additional morbidity associated with prolonged operative time, increased blood loss, and other potential complications inherent in the use of internal fixation devices. A variety of studies, which will be discussed further, have looked at the ability of osteoporotic bone to withstand the forces of different internal fixation devices as well as the effect of internal fixation on producing or aggravating spinal osteoporosis. The other question for which there is no definitive answer is which currently available fixation system is best for the osteoporotic spine.

Osteopenia simply means that there is less bone tissue present in any given bone than would normally be expected. The osteopenia may be caused by osteoporosis or osteomalacia. Although bone loss is a normal phenomenon during aging, it is this abnormally accelerated loss of bone that leads to the pathologic, radiographic, and clinical manifestations of osteoporosis.

Types of Osteoporosis

For most patients with osteoporosis there is no identifiable metabolic defect responsible for the osteoporosis. These patients fall into the broad category of involutional or age-related osteoporosis. It is generally agreed that there are two distinct types of involutional osteoporosis.[1,2]

Type I osteoporosis is more common in women and appears to be related to postmenopausal hormonal and physiologic changes. Symptoms and structural changes related to this type of osteoporosis begin to appear within 15 to 20 years after menopause.

Type II osteoporosis is seen in older patients, usually individuals who are 70 years of age or older.[1] Although still more frequent in females than males, the ratio decreases to approximately two to one. Although the etiology is not completely understood, the osteoporotic changes appear to result from an acceleration of the normal aging phenomenon involving the bone tissue.

The vertebrae are normally composed of both cortical and cancellous bone. Because the posterior elements are principally composed of cortical bone, these anatomic structures are usually spared the clinically evident effects of osteoporosis. However, the vertebral body is primarily composed of trabecular bone and typically manifests the radiographic changes so often associated with osteoporosis. Even though the cortex of the vertebral body is rather thin (0.5 to 1.0 mm), it is responsible for half of the compressive strength of the vertebral body.[3] In contact with the cortex are horizontal layers of trabecular bone, which form the vertebral endplate. These layers of trabecular bone, which may be several millimeters wide, are thickest in the central portion of the vertebral body, the area where the cortex is thinnest.[4]

Radiographically, 29% of women and 18% of men between the ages of 45 and 79 will demonstrate evidence of osteoporosis on plain radiographs.[5] One study, which used absorptiometry to assess bone density, found that 50% of women older than 65 years of age had a bone density below the predicted fracture threshold. Because type I osteoporosis affects trabecular bone loss more than cortical bone, vertebral compression fractures are seen more frequently than hip fractures in this younger age group.[6] Because of the significantly greater number of women with type I osteoporosis, the vertebral manifestations of osteoporosis and, ultimately, compression fractures are seen in a female-male ratio of almost six to one. In older patients, with predominantly type II osteoporosis, the percentage of women experiencing its detrimental effects is still higher, but only in a ratio of two to one.

Certain risk factors increase the tendency of some individuals to develop the vertebral manifestations of osteoporosis.[7,8] White females appear to be most at risk for developing type I osteoporosis. Premature menopause, whether the cause is metabolic, hormonal, or surgical, will increase the risk of type I osteoporosis. A wide variety of other physiologic and metabolic abnormalities can also hasten the onset of osteoporosis. Malnutrition, diabetes mellitus, Cushing's syndrome, hyperthyroidism, acromegaly, and homocystinuria can result in early osteoporosis. The use of excessive alcohol, tobacco, antacids, corticosteroids, and coffee have also all been implicated in an increased risk of osteoporosis.[5,9,10]

Vertebral compression fractures are quite common in patients with type I osteoporosis. In fact, it is estimated that from 5% to 40% of postmenopausal women will develop compression fractures.[11] Most of these fractures involve the vertebrae of the lower thoracic and lumbar spine. The vast majority of compression fractures heal uneventfully within two to three months with complete resolution of symptoms. However, with compression fractures that result in the loss of more than 33% to 50% of the normal vertebral body height, persistent pain can result from the ensuing mechanical and, ultimately, degenerative changes. A patient with several compression fractures of lesser degree of severity in adjacent vertebrae may also have disabling pain, if the normal articular mechanics are sufficiently altered.

Treatment

Unfortunately, for those few patients with persistent symptoms, there are not many therapeutic solutions to choose from. Physical therapy modalities, both passive and active, do little to alter the long-term course of symptoms. Bracing can give temporary immobilization and concomitant relief, but prolonged, particularly rigid, bracing is poorly tolerated by elderly patients. Medications should be non-narcotic, if at all possible, to avoid the addiction that can result from prolonged use, as well as the depressive side effects that many of these drugs have when used by elderly patients.

Surgery is indicated in these patients only if there is a significant and symptomatic structural deformity or neurologic involvement. In those few patients in which surgery is indicated, the surgery should attempt to correct or stabilize the deformity and, at the same time, alleviate any neurologic compression. Correction of the typical kyphotic deformity in these patients is often quite difficult because of the rigidity of the deformity as well as the inherent difficulty in maintaining firm fixation in the osteoporotic bone with internal fixation devices.

Because most patients with osteoporosis will not need surgical intervention, the vast majority of the surgical procedures involving osteoporotic bone will be performed on patients with degenerative disease resulting in motion segment instability. The indications for fusion in patients with degenerative lumbar spine disease are not universally agreed upon, particularly in patients with mild degenerative spondylolisthesis. However, with the increasingly sophisticated internal fixation devices designed specifically for use in the lumbar spine, lumbar spinal fusions for degenerative disease are becoming more popular. For most vertebrae, sublaminar hooks offer adequate fixation, even in osteoporotic vertebrae. However, the use of sublaminar hooks in the lower lumbar spine, particularly at L5 and S1, presents unique difficulties. The most obvious of these problems is the previously decompressed or presently stenotic patient in which a canal decompression eliminates the possibility of sublaminar fixation. Even in those patients with intact lower lumbar and first sacral lamina, sublaminar hook fixation is less than optimal because of the anatomic variations at these levels, which are accentuated by the lower lumbar lordosis. Thus, the rate of failure and dislodgement of sublaminar hooks is unacceptably high, particularly at L5 and S1.

Pedicle screw fixation has eliminated many of the problems inherent with sublaminar hook fixation. When pedicle screws were first introduced, the patient with significant osteoporosis seemed to be the ideal candidate for internal fixation with pedicle screws. Unfortunately, it soon became apparent that even with this markedly improved fixation system, there was a tendency for the pedicle screws to pull out of the osteoporotic bone or, worse, strip the pedicle on insertion, making fixation impossible. Laboratory studies have conclusively shown that pedicle screw fixation is significantly compromised by the presence of osteoporotic bone. A recent study has shown that the pull-out strength of a pedicle screw in normal bone with a bone mineral density of 1.7 per cm^2 was 1,534 N.[12] This figure contrasts sharply with the 210 N pull-out strength of a pedicle screw in osteoporotic bone with a bone mineral density of 0.82 per cm^2.[5] Thus, the need for a different type of fixation in these patients was clearly evident even with the improved and more rigid pedicle fixation devices.

As in other areas of the skeleton where bony fixation is tenuous, polymethylmethacrylate is now used to augment pedicle screw fixation in osteoporotic vertebrae. The use of polymethylmethacrylate to improve pedicle screw fixation has markedly improved the ability of the pedicle screws to resist pull-out and failure of fixation. Zindrick and associates[13] examined the use of polymethylmethacrylate to enhance pedicle screw fixation and have shown dramatic results. Optimal placement of the cement appears to be anteriorly at the tip of the screw to enhance increased surface area contact within the vertebral body. The use of 4 cc of polymethylmethacrylate to augment pedicle screw fixation (or 6 cc of polymethylmethacrylate in previously stripped pedicle fixation sites) increased pull-out strength by at least 2.5 times over control. Average pull-out strength with polymethylmethacrylate averaged 2,000 N. Cross-linking of the pedicle screws may further increase the strength of an already rigid system, as shown in other experimental studies.[14]

Despite these rather apparent advantages of polymethylmethacrylate augmentation, there are potential disadvantages and morbidity associated with this technique. Cement leakage through a penetrated pedicle wall can cause nerve root damage. Extra-pedicular cement, particularly in the retroperitoneal space, can cause significant problems of removal in the face of infection. Revision surgery in which the fixation device must be removed can render the previously instrumented pedicle useless for further fixation even with polymethylmethacrylate augmentation.

Although the use of the devices described above has been increasing, their true value in obtaining a solid fusion, particularly in the osteoporotic spine, has not been determined. Increased fusion rates with internal fixation are beginning to be reported in comparative studies in groups of patients fused with and without internal fixation.[15] Whether the presence or extent of osteoporosis affects fusion rate has not been specifically answered. Likewise, the question of which internal fixation system is best in the osteoporotic spine is still unanswered. There is no accepted answer as to whether a rigid or less rigid internal fixation system is best. Obviously, a major determinant in these patients is the osteoporosis itself, and whether a less rigid system can lower bone-fixation failure rates better than a more rigid system. Experimental studies have shown that rigid internal fixation systems can increase osteoporosis. One study showed a definite increase in osteoporosis in vertebrae instrumented in canine spinal fusions, although neither the fusion rate nor the mechanical stiffness appeared to be affected by these device-related bone density changes.[16]

Direct current electrical stimulation has been shown to improve the rate of fusion in both routine and high-risk fusion patients. However, its efficacy in patients with osteoporosis as a primary variable has not been investigated. Even though it is unclear whether electrical stimulation works as well or at all in markedly osteoporotic bone, its use may be advocated, because the morbidity associated with its use is so low that any potential benefit should outweigh the potential risk.

Because the effect of osteoporosis on fusion rate and quality is so poorly understood, it is difficult to design a postoperative program for these patients that differs from that used for any patient recovering from a lumbar spinal fusion. Postoperative bracing should be used routinely in patients with internal fixation to maximize postoperative immobilization and prevent instrumentation failure. Fusions to the sacrum with internal fixation should be protected with a thigh extension to avoid excessive stresses across the lumbosacral junction.

Patients whose significant osteoporosis was not previously evaluated should be referred for a thorough medical workup. This step avoids the risk of misdiagnosing one of the treatable causes of osteoporosis, even though these are much less common than types I and II described above. For those patients with advanced osteoporosis, appropriate treatment with calcium supplements, estrogen, vitamin D, and fluoride should be instituted as indicated. Once solid fusion is achieved, routine exercises should be begun.

References

1. Riggs BL, Melton LJ III: Evidence for two distinct syndromes of involutional osteoporosis. *Am J Med* 1983;75:899.
2. Riggs BL, Melton LJ III: Involutional osteoporosis. *N Engl J Med* 1986;314:1676.
3. Rockoff SD, Sweet E, Bleustein J: The relative contribution of trabecular and cortical bone to the strength of human lumbar vertebrae. *Calcif Tissue Res* 1969;3:163–175.
4. Lukert BP: Osteoporosis—A review and update. *Arch Phys Med Rehabil* 1982;63:480–487.
5. Riggs BL, Wahner HW, Dunn WL, et al: Differential changes in bone m ineral density of appendicular and axial skeleton with aging: Relationship to spinal osteoporosis. *J Clin Invest* 1981;67: 328–335.
6. Pagnini-Hill A, Ross RK, Gerkins VR: Menopausal estrogen therapy and hip fractures. *Ann Int Med* 1981;95:28–31.
7. Brown DM, Jowsey J, Bradford DS: Osteoporosis in ovarian dysgenesis. *J Pediatr* 1974;84:816–820.
8. Johansson BW, Kaij L, Kullander S, et al: On some late effects of bilateral oophorectomy in the age range 15–30 years. *Acta Obstet Gynecol Scand* 1975;54:449–461.
9. Heaney RP, Recker RR: Effects of nitrogen, phosphorus, and caffeine on calcium balance in women. *J Lab Clin Med* 1982;99: 46–55.
10. Seeman E, Melton LJ III, O'Fallon WM, et al: Risk factors for spinal osteoporosis in men. *A J Med* 1983;75:977–983.
11. Cummings SR: Epidemiology of osteoporotic fractures: Selected topics, in Roche AF (ed): *Osteoporosis: Current Concepts.* Columbus, OH, Ross Laboratories, 1987, pp 3–7.
12. Halvorson TL, Kelly L, Whitecloud T, et al: Effects of bone mineral density on pedicle screw pullout strength. Presented at the Annual Meeting of the Scoliosis Research Society, Dallas, TX, Sept 1990, p 96.
13. Zindrick MR, Knight BW, Patwardhan AG, et al: The effect of polymethylmethacrylate augmentation upon pedicle screw fixation in the spine. Presented at the Meeting of the International Society for the Study of the Lumbar Spine, Dallas, TX, June 5, 1986.
14. McAfee PC, Ruland CM, Warden KE, et al: Triangulation of pedicular instrumentation: A biomechanical analysis. Presented at the Annual Meeting of the Scoliosis Research Society, Dallas TX, Sept 1990, p 99.
15. Schwaegler P, Cram R, Lorenz M, et al: A comparison of single level fusions with and without hardware. Presented at the Meeting of the North American Spine Society, Carmel, CA, Aug 9, 1990.
16. Sutterlin CE, Warden KE, Farey ID, et al: Roentgenographic, biomechanical and quantitative histologic analysis of the influence of pedicle screw fixation in oopherectomized and nonoophorectomized canines. Presented at the Meeting of the North American Spine Society, Carmel CA, Aug 9, 1990.

Revision Surgery for Spinal Deformity

Ronald L. DeWald, MD

Introduction

The spinal deformity patient who has had previous surgery and who now has new or continuing problems and complaints may be a candidate for further surgical treatment. The clinical evaluation suggested for such a patient will be organized as follows: (1) initial assessment; (2) general evaluation; (3) indications; (4) goals of surgery; (5) considerations before undertaking surgery; (6) common forms of residual deformity; (7) common forms of pain syndrome in spinal deformity; (8) patient selection; (9) operative techniques; and (10) complications.

Initial Assessment

The spinal surgeon, unlike the neurosurgeon or the cardiovascular surgeon, has no medical counterpart. The spinal surgeon can't rely on a *spinologist*, as a neurosurgeon relies on a neurologist or cardiovascular surgeon relies on a cardiologist. There is no one to tell the patient "we have done all we can non-operatively now you should consider operative treatment."[1]

Initially for pain syndrome patients, general treatment, such as nonsteroidal anti-inflammatory agents, proper exercise, back school, and/or epidural steroid injections, may suffice. If the pain persists or is severe, further investigation, in addition to routine radiographs, may be indicated.[2]

History

In treating a patient who has had previous surgery for a deformity, a detailed and comprehensive history and physical examination is essential. Questions to be answered include the following: When did the patient first notice his deformity? How was it treated? How long was a brace worn? What type of brace was it? When was surgery performed? Was it in stages? What type of graft was used? Was anterior and posterior surgery performed?

Each part of the history helps the surgeon know the patient better. It also helps the surgeon determine how great an impact the physical disfigurement has upon the patient. This knowledge will help the surgeon understand how the patient deals with the disfigurement. The past medical history and social history also help the surgeon decide if the patient is a candidate for a one-, a two-, or a three-staged procedure.

General Evaluation

Physical Examination

In addition to the routine physical examination, special attention is given to the patient's stance and gait. Does the patient stand level? Are the knees straight or flexed? Is there an oblique pelvis? Are the leg lengths equal? Where is the sagittal vertical axis? Where does the plumb line fall?

Does the patient have good strength? Can the patient toe walk, heel walk, and squat? Are the deep tendon reflexes normal? Are there any abnormal reflexes? Is there good voluntary sphincter control and rectal tone?

Radiographic Examination

All old radiographs must be gathered and examined. What is the earliest radiograph? What was the deformity at that time? How supple was the deformity? Is there evidence of anterior fusion? Is there a pseudarthrosis currently? Are the disks degenerating? Is the deformity increasing?

New standing posteroanterior and lateral radiographs and bending radiographs, taken at a distance of 72 inches, are obtained on a 14 by 36-inch cassette as a measurement standard. If the patient's complaint is pain that has not responded to the usual nonsurgical treatment, a myelogram may reveal the cause. Because the presence of metal can interfere with the image gained by computed tomography or magnetic resonance imaging, myelography may provide better information (Fig. 1).

Rib Hump

Patients who complain of rib hump deformity should undergo evaluation to prove that the spine fusion is solid, stable, and balanced. Pulmonary function should be tested and arterial blood gases analyzed. A chest computed tomographic examination will reveal which ribs and how many ribs are to be excised (Fig. 2).

Indications

Revision surgery for spinal deformity is a major surgical undertaking. Most patients seek help because they are still deformed, because they are in pain, or because their spinal implant has failed.

Many patients seek help because an incidental radiograph has revealed a displaced or fractured rod or

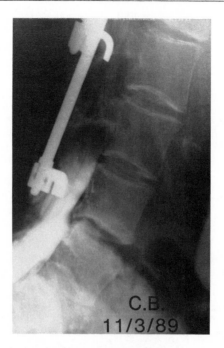

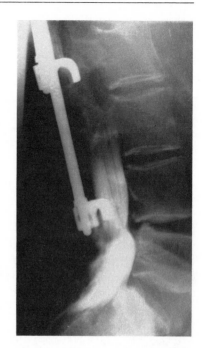

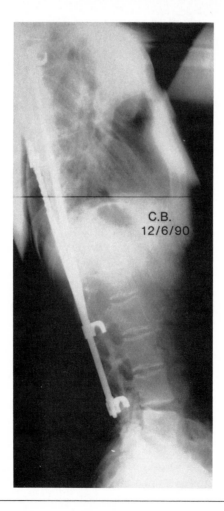

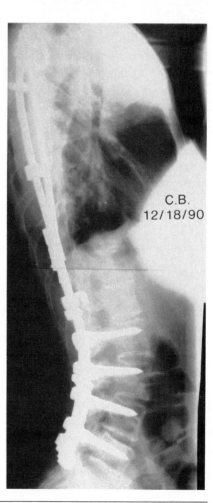

Fig. 1 Twelve years postoperative a pain syndrome developed and myelography (**top left** and **right**) revealed a defect at L4-L5 below the last fused level. Surgical decompression failed to relieve the pain. The flexion-extension myelogram shows instability at L4-L5. A lateral radiograph (**bottom left**) emphasizes the flat lumbar spine with instability at L4-L5. Implant removal, osteotomy, and reimplantation were performed (**bottom right**). Note the restitution of lumbar lordosis and the proper orientation of the individual vertebrae. L5 was included in this construction because of the instability between L4 and L5.

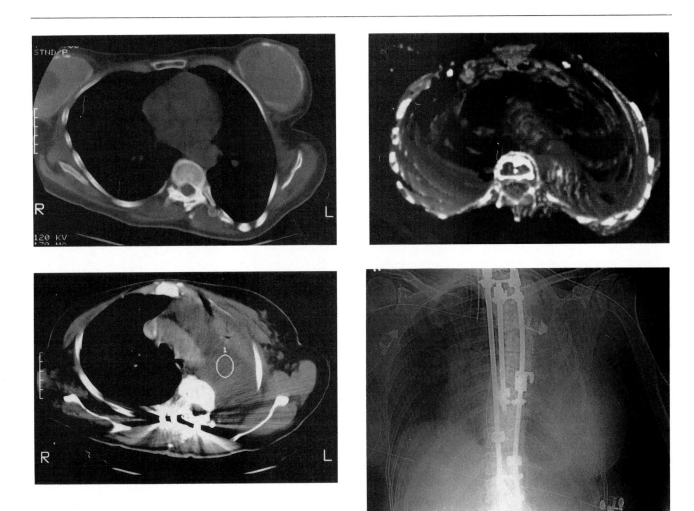

Fig. 2 Top left, This patient's major concern was the rib hump deformity. On the preoperative computed tomographic scans, note the rib deformity, the breast implants, and the location of the left scapula. **Top right,** Three-dimension computed tomography of the deformity. The spine must be stabilized before rib resection can be performed. **Bottom left,** The postoperative computed tomographic scan shows a large pleural effusion, the rib resection, and the better location of the left scapula. **Bottom right,** The postoperative radiographs illustrate the pleural effusion and the rib resection as well as control of the spine.

screw. If there is no pain or further deformity, there is no reason for surgery. If there is no pain but the surgeon can predict that severe problems will be forthcoming, it may be best to revise the surgery and perform preventive maintenance. Posterior implants usually fail because of a pseudarthrosis of the posterior fusion mass. Another reason posterior instruments can fail is because of insufficient anterior structural support.

The indications for revision surgery for spinal deformity are deformity, pain, and neuropathy, as well as fatigue fracture or dislocation of the implant.

Anterior surgery is indicated in the following situations: (1) if there has been previous anterior surgery; (2) if mobilization of the spine is needed and more mobility will be obtained if disk excision is performed; and (3) if circumferential fusion is desired.

Goals of Surgery

For revision surgery in spinal deformity, patency of the neural canal, alignment of the spine, stability of the spine, and support of the spine (sound anterior column) are the four principles of surgical spine care that must be kept foremost in considering spinal surgical conditions.

It is especially difficult to establish an indication for revision surgery when treating patients who complain of residual deformity. For this reason, it is imperative to make sure that patients understand the goals of surgery before undergoing an initial procedure to correct a deformity. The goals of spinal deformity surgery are, first, to prevent further deformity and, second, to safely correct the existing deformity.

Patients tend to believe that they will be normal or

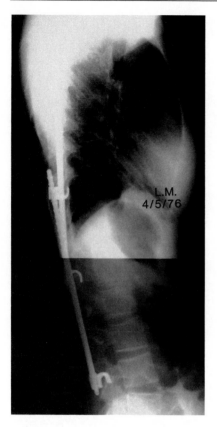
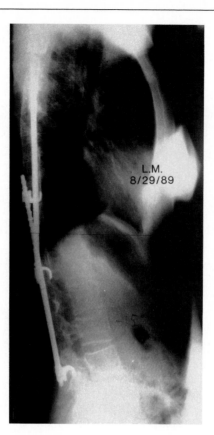
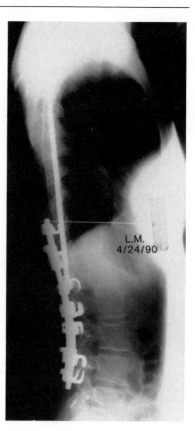

Fig. 3   **Left**, A flat back deformity was created by eliminating lumbar lordosis. Thirteen years later (**center**) lateral radiograph of the lumbar spine reveals probable pseudarthrosis between L3-L4, and L4 is tilted cephalad. The L3-L4 disk is not stable and instrumentation must include this motion segment. Osteotomy, realignment, and reimplantation were performed (**right**). The correct caudad position of L4 has now been obtained with a harmonious lumbar lordosis.

better than normal after their spinal deformity surgery. Throughout the years, this has not been possible. Twenty to 30 years ago, surgery for spinal deformity was reserved for the most severe cases and, because of the severity of the problems, full correction of deformity was impossible. Many fusions were too short, and without internal fixation immobilization was difficult. Even after the Harrington instruments became available, the importance of the sagittal plane contour was not appreciated and a flat back was often produced (Fig. 3). Luque spinal segmental fixation could not correct severe problems because of wire breakage and other problems (Fig. 4). Because techniques did not derotate the chest cage, rib deformities persisted. The outcome of revision surgery must be judged in terms of pain relief, correction of deformity, and improved function.[3]

Patients will undergo many operations if they think there is a reasonable chance for improvement of their deformity. Occasionally, a patient is happy with the result of revision surgery even though the surgeon is not. More often the patient is not happy, but the surgeon is satisfied with the result.

Pain syndromes are usually well defined, and their treatment will be dictated by the diagnosis. In general, it is best to remove the implant, decompress, realign, and reimplant. For deformity problems, the surgeon must be sure that he can improve the patient's balance. For implant problems, the treatment is to remove the implant, perform an osteotomy, realign, and reimplant.

The goals of surgery are to improve coronal and sagittal balance, relieve pain, and improve the neuropathy. These goals may be accomplished in one, two, or three operations.

The goal of surgery is to balance the spine. L3 should be in the neutral position, L4 is tilted caudad (flexion), and L2 is tilted cephalad (extension) (Fig. 5).

Considerations Before Undertaking Surgery

Diagnosis and Prognosis

Diagnosis and prognosis are of extreme importance when considering revision surgery. Congenital scoliosis is a very rigid defect, is difficult to correct, and carries with it a high risk of neurologic complication. Patients with paralytic scoliosis associated with amyotonia, hypotonia, cerebral palsy, or muscular dystrophy may not

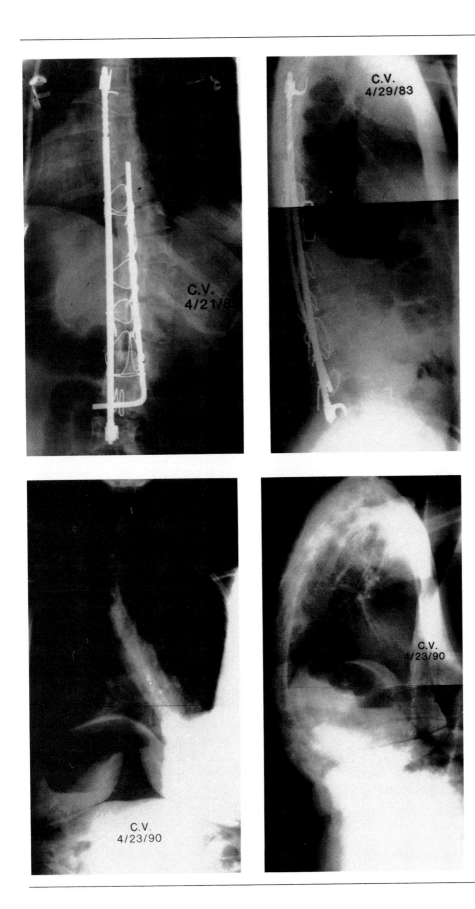

Fig. 4 This patient presented in 1983 with both coronal and sagittal plane decompensation. Correction by osteotomy and implantation gained good alignment although sagittal plane alignment is not ideal (**top left** and **right**). The fixation failed to control the spine. After bone and wire failure the implants were removed. Luque technique is not successful in revision surgery for spinal deformity (**bottom left** and **right**).

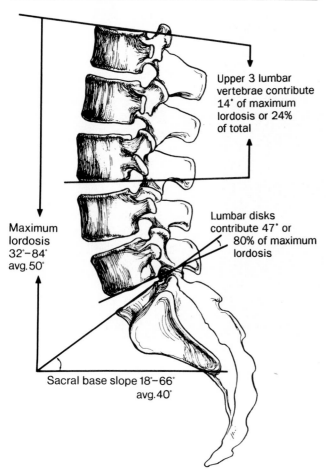

Upper 3 lumbar vertebrae contribute 14° of maximum lordosis or 24% of total

Maximum lordosis 32°–84° avg. 50°

Lumbar disks contribute 47° or 80% of maximum lordosis

Sacral base slope 18°–66° avg. 40°

Fig. 5 Average maximum lordosis as measured from superior L1 to superior S1; the average sacral slope as measured from superior S1 to the horizontal; the degree the disks contribute to lumbar lordosis; the degrees the upper three lumbar vertebrae contribute to maximum lordosis; and by inference the degrees the vertebral bodies contribute to maximum lordosis.

be good candidates for revision surgery. A patient with a diagnosis of idiopathic scoliosis usually has an excellent prognosis after revision.

Location of the Deformity

If only the rib hump is of concern, thoracoplasty may be all that is needed. If imbalance is a problem, the surgeon must judge how he can balance the spine and what will be involved in so doing. The sagittal plane imbalance is more noticeable than coronal plane imbalance.

The Number of Previous Operations

The number of previous operations is a factor in analyzing the patient's ability to withstand the rigors of spinal surgery. Deformity patients will go through severe surgical morbidity if they feel it will improve their physical disfigurement. Of course, if their expectation is not met, a depression might follow. For this reason, it is best to anticipate the patient's expected outcome.

Anterior or Posterior Osteotomies or Both

It has been our experience that the more osteotomies performed, the better the end result. If the spine has been fused both anteriorly and posteriorly then both sides must be osteotomized and at multiple levels.

Same-Day, Staged, or Simultaneous Surgery

These judgments must be made during a planning session. If osteotomy and intercurrent traction are required, staged surgery is necessary. Same-day surgery is preferable to staged surgery because the recovery is faster and the patient's nutrition better.[4] On occasion simultaneous surgery is needed. Most often this situation arises if both columns are to be osteotomized and fused. Generally this procedure is used when the spine is in kyphus and the desire is to place the lumbar segments into lordosis. The patient is placed in the lateral decubitus position to allow the surgeons to work simultaneously both anteriorly and posteriorly.

Predicted Blood Loss

Significant blood loss can be expected, and replacement with the patient's own blood is preferred. Correct positioning on a four poster frame with a free abdomen is valuable for control of blood loss as well as for correction of the osteotomized spine. We routinely use a cell saver. We always reinfuse the patient's cells as well as the patient's own fresh frozen plasma.

Length of Time of Surgery

The length of time required for surgery must be considered in planning the number of operations to be done. Surgical team fatigue is a consideration. Same-day surgery is preferred but to start a second stage after six to seven hours of surgery is not in the patient's best interest.

Rigidity of Deformity

If the surgeon can review all of the previous radiographs, he will be able to sense the rigidity of the deformity and to determine what can be accomplished by revision surgery. Although the surgeon will probably not be able to make the patient better than the improvement seen on the original side-bending films, sagittal plane balance may be improved regardless of the rigidity of the deformity.

Bone Quality and Bone Graft Availability

Bone quality and availability of bone graft is another consideration. Osteoporosis limits the amount of force that a surgeon can apply to correct the deformity. Allograft bone is suitable for spine fusions, and radiation of the graft reduces the risk of AIDS. Whether it is as good as autogenous bone is debatable.[5-7] However, if there is no autogenous bone available, the surgeon will have to use allograft bone.

Age and Health

Special attention must be paid to the age and health of the patient. Some chronic pain patients are addicted and have poor nutrition. It is better to rehabilitate these patients physically, mentally, and nutritionally before undertaking revision spinal surgery. In some cases, concurrent medical problems can rule out spinal surgery.

Common Forms of Residual Deformity

The most common forms of residual deformity dealt with by revision spinal surgery are imbalances in the coronal or sagittal plane. The surgeon must be cognizant of normal coronal and sagittal alignment. Normal coronal alignment is straight. The stable zone in the coronal plane extends superiorly from the two lumbosacral facets.[8,9] Sagittal alignment follows the sagittal vertical axis line. This line falls from C2 in front of T7, behind L3 and across S2 (Fig. 6).[10] The individual vertebrae are neutral or are ventrally or dorsally oriented. In addition, in the lumbar spine it is important to note such factors as maximum lordosis, sacral slope, and percent of disk contribution to the maximum lordosis.

Definitions of Deformity Terms

Too Short Fusion This particular situation can occur when the patient has been fused at an early age and the end vertebrae were not correctly identified. The usual result is a decompensated spine, not coronal or sagittal plane imbalance (Fig. 7).

The Spine Has "Fallen Over" This term generally refers to a sudden increase in the scoliotic or kyphotic deformity at the end of the fusion mass. This may be seen when the spine has not been balanced properly and is generally seen in the adult patient in whom the instrumentation did not go above the kyphus (Fig. 8).

Pseudarthrosis Pseudarthrosis represents a failure of fusion. Depending on the location, it may cause increasing deformity with implant failure (Fig. 9).

Coronal Plane Decompensation Coronal plane decompensation generally refers to the dorsal spine not being in line with the mid sacral line. In such cases, most of the spine lies outside of the Harrington stable zone (Fig. 7).

Sagittal Plane Decompensation Sagittal plane decompensation is generally seen when the sagittal vertical axis line does not fall in front of T7, behind L3, and across S2 (Fig. 7).

Flat Back Flat back is a clinical syndrome that results from the loss of lumbar lordosis and normal sacral slope. The patient stays bent forward, the knees are flexed, and the patient complains of pain and fatigue (Fig. 3).

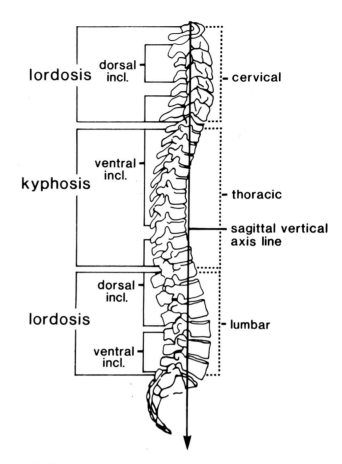

Fig. 6 The sagittal vertical axis line and the orientation of each individual vertebrae.

Rib Hump Deformity This term refers to an angular deformity of the ribs on the convex side of the scoliosis (Fig. 2).

Crankshaft Phenomenon This term refers to an increase in the rotation of a growing spine after posterior distraction and fusion caused by anterior spinal growth (Fig. 7).

Forward Head Thrust Head thrust is generally seen after kyphus correction when the cervical lordosis is rigid and cannot spontaneously correct.

Wrong Fusion Level Selection This situation generally causes decompensation because the end vertebra was not in the stable zone (Fig. 7).

"Add On" Phenomenon This problem generally occurs in a growing child when the incorrect end vertebrae were selected for the fusion and the scoliosis has progressed above and below the fusion zone (Fig. 7). The end vertebrae for fusion are selected conditionally on the posteroanterior radiograph. The lower end vertebrae must be in the stable zone on the concave bending film and preferably on the standing film. The stable zone is de-

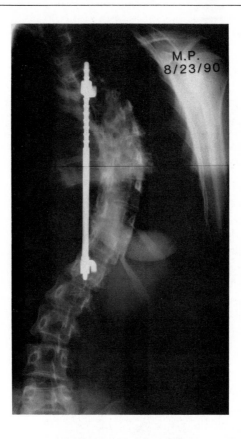
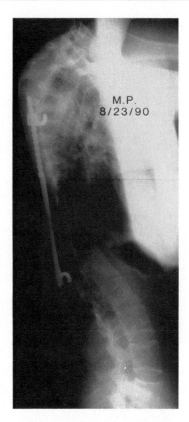
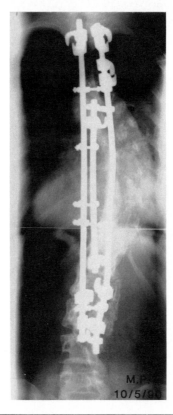
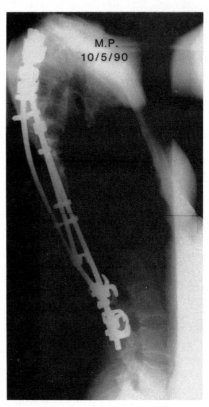

Fig. 7 Ten years after surgery, this patient complained of pain and deformity. Note the marked chest wall deformity, short fusion, and decompensation in both coronal and sagittal planes (**top left** and **right**). Treatment was by osteotomy at T4-T5 and T5-T6 and instrumentation from T2 to L3 with rib resection. Posteroanterior and lateral radiographs (**bottom left** and **right**) show restored balance of the spine.

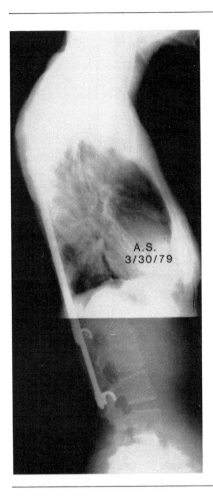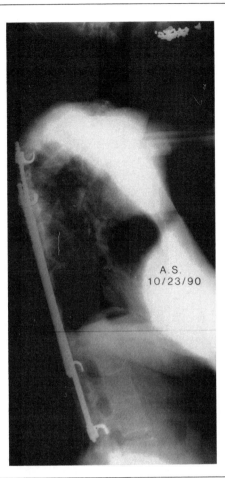

Fig. 8 Left, Postoperative lateral radiographs three years after fusion. Radiograph taken eleven years later (**right**) reveals fall off above Harrington rods because of poor sagittal balance.

fined by two parallel lines from the lumbosacral facets. The end vertebrae must be neutral on the concave bending film, and the disk below should be open on both sides on the bending radiographs. The definitive choice of the end vertebrae is determined by the standing lateral radiograph. If the lower vertebra determined in the frontal plane is at the apex of a junctional kyphosis, the instrumentation must be extended lower, and the hook is reversed to compress the kyphosis to restore the sagittal alignment and avoid decompensation. On the basis of a frontal radiograph, the instrumentation is extended to the next neutral vertebrae.

Failure to Recognize the Double Major Curve Failure to recognize a double major curve is generally seen when using the King classification for fusion end vertebrae selection.[11]

Failure to Recognize Double Thoracic Curve Pattern This situation is generally seen in the upper thoracic curve that does not correct fully on the side-bending radiograph.

Wrong Instrumentation Selected Generally seen with anterior instrumentation,[12] the spine may fall into kyphus (Fig. 10).

Common Forms of Pain Syndromes in Spinal Deformity

Pain syndromes are common and typical in spinal deformity patients.[13] If back pain is common in patients with straight unoperated spines, it must be at least as common or more common in patients with a previously operated spinal deformity. The pain complaints vary from mild burning hump pain to a rather specific low back and radicular pain. The pain can be located above the fusion mass but is most common below the fusion mass.[14]

Nachemson and associates[15] documented that low lumbar spine fusion with Harrington rods can cause pain problems in the segments below the fusion.

Low back pain syndrome can be caused by faulty alignment. Any attempt to alleviate the pain without restoring balance to the spine will usually fail. For this reason, in treating low back pain syndrome it is necessary to determine how best to align the spine, whether this can be done in one operation or two, and whether or not anterior surgery is needed. The same situation holds for deformity complaints, in which the cause of the patient's complaint usually has to do with a loss of either coronal or sagittal balance. Another source of complaint is residual rib hump deformity. Some pa-

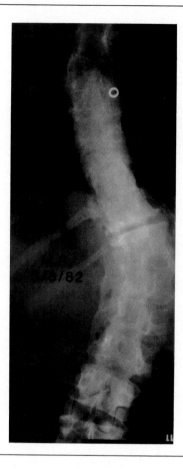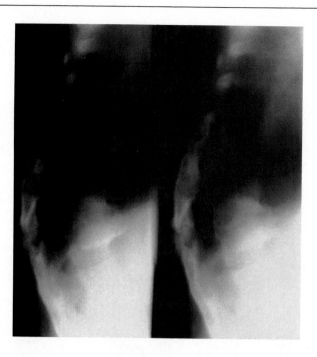

Fig. 9 Left, Posteroanterior radiograph demonstrates obvious pseudarthrosis at the apex of coronal and sagittal deformity. On tomograms (**right**), note large spurs anteriorly. This spur generally directs one to the posterior pseudarthrosis.

tients complain of neck fatigue and pain. This, too, is probably caused by poor sagittal or coronal alignment. On occasion, a spondylolysis will develop at L5, usually secondary to a flat lumbar spine.

Patients whose vertebrae are fused early in life generally have narrowed disks caused by continued growth of the vertebral body after solid posterior fusion. A pseudarthrosis can easily be identified by observing a normal disk height under the fusion mass in such a patient. If the last segment of spine is not fused, Harrington hooks may become dislodged. There is controversy regarding the best way to handle this situation, but perhaps opening that last level is in the patient's best interest (Fig. 11).

Pain syndromes in spinal deformity are generally localized in the lower lumbar area. They may be caused by degenerative disk disease, spinal stenosis, disk rupture, instability, or nerve root entrapment.

As Alf Nachemson reported in 1983, low lumbar spine surgery for deformity is associated with pain problems.[15] At that time, the problems were intensified because distortion of the normal lumbar sagittal anatomy caused undue stress and mechanical strain to the disks and facet joints. It is not yet known whether the new instrumentation now available, which maintains the normal sagittal contour of the lumbar spine, will still cause low back pain as a late sequelae.

The L4-L5 disk is at great jeopardy if the lumbar spine is straight and not in its normal sagittal contour. Degenerative disk disease or even disk ruptures are common. On occasion there may be such a severe encroachment on the canal that symptoms of spinal stenosis prevail and the patient constantly seeks a place to sit down (Fig. 1).

Instability may be demonstrated on flexion-extension radiographs. Myelograms can demonstrate nerve root entrapment. Myelograms are superior to other forms of imaging because the presence of metal interferes with magnetic resonance or computed tomographic imaging. Surgery for pain syndromes in spinal deformity must include: (1) removal of the implant; (2) decompression; (3) osteotomy; (4) realignment of the spine; and (5) reimplantation. Any attempt to merely decompress the problem without realignment will usually prove fruitless and, in fact, can complicate the eventual realignment and reimplantation.

Instrumentation failure or dislocation can be painful. If revision is to be undertaken it must include removal of the instruments, osteotomy of the spine, reimplan-

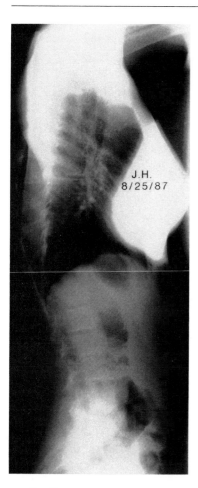 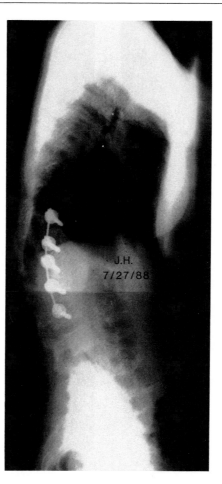 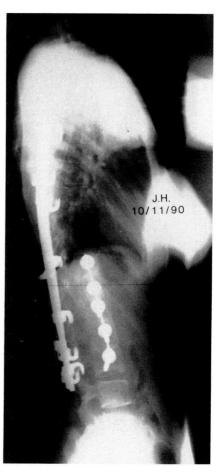

Fig. 10 Preoperative lateral radiograph (**left**) of a patient with a supple thoracolumbar scoliosis. The upper curve corrected, and there was little rotation on the side-bending radiograph. Zielke instruments were chosen to save levels (**center**). Postoperatively the spine is in more kyphus than preoperatively despite anterior grafts. Posterior instrumentation and fusion were needed to correct the situation (**right**). Although Zielke instrumentation can save levels, its tendency to create a kyphus must be respected.

tation in correct coronal and sagittal plane balance, and anterior strut graft support (Fig. 12).

Patient Selection

With all of these variables to consider, it is a challenge for the spine surgeon to select the patient he is able to help.

If a patient with low back pain below fusion sees a surgeon who is unfamiliar with deformity surgery and coronal and sagittal plane balance, the surgeon may decompress the problem only to have the pain syndrome recur very quickly. The spinal surgeon must analyze his ability to correct any particular situation. The best candidates for revision surgery are those patients with sagittal plane deformities. These patients are helped greatly by creating a harmonious lumbar lordosis (Fig. 13). Sometimes it is possible to connect the reimplantation instruments to the former instrumen-

tation without replacing the entire instrumentation. To do so saves the patient time in surgery and reduces blood loss.

Other patients that can be helped greatly are the rib hump deformity patients. If the spine is stable and the pulmonary function tests and arterial blood gases are satisfactory, excision of the deformity can provide a marked cosmetic improvement. The surgery can be performed through the old midline scar for better cosmesis with dissection out to the rib prominences. Computed tomographic (CT) scans of the chest done before surgery will help locate which ribs and which part of the ribs must be resected. Rib deformities are easily seen on a chest CT scan. The angular deformity of the rib is noted, and this is the area to be resected. As many ribs as necessary are resected, which is generally rib 4 or 5 through rib 11.

Patients with pain caused by instability generally can be helped quickly by creating a more harmonious lordosis and by including the unstable segment in the new

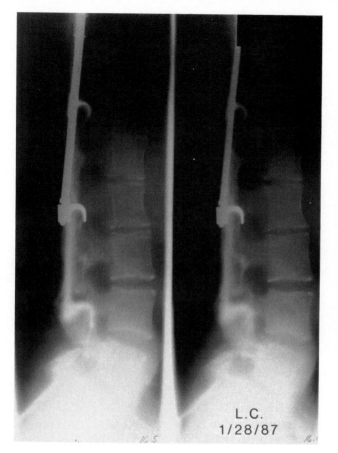 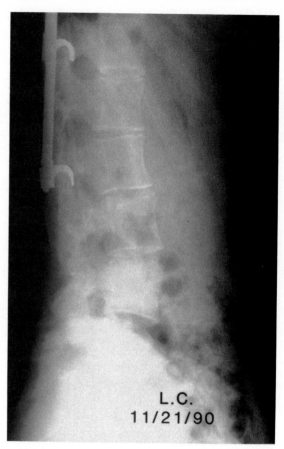

Fig. 11 A pain syndrome developed two years after fusion for scoliosis, and a computed tomogram (**left**) revealed a pseudarthrosis at L3-L4 and a spondylolysis of L5 that was not present previously. Note the disk height has not narrowed as compared with the disks above the pseudarthrosis in the area of solid fusion. The treatment was removal of the right Harrington rod, facet arthroplasty at L3-L4 through the pseudarthrosis, and autograft to the pars interarticularis at L5. At three years after the last surgery (**right**), this patient is free of pain.

instrumentation and fusion. Pain associated with pseudarthrosis can also be relieved, but alignment must be achieved so that the pseudarthrosis will unite.

Coronal plane deformities are difficult to improve, and usually require intercurrent traction in order to gain correction after osteotomy. The traction, consisting of halo gravity traction, generally starts slowly by adding a pound per day. Constant neurologic vigilance is necessary and requires daily neurologic examinations by the same examiner. In many cases, patients with coronal plane deformities were previously fused early and short. As a consequence, the spine is now rotated and decompensated. The problem is almost always in the coronal plane.

Patients with implant failure may be helped, but the cause of failure must be identified and corrected. In most cases, either there is no anterior column support or there is posterior pseudarthrosis. The surgeon must change the instrumentation, balance the spine, and support the anterior column.

Operative Techniques

Techniques of revision surgery for spinal deformity include: (1) removal of implants anteriorly, posteriorly, or both; (2) osteotomy of the spine either anteriorly or posteriorly or both; (3) reimplantation with modern implants to allow better sagittal and coronal balance; and (4) possible intercurrent skeletal traction, especially for coronal plane deformity.

Revision surgery may be done anteriorly, posteriorly, or both.[16] The surgery may be staged days apart, may be performed the same day, or may be simultaneous.

Anterior Surgery

If anterior surgery is needed for mobilization or circumferential fusion, the standard thoracoabdominal approach is used. The appropriate rib, which is usually the rib that leads to the interspace two levels above the most superior vertebra to be operated, is selected for entry, and the incision begins 3 to 4 cm from the spinous process and follows the rib to the costal chondral

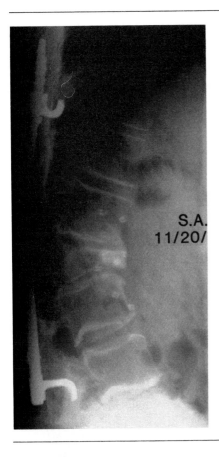

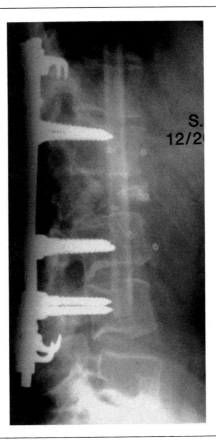

Fig. 12 This patient had a L3 hemangiopericytoma tumor removed anteriorly and posteriorly, and was irradiated. Harrington instrumentation and attempted fusion were performed (**left**). The anterior column reconstruction was not sufficient and the Harrington rods fractured. Osteotomy, realignment, and reimplantation, along with anterior strut fibula graft, were performed (**right**). Note embolization of segmental vessels bilaterally.

junction. The incision then proceeds down the abdomen midway between the umbilicus and the anterior superior iliac spine. It usually ends just caudad to the anterior superior iliac spine unless the L5-S1 disk space is to be included in the procedure, in which case it must continue more inferiorly.

The diaphragm is incised close to its insertion down to the spine. The segmental vessels are divided and disks are removed. Care is taken to preserve the end plates. The end plates are important if the surgeon wants to use a graft anteriorly to extend the motion segment or to prevent it from falling into kyphus. If the end plate is injured and the graft sinks into the vertebral body, realignment will be lost.

A spine previously fused anteriorly must be osteotomized and mobilized if correction is to be obtained. The approach is through the old incision, which is generally easy to accomplish because the vessels have been previously ligated and, in most cases, a bursa will have formed over any implant that was placed anteriorly.

Anteriorly, the implants are removed and the old disk spaces are identified. The graft and the union of bone are osteotomized. Bone is removed back to the posterior longitudinal ligament.

Osteotomies in the dorsal spine, which are necessary for coronal plane correction, are more hazardous because of the spinal cord. The spine is rotated and is in lordosis. The osteotomies are performed as above, but they are dangerous because of the spinal cord. Furthermore, the presence of the ribs limits mobility. The location of the osteotomy must be chosen carefully, because in many cases one segment of thoracic spine is straight and does not require osteotomy.

Posterior Surgery

The operation begins with excision of the old scar. The dissection is directly down to the spine. The usual method is to expose only the lower one-half of the spine in order to save blood. The instrumentation is identified and the spine stripped. Usually the instruments are helpful in identifying spinal levels. Harrington hooks identify levels of the spine. The sublaminar wires will identify the superior and inferior limits of the lamina.

The removal of wires requires a special technique. A 1/4-inch osteotome is used to remove the bone that grows around the wire both superiorly and inferiorly. The wire is then pulled taut against the anterior surface of the lamina, cut close to the lamina, and removed. It is important that the wire be freely moveable before it is removed, to avoid injuring the dura.

The old rods are cut and removed. Sometimes the hooks adhere to the dura below, causing a leak to develop. Such leaks must be closed either primarily or with a graft. The surgeon must be prepared to repair the dura, because these tears and leaks occur frequently (Fig. 14).

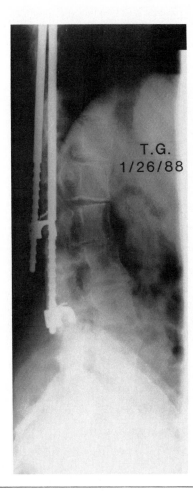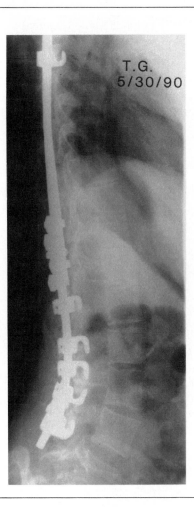

Fig. 13 This patient, who had a fusion for scoliosis 12 years before, presented with low back pain (**left**). Note the lumbar kyphosis and the subluxation of L4 on L5. Rod removal, multiple lumbar osteotomies, and creation of harmonious lordosis were performed (**right**). Note how the Cotrel-Dubousset instrumentations have been joined to the remaining Harrington rod.

After the levels have been identified and the instruments removed, the transverse processes must be identified. The osteotomy should be at the level of the disk. The osteotomies are then performed in a chevron fashion through what were previously the facet joints of the spine. Chevron osteotomies are desirable because they provide medial, lateral, and rotational stability. A trough approximately 6 to 7 mm wide is cut. Care is taken to preserve the nerve root directly below the osteotomy and, of course, the osteotomy sites must be undercut to prevent nerve root pinching when the osteotomy is closed. If there is scoliosis, the spine fusion must be cut wider on the side of the convexity to allow straightening during derotation and lordosing (Fig. 15).

The distorted anatomy makes this surgery difficult. The surgeon must use all available sources to become and stay oriented. If the patient has had a previous laminectomy it is imperative that the surgeon find the pedicles and the roots, because it will be necessary to use pedicle screws for fixation. Often, after the osteotomy is complete, it is possible to probe for the pedicle and to be sure that the screw is in the right position.

Usually the lower lumbar spine must be osteotom-ized, because these vertebrae are the ones that must be moved considerably to correct the sagittal plane and achieve balance. The actual technique of osteotomy varies, depending on the situation. Sometimes it is possible to use a hook site for a beginning or to begin where the sublaminar wires were removed. At other times the surgeon simply uses a rongeur until the flavum is identified. The Kerrison is then used to continue to take bone out to the foramen. I always dissect the dura away before using the Kerrison. As the osteotomy is completed, the motion segment will fall into lordosis. It is important to use a spreader to obtain room to undercut the osteotomy so that the nerve roots will be free after correction. It is very important to do as many osteotomies as possible (Fig. 15). Osteotomies of the lumbar spine are valuable for correction of a flat back problem. Positioning the patient on a four poster frame allows the spine to fall into lordosis after osteotomy. The patient's chest is supported on the superior two posts of the four poster frame, and the inferior two posts support the pelvis and thighs.

With the Cotrel-Dubousset instrumentation, it is possible to rotate the scoliosis deformity into lordosis by

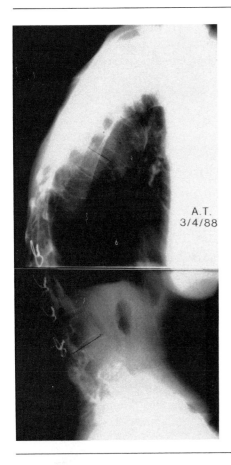
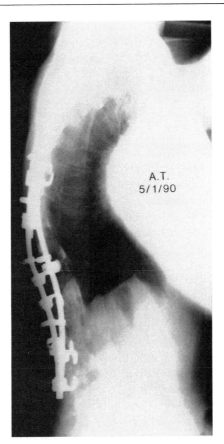

Fig. 14 Left, Progressive kyphus developed after decompression and rod removal for pain after attempted fusion for scoliosis. Sublaminar wires help locate sites for osteotomy. **Right**, This patient underwent anterior diskectomy and mobilization followed by posterior osteotomy and reimplantation. The last instrumented vertebra is L3, and dominos were used to extend the of instrumentation above the apex of the kyphus.

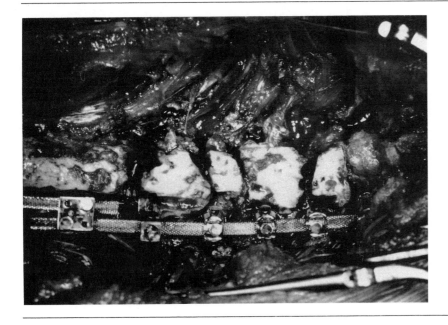

Fig. 15 Illustrates multiple osteotomies in the lumbar spine. The head is to the left and the feet are to the right in this photograph. Note the chevron shaped osteotomies. Note the pedicle screws and the domino. Cotrel-Dubousset instrumentation is best for revision surgery, because it is versatile and universal. One can compress, distract, use hooks or screws, all with the same system and on the same rod.

placing the rod onto the convexity and rotating it 90 degrees into lordosis. This is best done using pedicle screws, which place the rotation force more laterally than do hooks, which are situated closer to the midline.

In correcting the lumbar spine after osteotomy, it is particularly important to deal with sagittal plane deformities.[16–18] Reinstrumentation is always performed from the last motion segment in the Harrington stable zone with a good disk below to the highest motion segment in the mid sacral line above the kyphus. This arrangement balances the coronal plane. In the sagittal plane the amount of thoracic kyphosis must equal the amount of lumbar lordosis to balance the spine.

Rib Hump

Depending upon the amount of rotation, the ribs can be excised either at their articulation or in the middle of the rib, at the site of the major deformity (Fig. 2).

These ribs usually do not aid in respiration and their removal does not decrease pulmonary function. Insertion of a chest tube is necessary. After surgery, a flail chest does not develop, because the chest wall is stabilized by chest tube suction and the patient is supine.

The Entrapment Syndromes

The surgical technique is similar to that described above but includes additional surgery to decompress the entrapment syndromes. It may be necessary to remove lamina, to remove facet joints, or to extend the instrumentation inferiorly one level. The need to extend the instrumentation one level is most common in cases of instability. If the lamina is to be removed, a pedicle screw is needed at that level. If the disk is healthy, it is sometimes possible to end the fusion one level higher by performing a facet arthroplasty through the old facet joint. A facet arthroplasty is a technique developed for facets when the disk above is normal. The disk is considered normal if it has normal height, no vertebral body spurs, and is hydrated on magnetic resonance imaging scans. The arthroplasty is accomplished through the old joint by removing the fibrous scar and replacing it with fat; in essence performing a fat facet arthroplasty. Fusion to the sacrum is difficult to achieve.[19] Because of the high failure rate and the difficulty in achieving balance control, we prefer to avoid fusion to the sacrum if at all possible.

Complications

A common complication after surgery is dissatisfaction on the part of the patient or the surgeon in regard to cosmesis. Patients with deformities tend to believe that one more operation will make them normal. The surgeon must know what he can accomplish safely, and he must be able to transmit that information to his patient.

Pain syndromes can be relieved. However, after three or four procedures there are diminishing returns and a good result is less likely. Arachnoiditis is always a possible risk. There is also the danger of further neuropathy or paralysis, and the risk is likely to be greater than at the original surgery. Wake-up tests and spinal-cord monitoring are standard. Nevertheless we are dealing with a population of patients whose risk is much higher than that of the average adolescent patient with idiopathic scoliosis.

Bone grafts do not always heal. Autografts are preferable to allografts, but many patients have no bone left for graft. Pseudarthrosis is still possible and implant failure can still occur. Revision surgery for spinal deformity patients is demanding, difficult, dangerous, and emotionally draining for both the surgeon and the patient. To achieve the best result, the surgeon must be meticulous in planning and must execute a demanding surgical procedure with precision and care.

References

1. Bradford DS: Adult scoliosis: Current concepts of treatment. *Clin Orthop* 1988;229:70–87.
2. Macnab I: *Backache*. Baltimore, Williams and Wilkins, 1977.
3. Kostuik JP: Decision making in adult scoliosis. *Spine* 1979;4:521–525.
4. Mandelbaum BR, Tolo VT, McAfee PC, et al: Nutritional deficiencies after staged anterior and posterior spinal reconstructive surgery. *Clin Orthop* 1988;234:5–11.
5. Aurori BF, Weierman RJ, Lowell HA, et al: Pseudarthrosis after spinal fusion for scoliosis. A comparison of autogeneic and allogeneic bone grafts. *Clin Orthop* 1985;199:153–158.
6. Buck MD, Malinin TI, Brown MD: Bone transplantation and human immunodeficiency virus. An estimate of risk of acquired immunodeficiency syndrome (AIDS). *Clin Orthop* 1989;240:129–136.
7. McCarthy RE, Peek RD, Morrissy RT, et al: Allograft bone in spinal fusion for paralytic scoliosis. *J Bone Joint Surg* 1986;68A:370–375.
8. Harrington PR: Treatment of scoliosis: Correction and internal fixation by spine instrumentation. *J Bone Joint Surg* 1962;44A:591–610.
9. Harrington PR: Technical details in relation to the successful use of instrumentation in scoliosis. *Orthop Clin North Am* 1972;3:49–67.
10. Stagnara P, De Mauroy JC, Dran G, et al: Reciprocal angulation of vertebral bodies in a sagittal plane: Approach to references for the evaluation of kyphosis and lordosis. *Spine* 1982;7:335–342.
11. King HA, Moe JH, Bradford DS, et al: The selection of fusion levels in thoracic idiopathic scoliosis. *J Bone Joint Surg* 1983;65A:1302–1313.
12. Zielke K: Ventral derotation spondylolisthesis. Results of treatment of cases of idiopathic lumbar scoliosis. Author's translation. *Z Orthop* 1982;120:320–329.
13. Jackson RP, Simmons EH, Stripinis D: Incidence and severity of back pain in adult idiopathic scoliosis. *Spine* 1983;8:749–756.
14. Grubb SA, Lipscomb HS, Conrad RW: Diagnostic findings in painful adult scoliosis. Presented at the Meeting of the Scoliosis Research Society, Amsterdam, The Netherlands, September 1989.
15. Cochran T, Irstam L, Nachemson A: Long-term anatomic and functional changes in patients with adolescent idiopathic scoliosis treated by Harrington rod fusion. *Spine* 1983;8:576–584.
16. Doherty JH: Complications of fusion in lumbar scoliosis. *J Bone Joint Surg* 1973;55A:438.
17. Grobler LJ, Moe JH, Winter RB, et al: Loss of lumbar lordosis following surgical correction of thoracolumbar deformities. *Orthop Trans* 1978;2:239.
18. Lagrone MO, Bradford DS, Moe JH, et al: Treatment of symp-

Adult Scoliosis: Evaluation and Nonsurgical Treatment

James W. Ogilvie, MD

Scoliosis is defined as a coronal plane deformity that is greater than 10 degrees as measured by the Cobb method and that has structural rotation at the apical segment. If the curvature is present before skeletal maturity and has no other diagnostic features that categorize it as neuromuscular, congenital, traumatic, infectious, postinfectious, or syndrome-related, then it is regarded as idiopathic in etiology. Kostuik and Bentivoglio[1] reviewed 5,000 intravenous pyelograms taken in adults. They noted that in these films the incidence of lumbar or thoracolumbar scoliosis was 2.9%. De novo scoliosis, a coronal plane deformity greater than 10 degrees that arises after skeletal maturity, is the most frequent type of scoliosis in patients older than 50 years of age. Robin and associates,[2] who reviewed 554 patients between the ages of 50 and 84, noted that 30% had a curvature greater than 10 degrees. This is an age-related phenomenon, and at a five-year follow-up an additional 10% were noted to have this scoliosis. Osteoporosis and age-related changes in the disk explain this pathogenesis. These figures indicate that a significant number of patients have scoliosis deformities, and that their number increases as the mean age advances.[3]

Before assigning therapeutic priorities for this age group, it is necessary to review the natural history of adult scoliosis in order to understand the disease process and to identify certain groups at risk for complications. Natural history studies, however, should not foster complacency on the basis of statistical probability, and in no case should a treatment plan be instituted that is not based on individualized follow-up.

The first natural history consideration is progression of an idiopathic curve. Collis and Ponsetti[4] noticed at follow-up that 65% of idiopathic curves had progressed more than 5 degrees. The average progression was 15 degrees. Deformities of the thoracic spine between 60 and 80 degrees were at greatest risk for progression. Based on a 40.5-year followup of 102 patients with idiopathic scoliosis, Weinstein and associates[5] reported that 50- to 75-degree thoracic curves were the ones that had progressed most commonly, but that no curve had progressed more than 18 degrees. Noting no increase in incidence of pain in those who had progression, they concluded that this was not a significant medical problem. While these data are useful in that they provide statistical information regarding the probability of progression, no curve can be diagnosed as progressive until there has been a 5-degree progression

documented on successive radiographs of identical technique (Fig. 1).

The effect of pregnancy on scoliosis progression has been reviewed by numerous authors.[6,7] Several authors have noted the association of early or multiple pregnancies with curve progression. A report by Betz and associates[6] on 221 pregnancies indicated that in 25% of cases the curve progressed by more than 5 degrees, and in 10% it progressed by more than 10 degrees. These researchers noted no difference between those who experienced pregnancies and another, nonpregnant group. They also reported a 7.6% incidence of cesarean section, which was unrelated to the scoliosis and was one half the national average for that time. Their conclusion was that pregnancy, age, number of pregnancies, and curve stability at maturity bore no relation to progression.

Curve progression varies enough that no one can predict with any degree of statistical certainty which curves will or will not progress. Carefully documented followup remains the only method for establishing the diagnosis for progressive idiopathic scoliosis in the adult.

Pulmonary compromise has been the subject of misinformation and apprehension in the nonmedical public and even among certain medical specialties not thoroughly familiar with scoliosis. Zorab[8] reported that the total lung capacity, vital capacity, and forced respiratory capacity were lower in paralytic than in nonparalytic curves. Information obtained for the pulmonary complication rate in neuromuscular curves and those associated with kyphoscoliosis does not apply to patients with idiopathic curvatures.[9] The likelihood of respiratory distress is greater in these patients than it is in patients with idiopathic curves. The number of alveoli in the developing lung increases until the age of 7 years; after that time, the alveolar size increases. Zorab[8] reported that of 11 patients who died of pulmonary insufficiency, ten had significant scoliosis curvatures before they were 5 years of age. The eleventh patient had asthma. The point should be emphasized that pulmonary insufficiency is rare in adults with adolescent idiopathic curvatures.

Some patients with scoliosis experience subjective dyspnea. A study by Cooper and associates,[10] in 1984, noted a decrease in maximum inspiratory pressures and normal expiratory pressures in patients with idiopathic scoliosis. These researchers also noted a marked increase in breathing effort and a five-fold increase in

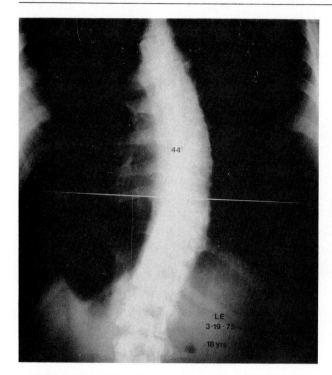 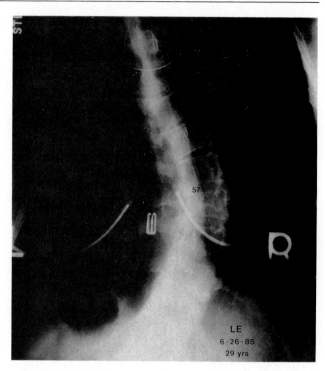

Fig. 1 **Left**, This 18-year-old woman with a 44-degree curve was asymptomatic following Milwaukee brace treatment in 1975. **Right**, In 1985 the curve had progressed to 57 degrees with back pain that was resistant to conservative treatment. She ultimately underwent surgical correction of her scoliosis.

chest wall compliance in scoliotics.[11] The subjective dyspnea, therefore, experienced by patients with curves in the 90- to 100-degree range, who exhibit normal arterial blood gases, may be accounted for by this mechanical chest wall dysfunction. In summary, although subjective dyspnea is not uncommon in patients with idiopathic scoliosis, spirometric pulmonary function tests are seldom abnormal until coronal plane deformity exceeds 60 degrees.[12,13] Parenchymal dysfunction is present only in those with advanced scoliosis exceeding 100 degrees. Other forms of pulmonary disease, including asthma, chronic obstructive pulmonary disease caused by tobacco use, and pneumoconiosis secondary to environmental pollution, are frequently more important clinically than the scoliosis deformity.

In patients with idiopathic scoliosis, pain is controversial but common. Nachemson[14] reported that only 39 of 97 scoliotics had mild back pain and that prophylactic surgery for pain was unjustified. Fowles and associates,[15] however, reported in 1979 that most adults with scoliosis experience pain and that one in four may be disabled by pain. Jackson and associates[16] found that 83% had progressive or persistent pain and that pain increased with age and with the degree of deformity. Briard and associates[17] observed that pain in adults with scoliosis is frequently resistant to conservative treatment and is persistent.

When evaluating an adult with painful scoliosis, it is necessary to understand the origin of that pain. Spinal fatigue, one common complaint, consists of vague aching in the area of the scoliosis. Sometimes it is only fully appreciated after spinal reconstructive surgery, when the pain is gone and the patient feels an increased sense of well-being at having lost this spinal fatigue. In a personal series of 61 adults undergoing spinal reconstructive surgery for idiopathic deformities, 53 of 61 exhibited symptoms of spinal fatigue.

With the uneven loading of facets and disks in the scoliotic deformity, premature degeneration can take place on either the concave or the convex side of the scoliosis.[5,18] Computed tomography with myelography demonstrates this, as well as possible subarticular stenosis caused by facet hypertrophy. In patients with right thoracic curves and sharp rib rise, there may be scapular thoracic pain caused by fatigue of the parascapular muscles and the abnormal articulation of the shoulder girdle with the thorax.

Although scoliotic deformities are often easily documentable, the surgeon must be alert for other sources of pain, including herniated nucleus pulposus, spondylolysis, and primary and metastatic tumors of the spinal column or the neural elements (Fig. 2). In summary, pain is common, particularly in the lumbar spine. It is incumbent on the physician to accurately determine and understand that source of pain. This pain is frequently resistant to treatment and, in a general

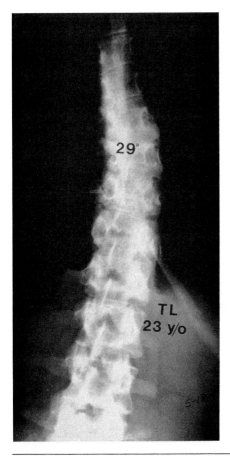

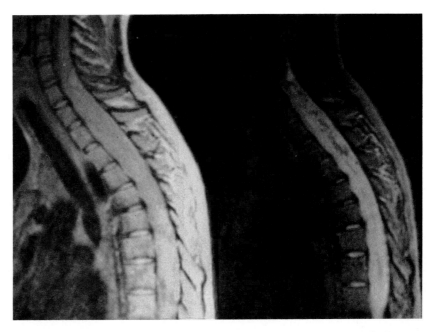

Fig. 2 **Left**, This 23-year-old woman had been treated for 10 years for a painful scoliosis. When first examined by the author she had a mild curvature with no focal physical finding except for mild clonus in both lower limbs. **Right**, An MRI of her thoracic spine revealed a large cystic glioma of the thoracic spinal cord, which required multiple level laminectomy and myelotomy.

sense, seems to be related to the age of the patient and curve severity.

Psychologic considerations are variable in scoliosis. Collis and Ponsetti[4] acknowledged the existence of these considerations, but felt them to be unimportant in the overall personal and professional lives of their patients. Nachemson,[9] however, reported that patients with spine deformities tended to have a poor body image, often remained unmarried, and, in general, had significant self-image problems as a result of their spine deformity.

The nonsurgical treatment of scoliosis generally attempts to relieve symptoms of spondylosis resulting from the spine deformity. A low-impact aerobic exercise program can help improve cardiopulmonary reserve, promote endorphin production, control weight, and possibly delay or retard the onset of age-related osteoporosis. Such low-impact aerobic exercise may include walking, swimming, cycling, and selected weight-lifting maneuvers. While this program may be initiated in a hospital setting or by a professional physical therapist, it is important for patients to make these activities a part of their regular routine on a life-long basis. If the exercises have some recreational value, adherence to the regime will be easier.

Nonsteroidal anti-inflammatory agents are commonly prescribed for pain relief. Primarily prostaglandin antagonists with an anti-inflammatory, antipyretic, and analgesic effect, these drugs have the negative effect of generally forming an acidic environment in the stomach, which may promote gastric hyperacidity and even peptic ulcer disease. On a systemic basis they inhibit gastric mucus production and, even if they are not locally irritative to the stomach, may promote peptic or gastric ulceration. Patients with marginal renal function, who depend on renal prostaglandins for renal blood flow, can have a significant increase in creatinine when taking certain nonsteroidal agents. For those who are on chronic anti-inflammatory agents, appropriate hematologic evaluation should be performed.

Antidepressants, such as amitriptyline, are used to help patients sleep more soundly and can have value in treating chronic pain symptoms. They frequently have unacceptable side effects, such as drowsiness, increased appetite, or dry mouth, however, which can be intolerable for some patients. It is important that opioids not be used for chronic pain patterns. They can be used on selected occasions for periods not to exceed 72 hours when exacerbation of pain is present, but the

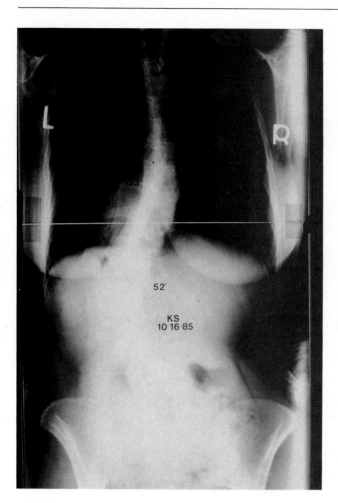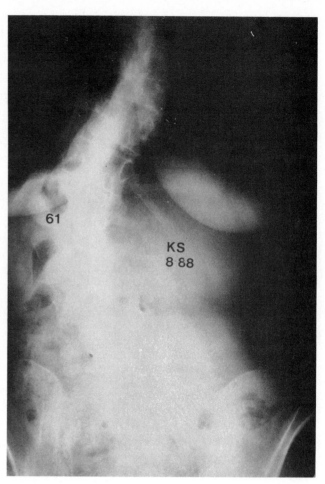

Fig. 3 **Left**, This 55-year-old woman had a painful left lumbar scoliosis. **Right**, Despite the use of a brace, three years later her curve had progressed to 61 degrees and the pain was no longer controlled by the use of a brace. She ultimately required surgical correction of her curvature.

patient must understand that primary pain control does not involve the use of controlled substances.

The use of orthotics is variable. Unlike adolescents, who wear a brace with the anticipation that the curve will be controlled and the brace will be discontinued at skeletal maturity, orthotic use in adults is for pain control. There is no evidence that the prolonged wearing of a brace in adult scoliosis changes the natural history of progression (Fig. 3).[19] Generally, braces are used for pain control in those patients where surgery is not indicated or where medical contraindications preclude surgical treatment. They are used on an as-needed basis, and patients should be encouraged to engage in activities without the brace in order to avoid undesirable deconditioning of the trunk and abdominal musculature.

General medical evaluation and treatment is indicated in those who seek treatment for scoliosis. Laboratory evaluation should be done to screen for treatable causes of osteopenia, such as osteomalacia,

estrogen-dependent osteoporosis, and hypothyroidism. A normal sedimentation rate rules out such diseases as multiple myeloma. Fluoride, used to treat postmenopausal osteoporosis, was noted to result in an increase in peripheral fractures while not decreasing vertebral fractures.[20] Although some questions remain regarding dosage regimens and type of preparation and duration, in general, the use of fluoride supplements has not proven to be of value in treating osteoporosis. Antiresorptive agents, such as estrogen, calcitonin, or diphosphonates, can help retard postmenopausal osteopenia and can negate its contribution to progressive or painful adult spinal deformities.[21]

Activity modifications are also important in controlling pain from adult spine deformities. Such recreational activities as golf and softball and some domestic chores can exacerbate pain. Patients may have to discontinue these activities.

Other empirical pain management techniques, such as transcutaneous electrical nerve stimulation, acupuncture, and epidural, facet, or trigger-point injections, may also help relieve certain localized symptoms. Their value, however, has not been very predictable and, at best, there is only empirical justification for their use. They do not alter the course of painful adult spine deformities.

Summary

Adult spine deformities may result from idiopathic and degenerative etiologies.[8] These two entities may have superimposed on them an iatrogenic component from diskectomies or laminectomies done to relieve localized stenosis or disk herniations. The cumulative effect on the spine may result in painful and even crippling spine deformities. These are common, and their incidence in the adult population ranges from 3% to 30%, depending on the age group. Spine deformities are commonly painful and can be disabling, but they are rarely fatal.[19] It is incumbent on the surgeon to understand the pathology involved in painful spine disorders and to have a reasonable understanding of the prognosis before attempting invasive therapy. An understanding of the risk/benefit ratio to the patient is also necessary. The decision to proceed with surgical treatment is justified in many cases, but it must be based on a thorough understanding of the anticipated benefits from surgical treatment and the risk of serious complications leading to multiple surgeries and results that can be less desirable than the original condition.

References

1. Kostuik JP, Bentivoglio J: The incidence of low-back pain in adult scoliosis. *Spine* 1981;6:268–273.
2. Robin GS, Span Y, Steinberg RL, et al: Scoliosis in the elderly: A follow-up study. *Spine* 1982;7:355–359.
3. Thevenon A, Pollez B, Cantegrit F, et al: Relationship between kyphosis, scoliosis and osteoporosis in the elderly population. *Spine* 1987;12:744–745.
4. Collis DK, Ponsetti IV: Long-term follow-up of patients with idiopathic scoliosis not treated surgically. *J Bone Joint Surg* 1969, 51A:425–445.
5. Weinstein SL, Zavala DC, Ponsetti I: Idiopathic scoliosis: Long-term follow-up and prognosis in untreated patients. *J Bone Joint Surg* 1983;63A:702–712.
6. Betz RR, Bunnell WP, Lambrecht-Mulier E, et al: Scoliosis and pregnancy. *J Bone Joint Surg* 1987;69A:90–96.
7. Blount WP, Mellencamp DD: The effect of pregnancy on idiopathic scoliosis. *J Bone Joint Surg* 1980;62A:1083–1087.
8. Zorab PA: Assessment of cardio-respiratory function, in Zorab PA (ed): The National Fund for Research into Poliomyelitis and Other Crippling Diseases; *Proceedings of a Symposium on Scoliosis.* London, Vincent House, 1964, p 54.
9. Nachemson A: A long-term follow-up study of non-treated scoliosis. *J Bone Joint Surg* 1969;51A:302–304.
10. Cooper DM, Rojas JV, Mellins RB, et al: Respiratory mechanics in adolescents with idiopathic scoliosis. *Am Rev Respir Dis* 1984; 130:22.
11. Bergofsky EH: Respiratory failure in disorders of the thoracic cage. *Am Rev Respir Dis* 1979;119;643–669.
12. Gagnon S: Pulmonary function test study before and after spinal fusion in young idiopathic scoliosis. *Spine* 1989;14:620–624.
13. Primiano FP Jr, Nussbaum E, Hirschfeld SS, et al: Early echocardiographic and pulmonary function findings in idiopathic scoliosis. *J Pediatr Orthop* 1983;3:475–481.
14. Nachemson A: Adult scoliosis and back pain. *Spine* 1979;4:513–517.
15. Fowles JV, Drummond DS, L'Ecuyer S, et al: Untreated scoliosis in the adult. *Clin Orthop* 1978;134:212–217.
16. Jackson RP, Simmons EH, Stripinis D: Incidence and severity of back pain in adult idiopathic scoliosis. *Spine* 1983;8:749–756.
17. Briard JL, Jegou D, Cauchoix J: Adult lumbar scoliosis. *Spine* 1979;4:526–432.
18. Simmons EH, Jackson RP: The management of nerve root entrapment syndromes associated with the collapsing scoliosis of idiopathic lumbar and thoracolumbar curves. *Spine* 1979;4:533–541.
19. Ascani E, Bartolozzi P, Logroscino CA, et al: Natural history of untreated idiopathic scoliosis after skeletal maturity. *Spine* 1986; 11:784–789.
20. Riggs BL. Hodgson SF, O'Fallon WM, et al: Effect of flouride treatment on the fracture rate in postmenopausal women with osteoporosis. *N Engl J Med* 1990;322:802–809.
21. Storm T, Thamsborg G, Steiniche T, et al: Effect of intermittent cyclical etidronate therapy on bone mass and fracture rate in women with postmenopausal osteoporosis. *N Engl J Med* 1990; 322:1265–1271.

Clinical Applications for Magnetic Resonance Imaging of the Spine

Howard B. Cotler, MD

Introduction

Since its introduction, magnetic resonance imaging (MRI) has provided a wealth of scientific information about the human spine. MRI is useful not only in demonstrating pathologic abnormalities, but also in augmenting knowledge of changes that occur in the spine during normal aging. In addition to anatomic information, this technology can also give molecular based, physiological information about the tissue being studied.[1,2] It is nonetheless important to remember that MRI is essentially a diagnostic test ordered by a physician to assist in making a diagnosis by augmenting information already gained through an appropriate history, physical examination, and routine radiographs.

Indications

The primary advantages of MRI of the spine are that it does not expose the patient to ionizing radiation, it is noninvasive, and it provides excellent visualization of such spinal soft tissues as the spinal cord, nerve roots, and ligaments. Thus, MRI is indicated when it can provide information needed for diagnosis in a less invasive manner, and at a cost lower than that of other imaging modalities. MRI is currently very helpful for detecting intraspinal tumors, bone and soft-tissue tumors of the spine (including primary and metastatic tumors), disk pathology, Arnold-Chiari malformations, syringomyelia, spinal infections, demyelinating disorders, and C1-2 instabilities (Fig. 1), and for assessing the results of spinal surgery.

Limitations

MRI has several limitations compared with computerized tomography (CT). Magnetic resonance (MR) images lack a digitalized scout image for slice selection. The high cost of the study is a relative limitation. Because most spinal implants and orthoses used in orthopaedics are weakly ferromagnetic, they can generate some artifact, but this problem can be reduced by spine echo sequencing (Fig. 2) or by using other materials, such as titanium.[3] A few metallic devices that have demonstrated metallic properties are contraindicated for MRI. Because of their ferromagnetic nature, Mayfield and Heifetz aneurysm clips will undergo torquing during MRI.[4] Federal guidelines exclude the use of MRI for patients with cardiac pacemakers. Patients with dorsal column and bone growth stimulators are also excluded, because of the ferromagnetic effect of MRI on the telemetry devices. Patients known to have ocular metallic foreign bodies are excluded for fear that migration of the ferromagnetic body will decrease visual acuity. Lastly, because MRI affords poor visualization of bony detail, it has limited use in diagnosing traumatic injuries (Fig. 3).

Complications

There have been no known complications from the use of MRI so long as the contraindications were fol-

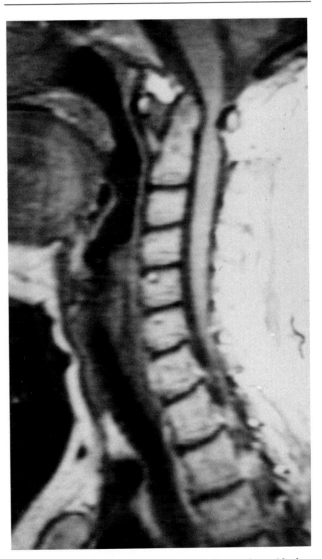

Fig. 1 Sagittal MRI of the cervical spine in a patient with rheumatoid arthritis. Note the increased space at the atlanto-dens interval and the spinal cord narrowing.

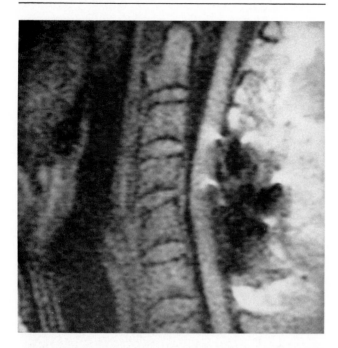

Fig. 2 Postoperative sagittal MRI of the cervical spine after posterior fusion and internal fixation with stainless steel wire.

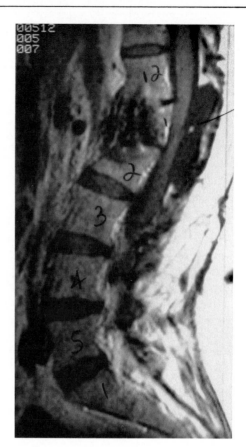

Fig. 4 Sagittal T$_1$-weighted image of an extradural arachnoid cyst. The patient had previously undergone anterior and posterior fusions for an L1 fracture.

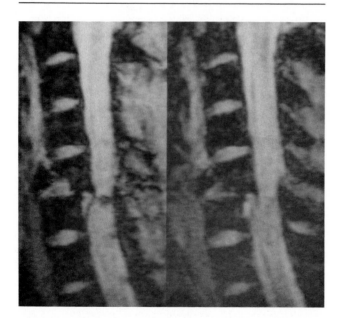

Fig. 3 Sagittal T$_2$-weighted images of a C5 compressive flexion injury. The anterior teardrop fracture and C5-6 disk herniation are apparent. Anterior vertebral body comminution and posterior fractures are difficult to interpret.

lowed. There are, however, many difficulties in obtaining a MRI, and these can lead to complications if precautions are not taken. Monitoring vital signs and maintaining life support in a magnetic field is one problem that must be overcome before evaluating critically ill patients. When working in a magnetic field, remembering to eliminate such items as handbags, credit cards, traction weights, scissors, hair pins or clips, and watches can be a problem for the patient or staff. Patient claustrophobia is another significant difficulty that must be overcome if an accurate study is to be obtained.

MRI of the Normal Spine

In the normal spine, the sequence of signal intensities in descending order are fat, nucleus pulposus, bone marrow, cancellous bone, spinal cord, muscle, cerebrospinal fluid, annulus fibrosus, ligaments, and compact cortical bone when spin-echo sequencing is used.[5] The spinal cord and medullary or cancellous bone are best visualized on T$_1$-weighted imaging. Ligamentous structures, subarachnoid space, and intervertebral disks are visualized more clearly using T$_2$-weighted imaging.

MRI of the Aging Spine

MRI provides a unique opportunity for noninvasive visualization of the aging spine. In the aging process,

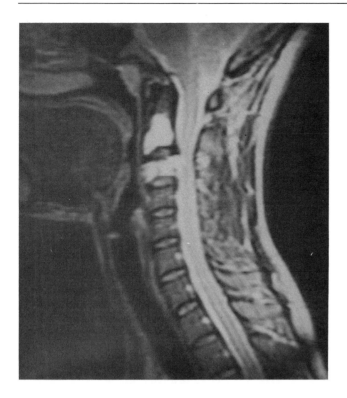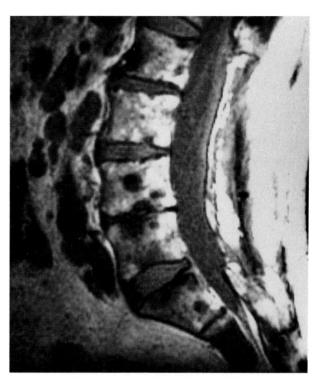

Fig. 5   **Left,** Sagittal T_2-weighted image of hemangioendothelioma of C2 and C3. **Right,** Sagittal T_1-weighted image of the lumbar spine of a patient with metastatic prostate carcinoma. The blastic lesions are of the same signal intensity as cortical bone.

discussion commonly focuses on disk degeneration. It is known that during aging the disk gradually loses water content and proteoglycan content, and that there is an increase in the ratio of keratan sulfate to chondroitin sulfate.[6-8] MRI has shown the aging disk to have a decreased signal on the T_2-weighted image. This decrease is believed to represent a change in the water content.[5,9,10]

Boden and associates[11] have performed two prospective studies in which they evaluated asymptomatic subjects in order to determine the prevalence of abnormal findings in the cervical and lumbar spine. In these studies, MRI showed that 19% of the subjects had an abnormality in the cervical spine and 28% of the subjects had an abnormality in the lumbar spine. The researchers concluded that these abnormalities on MRI are probably a result of the natural aging process. In order for such abnormalities to be considered pathologic and, hence, candidates for surgical treatment, the MRI findings must be correlated with clinical signs and symptoms.

MRI of Spinal Pathology

MRI can be very accurate in evaluating various pathologic conditions of the spine. A T_1-weighted image is particularly useful in evaluating intramedullary lesions, cystic cord lesions, and destructive bone lesions. T_2-weighted images are used to evaluate osteophytic bone spurs, degenerative disk disease, and acute spinal cord injury.

Syringomyelia, syrinx cavities containing cerebrospinal fluid within the spinal cord, and other arachnoid cysts (Fig. 4), whether intra- or extra-dural, are easily demonstrated on a T_1-weighted imaging sequence.[12-16] Soft-tissue fibroma, dural estasia, meningocele, lipoma, cystic astrocytoma, ependymoma, and metastasis to the cord can be detected without the use of intrathecal contrast agents.[17,18] Demyelinating disorders, as seen in the plaques of multiple sclerosis, may be detected in the brain and upper cervical spinal cord by MRI.[19] MRI is also used to detect hydromyelia and Arnold-Chiari malformation.[14]

Various conditions, including primary bone tumors and tumor-like conditions, metastatic disease, and infections, can be determined easily by the characteristic appearance on MRI of the osseous structures.[20] Normal cancellous bone demonstrates a characteristically high spinal intensity and is best seen on T_1-weighted images. In contrast, vertebral hemangiomas or hemangioendotheliomas (Fig. 5, *left*) show a bright signal on both T_1- and T_2-weighted images. Lytic metastatic disease usually demonstrates bright signals on T_2-weighted images and dark signals on T_1-weighted images. Blastic metastatic disease (Fig. 5, *right*) shows a low signal in-

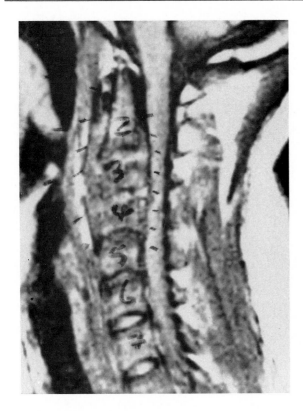

Fig. 6 Anterior C3-4 disk excision and fusion resulted in staphylococcus osteomyelitis with epidural abscess. T$_1$-weighted image demonstrates the extent of the infection.

tensity on T$_1$-weighted images and has the same appearance as cortical bone. MRI may also be of use in detecting disorders such as thalassemia, marrow iron deposition, and osteopetrosis,[21] in which disease tissue replaces normal marrow.

MRI has also been proven to be of benefit in diagnosing pyogenic osteomyelitis (Fig. 6),[22] tuberculous osteomyelitis (Fig. 7),[23] and diskitis (Fig. 8, *left*).[24] Pyogenic infections demonstrate a low signal intensity on T$_1$-weighted images and a bright signal intensity on T$_2$-weighted images. MRI is particularly useful in evaluating tuberculous osteomyelitis, because visualization of the abscess formation aids preoperative planning.

MRI is also used to evaluate spinal dysraphism,[25] Arnold-Chiari malformations, tethered cord, diastematomyelia, lipomyelomeningocele, and congenital spinal stenosis as seen in achondroplastic dwarfism (Fig. 8, *right*). Craniovertebral anomalies can be evaluated easily in a noninvasive fashion.

The use of MRI in evaluating acute spinal cord trauma provides excellent soft-tissue visualization. T$_1$-weighted images demonstrate injuries to bone (Fig. 9), and T$_2$-weighted images display injuries to ligament (Fig. 10), disk (Fig. 11), and spinal cord (Fig. 12). In evaluating acute spinal cord injuries, we have demonstrated three patterns of signal intensities, as seen on MRI, and have correlated those patterns with neurologic recovery.[26]

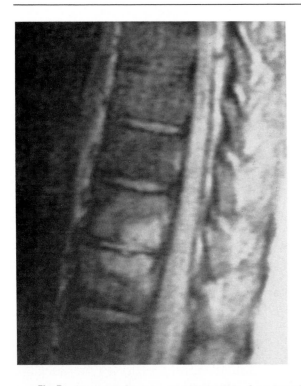
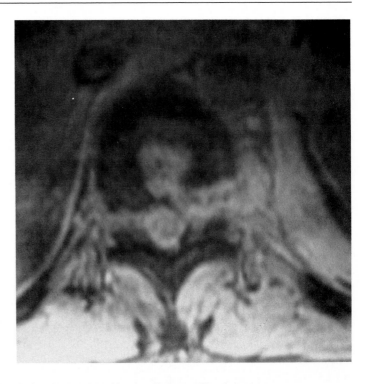

Fig. 7 Sagittal (**left**) and axial (**right**) MRIs of a tuberculous lesion show early epidural and paramedian abscesses.

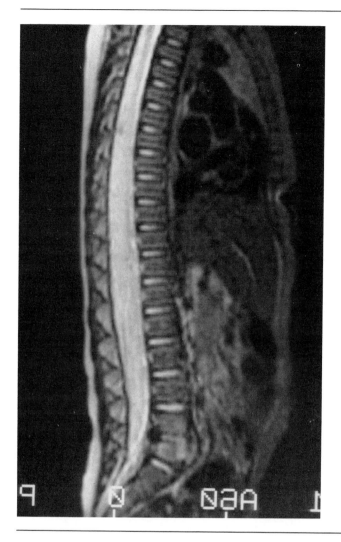

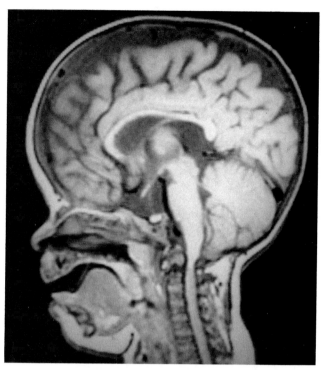

Fig. 8 **Left**, Sagittal T_2-weighted image of a 15-month-old infant who stopped walking because of the L4-5 diskitis. **Right**, Sagittal T_1-weighted image of a child with achondroplastic dwarfism and C1 spinal stenosis.

MRI of the disk (Fig. 13) is highly sensitive for detecting abnormalities.[27] On T_1-weighted images the normal disk has a central portion of intermediate signal intensity and a peripheral portion of decreased signal intensity, but on T_2-weighted images the central portion becomes hyperintense and the peripheral portion is of low signal intensity. MRI can be used to diagnose the degenerative disk by noting the loss of signal intensity of T_2-weighted images, whether or not the disk degeneration is the source of the clinical syndrome. In order to determine the source of pain in degenerative disk disease, provocative testing (diskography)[28,29] is often used to identify the source of the pain. MRI is extremely useful in evaluating a herniated disk and, when correlated with a clinical radiculopathy or myelopathy, it can clearly identify the pathologic source of the pain syndrome. Recently, the introduction of an exogenously administered paramagnetic contrast agent, gadolinium diethylenetriamine pentaacetic acid (Gd-DTPA), has been found to be extremely useful in distinguishing disk from scar in patients with failed back surgery syndrome.[27,30] Compared with a normal disk, a

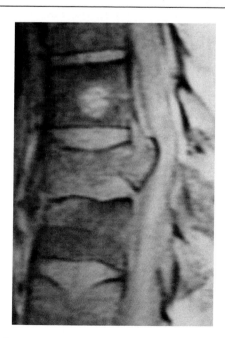

Fig. 9 Sagittal MRI of a T12 burst fracture.

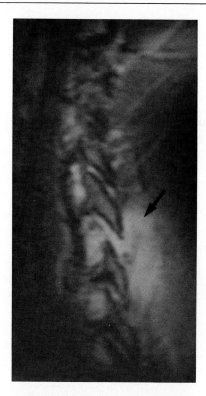

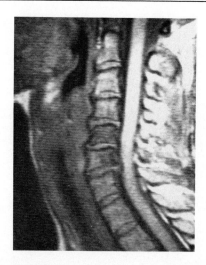

Fig. 11 Sagittal MRI of the cervical spine shows a C6-7 herniated disk with cord compression.

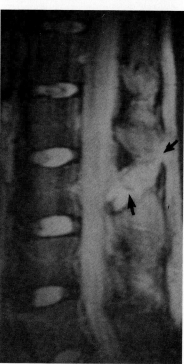

Fig. 10 **Top**, Sagittal MRI of a cervical joint capsule disruption and associated hematoma (arrow). **Bottom**, Sagittal MRI of a lumbar interspinous disruption and associated hematoma (arrows).

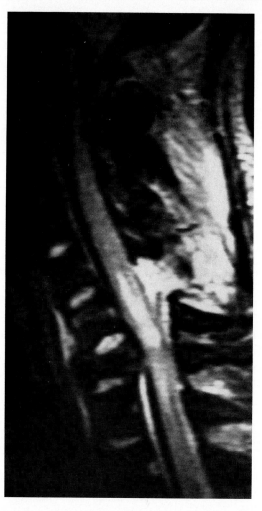

Fig. 12 Sagittal T_2-weighted MRI of a C7 compressive flexion injury with a significant kyphosis, interspinous ligament disruption, and a type II (hyperintensity = edema) cord injury.

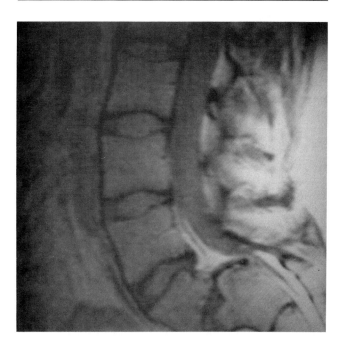

Fig. 13 Sagittal MRI of the lumbar spine in a patient with a grade III L5 spondylolisthesis. Note the disrupted disk at L4-5.

recurrent or persistent disk herniation is isointense on a T_1-weighted image and hypointense to hyperintense on a T_2- or T_2*-weighted image. After Gd-DTPA injection, there is minimal enhancement of the disk on T_1-weighted images made within six to ten minutes. After a delay of 30 to 40 minutes, T_1-weighted imaging shows

signal enhancement of the disk. Postoperative scar, when imaged following injection of Gd-DTPA, demonstrates enhancement or a hyperintensity in both early and delayed T_1-weighted images (Fig. 14). To avoid confusion, early imaging after injection is recommended to differentiate scar from recurrent disk, because it appears that the late enhancement of disk is caused by the diffusion of the contrast agent from surrounding vascular tissues. Thus, the enhancement of a tissue is based on its vascularity. A disk has negligible intravascular space, young scar is made up of capillaries interspersed through collagen and fibroblasts, and old scar is predominantly fibrous in nature. Thus, to differentiate persistent or recurrent disk herniation from postoperative scar, it is necessary to consider early Gd-DTPA enhancement, location, morphology, and mass effect.

Recently MRI has been used to assess functional stability after lumbar spinal fusion.[30,31] Stable fusions of greater than 12 months duration demonstrate subchondral bands of hyperintensity on T_1-weighted images, reflecting a conversion of red to yellow marrow because of a decrease in biomechanical stress. Unstable fusions are characterized by a hypointense subchondral band on T_1-weighted images, but they have a hyperintense subchondral band on T_2-weighted images. This band reflects inflammation, hyperemia, and/or granulation tissue resulting from increased biomechanical stress.

The introduction of MRI has provided an excellent opportunity to visualize anatomic and pathophysiologic aspects of the spine. The clinician can use this valuable scientific information to develop improved modes of treatment.

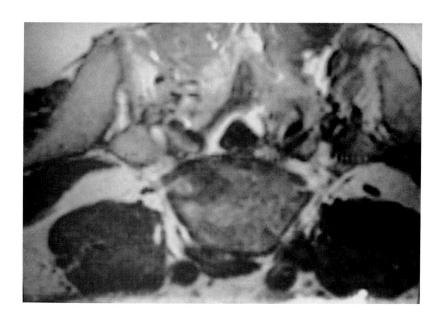

Fig. 14 Axial T_1-weighted image at L5-S1 with a persistent or recurrent disk herniation after previous spinal surgery. Note the enhancement (hyperintensity) surrounding the posterior aspect of the dura after the administration of Gd-DTPA.

References

1. Fitzgerald RH Jr, Berquist TH: Editorial: Magnetic resonance imaging: Editorial. *J Bone Joint Surg* 1986;68A:799–801.
2. Brand-Zawadzki M, Mills CM, Davis PL: CNS application of NMR imaging. *Appl Radiol* 1983;12:25–30.
3. Savoloine ER, Ebraheim NA, Andreshak TG, et al: Anterior and posterior cervical spine fixation using titanium implants to facilitate magnetic resonance imaging evaluation. *J Orthop Trauma* 1989;3:295–299.
4. Berquist TH: Magnetic resonance imaging: Preliminary experience in orthopedic radiology. *Magn Reson Imaging* 1984;2:41–52.
5. Modic MT, Weinstein MA, Pavlicek W, et al: Magnetic resonance imaging of the cervical spine: Technical and clinical observations. *AJR* 1983;141:1129–1136.
6. Gower WE, Pedrini V: Age-related variations in proteinpolysaccharides from human nucleus pulposus, annulus fibrosis, and costal cartilages. *J Bone Joint Surg* 1969;51A:1154–1162.
7. Hendry NGC: The hydration of the nucleus pulposus and its relation to intervertebral disc derangement. *J Bone Joint Surg* 1958;40B:132–144.
8. Lipson SJ, Muir H: Experimental intervertebral disc degeneration: Morphologic and proteoglycan changes over time. *Arthritis Rheum* 1981;24:12–21.
9. Chafetz NI, Genant HK, Moon KL, et al: Recognition of lumbar disk herniation with NMR. *AJR* 1983;141:1153–1156.
10. Edelman RR, Shoukimas GM, Stark DD, et al: High-resolution surface-coil imaging of lumbar disk disease. *AJR* 1985;144:1123–1129.
11. Boden SD, Davis DO, Dina TS, et al: Abnormal magnetic-resonance scans of the lumbar spine in asymptomatic subjects: A prospective investigation. *J Bone Joint Surg* 1990;72A:403–408.
12. DeLa Paz RL, Brady TJ, Buonanno FS, et al: Nuclear magnetic resonance (NMR) imaging of Arnold-Chiari type I malformation with hydromyelia. *J Comput Assist Tomogr* 1983;7:126–129.
13. Kokmen E, Marsh WR, Baker HL Jr: Magnetic resonance imaging in syringomyelia. *Neurosurgery* 1985;17:267–270.
14. Lee BCP, Zimmerman RD, Manning JJ, et al: MR imaging of syringomyelia and hydromyelia. *AJR* 1985;144:1149–1156.
15. Sherman JL, Barkovich AJ, Citrin CM: The MR appearance of syringomyelia: New observations. *AJR* 1987;148:381–391.
16. Yeates A, Brant-Zawadzki M, Norman D, et al: Nuclear magnetic resonance imaging of syringomyelia. *AJNR* 1983;4:234–237.
17. Han JS, Kaufman B, El Yousef SJ, et al: NMR imaging of the spine. *AJR* 1983;141:1137–1145.
18. Kucharczyk W, Brant-Zawadzki M, Sabel D, et al: Central nervous system tumors in children: Detection by magnetic resonance imaging. *Radiology* 1985;155:131–136.
19. Marovilla KR, Weinreb JC, Suss R, et al: Magnetic resonance demonstration of multiple sclerosis plaques in the cervical cord. *AJR* 1985;144:381–385.
20. Moon KL Jr, Genant HK, Helms CA, et al: Musculoskeletal applications of nuclear magnetic resonance. *Radiology* 1983;147:161–171.
21. Rao VM, Dalinka MK, Mitchell DG, et al: Osteopetrosis: MR characteristics at 1.5T. *Radiology* 1986;161:217–220.
22. Modic MT, Feiglin DH, Piraino DW, et al: Vertebral osteomyelitis: Assessment using MR. *Radiology* 1985;157:157–166.
23. Bell GR, Stearns KL, Bonutti PM, et al: MRI diagnosis of tuberculous vertebral osteomyelitis. *Spine* 1990;15:462–465.
24. Modic MT, Pavlicek W, Weinstein MA, et al: Magnetic resonance imaging of intervertebral disk disease: Clinical and pulse sequence considerations. *Radiology* 1984;152:103–111.
25. Hans JS, Benson JE, Kaufman B, et al: Demonstration of diastematomyelia and associated abnormalities with MR imaging. *AJNR* 1985;6:215–219.
26. Bondurant FJ, Cotler HB, Kulkarni MV, et al: Acute spinal cord injury: A study using physical examination and magnetic resonance imaging. *Spine* 1990;15:161–168.
27. Berns DH, Blaser SI, Modic MT: Magnetic resonance imaging of the spine. *Clin Orthop* 1990;244:78–100.
28. Linson MA, Crowe CH: Comparison of magnetic resonance imaging and lumbar discography in the diagnosis of disc degeneration. *Clin Orthop* 1990;250:160–163.
29. Schneiderman G, Flannigan B, Kingston S, et al: Magnetic resonance imaging in the diagnosis of disc degeneration: Correlation with discography. *Spine* 1987;12:276–281.
30. Djukic S, Lang P, Morris J, et al: The postoperative spine: Magnetic resonance imaging. Radiographic imaging in orthopaedics. *Orthop Clin North Am* 1990;21:603–624.
31. Lang P, Chafetz N, Genant HK, et al: Lumbar spinal fusion: Assessment of functional stability with magnetic resonance imaging. *Spine* 1990;15:581–588.

Magnetic Resonance Imaging of Acute Spinal Injury

John H. Harris, Jr, MD, DSc

Larry A. Kramer, MD

Joel W. Yeakley, MD

Magnetic Resonance Imaging of Acute Spinal Injury

Of the various imaging modalities presently available, magnetic resonance imaging (MRI) provides the most accurate depiction of the soft-tissue structures of the spine and spinal cord. The unprecedented ability of MRI to assess the histopathology and extent of spinal cord injury and to identify acute traumatic disk injuries provides information not heretofore available for patient management decisions. These advantages make MRI an invaluable addition to the traditional methods of imaging acute spinal trauma and have added a new step to the algorithm of patient management.

This chapter discusses the role of MRI in evaluating acute spinal trauma and illustrates examples of its application to the diagnosis of ligamentous, disk, and spinal cord injuries.

The radiographic evaluation of the acutely injured spine must be based on the clinical evaluation of the patient and begins with plain-film studies to delineate the location(s) and type(s) of the spinal injury.[1-4]

The role of MRI in evaluating acute spinal trauma is based on a relatively limited experience to date. A review of the English-language literature relative to MRI evaluation of acute[5-14] or recent[7] spinal injury reveals only 78 patients scanned within the first seven days following injury. Of the 78, a total of 53 were reported from our institution.[8,10,13] This limited experience is due, in part, to the relatively small number of patients with spinal injuries seen in centers capable of evaluating the injury with MRI, the difficulty in placing patients with spinal injuries (many of whom also have other injuries) in the magnet, and the frequent requirement for magnetically compatible and/or remote life-support, monitoring, and traction systems. However, based on this experience and the experience related in at least one review article,[15] a consensus has developed regarding the role of MRI in the evaluation of acute spinal trauma.

It is generally agreed that MRI is superior to any other imaging modality in detection of the site and extent of spinal cord injury and is the only method available to characterize its histopathology. MRI is the only imaging modality by which epidural hemorrhage and the integrity of major vessels of the spine and neck can be accurately demonstrated noninvasively. Ligamentous and disk injuries are more accurately demonstrated by MRI than by computed tomography (CT) or CT myelography. All this critically important diag-

nostic information accrues noninvasively, without the use of ionizing radiation, and without requiring patient motion. Conversely, MRI does not display spinal skeletal injuries as accurately as CT, three-dimensional CT, or polydirectional tomography.

MRI of the acutely injured spine is optimally performed with a high field strength system.[7,16,17] Image resolution is enhanced by the use of surface coils and cardiac or motion compensating gradients[15] for the suppression of cerebrospinal fluid flow artifacts.

A consensus regarding standard MRI sequences has not yet evolved because of inherent differences related to magnetic field strength and manufacturer differences in pulse sequence design. However, the proper selection of pulse sequence parameters provides the flexibility to demonstrate optimally not only the anatomic part being examined, but also the type of pathologic condition being imaged. In general, the three pulse sequence parameters that are modified to produce tissue contrast are pulse repetition time, echo time, and flip angle. Spin-echo sequences are used to produce the classic relatively T_1-weighted, proton density-weighted, or T_2-weighted images. More recently, gradient echo techniques have been employed in the MRI evaluation of acute spinal trauma.

Using spin-echo technique, T_1-weighted, proton density-weighted, and T_2-weighted images are obtained by altering both repetition time and echo time while flip angle remains constant at 90 degrees. T_1-weighted images (Fig. 1), which are produced by short repetition time and echo time (600–800 msec, 20 msec, respectively), demonstrate bone marrow, fat, subacute hemorrhage, and the spinal cord to best advantage.

Proton density-weighted images are obtained simultaneously with T_2-weighted images and are produced by a long repetition time and a short echo time (2000–3000 msec, 20 msec, respectively). Cerebrospinal fluid and spinal cord are relatively isointense on proton density-weighted images (Fig. 2, *left*).

T_2-weighted images are produced by a long repetition time and a long echo time (2000–3000 msec, 70–100 msec, respectively). On T_2-weighted images, cerebrospinal fluid is bright relative to the spinal cord, which gives the image a myelographic appearance (Fig. 2, *right*). Although they have a poor signal-to-noise ratio, T_2-weighted images are sensitive to such spinal cord problems as edema and acute hemorrhage.

Gradient echo pulse sequences (Fig. 3), which employ partial flip angle (20 degrees) and a short repetition

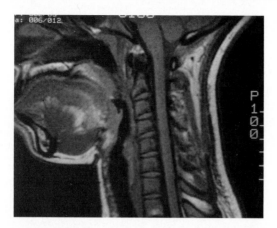

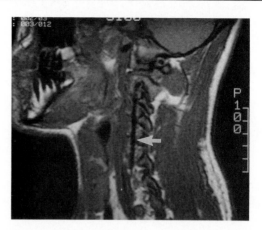

Fig. 1 T₁-weighted and mid-sagittal (**left**) and para-sagittal (**right**) MR images of a normal adult cervical spine. The bright (high intensity) signal represents fat. The cerebral spinal fluid is low signal intensity and spinal cord is intermediate signal intensity. In the para-sagittal image (**right**), the vertebral artery (arrow) is clearly delineated as a tubular structure of signal void.

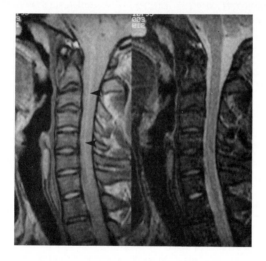

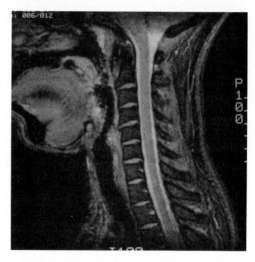

Fig. 2 Proton density-weighted and T₂-weighted images. Spin echo sequences were used to obtain these proton density-weighted "first" (**left**) and T₂-weighted "second" (**right**) images, simultaneously, of a normal adult cervical spin. In the "first" echo, or protein density-weighted image (**left**), ligamentous and skeletal anatomy is sharply defined, whereas the cord and cerebral spinal fluid are isointense. The thin, high intensity signal within the cord (arrow heads) is an artifact. In the "second" echo, or T₂-weighted image, there is poor ligamentous-skeletal definition, while the high intensity cerebral spinal fluid signal is in sharp contrast to the isointense cord, which gives the image its myelographic appearance.

Fig. 3 Gradient echo mid-sagittal (flip angle = 20 degrees) image of a normal adult cervical spine. Ligamentous and skeletal anatomy and the "myelographic" appearance of the cerebral spinal fluid and spinal cord both occur on the same image.

time and echo time, achieve the myelographic image appearance in relatively shorter acquisition times. Gradient echo pulse sequence has the additional advantage of being particularly sensitive to the detection of evolving hemorrhage (Fig. 4).

Although other imaging sequences are available, they are manufacturer specific and are beyond the scope of this chapter.

T₁-weighted, T₂-weighted, proton density-weighted,

and gradient echo sequences in axial and sagittal planes with 5 mm slices are routinely obtained in our department for the evaluation of acute spinal trauma. Gradient echo sequence is being used with increasing frequency because of its inherent sensitivity to hemorrhage, reduction of pulsation artifacts, and shorter data acquisition times. The gradient echo sequence is also commonly employed for axial imaging. While cord abnormalities are visible in both axial and sagittal images, the initial and temporally related changes in intramedullary signal characteristics, as well as the extent and nature of cord injury, are best seen in the sagittal plane.[11]

Indications for MRI of Acute Spinal Trauma

Clinical indications for MRI of patients with acute spinal trauma include myelopathy, central radiculopathy, or persistent, inappropriate pain that may be secondary to acute disk protrusion or herniation.

Clinical signs of spinal cord damage require evaluation by MRI to determine not only the site and extent of the cord injury, but the histopathologic details of the intramedullary injury as reflected by the MRI characteristics.

The histopathology of experimental spinal cord injury has been extensively studied.[18] Mongrel dog,[19] primate,[20-22] and rat[23,24] experiments have all demonstrated a similarity between experimentally induced spinal damage and that observed in humans.[25,26] The MRI characteristics of the experimental dog[19] and rat[23,24] injuries are similar to those observed in living human patients with cord injury[5,8,10,13,17] and confirmed at autopsy in one patient. Acutely, intramedullary hemorrhage results in a hypointense signal, and edema produces a hyperintense image on T_2-weighted images.[10,11,23,24]

Specific radiologic indications for MRI evaluation of the acutely injured spine include hyperextension dislocation of the cervical spine,[27] not only because of the invariably present myelopathy, but in order to evaluate the disk and associated ligamentous injuries. MRI is indicated in the evaluation of occipito-atlantal disassociation, particularly occipito-atlantal subluxation in children, and in anterior subluxation of the cervical spine,[28] when the plain-film study is equivocal or when a history of prior neck injury makes the acuity of plain-film signs of anterior subluxation ambiguous.

MRI of the acutely injured spine should be seriously considered in any patient with fracture or fracture-dislocation involving the spinal canal or any injury resulting in discontinuity of the longitudinal axis of the canal. Finally, a disparity between the radiologic and clinical findings, particularly with respect to significant and/or persistent pain or the presence of a neurologic deficit, should prompt consideration of MR evaluation.

Clinical Application of MRI in Acute Spinal Trauma

Although MRI provides unique and clinically essential information not available by any other imaging modality, it is not indicated in every patient with acute spinal trauma. The principle indications for MRI in evaluating acute spinal trauma have been cited earlier. Similarly, it is important to re-emphasize that the imaging evaluation of all patients with acute spinal trauma begins with the appropriate plain-film examinations.

With respect to spinal cord injury, Kulkarni and associates[8] described three patterns of spinal cord signal characteristics seen on relatively T_2-weighted images. They postulated that these patterns represented hemorrhage (type I), edema (type II), and mixed hemorrhage and edema (type III). The type I pattern was described as a large central hypointense area, representing intracellular deoxyhemoglobin surrounded by a thin peripheral rim of high intense signal of edema (Fig. 4); type II, exemplified and illustrated in Case 4, below, as a homogeneous high intensity signal; and type III as being centrally isointense, surrounded by a thick hypointense rim. Our review of the 27 patients in the study of Kulkarni and associates,[8] plus an additional 46 patients, confirmed the definition of types I and II. However, the type III spinal cord injury is best defined as being an inhomogeneous mixture of hypo- and hyperintense signals as is shown in Case 7, below.

Kadoya and associates,[6] Kulkarni and associates,[8,10] Mirvis and associates,[11] and Bondurant and associates[13] implied a relationship between the histopathologic findings in acute cord injury and the MR signal characteristics in human patients. This implication was based on extrapolation of the MR signal characteristics of brain trauma and a correlation between the MR signal characteristic of acute spinal cord injury and patient outcome.

Weirich and associates,[24] from our institution, and Wittenberg and associates[17] have established a direct correlation between the MR signal characteristics and the histopathologic findings in acute spinal cord injury. Based on this data, we have reviewed the MR images of 73 patients, to date, who had MR examinations of the spine between three and 24 hours after trauma. We then classified the injuries according to the signal characteristics described by Kulkarni and associates[8,10] for type I and II injuries and an inhomogeneous hyper- and hypointense pattern for type III. Finally, we compared the admission neurologic Frankel status with that after a follow-up period of from three to 40 months. This patient population includes the 27 patients previously reported by Kulkarni and associates[8] and Bondurant and associates.[13] The results of this review are shown in Tables 1 through 4.

Of the 73 patients, 20 (27%) had MR type I (hemorrhagic) injuries (Figs. 4 to 6) on admission MR scan (Table 1). None of the 20 had an admission Frankel grade greater than C and only four of twenty (20%) experienced clinically significant neurologic improvement, with neurologic improvement being defined as a positive change of at least one Frankel class. Sixteen of the 20 (80%) had no neurologic improvement.

Another 32 patients (44%) had type II (edema) injuries (Figs. 7 to 9) on admission MR scan (Table 2). Of the 32, 28 (87%) had admission Frankel grades of C or D. Of the 32 patients with type II cord injuries, 20 (63%) experienced significant neurologic improvement, whereas 12 (37%) did not.

Another 22 patients (30%) had type III (mixed) injuries (Fig. 10) on admission MR scan (Table 3). One

Table 1
Frankel class type I (hemorrhage) (N = 20)

Admission Diagnosis	No.	Follow-up Diagnosis (3 to 4 months)
A	8	7A, 1B
B	6	6B
C	6	1B, 1C, 4D

4/20 (20%)—significant neurological improvement (C to D)
16/20 (80%)—no significant neurological improvement (A or B)

Table 2
Frankel class type II (edema) (N = 32)

Admission Diagnosis	No.	Follow-up Diagnosis (1 to 12 months)
A	2	1A, 1B
B	2	none B, 2C
C	13	4C, 7D, 2E
D	15	4D, 11E

20/32 (63%)—significant neurological improvement (D or E)
12/32 (37%)—no significant neurological improvement (A or B)

Table 3
Frankel class type III (mixed) (N = 22)*

Admission Diagnosis	No.	Follow-up Diagnosis (3 to 40 months)
A	7	3A, 2B, 1C
B	3	1B, 1C, 1D
C	6	1C, 4D, 1E
D	5	3D, 2E

8/21 (38%)—significant neurological improvement (D or E)
13/21 (62%)—no significant neurological improvement
*1 patient lost to follow-up.

Table 4
Frankel class summary comparison (N = 73)

	Admission (3 to 24 hours)		Follow-up (3 to 40 months)	
Type	No. (%)		Significant Improvement	No Significant Improvement
I	20 (27%)		4 (20%)	16 (80%)
II	32 (43%)		20 (63%)	12 (37%)
III	21 (29%)		8 (38%)	13 (62%)

of these patients was lost to follow-up and was excluded from the study. In this group, admission Frankel grades were divided almost equally between those with A or B (10/21) and C or D (11/21). Of the 21 patients with type III cord injuries, eight (38%) experienced significant neurologic improvement, while 13 (62%) did not.

The results of this ongoing study suggest a better prognosis and improved response to an aggressive treatment regimen for patients with nonhemorrhagic cord injury.

The following cases have been selected to illustrate the MRI appearance of various types of acute spinal and spinal cord injury. It is beyond the scope of this chapter to discuss the MRI characteristics of late sequelae or complications of spinal injury.

Case Studies

Case 1 This case (Fig. 4) illustrates hyperextension dislocation of the cervical spine with type I spinal cord injury. The T$_2$-weighted image (Fig. 4, *left*) demonstrates all the MR signs of hyperextension dislocation, including posterior displacement of the involved vertebra, disrupted anterior longitudinal ligament and annulus (curved arrow), widened disk space with hypointense signal of hemorrhage (arrow), disruption of the posterior annulus with extruded nucleus material (arrow head) between the subjacent vertebral body and the intact, but separated, posterior longitudinal ligament (stemmed arrow), disruption of the ligamentum flavum (open arrow), and anteroposterior compression of the spinal cord. The asterisk indicates hemorrhage in the retropharyngeal fascial space.

The swollen cord with hypointense signal of central hemorrhage (arrow head) and surrounding hyperintense signal of peripheral edema, while visible in the T$_2$-weighted image (Fig. 4, *left*), is more obvious in the gradient echo image (Fig. 4, *center*). The axial gradient echo image (Fig. 4, *right*) demonstrates the typical appearance of the type I cord injury, that is, central hypointense hemorrhage with thin surrounding hyperintense edema (arrow).

Case 2

In this case, shown in Figure 5, the injury was a simple wedge compression fracture of T12 with retropulsion of fragments associated with a type I cord injury and an epidural hematoma. The T$_2$-weighted sagittal image (Fig. 5, *left*) demonstrates the wedge compression fracture of T12 with retropulsion of body fragments. The central hypointense signal of hemorrhage (arrow) with surrounding hyperintense edema signal is seen on both the sagittal and axial (Fig. 5, *center*) image. Axial gradient echo image at a slightly caudal level (Fig. 5, *right*) demonstrates a small caudal extension of the central hemorrhage (arrow) and an epidural hematoma (arrow heads).

Case 3

The injury in Case 3 (Fig. 6) was a bilateral interfacetal dislocation with type I cord injury. Both the T$_2$-weighted (Fig. 6, *top left*) and gradient echo (Fig. 6, *top right*) sagittal images demonstrate the bilateral inter-

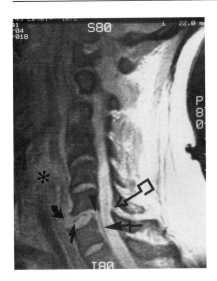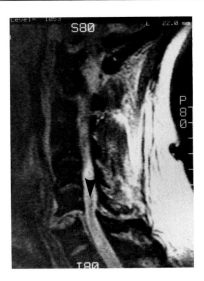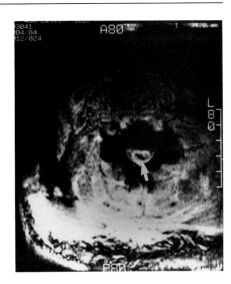

Fig. 4   MR images of acute herniated disk with type I cord injury.

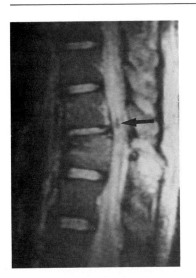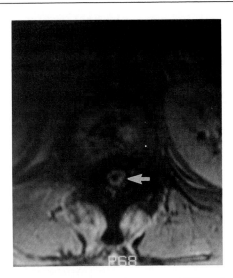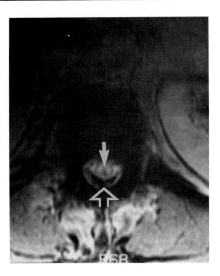

Fig. 5   Type I cord injury secondary to retropulsed posterior fragments of T12 wedge compression fracture.

facetal dislocation with anteroposterior cord compression at the level of the dislocation. Disruption and separation of the posterior longitudinal ligament (arrow) and the ligamentum flavum (curved arrow) are clearly shown on the T$_2$-weighted image (Fig. 6, *top left*), while the central hypointense signal of the type I cord injury (arrow head) is only faintly seen. The true extent of the type I cord injury, which involves two levels (arrow heads), is more accurately reflected on the sagittal gradient echo image (Fig. 6, *top right*). The more rostral axial image (Fig. 6, *bottom left*) and that obtained at the level of dislocation (Fig. 6, *bottom right*), both show the

typical central hypointense signal of blood (arrow) with surrounding and hyperintense signal of edema.

Case 4

Case 4 (Fig. 7) illustrates a typical MR signal of a type II cord injury (edema) in gradient echo sagittal (Fig. 7, *left*) and axial (Fig. 7, *right*) images of a patient with severe wedge compression fracture of T7 and retropulsion of fragments. The hyperintense cord signal makes the cord isointense with surrounding cerebrospinal fluid, hence the "absent cord sign." In the axial image (Fig. 7, *right*) the central hyperintensity (arrow)

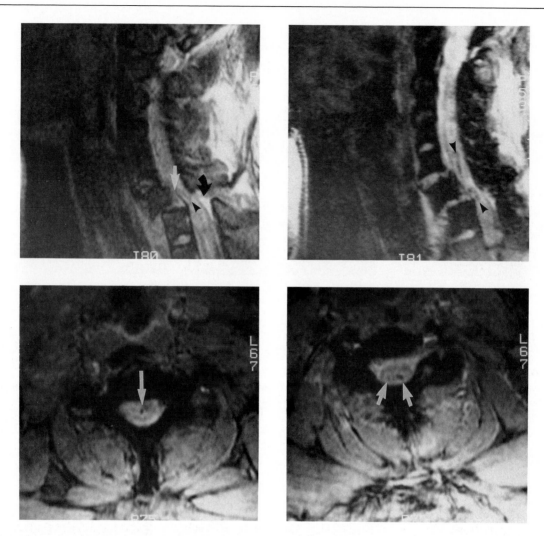

Fig. 6 Type I cord injury associated with bilateral interfacetal dislocation.

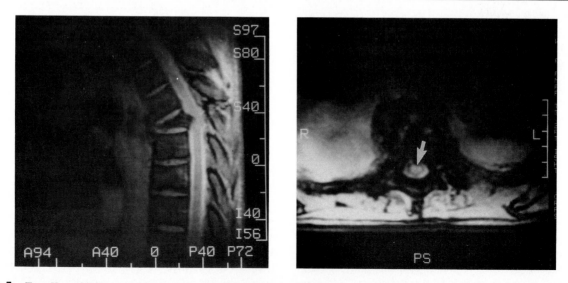

Fig. 7 Type II cord injury secondary to retropulsed posterior fragments of a severe wedge compression fracture of T7.

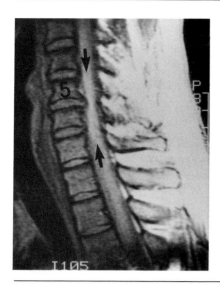

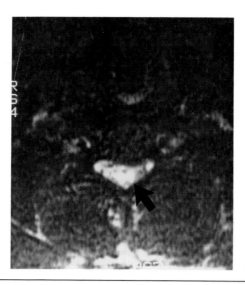

Fig. 8 Type II cord injury secondary to cervical spondylosis ("the Taylor mechanism").

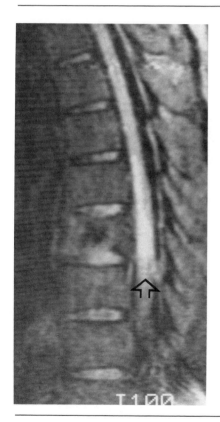

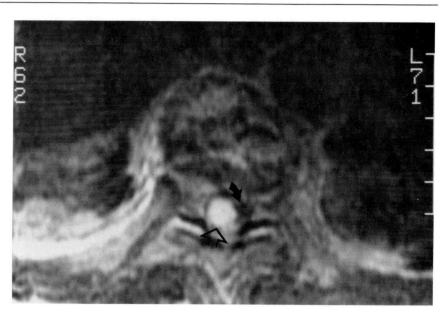

Fig. 9   Type II cord injury secondary to bursting fracture, T9.

is surrounded by less intense signal of the peripheral cord and the hyperintense cerebrospinal fluid.

Case 5

This case shows a Taylor mechanism of the cervical spine with type II cord injury. Impingement of the cord between the posterior osteophytes at the fifth disk and the lamina and ligamentum flavum resulted in cord edema, characterized by the uniform, diffuse, hyperintense signal (arrows) in sagittal (Fig. 8, *left*) and axial

(Fig. 8, *right*) T₂-weighted images. The absence of ligamentous injury or prevertebral hematoma are characteristic of the Taylor mechanism and distinguish it from hyperextension dislocation.

Case 6

Case 6 (Fig. 9) shows a burst fracture of T9 with type II cord injury. The homogeneous high intensity signal of the swollen, edematous cord (open arrow) seen at the level of the fracture in sagittal T₂-weighted (Fig. 9,

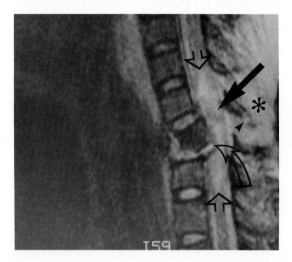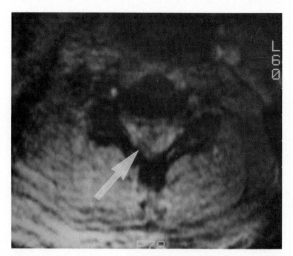

Fig. 10 Type III cord injury associated with flexion teardrop fracture, C6.

left) and axial (Fig. 9, *right*) gradient echo images is characteristic of the type II cord injury. In the axial image (Fig. 9, *right*), the edematous cord is displaced to the right by a hypointense epidural hematoma (curved arrow).

Case 7

In Case 7 (Fig. 10), there is a type III cord injury associated with a flexion tear-drop fracture of C6. In both the sagittal (Fig. 10, *left*) and axial (Fig. 10, *right*) gradient echo images, the spinal cord injury is characterized by inhomogeneous, mottled hypo- and hyperintense signals. In the sagittal T_2-weighted image (Fig. 10, *left*), the type III pattern is located posterior to the vertebral body (arrow). Hyperintense signal of edema extends rostrally and caudally (open arrows) from the area of maximum cord injury.

The sagittal image (Fig. 10, *left*) shows a large area of mixed signal secondary to disruption of the posterior ligament complex (*) surrounding the spinous process of C5, which is the site of a concomitant clay-shovelers's fracture (arrow head). The posterior longitudinal ligament and posterior annulus at C6-7 are disrupted and the disk material is herniated posteriorly (curved open arrow). The anterior annulus and anterior longitudinal ligament remain attached to the teardrop fragment.

Case 8

The high intensity signal (Fig. 11) in the seventh intervertebral foramen (arrow) in this patient with acute cervical spine trauma represents cerebrospinal fluid leakage secondary to root sleeve tear and cervical root avulsion.

Fig. 11 Avulsion of cervical root with cerebral spinal fluid leak into the intervertebral foramen.

References

1. Harris JH Jr, Edeiken-Monroe B: *Radiology of Acute Cervical Spine Trauma*, ed 2. Baltimore, Williams & Wilkins, 1987.
2. Harris JH Jr: Acute spinal injury: Radiographic evaluation of spinal trauma. *Orthop Clin North Am* 1986;17:1,75–86.
3. Cohen W: Recent developments in the imaging of neuraxis trauma. *Curr Opin Radiol* 1990;22:34–39.
4. Green BA, Callahan RA: A radiological approach to acute spinal-cord injury in radiographic evaluation of the spine, in Post MJD (ed): *Radiographic Evaluation of the Spine*. New York, Masson Publishing USA, chap 34, 1980.
5. McArdle CB, Wright JW, Prevost WJ, et al: MR imaging of the acutely injured patient with cervical traction. *Radiology* 1986;159:273–274.
6. Kadoya S, Nakamura T, Kobayashi S, et al: Magnetic resonance imaging of acute spinal cord injury: Report of three cases. *Neuroradiology* 1987;29:252–255.
7. Tart RW, Drolshagen LF, Kerner TC, et al: MR imaging of recent spinal trauma. *J Comput Assist Tomogr* 1987;11:412–417.

8. Kulkarni MV, McArdle CB, Kopanicky D, et al: Acute spinal cord injury: MR imaging at 1.5T[1]. *Radiology* 1987;164:837–843.

9. Quencer RM, Sheldon JJ, Post MJD, et al: MRI of the chronically injured cervical spinal cord. *AJNR* 1986;14:125–132.

10. Kulkarni MV, Bondurant FJ, Rose SL, et al: Tesla magnetic resonance imaging of acute spinal trauma. *Radiographics* 1988;8:1059–1082.

11. Mirvis SE, Geisler FH, Jelinek JJ, et al: Acute cervical spine trauma: Evaluation with 1.5-T MR imaging. *Radiology* 1986;166:807–816.

12. Goldberg AL, Daffner RH, Schapiro RL: Imaging of acute spinal trauma: An evolving multi-modality approach. *Clin Imaging* 1990;14:11–16.

13. Bondurant FJ, Cotler HB, Kulkarni MV, et al: Acute spinal cord injury: A study using physical examination and magnetic resonance imaging. *Spine* 1990;15:161–168.

14. Deeb ZL, Rothfus WE, Goldberg AL, et al: Absent cord sign in acute spinal trauma. *Clin Imaging* 1990;14:138–142.

15. Quencer RM: The injured spinal cord: Evaluation with magnetic resonance and intraoperative sonography. *Radiol Clin North Am* 1988;26:1025–1045.

16. Goldberg AL, Rothfus WE, Deeb ZL, et al: The impact of magnetic resonance on the diagnostic evaluation of acute cervico-thoracic spinal trauma. *Skeletal Radiol* 1988;17:89–95.

17. Wittenberg RH, Boetel U, Beyer H-K: Magnetic resonance imaging and computer tomography of acute spinal cord trauma. *Clin Orthop* 1990;260:176–185.

18. De La Torre JC: Spinal cord injury: Review of basic and applied research. *Spine* 1981;6:315–335.

19. Chakeres DW, Flickinger F, Bresnahan JC, et al: MR imaging of acute spinal cord trauma. *AJNR* 1987;8:5–10.

20. Wagner FC Jr, Dohrmann GJ, Bucy PC: Histopathology of transitory traumatic paraplegia in the monkey. *J Neurosurg* 1971;35:272–276.

21. Yashon D, Bingham WG Jr, Faddoul EM, et al: Edema of the spinal cord following experimental impact trauma. *J Neurosurg* 1973;38:693–697.

22. Bresnahan JC, King JS, Martin GF, et al: A neuroanatomical analysis of spinal cord injury in the Rhesus monkey (Macaca mulatta). *J Neurol Sci* 1976;28:521–542.

23. Hackney DB, Asato R, Joseph PM, et al: Hemorrhage and edema in acute spinal cord compression: Demonstration by MR imaging. *Radiology* 1986;161:387–390.

24. Weirich SD, Cotler HB, Narayana PA, et al: Histopathologic correlation of magnetic resonance imaging signal patterns in a spinal cord injury model. *Spine* 1990;15:630–638.

25. Ducker TB: Experimental injury of the spinal cord, in Vinken PJ, Bruyn GW (eds): *Handbook of Clinical Neurology.* New York, American Elsevier, 1976.

26. Jellinger K: Neuropathology of cord injuries, in Vinken PJ, Bruyn GW (eds): *Handbook of Clinical Neurology.* New York, American Elsevier, 1976.

27. Edeiken-Monroe B, Wagner LK, Harris JH Jr: Hyperextension dislocation of the cervical spine. *AJNR* 1986;7:135–140.

28. Green JD, Harle TS, Harris JH Jr: Anterior subluxation of the cervical spine: Hyperflexion sprain. *AJR* 1981;2:243–250.

Magnetic Resonance Imaging of the Spine

Joel W. Yeakley, MD

John H. Harris, Jr, MD, DSc

Fundamentals of Magnetic Resonance Imaging (MRI)

This paper describes the physics of magnetic resonance imaging so that the clinician may understand the basics of the process by which the image is produced. Examples of application will be drawn from the lumbar spine.

Magnetic resonance imaging (MRI) produces images by subjecting the body to radiofrequency sound waves while the patient is in a strong magnetic field. Energy emitted by the body is recorded and analyzed by computer to produce an electronic image.

In order for magnetism to exist there must be a difference in energy states. Resonance is the exchange of energy between two systems with the same natural frequency.

The hydrogen nucleus (proton) is a spinning charged particle, and because moving charges produce magnetic fields, each hydrogen nucleus has its own minute magnetic field, called a magnetic dipole moment. An externally applied magnetic field causes the dipole moments of the majority of the hydrogen nuclei (protons) to align with the longitudinal (z) axis of the magnetic field. The protons that align antiparallel to the magnetic field are in a higher energy state than those that align with the magnetic field resulting in a difference in energy states (magnetism) along the (z) axis (Fig. 1).

A radiofrequency (RF) pulse of sufficient power and duration will raise the energy level of the protons. When this occurs, all the proton dipole moments are brought to the same energy level relative to the z axis, and magnetization in the z axis ceases (Fig. 2).

The induced energy will dissipate to adjacent molecules by means of a thermal interaction similar to Brownian motion. As this occurs, the excited protons return to their original ground state or equilibrium state, reestablishing magnetization on the longitudinal or z axis (Fig. 3). The change in size and direction of the magnetization vector induces an electrical signal in the recording coil. This return to equilibrium once the RF pulse is turned off is called "relaxation." T_1 relaxation time is the time required for 63% of the original ground state magnetism to reform in the longitudinal or z axis. Ninety-five percent of the magnetization in the z axis is reformed in three T_1. The restoration of magnetization in the z axis is therefore exponential (Fig. 4).

The magnetic dipole moment also has a motion, called precession, which is similar to the wobbling mo-

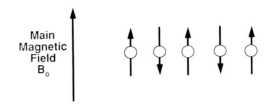

Fig. 1 Alignment of proton magnetic dipole moments in a strong magnetic field.

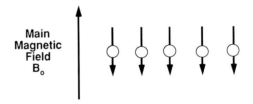

Fig. 2 Alignment of proton magnetic dipole moments following absorption of radiofrequency pulse energy.

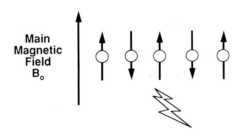

Fig. 3 Realignment of proton magnetic dipole moments with energy release to "lattice" by thermal energy interactions.

tion of a spinning top. The precession of the dipole moment forms a cone, the tip of which is the spinning hydrogen nucleus. The angle of precession (θ) is the angle the axis of the precessing dipole moment forms with the z axis (Fig. 5) of the magnetic field.

An applied RF excitation pulse will change the precession of the magnetic dipole moment. When the RF pulse is applied perpendicular to the z axis, the

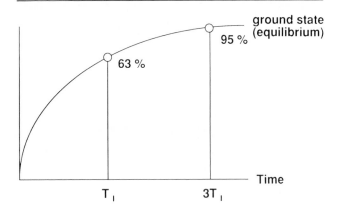

Fig. 4 T_1 buildup curve. Vertical axis = the degree of magnetization in the longitudinal (z) plane.

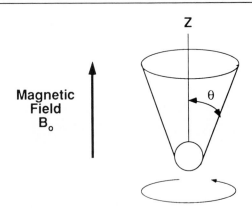

Fig. 5 Proton precession (Theta = angle of precession)

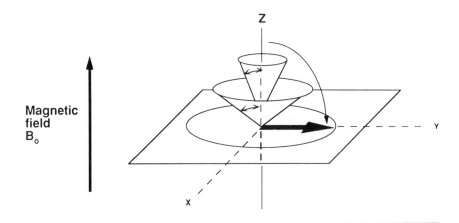

Fig. 6 Ninety degree "flip" of net magnetization vector

energy of the RF pulse causes the dipole moments to precess coherently, in phase. As energy is absorbed by the protons and phasing becomes coherent, a magnetization vector is produced in the x,y plane that is perpendicular to the original z axis (Fig. 6). The RF pulse that causes the magnetization vector to rotate 90 degrees into the x,y plane is referred to as the 90-degree pulse.

The change in amplitude and direction of the magnetic vector induces an electrical current in the receiver coil. The amplitude of this current decreases as precessional coherence is lost. The progressive loss of the strength of the electrical current is known as free induction decay.

Free induction decay is transient and difficult to measure. Therefore an echo of the free induction decay is produced by reversing the RF pulse and applying it in a direction 180 degrees to the original pulse. Rephasing recurs in the x,y plane, but the resultant magnetization

vector, or echo, is reformed 180 degrees away from the original. The echo builds up like a mirror image of the original free induction decay and then decays again. The rephasing vector in the x,y plane is referred to as a 180-degree RF pulse (Fig. 7).

T_2 relaxation time is the time it takes for 63% of the protons to dephase or lose coherence (loss of magnetization) in the transverse (x,y) plane. The time it takes for 95% of the protons to dephase is three T_2 (Fig. 8). The loss of magnetization occurring during T_2 causes an exponential decay of the strength of the electrical current induced.

The energy added to the system to produce the change in magnetization vector (excitation) must be at the specific precessional frequency of the molecule to be imaged, i.e., hydrogen. The resonant frequency is also called the Lamor frequency.

The return to equilibrium is achieved through energy dissipation called relaxation, which can occur by two

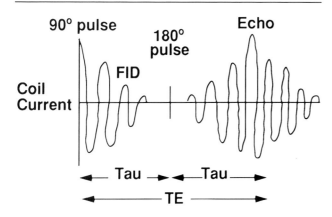

Fig. 7 Free induction decay (FID) and echo production (TE = echo time)

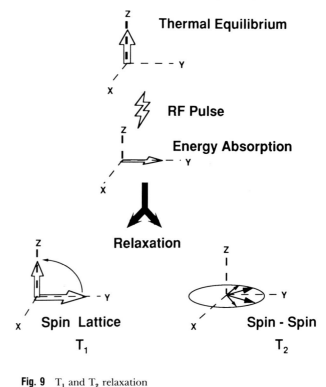

Fig. 9 T_1 and T_2 relaxation

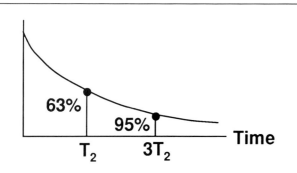

Fig. 8 T_2 decay curve. Vertical axis = the degree of magnetization on the transverse (x, y) plane.

mechanisms. In the first of these mechanisms, energy is dissipated to the adjacent environment or molecular lattice by means of thermal interaction related to Brownian motion. This type of energy dissipation is called spin lattice or T_1 relaxation. In the second mechanism, an excited molecule dissipates energy by inducing spin in unexcited molecules. This type of energy dissipation, which is similar to the effect that spinning planets or stars exert on each other, is called spin-spin or T_2 relaxation (Fig. 9). The T_1 and T_2 relaxation mechanisms occur simultaneously but are independent of each other.

Protons associated with large molecules, such as fat or protein, are efficient in dissipating energy by thermal equilibrium and have a short T_1 (white) signal whereas pure fluid molecules, like spinal fluid, dissipate energy poorly by thermal equilibrium resulting in a long T_1 (black) signal on T_1-weighted images. Similarly, protons associated with larger molecules, such as fat, readily dissipate energy by inducing spin in unexcited protons, resulting in short T_2 (black) signal, and protons in a pure fluid, such as spinal fluid, induce spins in other protons poorly, resulting in long T_2 (white) signal on T_2-weighted images.

Paramagnetic contrast materials, such as gadolinium diethylenetriamine pentaacetic acid (Gd-DTPA), act by enhancing relaxation. This relaxation enhancement has a greater effect on T_1 (thermal equilibrium) than it does on T_2 (induced spin). For this reason, Gd-DTPA shortens T_1, creating a bright signal, or enhancement, on a T_1-weighted image.

A typical spin-echo pulse sequence consists of a 90-degree RF pulse followed by a 180-degree refocusing pulse, which produces an echo. The interval between repetitive 90-degree RF pulses is the repetition time (TR). Multiple 180-degree refocusing pulses may be applied, producing multiple echoes that decrease progressively in amplitude as transverse magnetization is lost through spin-spin (T_2) relaxation. Each successive echo therefore becomes harder to record as the signal amplitude progressively decreases. This is why the second echo (T_2-weighted image) has more noise or grain than the first echo (proton density-weighted image) (Fig. 10).

T_1 contrast depends primarily on repetition time. If the repetition time (TR) is longer, the contrast between two tissues with differing T_1 is less (Fig. 11). Therefore, if T_1-weighting is desired, the repetition time must be kept short. However, the time when the signal is mea-

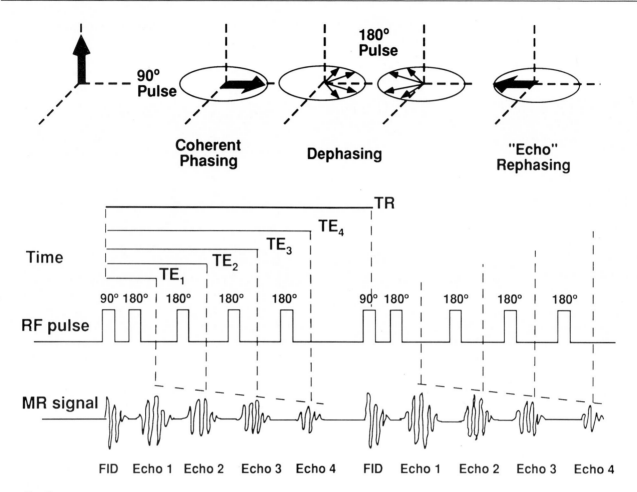

Fig. 10 **Top,** Spin echo. **Bottom,** Repetition time (TR) and echo time (TE).

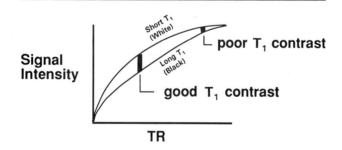

Fig. 11 T_1 contrast curve (TR = repetition time)

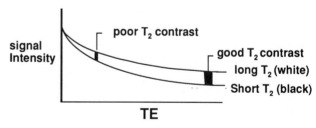

Fig. 12 T_2 contrast curve (TE = echo time)

sured, the echo time, must also be short to take advantage of greater separation of the signal intensity (contrast) between substances of different T_1. The short echo time also deemphasizes T_2-weighting, because T_2 contrast is less when the echo time is shorter, as will be seen in the next paragraph. An average pulse sequence that has a repetition time of 400 to 800 msec and an echo time of 20 msec is referred to as a short repetition time, short echo time (short TR-TE) sequence.

On the other hand, T_2 contrast depends primarily on

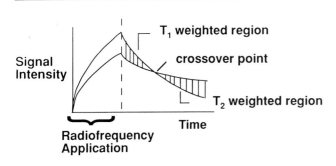

Fig. 13 Combined T_1 and T_2 contrast curves (Refer to Figs. 11 and 12.)

the echo time (TE) (Fig. 12). At constant repetition time, the longer the echo time, the better the contrast, as a result of T_2 relaxation. To produce a T_2-weighted image, a long repetition time (TR) is chosen to deemphasize T_1-weighting. A long echo time (TE) is chosen to produce better T_2 contrast. A long repetition time is considered to be greater than 1,500 msec. An average pulse sequence for T_2-weighting would have a repetition time (TR) of 2,000 to 3,000 and an echo time (TE) of 80 to 160 msec. This is often referred to as a long repetition time, long echo time (long TR-TE) sequence, or the second echo.

If proton density or balanced weighting is desired, it is necessary to deemphasize T_1-weighting by lengthening the repetition time, and also necessary to deemphasize T_2-weighting by shortening the echo time. An average pulse sequence would have a repetition time (TR) of 2,000 to 3,000 and an echo time (TE) of 20 msec. This is often referred to as a long repetition time, short echo time (long TR-short TE) sequence or first echo.

To get a better understanding of T_1- and T_2-weighting on a spin echo sequence, it is necessary to superimpose the T_1 and T_2 relaxation curves (Fig. 13). The T_1 recovery process and the T_2 decay process occur simultaneously but are independent of each other. The signal intensity resulting from T_1 or T_2 relaxation will vary, depending on where on the curve the signal is measured (echo time). The crossover point, where T_1 and T_2 relaxation are balanced, produces proton density-weighted images, which are neither purely T_1- nor T_2-weighted, but instead are relatively T_1- or T_2-weighed. Spinal fluid can serve as an example. Because spinal fluid has a long T_1, it will be black or dark on a T_1-weighted image. Because it has a long T_2, it will be white on a T_2-weighted image. It will usually be gray on a proton density-weighted image, but it can be darker or lighter depending on exactly where it is measured relative to the crossover point, where T_1 and T_2 factors are balanced.

We have noted previously that the longer the echo time, the lower all of the signals are and, therefore, the poorer the quality of the image. This explains why T_2-weighted images often have more noise or grain than other images. Long repetition time images give greater signal than short repetition time images, because the net magnetization vector in the z axis has longer to recover. When the magnetization vector is subsequently flipped, it produces more relative change in the magnitude of the net magnetization, which is what produces current in the detector coil that produces the signal. Hence, a long repetition time and a short echo time gives images (proton density-weighted or balanced images) with the strongest signal and the least graininess or mottle.

Another pulse sequence frequently used now is the gradient echo (GRE) partial flip angle of less than 90 degrees. Because these are used in order to decrease scan time, they are called "fast scans." They use a quickly reversible gradient energy application to the system rather than a 180-degree refocusing pulse.

The GRE pulse sequence has no 180-degree pulse to correct for inhomogeneity in the external magnetic field. Because of this, GRE images reflect not only the inherent properties of the tissues themselves, but also the ratio of focally induced magnetic field distortions to the externally applied field, known as magnetic susceptibility. Thus, what is measured is not a true T_2, but a T_2^*, which is the result both of T_2 relaxation and of magnetic susceptibility. A "boundary effect" is produced by magnetic inhomogeneities. These inhomogeneities are seen at the interfaces of tissues of far different make up. The interface between spinal fluid and fibrous tissue, such as dura, posterior longitudinal ligaments, and the outer fibers of annulus, is an example. This boundary effect may be useful in identifying lack of continuity of these structures.

Like T_2-weighted spin-echo images, GRE images produce a good "myelographic effect," because the spinal fluid has a high signal. However, because intervertebral disks that are still hydrated also possess a bright signal, the identification of disk herniation may depend on the presence of a black rim between the disk substance and spinal fluid, as well as distortion of the spinal cord in the cervical and thoracic areas. GRE images also tend to exaggerate the size of osteophytes and minimize the size of the spinal cord. For this reason, it is possible to overestimate the degree of spinal stenosis and cord compression. The true amount of compression can be estimated more accurately on T_1-weighted images.

However, because GRE images allow more sensitive identification of blood products than is possible with conventional T_2 images, they are more accurate in identifying spinal cord hemorrhage.

Motion phenomena are quite complex. The usual flow void in blood vessels in conventional MR images results when the excited nuclei move out of the imaging plane before a change in the direction or magnitude of the net magnetization vector can be recorded. When this happens, no signal is recorded. Stated another way, a nucleus must receive both the 90-degree and the 180-degree pulse in order to be imaged. The 180-degree pulse is not received because the nuclei receiving the 90-degree pulse in one plane have moved to another plane before the 180-degree pulse is applied. This is called the "time of flight" effect. Motion may also cause nuclei to be out of phase with their stationary neighbors. With newer techniques that use volume stimulation and acquisition, a three-dimensional "slab" may be excited and imaged. This allows MR angiography, where only the moving protons are imaged, by either time-of-flight or phase techniques. In the spine, motion phenomena in the cerebrospinal fluid may be confusing and may be mistaken for arteriovenous malformations or tumors. Motion phenomena tend to vary in location and signal intensity from one pulse sequence to another. They are frequently located anterior to the brain stem and the upper cervical spine, and posteriorly in the thoracic spinal cerebrospinal fluid. Paradoxical enhancement, or bright signal, can occur in blood vessels, particularly veins, that have a slow rate of flow. The mathematical method that the computer uses to produce an image called Fourier transform uses phase as one digital matrix and frequency as the other. Uncorrected signal caused by moving protons can lead the computer to assign a different signal intensity, or a false

location (misregistration artifact) along the phase-encoding axis.

The evolution of blood products in tissues, such as brain or spinal cord, that have an intact blood-brain barrier allows fairly accurate estimation of the age of a hematoma. Deoxyhemoglobin in an acute hematoma will be isointense to brain tissue with no contrast to slightly hypointense on a T_1-weighted image, but very hypointense on a T_2-weighted image. Later in subacute hematoma, methemoglobin formation produces bright signal at the periphery of the hematoma, which moves centrally, first on a T_1-weighted image and then on a T_2-weighted image. As the hematoma becomes chronic, macrophages at the periphery of the hematoma produce a hemosiderin ring, which is low signal on a T_2-weighted image. As the hematoma ages, it may assume the signal characteristics of spinal fluid, but the hemosiderin rim remains. Sometimes a hemosiderin scar, which has a low signal on a T_2-weighted image, is all that remains.

The final MR image is produced by a combination of factors including T_1 relaxation, T_2 relaxation, proton density, flow phenomena, artifacts, and paramagnetic contrast enhancement. Thinking in terms of classical radiographic densities does not work with MRI. A summary of the signal intensities of various tissue types produced by conventional pulse sequences is shown in Outline I. Sources of general information on MRI fundamentals are included in the reference list.[1-10]

Application of MRI Fundamentals to Image Interpretation

Various factors, including imaging sequence, proton density, flow phenomena, artifacts, magnetic susceptibility, and paramagnetic contrast enhancement, affect signal intensity and, therefore, image interpretation. This chapter is intended to describe and illustrate the basis of various MR images and the way in which pathologic states are depicted by MRI. It is not intended to be an encyclopedic compendium of the magnetic resonance appearance of all pathologic conditions affecting the spine. Images shown are primarily of the lumbar spine.

The effect of various imaging sequences upon various normal tissues of the lumbar spine are illustrated in Figure 14. The low intensity (dark) signal of blood (hematopoietic marrow), as compared to the high intensity (white) signal of fat on T_1-weighted images is contrasted in the sagittal images of the spine of a 14-year-old (Fig. 14, *top left*) and an older adult (Fig. 14, *top center*).[11,12] The intervertebral disks of both are of lower signal intensity than the marrow. The spinal fluid has a low (dark) signal, while the subcutaneous fat has the highest (white) signal.

The characteristics of a proton-density image are depicted in Figure 14 (*top right*). Because of their fluid

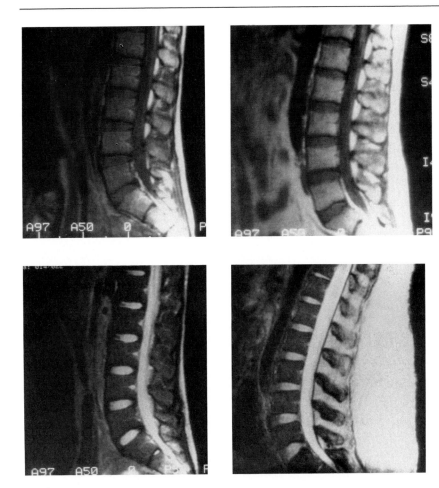

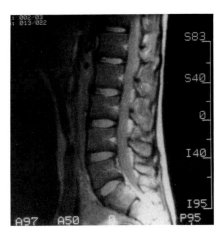

Fig. 14 Normal sagittal lumbar spine MRIs are: T$_1$-weighted images (**top left** and **center**), proton-density image (**top right**), conventional T$_2$-weighted (spin-echo) image (**bottom left**), and gradient echo gradient refocused (GRE) image (**bottom center**).

content, the intervertebral disks have a relatively higher signal intensity than the fat-containing bone marrow, and the spinal fluid has an intermediate (gray) signal. The outer fibers of the annulus fibrosis have the lowest signal because of their fibrous content.[13]

Figures 14, *bottom left* and *bottom center*, compare a conventional T$_2$-weighted (spin-echo) image (Fig. 14, *bottom left*) with a gradient echo (T$_2$* or "T$_2$-like") gradient refocused or GRE image (Fig. 14, *bottom center*). Both have a "myelographic effect" in that the spinal fluid has a very bright signal. The intervertebral disks now also have a bright signal because of their fluid content. The outer fibers of the annulus are not as clearly distinguished as in the proton density-weighted image. In both, the fatty bone marrow now has a relatively low signal (dark). The thick dark line at the posterior aspect of the spinal canal on the GRE image (Fig. 14, *bottom center*) is a "boundary effect" caused by artifactual accentuation of the dura—the result of magnetic susceptibility at the interface between substances of very different nature, in this case spinal fluid and fibrous tissue.

Our lumbar spine scan protocol generally calls for para-axial oblique images slanted through the interspaces. Nonslanted "stacked" contiguous axial images are used to evaluate fractures, fusions, and sometimes spinal stenosis. Both T$_1$-weighted para-axial oblique images and T$_2$*-weighted GRE para-axial oblique images are used. The combination of these two types of axial images has been shown to be superior to either type of axial image alone in the detection of various types of abnormalities.[14,15] The axial images must always be correlated with the sagittal images to insure detection of any abnormality in two planes.

Modic and associates[16] and deRoos and associates[17] have described three types of change (Figs. 15, 16, 17, and 18) that take place in the bone marrow adjacent to the vertebral endplates on either side of degenerated intervertebral disks and which must not be misinterpreted as diskitis or metastatic disease. The disk space may be narrowed with low signal in the disk itself on all pulse sequences as the result of degeneration and water loss (desiccation).[18-26]

Figure 19 demonstrates an area of focal fat within

Fig. 15 Modic type I changes. The T_1-weighted spin-echo image (**left**) shows a degenerated disk with intact endplates. The adjacent bone marrow on either side of the disk has a low signal (arrows). The T_2-weighted image (**right**) shows that the marrow adjacent to the degenerated disk is slightly increased in signal relative to the signal in the remainder of the bone marrow (arrows). These changes are related to vascularized immature fibrous tissue (granulation tissue). Paramagnetic contrast may enhance these marrow areas. (Courtesy of Mauricio Castillo, MD.)

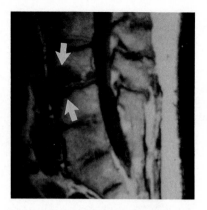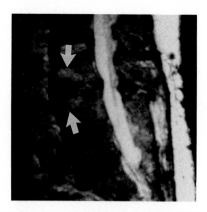

Fig. 16 Modic type II changes, primarily related to fatty degeneration of the marrow surrounding a degenerated disk. The T_1-weighted image (**left**) shows that the signal is higher adjacent to the degenerated disk than it is in the remainder of the marrow. The T_2-weighted image (**right**) shows that the signal adjacent to the disk is less intense than on the T_1-weighted image, but it is still slightly higher in signal intensity than the remainder of the marrow. Note that, as expected, the degenerated disk retains low signal on both pulse sequences, which distinguishes disk degeneration from diskitis.

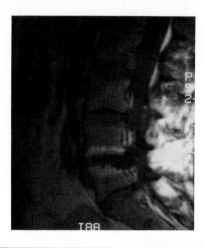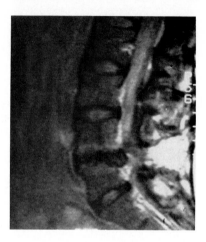

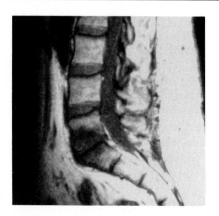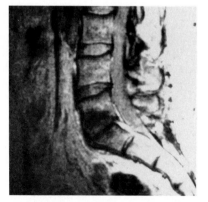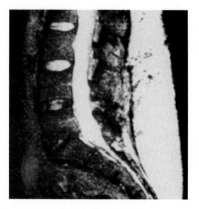

Fig. 17 Modic type III changes. The T_1-weighted image (**left**) shows low signal on either side of a degenerated disk at L5-S1. The proton density-weighted image (**center**) and T_2-weighted image (**right**) show that the bone marrow on either side of the degenerated disk has a low signal on all pulse sequences. Note that the degenerated disk also has a low signal on all pulse sequences. Type III changes are related to sclerosis in the bone marrow adjacent to narrow degenerated disks, a phenomenon commonly seen on plain film of the spine. (Courtesy of Mauricio Castillo, MD.)

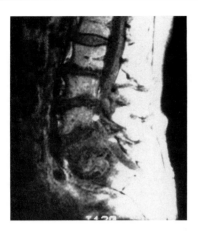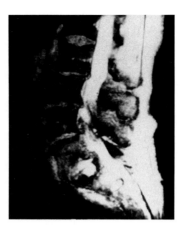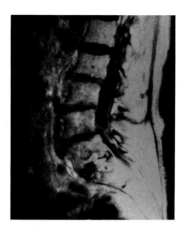

Fig. 18 L5-S1 diskitis. The T₁-weighted image (**left**) shows that the endplates at L5-S1 are no longer intact. An irregular area of mixed signal is seen there. Ordinarily, with diskitis one would expect very low signal within the disk on T₁-weighted images. In this case, the areas of higher signal may be related to necrosis and proteinaceous debris with bound water (see Outline 1). Far different from degenerative change, however, is the T₂-weighted image (**center**), which shows a very high signal in the area of the disk and destroyed endplates. A repeat T₁-weighted image (**right**) following paramagnetic contrast enhancement (Gd-DTPA), when compared with the noncontrast T₁-weighted image, shows contrast enhancement (bright signal) caused by T₁ shortening in the area of the inflammatory abnormality.

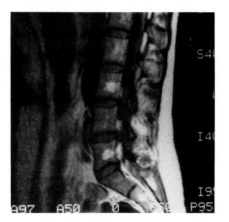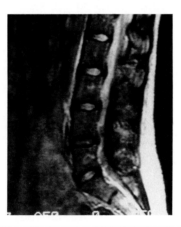

Fig. 19 An area of focal fat within the bone marrow. The T₁-weighted image (**left**) shows a rounded area in L5 that has a relatively high signal compared with the surrounding marrow. On the T₂-weighted image (**right**), this area produces relatively lower signal intensity than it did on the T₁-weighted image, although its signal still remains slightly higher than that of the surrounding marrow. A second, less conspicuous area of the same process is seen in L3.

the bone marrow.[26] The T₁-weighted image (Fig. 19, *left*) shows a rounded area in L5 that has a relatively high signal compared with the surrounding marrow. On the T₂-weighted image (Fig. 19, *right*), this area produces relatively lower signal intensity than it did on the T₁-weighted image, although its signal still remains slightly higher than that of the surrounding marrow. A second, less conspicuous area of the same process is seen in L3.

Hemangioma of bone generally has a high signal on all pulse sequences.[27-29] The high signal in the second thoracic vertebra on the T₁-weighted image (Fig. 20, *left*) is related to fat content. Because hemangioma of bone is a neoplasm and its water content is relatively higher than that of adjacent tissues, it will produce a

high signal on both proton-density and T₂-weighted images (Fig. 20, *right*). The incidental finding of focal fat deposition in a vertebral body is characterized by high signal on T₁-weighted images and lower signal on T₂-weighted images.

Metastatic disease, like most nonfat-containing neoplasms, shows low signal on T₁-weighted images and high signal on T₂-weighted images. An unusual variation of metastatic disease is illustrated in Figure 21 in which, on the T₁-weighted image, the intervertebral disks are higher in signal than the bone marrow. This should not be the case on a T₁-weighted image unless the bone marrow is abnormally low in signal.[30] Paramagnetic contrast material produced abnormal enhancement of virtually the entire marrow indicating

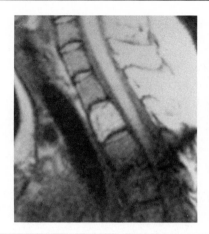

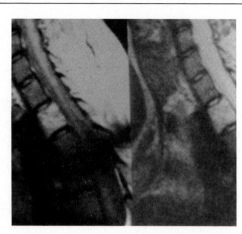

Fig. 20 Hemangioma: T$_1$-weighted (**left**), protondensity, and T$_2$-weighted images (**right**). (Courtesy of Mauricio Castillo, MD)

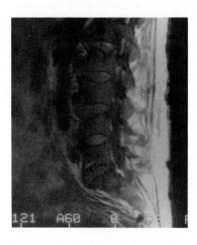

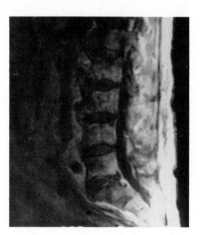

Fig. 21 Unusual magnetic resonance manifestation of vertebral body metastases. In the T$_1$-weighted image (**left**), the marrow is of lower intensity signal than the disks. Contrast enhancement (**right**) confirms diffuse carcinomatous infiltration in a patient with known malignancy.

diffuse carcinomatous infiltration in a patient with known malignancy.

Paramagnetic contrast enhancement permits demonstration of certain annular tears noninvasively by MRI.[31-33] Because the magnetic resonance findings of an annular tear and a diskectomy scar are very similar in appearance, the distinction is commonly made on the basis of prior surgery.[34]

MRI[35-38] and especially MRI before and after administering Gd-DTPA[39-46] is the imaging modality of choice in the distinction between scar and recurrent disk herniation in postoperative patients (Fig. 22). Usually scar tissue will be enhanced, whereas the disk material will not. The postgadolinium images must be performed immediately after contrast administration, because delayed imaging may result in some enhancement of the disk fragment.

Although arachnoidal adhesions within the thecal sac may be defined on noncontrast images,[47] occasional enhancement with paramagnetic contrast can occur, but usually not to the same degree as is seen in extradural scar tissue and fibrosis (Fig. 23).[48]

Magnetic susceptibility artifacts are caused by retained postoperative microscopic metallic foreign bodies, such as from drill bits, instruments, or suction tips. These result in a relatively unrevealing T$_1$-weighted image, but produce a large black artifact on T$_2$*-weighted GRE images. This combination of poor definition on T$_1$-weighted images and a disproportionally large area of distortion on GRE images would not be expected with disk material but is fairly characteristic of magnetic susceptibility artifacts.

In trauma cases, signal intensity changes caused by blood products and magnetic susceptibility phenomena can be used to evaluate the relative proportions of edema and hemorrhage within an injured spinal cord.[49] This application of magnetic resonance to spinal and spinal cord trauma is discussed in Chapter 29.

Signal characteristics of magnetic resonance images may also be valuable in the identification of certain

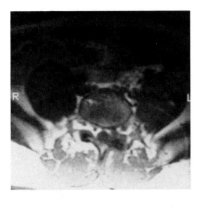
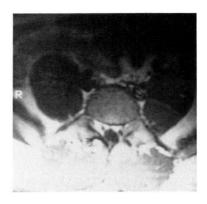

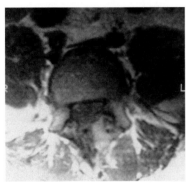
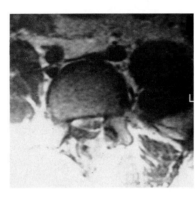

Fig. 22 T$_1$-weighted axial images before and after administration of gadolinium in a postoperative spine with left-sided scar tissue. The pregadolinium image (**top left**) shows the nerve root and proximal neural foramen on the left obscured by low-signal scar tissue, which is also inseparable from the thecal sac. The postgadolinium image (**top right**) indicates enhancement of the scar tissue, which is now higher in signal and clearly demonstrates the nerve root itself as well as the thecal sac. The bottom two figures demonstrate recurrent disk herniation surrounded by scar tissue following surgery. Before gadolinium administration (**bottom left**), low-signal material obliterates the anterior epidural fat on a T$_1$-weighted axial image. After gadolinium administration (**bottom right**), the enhanced scar tissue has a high signal, revealing the nonenhanced disk fragment contained within it. The distorted thecal sac is now clearly delineated posteriorly.

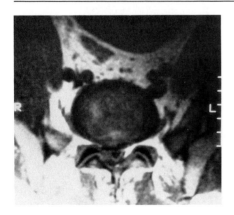
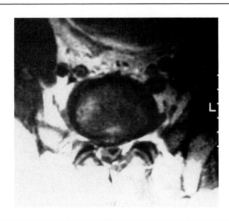

Fig. 23 Arachnoidal adhesion. Before contrast administration (**left**), a triangular pocket of low-signal cerebrospinal fluid is seen within the thecal sac, which contains peripheral adhesions of slightly higher signal. After administration of contrast (**right**), the adhesions show a slightly enhanced signal, whereas the cerebrospinal fluid remains unchanged.

types of neoplasms. An intradural lipoma, for example, will produce a high signal on the T$_1$-weighted image in contrast with the low-signal cerebrospinal fluid and intermediate signal spinal cord (Fig. 24, *left*). On T$_2$-weighted images (Fig. 24, *right*) the tumor signal should be lower than that of the surrounding high-signal cerebrospinal fluid. This combination of T$_1$ and T$_2$ signal characteristics is compatible with a fairly homogeneous fat-containing tumor (lipoma).[50] Conversely, the high fluid content of the cells of most neoplasms will have

low signal on T$_1$-weighted images and high signal on T$_2$-weighted images (Fig. 25).

Calcified lesions, such as a filum terminale ependymoma (Fig. 26), demonstrate another type of signal pattern, with the lesion being relatively isointense with the lower spinal cord on the T$_1$-weighted sagittal image (Fig. 26, *left*), but having a very low signal on the T$_2$*-weighted GRE sagittal image (Fig. 26, *right*).

Motion phenomena can be used as an aid in magnetic resonance as in the example of an arteriovenous fistula

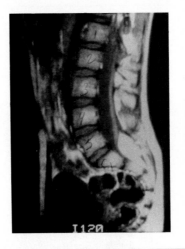
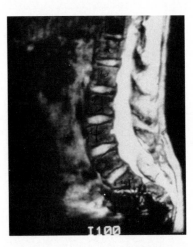

Fig. 24 Intradural lipoma with tethered cord. **Left**, T₁-weighted and (**right**) T₂-weighted images.

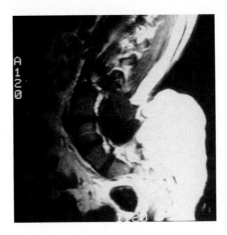
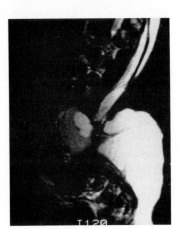

Fig. 25 Epidermoid "cyst". **Left**, T₁-weighted and (**right**) T₂-weighted images.

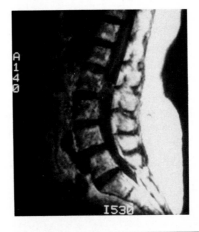
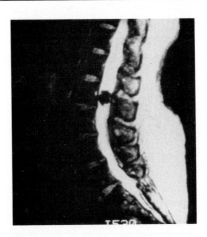

Fig. 26 Calcified filum terminale ependymoma. **Left**, T₁-weighted and (**right**) T₂-weighted images.

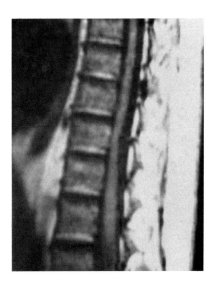
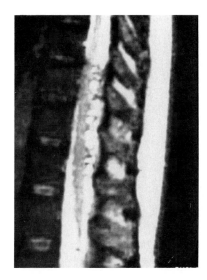

Fig. 27 Arteriovenous malformation. **Left**, T₁-weighted and (**right**) T₂-weighted images. (Courtesy of Mauricio Castillo, MD)

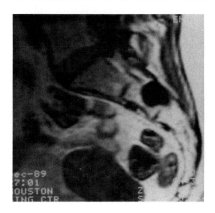
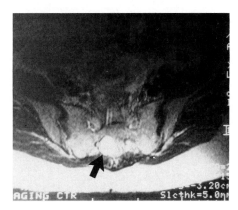

Fig. 28 Nerve root sheath cyst. **Left**, T₁-weighted sagittal and (**right**), T₂-weighted axial images.

when faint areas of low intense signal on T₁-weighted images (Fig. 27, *left*) suggest areas of high velocity flow void. In this instance, the T₂-weighted image (Fig. 27, *right*) will demonstrate multiple serpiginous areas of high-velocity flow void consistent with arteriovenous malformation.[51,52]

Motion phenomena also result from cerebrospinal fluid pulsation in a normal patient. These areas of normal flow-related phenomena are usually seen anteriorly in the upper cervical spine and brain stem and posteriorly in the thoracic spine.[53] They are usually inconstant and vary from one pulse sequence or imaging plane to another. Linear-flow phenomena caused by a higher velocity jet effect can also be seen in the cerebrospinal fluid near areas where the subarachnoid space narrows (spinal stenosis). Such cerebrospinal

fluid flow artifacts can be reduced by the use of special MR flow-compensation techniques.[54]

Finally, signal characteristics may also be important in assessing developmental or congenital abnormalities such as a sacral nerve root sheath cyst (Tarlov cyst).[55] These signal characteristics follow those of cerebrospinal fluid on all pulse sequences, including the T₁-weighted sagittal image (Fig. 28, *left*) and the T₂*-weighted GRE axial image (arrow in Fig. 28, *right*).

In diastematomyelia, the small high-signal area seen on T₁-weighted images is caused either by associated small lipomas or by fatty marrow within the bony spicule adjacent to the two hemicords. The T₁-weighted sagittal view (Fig. 29, *top left*) and coronal view (Fig. 29, *top right*) demonstrate a tethered cord and a small linear high-signal area posteriorly. The T₁-weighted axial view

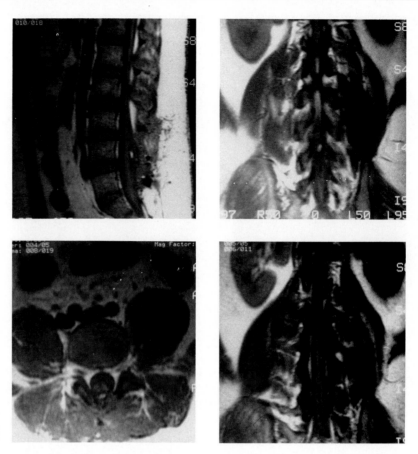

Fig. 29 Diastematomyelia. T_1-weighted sagittal view (**top left**); and coronal view (**top right**), T_1-weighted axial view (**bottom left**); and coronal view (**bottom right**).

(Fig. 29, *bottom left*) and coronal view (Fig. 29, *bottom right*) clearly demonstrate the two hemicords.

In summary, the purpose of this portion of the course is to demonstrate how fundamental MRI principles can be applied to image interpretation.

References

1. Brant-Zawadzki M, Norman D: *Magnetic Resonance Imaging of the Central Nervous System.* New York, Raven Press, 1987.
2. Enzmann DR, DeLaPaz RL, Rubin JB: *Magnetic Resonance of the Spine.* St. Louis, CV Mosby, 1990.
3. Friedman BR, Jones JP, Chaves-Munoz G, et al: *Principles of MRI.* New York, McGraw-Hill, 1989.
4. Heiken JP, Glazer HS, Lee JKT, et al: *Manual of Clinical Magnetic Resonance Imaging.* New York, Raven Press, 1986.
5. Horowitz AL: *MRI Physics for Physicians.* New York, Springer-Verlag, 1989.
6. Lufkin RB: *The MRI Manual.* Chicago, Year Book Medical Publishers, 1990.
7. Modic MT, Masaryk TJ, Ross JS: *Magnetic Resonance Imaging of the Spine.* Chicago, Year Book Medical Publishers, 1989.
8. Newton TH, Potts D: *Modern Neuroradiology, Advanced Imaging Techniques.* San Anselmo, CA, Clavadel Press, vol 2, 1983.
9. Nuclear magnetic resonance: Principles of imaging, pulse sequences, equipment, clinical applications. *Radiographics* 1984; 4(Special edition).
10. Smith HJ, Ranallo FN: *A Non-Mathematical Approach to Basic MRI.* Madison, WI, Medical Physics Publishing, 1989.
11. Ricci C, Cova MC, Kang YS, et al: Normal age-related patterns of cellular and fatty bone marrow distribution in the axial skeleton: MR imaging study. *Radiology* 1990;177:83–88.
12. Dooms GC, Fisher MR, Hricak H, et al: Bone marrow imaging: Magnetic resonance studies related to age and sex. *Radiology* 1985;155(2):429–432.
13. Yu S, Haughton VM, Lynch KL, et al: Fibrous structure in the intervertebral disk: Correlation of MR appearance with anatomic sections. *AJNR* 1989;10:1105–1110.
14. Murayama S, Numaguchi Y, Robinson E: Degnerative lumbar spine disorders in gradient refocused echo axial magnetic resonance images. *Clin Imaging* 1990;14(3):198–203.
15. Murayama S, Numaguchi Y, Robinson AE: The diagnosis of herniated intervertebral disks with MR imaging: A comparison of gradient-refocused echo and spin-echo pulse sequences. *AJNR* 1990;11:17–22.
16. Modic MT, Steinberg PM, Ross JS, et al: Degnerative disk disease: Assessment of changes in vertebral body marrow with MR imaging. *Radiology* 1988;166:193–199.
17. deRoos A, Kressel H, Spritzer C, et al: MR imaging of marrow changes adjacent to end plates in degenerative lumbar disk disease. *Am J Roentgenol* 1987;149:531–534.
18. Yu S, Haughton VM, Sether LA, et al: Criteria for classifying normal and degenerated lumbar intervertebral disks. *Radiology* 1989;170:523–526.

19. Yu S, Haughton VM, Ho PSP, et al: Progressive and regressive changes in the nucleus pulposus: Part II: The adult. *Radiology* 1988;169:93–97.

20. Sobel DF, Zyroff J, Thome RP: Diskogenic vertebral sclerosis: MR imaging. *J Comp Assist Tomogr* 1987;11(5):855–858.

21. Aguila LA, Piraino DW, Modic MT, et al: The intranuclear cleft of the intervertebral disk: Magnetic resonance imaging. *Radiology* 1985;155:155–158.

22. Modic MT, Pavlicek W, Weinstein MA, et al: Magnetic resonance imaging of intervertebral disc disease: Clinical and pulse sequence considerations. *Radiology* 1984;152:103–111.

23. Sharif HS, Clark DC, Aabed MY, et al: Granulomatous spinal infections: MR imaging. *Radiology* 1990;177:101–107.

24. Sharif HS, Aideyan OA, Clark DC, et al: Brucellar and tuberculous spondylitis: Comparative imaging features. *Radiology* 1989;171:419–425.

25. Thrush A, Enzmann D: MR imaging of infectious spondylitis. *AJNR* 1990;11:1171–1180.

26. Hajek PC, Baker LI, Goobar JE, et al: Focal fat deposition in axial bone marrow: MR characteristics. *Radiology* 1987;162:245–249.

27. Ross J, Masaryk TJ, Modic MT, et al: Vertebral hemangiomas: MR imaging. *Radiology* 1987;165:165–169.

28. Laredo JD, Assouline E, Gelbert F, et al: Vertebral hemangiomas: Fat content as a sign of aggressiveness. *Radiology* 1990;177:467–472.

29. Baker LL, Goodman SB, Perkash I, et al: Benign versus pathologic compression fractures of vertebral bodies: Assessment with conventional spin-echo, chemical-shift and STIR MR imaging. *Radiology* 1990;174:495–502.

30. Castillo M, Malko JA, Hoffman JR: The bright intervertebral disk: An indirect sign of abnormal spinal bone marrow on T1-weighted MR images. *AJNR* 1990;11:23–26.

31. Ross JS, Modic MT, Masaryk TJ: Tears of the annulus fibrosis: Assessment with Gd-DTPA-enhanced MR imaging. *AJNR* 1989;10:1251–1254.

32. Yu S, Haughton VM, Sether LA, et al: Comparison of MR and diskography in detecting radial tears of the annulus: A postmortem study. *AJNR* 1989;10:1077–1081.

33. Yu SW, Sether LA, Ho PS, et al: Tears of the anulus fibrosus: Correlation between MR and pathologic findings in cadavers. *AJNR* 1988;9:367–370.

34. Nguyen CM, Ho K-C, Yu S, et al: An experimental model to study contrast enhancement in MR imaging of the intervertebral disk. *AJNR* 1989;10:811–814.

35. Mikhael M, Ciric IS, Kudrna JC, et al: Recognition of lumbar disc disease with magnetic resonance imaging. *Comput Radiol* 1985;9(4):213–222.

36. Ross JS, Masaryk TJ, Modic MT, et al: Lumbar spine: Postoperative assessment with surface-coil MR imaging. *Radiology* 1987;164(3):851–860.

37. Frocrain L, Duvauferrier R, Husson J-L, et al: Recurrent postoperative sciatica: Evaluation with MR imaging and enhanced CT. *Radiology* 1989;170:531–533.

38. Ross JS, Modic MT, Masaryk TJ, et al: The postoperative lumbar spine. *Semin Roentgenol* 1988;23(2):125–136.

39. Hueftle MG, Modic MT, Ross JS, et al: Lumbar spine: Postoperative MR imaging with Gd-DTPA. *Radiology* 1988;167:817–824.

40. Bundschuh CV, Stein L, Slusser JH, et al: Distinguishing between scar and recurrent herniated disk in postoperative patients: Value of contrast-enhanced CT and MR imaging. *AJNR* 1990;11:949–958.

41. Sotiropoulos S, Chafetz NI, Lang P, et al: Differentiation between postoperative scar and recurrent disk hernation: Prospective comparison of MR, CT, and contrast-enhanced CT. *AJNR* 1989;10:639–643.

42. Ross JS, Delamarter R, Hueftle MG, et al: Gadolinium-DTPA-enhanced MR imaging of the postoperative lumbar spine: Time course and mechanism of enhancement. *AJNR* 1989;10:37–46.

43. Ross JS, Blaser S, Masaryk TJ, et al: Gd-DTPA enhancement of posterior epidural scar: An experimental model. *AJNR* 1989;10:1083–1088.

44. Bundschuh CV, Modic MT, Ross JS, et al: Epidural fibrosis and recurrent disk herniation in the lumbar spine: MR imaging assessment. *AJR* 1988;150:923–932.

45. Djukic S, Genant HK, Helms CA, et al: Magnetic resonance imaging of the postoperative lumbar spine. *Radiol Clin North Am* 1990;28(2):341–360.

46. Ross JS, Masaryk TS, Schrader M, et al: MR imaging of the postoperative lumbar spine: Assessment with gadopentetate dimeglumine. *AJNR* 1990;11:771–776.

47. Ross JS, Masaryk TJ, Modic MT, et al: MR imaging of lumbar arachnoiditis. *AJNR* 1987;8:885–892.

48. Johnson CE, Sze G: Benign lumbar arachnoiditis: MR imaging with gadopentetate dimeglumine. *AJNR* 1990;11:763–770.

49. Kulkarni MV, McArdle CB, Kopanicky B, et al: Acute spinal cord injury: MR imaging at 1.5 T. *Radiology* 1987;164:837–843.

50. Raghavan N, Barkovich AJ, Edwards M, et al: MR imaging in the tethered spinal cord syndrome. *AJNR* 1989;10:27–36.

51. Kulkarni MV, Burks DD, Price AC, et al: Diagnosis of spinal arteriovenous malformation in a pregnant patient by MR imaging. *J Comput Assist Tomogr* 1985;9:171–173.

52. Masaryk TJ, Ross JS, Modic MT, et al: Radiculomeningeal vascular malformations of the spine: MR imaging. *Radiology* 1987;164:845–849.

53. Enzmann DR, Rubin JB, DeLaPaz R, et al: Cerebrospinal fluid pulsation: Benefits and pitfalls in MR imaging. *Radiology* 1986;161:773–778.

54. Rubin JB, Wright A, Enzmann D: Lumbar spine: Motion compensation for cerebrospinal fluid on MR imaging. *Radiology* 1988;166:225–231.

55. Altman NR, Altman DH: MR imaging in spinal dyraphism. *AJNR* 1987;8:533–538.

Pathological Fractures and Metastatic Bone Disease

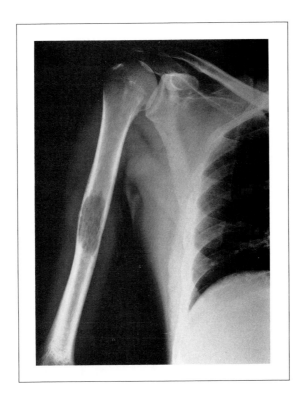

Metastatic Bone Disease: General Principles, Pathophysiology, Evaluation, and Biopsy

Frank J. Frassica, MD

Steven Gitelis, MD

Franklin H. Sim, MD

Introduction

Metastasis to bone with destruction of the skeletal system is a common problem in patients older than 40 years of age. Knowledge of the pathogenesis and pathophysiology of metastasis to bone enables the clinician to establish a diagnosis early and to plan effective treatment. The patient with metastases to bone may present many different and challenging diagnostic and therapeutic problems for the orthopaedic surgeon.

Each year in the United States there are more than one million new cases of malignancies outside the musculoskeletal system.[1] Of these million cases, almost half are the common primary tumors that metastasize to bone (Table 1). The large number of cases of metastatic bone disease is in sharp contrast to the small number of primary bone and soft-tissue sarcomas (fewer than 10,000).

Destruction of the musculoskeletal system compromises its three major functions: (1) structural support, (2) hematopoiesis, and (3) mineral metabolism.

Bone is the third most common site of metastatic disease. Although metastases to the lung and liver are more common, they are often asymptomatic until shortly before the patients succumb to their disease. In contrast, metastases to bone pose major problems for the cancer patient, including uncontrollable pain, forced immobilization, pathologic fractures, anemias, and hypercalcemia. Prompt and accurate diagnosis allows the clinician to formulate a logical treatment plan.

As advances in the systemic treatment of malignancies continue, it is especially important for the orthopaedic surgeon to design a durable reconstructive procedure for the patient with metastatic bone disease. During the past 20 years there have been significant increases in the 5-year survival rates for three of the five common carcinomas (breast, lung, and prostate) that metastasize to bone.[1] The 5-year survival for breast and prostate cancer now exceeds 75%. The probability of implant failure (Fig. 1) approaches 30% to 40% in patients who survive five years after operation for impending or pathologic fracture.[2]

Pathogenesis

The majority of metastases to bone originate from carcinomas in five major visceral organs:[3] breast, prostate, lung, kidney, and thyroid. The skeletal distribution of bone metastases commonly involves the spine, pelvis, ribs, skull, and proximal long bones. These particular locations correspond to the sites of erythrocyte production. There are two major theories concerning the affinity of certain primary tumors to metastasize to bone and their fairly selective skeletal distribution: the "soil hypothesis" and the "circulation theory."

The "soil hypothesis" was first formulated by Paget[4] who proposed that the cancer cells are seeds scattered in soils of different fertility. The "soil hypothesis" suggests that local factors may be present in certain organs that favor the implantation of metastatic cells. One cannot explain the distribution of metastatic cells solely on the basis of the arterial blood supply because some tissues with rich blood supplies, such as skeletal muscle and spleen, seldom harbor metastatic cells. Implantation factors might include proper nutrients, oxygen tension, hydrogen ion concentration, immune system cells and humeral factors, hormonal environment, cell surface properties, and many unrecognized factors.

Ewing[5] postulated that the unique features of the venous systems of the body account for affinity of certain tumors to metastasize to bone and for the selective distribution of tumors. He proposed that the "mechanism of the circulation will doubtless explain most of these peculiarities [of metastatic distribution], for there is as yet no evidence that any one parenchymatous organ is more adapted than others to the growth of . . . tumor-cells." The major pathways of metastatic tumor cells are shown in Table 2. The most common sites of metastatic disease are the lungs and the liver. Both of these organs receive their afferent blood from the two main venous systems, the systemic (inferior and superior vena cava) and the portal venous systems. Lung carcinomas can enter the circulation through the pulmonary veins or arteries through direct invasion and can then be distributed via the arterial system to bone and other organs. Passage through the pulmonary veins might explain the high rate of bone metastases distal to the knee and elbow in patients with carcinomas of the lung.

The distribution of metastatic cells to the vertebrae, skull, ribs, pelvis, and proximal long bones closely follows the anatomic features of the vertebral vein system. The importance of the vertebral vein system in the spread of metastatic cells was first fully appreciated by Batson.[6] He studied the vertebral vein system extensively by using contrast agents in human cadavers and live monkeys. He characterized the six major anatomic

Table 1
Estimated new cases of cancer in the United States in 1991

Types	No. of Cases
Tumors that commonly metastasize to bone	
Breast carcinoma	175,900
Lung carcinoma	161,000
Prostate carcinoma	122,000
Kidney carcinoma	25,300
Thyroid carcinoma	12,400
Primary malignancies of the musculoskeletal system	
Bone sarcoma	2,000
Soft-tissue sarcoma	5,800

and physiologic features of the system: (1) an inter-communicating network of thin-walled veins with a low intraluminal pressure; (2) a longitudinal course with a segmental distribution according to the vertebrae that extend from the dural venous sinuses of the skull to the sacrum; (3) location outside the thoracoabdominal cavity where veins are not subject to compression or collapse by increases in intra-abdominal pressure; (4) a valveless system that allows retrograde embolism; (5) connections to major organs, such as the breast, prostate, lung, kidney, and thyroid; and (6) connections to the proximal long bones. The anatomic features of the vertebral vein system help explain the affinity of the common carcinomas for metastatic sites in bone and their anatomic distribution.

Coman and deLong[7] studied the role of increases in intra-abdominal pressure in determining whether tumor cells enter the systemic or portal venous system or the vertebral vein system. In their animal model, they found that abdominal compression, which favors the collapse of the systemic and portal veins with a shunting of blood into the vertebral vein system, resulted in an 86% rate of metastases to the vertebral vein system, whereas in the absence of abdominal compression there was only a 6% incidence of vertebral vein metastases and a 100% incidence of pulmonary metastases.

A simple diagrammatic depiction of the vertebral vein system, along with the major organs that drain venous blood into the system, is shown in Figure 2. Both anatomic and experimental studies have supported the role of the vertebral vein system in the spread of metastatic cells from carcinomas to bone.

Pathophysiology

The biologic behavior of tumor cells and the response of the host bone after implantation and growth of the tumor cells are variable. The tumor cells may remain indolent, multiply slowly, or multiply rapidly. The host bone probably modulates the tumor cells' activity through the immune system and other, unknown, factors. There may be extensive bone production within a metastatic focus or there may be scant or no new bone.

The radiographic features of skeletal metastases can be explained on the basis of the amount of bone destruction and bone formation. When bone destruction greatly exceeds new bone formation, the lesion has a lytic appearance on the plain radiograph. When the tumor cells are particularly aggressive and there is little or no new bone formation, the lack of technetium up-

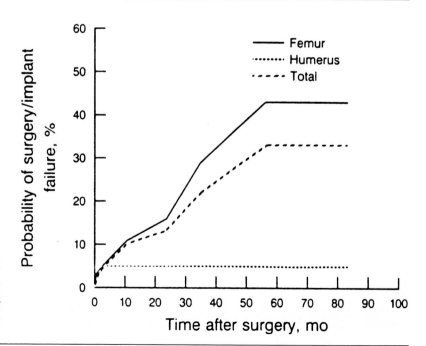

Fig. 1 Probability of implant failure after surgical reconstruction of metastatic lesions of femur and humerus. (Reproduced with permission from Yazawa Y, Frassica FJ, Chao EYS, et al: Metastatic bone disease: A study of the surgical treatment of 166 pathologic humeral and femoral fractures. *Clin Orthop* 1990;251:213–219.)

Table 2
Major vascular pathways of metastatic spread

Vascular System	Organ
Systemic venous circulation, main lymphatic trunks	Lungs
Portal venous system	Liver
Vertebral vein system	Bone
Pulmonary veins	All organs and bone

take by the osteoblast results in either a negative bone scan or one in which the technetium uptake is low. The same mechanism is seen in myeloma lesions of bone, in which there is no new bone formation. In contrast, when bone formation greatly exceeds bone destruction, the lesion will be extremely "hot" on the technetium bone scan.[8] Plain radiographs may show a mixed pattern of bone destruction and formation or the pattern may be profoundly blastic. Tumors with a desmoplastic reaction within the primary tumor (such as breast and prostate cancer) often have blastic metastases.

After implantation of the metastatic cells, the host bone is destroyed by two mechanisms: osteoclast-dependent and osteoclast-independent bone lysis. Osteoclast-dependent mechanisms are probably related to production of several agents that stimulate the osteoclast: osteoclast activating factor, parathyroid hormone, prostaglandins, tumor growth factors, and many uncharacterized factors. In a set of elegant experiments, Galasko[9] demonstrated that osteoclasts destroy bone within 24 hours of metastatic implantation. Interestingly, the osteoclasts are not found within the tumor cells themselves but are separated from them by a fibrous stroma. Prostaglandin and other substances influence bone destruction and the activity of osteoclasts.[10,11] Other investigators[12] showed that the tumor cells themselves may destroy bone.

Bone formation may occur within a fibrous stroma or may be a reactive process occurring at the periphery of the tumor cells. Periosteal new bone formation may occur where the tumor cells have perforated the cortex or caused a pathologic fracture. New bone formation occurs in virtually all metastatic tumors of the skeleton with the exception of myeloma, lymphoma, leukemia, and highly anaplastic, large lytic lesions associated with rapid gross destruction of bone. The early osteoblastic activity of new bone formation is usually detected by technetium bone scans. The osteoblasts readily pick up the technetium. The technetium bone scans have a greater than 90% sensitivity.[13]

Disordered Function

The primary functions of the skeletal system—structural support; production of erythrocytes, leukocytes, and platelets; and mineral homeostasis—often become

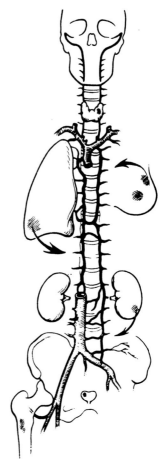

Fig. 2 Schematic diagram of Batson's vertebral vein system and five common visceral organs that drain cancer cells into system. (Reproduced with permission from Frassica FJ, Sim FH: Pathogenesis and prognosis, in Sim FH (ed): *Diagnosis and Management of Metastatic Bone Disease: A Multidisciplinary Approach.* New York, Raven Press, 1988, pp 1–16. By permission of Mayo Foundation.)

severely compromised by the implantation and growth of metastatic cells.

Structural Support

The structure of the skeleton is weakened by the resorption of the two-phase structure of bone: the collagen fibrils and the hydroxyapatite crystals. Plain radiographs always underestimate the degree of bone destruction. Pugh and associates[14] described the biomechanical considerations as threefold: (1) estimation of stress concentration due to the configuration of the edges of bony defect (stress-riser effect), (2) estimation of extent of weakening caused by frank bone loss (open-section effect), and (3) considerations of stress transmission and shock absorption. The mechanical considerations are not precise and future studies will probably change the method used to assess the risk of fracture.

In general, stress risers are defects less than one-half the diameter of the bone. There is an abrupt change in modulus of the bone between the intact cortices and the area of the destroyed cortical bone. Stress concentrates at points within the bone where less material is present to transmit the forces. As the extremity is further loaded, the forces exceed the ultimate strength of the bone and a fracture occurs. Bone is a viscoelastic material that is able to store more energy if it is loaded slowly. When the patient with a metastatic lesion has a relatively minor fall or twists the extremity rapidly, such as when pivoting, the bone is loaded rapidly. The bone is not able to store as much energy as when the patient places the foot on the ground slowly, and the weakened cortices often fracture at the site of the bone destruction. An open-section effect occurs when there is a defect in the bone in which the length of the defect exceeds 75% of the diameter of the bone. When an open section exists, the torsional strength of the bone is decreased by up to 90%.

The "fracture risk" with metastatic lesions is a complex concept that depends on the size of the defect, the interface of intact bone and diseased bone, and the location of the lesion. The ability of the patients to modify their activities is also important. Heavy torsional loads on the affected bone, as occur in pivoting on one leg or changing a car tire, must be avoided. The histologic appearance of the primary lesion is also important. For example, renal cell tumors produce large lytic lesions with minimal new bone formation. These lesions are at especially high risk for fracture.

Significant destruction of the skeletal system results in pain, forced immobilization, and pathologic fractures. Although metastases to bone are third in frequency of occurrence behind metastases to lung and liver, they often become the most painful site of metastatic disease.

Hematopoiesis

Widespread metastases to bone often result in suppression of erythrocyte, leukocyte, and platelet production. The suppression of the hematopoietic stem cells results from three principal causes: (1) marrow replacement with tumor cells, (2) external-beam irradiation, and (3) cytotoxic systemic chemotherapy. In addition, there may be decreased iron utilization as is seen in anemias of chronic disease. The most common primary tumors that result in marrow replacement include carcinomas of the breast, prostate, lung, and thyroid. Erythrocyte and platelet production are usually more severely affected than is leukocyte production.

Replacement of the bone marrow stem cells with tumor cells results in a normochromic, normocytic anemia with immature erythrocytes appearing in the peripheral blood smear. The anemia can vary from mild to severe. The peripheral blood smear often shows teardrop and fragmented cells. The leukocyte count may be increased, with a left shift. The combination of immature cell types and a normochromic, normocytic anemia is often termed a "leukoerythroblastic" reaction.

Marrow aspirates often yield a "dry tap" because of extensive infiltration, whereas marrow biopsy specimens are more diagnostic, demonstrating replacement by metastatic cells.

Hematologic support is a prerequisite to a successful outcome. If significant intraoperative bleeding is anticipated, one should consider preoperative blood transfusions to achieve a hematocrit of approximately 30%. Surgery should be avoided when the patient's neutrophil count is less than 500 cells/mm³. Although platelet counts less than 50,000/mm³ are not an absolute contraindication to surgery; one should be prepared for the possibility of excessive bleeding in the operating room.

Mineral Metabolism: Hypercalcemia

Hypercalcemia can occur in patients with extensive bone metastases or, less commonly, as a result of humeral mechanism (for example, paraneoplastic syndromes, in which the tumor secretes a parathormone-type polypeptide that activates osteoclasts to resorb bone). One should monitor the serum calcium level closely in the cancer patient with bone metastases who is immobilized or in the perioperative period.

The symptoms of hypercalcemia are related to the absolute serum calcium level and to the rate of increase. When the serum calcium level increases rapidly, severe symptoms may result, whereas slow increases produce milder symptoms at a high absolute serum calcium level. Early symptoms of hypercalcemia include polyuria, polydipsia, anorexia, nausea/vomiting, easy fatigability, and weakness. Late symptoms include confusion, coma, muscle weakness, and paralysis.

Hypercalcemia must be treated before undertaking surgery. Adequate hydration and saline diuresis are the mainstays of treatment and prevention. Plicamycin, diphosphonates, and calcitonin are effective in refractory cases but clinicians should be familiar with their side effects.

Clinical Manifestations

There are usually several clues in the patient's history to alert the clinician that metastases to bone may be the source of the patient's musculoskeletal pain. Pain secondary to tumor destruction of bone is usually dull at onset and there is a steady progression in intensity. Nocturnal pain is one of the hallmarks of destruction of bone by metastatic tumors and primary bone tumors. It is not unusual for patients to awaken at night with severe pain and require narcotics for comfort. As the destruction of bone progresses, narcotics given orally often will not control the pain. Patients with compression of the spinal cord, nerve roots, or the cauda equina (secondary to vertebral involvement or epidural deposits) often have an unrelenting and intense burning

Destructive Lesions of Bone

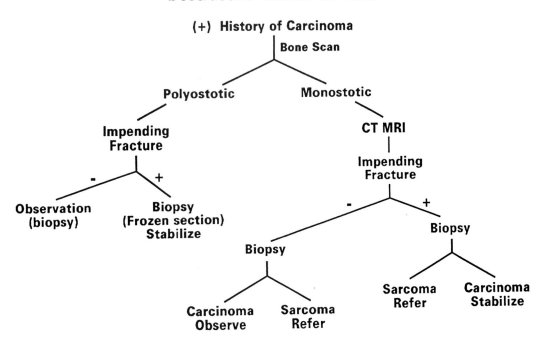

Fig. 3 Algorithm for evaluation of destructive lesions of bone in patients with history of cancer.

pain. Caution should be exercised to avoid missing spinal cord or cauda equina compression, because neurologic deficits can progress rapidly and patients seldom recover from the neurologic loss. Pain that occurs at night and progresses in intensity and duration should alert the physician to the possibility of metastatic bone disease or a primary bone tumor.

General Principles: Evaluation and Biopsy

The evaluation and ultimate biopsy of destructive lesions of bone are critical parts of patient management. If done improperly, significant morbidity can result that would otherwise have been avoidable. In addition, the proper recognition of primary bone tumors is critical to facilitate limb salvage procedures.[15]

It has been suggested recently that an improperly performed biopsy of primary bone tumors can lead to amputation that is otherwise unnecessary. Although biopsy is a simple technical skill, it is a complex cognitive skill that requires a thoughtful surgeon who anticipates every possible scenario.

Statistically, most destructive lesions of bone are secondary to metastatic carcinoma. The average orthopaedic surgeon, however, will see one primary bone sarcoma every 5 years. It is important that this tumor be recognized prior to biopsy.

There are clinical and radiographic features that should alert the clinician that a primary bone tumor is present. These features can be elicited by a careful history, physical examination, routine laboratory studies, and such simple imaging procedures as radiographs and technetium bone scans.

Primary bone tumors must be evaluated anatomically by magnetic resonance imaging (MRI) scans, computed tomography (CT) scans, and, at times, angiography before biopsy.[16] The biopsy can alter these studies and provide erroneous information. It would be unrealistic and exceedingly costly to perform these more sophisticated studies (for example, MRI, CT, and angiography) on all patients with destructive lesions of bone. Secondary lesions, for example, metastatic carcinoma or myeloma, frequently need only two plain radiographs before undertaking surgical intervention.

A strategy for the evaluation and biopsy of destructive lesions of bone is necessary to facilitate limb salvage, obtain appropriate diagnostic tissue, and provide for timely and cost-effective care.

General Guidelines

The evaluation of the patient with a destructive lesion in bone can often be expedited by the use of a systematic plan. Simple but effective algorithms for patients with destructive lesions of bone with and without a history of carcinoma are shown in Figures 3 and 4. It

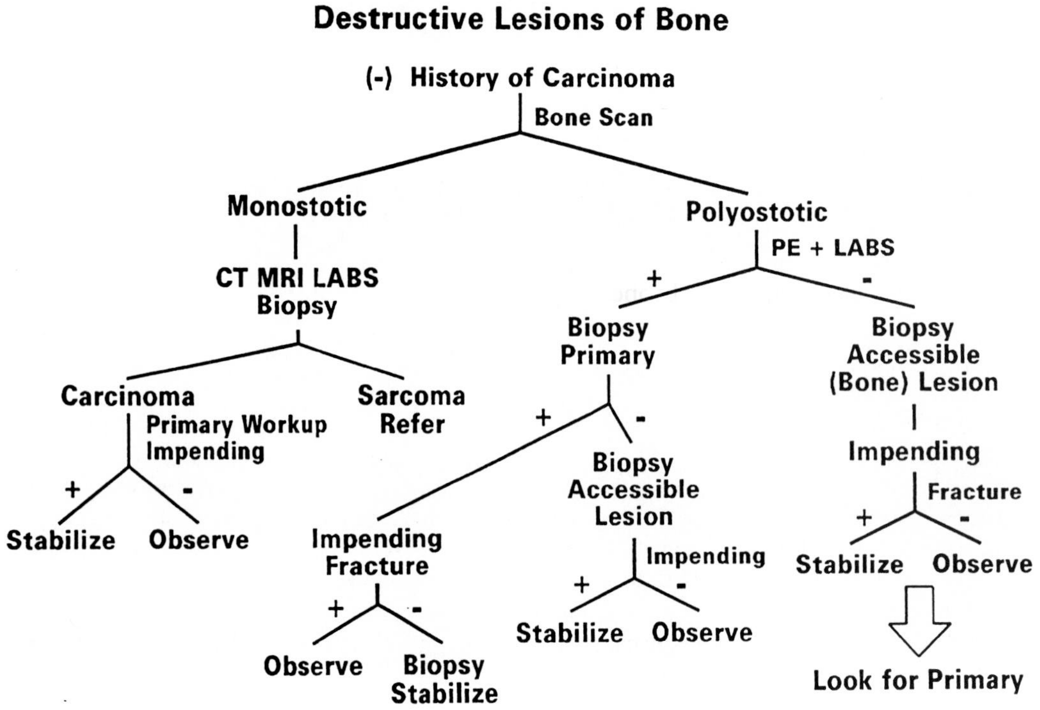

Destructive Lesions of Bone

(-) History of Carcinoma
Bone Scan

```
                    Monostotic                              Polyostotic
                        |                                    PE + LABS
                   CT MRI LABS                            +            -
                     Biopsy                         Biopsy          Biopsy
                                                   Primary         Accessible
           Carcinoma              Sarcoma        +        -       (Bone) Lesion
        Primary Workup             Refer                              |
          Impending                              Biopsy          Impending
       +           -                            Accessible              Fracture
   Stabilize     Observe          Impending      Lesion          +          -
                                   Fracture              Impending  Stabilize  Observe
                                +         -           +         -
                            Observe     Biopsy     Stabilize   Observe      ⇩
                                        Stabilize
                                                              Look for Primary
```

Fig. 4   Algorithm for evaluation of destructive lesions of bone in patients without history of cancer (PE = physical examination).

is recommended that patients diagnosed as having sarcoma be referred to an orthopaedic oncologist.

The age at presentation is an important feature that suggests the presence of a primary bone lesion. Patients older than 40 years are more likely than younger patients to have metastatic carcinoma or myeloma. This is especially true if they have a prior history of carcinoma, for example, breast, lung, prostate, renal, or thyroid carcinomas.

A useful screening examination to evaluate a destructive lesion of bone is a technetium bone scan.[13,16–18] This scan will, in most instances (except myeloma), determine whether the process is monostotic or polyostotic. Monostotic destructive lesions, regardless of age, need to be evaluated as primary bone tumors. Serum laboratory tests can be useful in some lesions. Primary hyperparathyroidism can be detected by serum calcium, phosphate, alkaline phosphatase, or a direct measurement of parathyroid hormone level.

Myeloma will usually manifest a dysproteinemia. Serum or urine immunoglobulin electrophoresis is effective in screening for myeloma of bone.

In male patients older than 40 years of age, a serum prostatic phosphatase level should be measured to evaluate for the presence of prostate carcinoma. This test is especially important when osteoblastic lesions are present. Physical examination of the prostate is another important component of patient evaluation.

A urinalysis is a simple and inexpensive laboratory screen for occult cancers. A dysproteinuria is frequently present in myeloma. Hematuria may be present in patients with occult renal or bladder cancers. The bone scan will, at times, detect an occult renal cell carcinoma because of collection of the radioisotope in the tumor. Better studies for renal screening include ultrasonograms, intravenous pyelograms, and CT. It is particularly important to be aware of a renal cell carcinoma before biopsy because of the risk of excessive hemorrhage.

Plain chest radiographs should be performed on all patients to evaluate the presence of intrathoracic abnormality. A careful history for exposure to known carcinogens, such as cigarette smoke, should be done.

Patients older than 40 years of age who present with a destructive lesion of bone without a prior history of carcinoma should be carefully examined for a primary site. The easiest sites of detection are prostate, thyroid, and breast. Masses in these locations should prompt further evaluation and biopsy. The prostate can be further evaluated by measurement of serum prostatic acid phosphatase, CT, or transrectal ultrasonography. A needle biopsy of the mass undertaken before addressing the bone lesion may provide useful information. Breast tumors are best evaluated by mammography, and they, too, can undergo biopsy before management of the bone lesion. Thyroid nodules can be evaluated by a thyroid radioisotope scan and ultrasonography before obtaining tissue. If no primary site is obvious, and if the process is polyostotic, suggesting metastatic carcinoma, the best source of diagnostic tissue may be bone.

The bone biopsy can sometimes direct the pathologist to the primary site. This is especially true for clear cell carcinoma (renal) and follicular carcinoma (thyroid). A periodic acid-Schiff stain for glycogen will aid in the diagnosis of renal carcinoma. Thyroglobulin stain or immunohistochemistry for thyroglobulin will further confirm the thyroid as the primary site.

Carcinoembryonic antigen suggests a bronchial or prostatic primary site. Prostate-specific antigen strongly suggests the prostate as the primary site. Melanoma can at times be diagnosed by its typical pigment. Metastatic squamous cell carcinoma is problematic because of its histologic similarities to bone cancer regardless of tissue of origin.

Metastatic breast carcinoma can at times be diagnosed by the bone biopsy if the histologic pattern is typical. If the bone biopsy does not direct the pathologist to the primary site, then a work-up in search of the primary tumor will be necessary. In many cases, the primary site of carcinoma is never found.

Bone biopsy of suspected metastatic carcinoma can be accomplished in several ways. If the tumor is polyostotic and will be treated surgically (for example, impending or pathologic fracture), a biopsy with frozen section evaluation can be performed at the time of definitive surgery.[19-23] Most metastatic carcinomas can be easily diagnosed in this way with little error. Although the primary site may not be determined until permanent sections or later work-up, enough information can be obtained to proceed with planned stabilization or reconstruction. Enough tissue should be obtained to establish the diagnosis and aid in management.

Hormonal evaluations of metastatic breast carcinoma for progesterone and estrogen receptors are useful for oncologic management. Tissue culture with in vitro chemotherapeutic sensitivity testing is also showing more promise with certain cancers. In polyostotic cancers in which a fracture or impending fracture does not exist but tissue is necessary, a closed needle biopsy is a useful technique.[24,25] Even though only a small amount of tissue can be obtained with a 3-mm core needle, it is usually sufficient to make the diagnosis. This biopsy technique is especially useful for pelvic and spinal lesions, in which open biopsy is an extensive procedure. It does carry the risk of fracture in long-bone lesions and of neurologic injury in vertebral body lesions. Thin needles (18 or 20 gauge) can be used where the risk is excessive with core needles. This technique requires an experienced pathologist who can interpret cytologic appearance.

Monostotic destructive lesions, especially in patients younger than 40 years of age, must be respected.[16] These tumors should be assumed to be primary until proved otherwise. Even with a history of a prior carcinoma, the lesion may represent a second primary malignancy. Proper prebiopsy imaging is important.[26]

The biopsy should be performed with care so as not to preclude limb salvage for primary bone sarcomas. Longitudinal incisions, careful hemostasis, avoidance of neurovascular bundles, and proper sampling are well established principles that need to be followed during biopsy.[15,27] Internal fixation of primary bone sarcomas should be avoided because it may interfere with later limb salvage.

Although there are some similarities between traumatic fractures and pathologic fractures, it is the differences between the two that require discussion and that make the latter group a challenging orthopaedic problem. Pathologic fractures, especially of the hip, have a high morbidity and mortality. Medical stabilization before surgical intervention is an important principle when dealing with these patients.[19-21]

Patients with metastatic carcinoma are at risk for a host of problems, some of which can be improved or reversed before surgery. The most serious problem is pulmonary dysfunction. Parenchymal involvement by carcinoma will cause diminished pulmonary capacity and hypoxemia. Decreased ventilatory function may also be secondary to a malignant pleural effusion, pain medications with central depression, atelectasis, and pulmonary embolism. The last is the result of stasis secondary to bed rest and hypercoagulation frequently seen in patients with metastatic carcinoma. Some of these problems can be reversed before surgery. Careful monitoring of arterial oxygenation should be routine. Procedures such as thoracentesis, insertion of chest tubes, and even endotracheal intubation should be considered before surgery to improve pulmonary function.

Anemia and thrombocytopenia should also be anticipated and reversed. These problems may be the result of diffuse bone marrow involvement by metastatic carcinoma as well as the effect of cytotoxic drugs frequently used to treat these patients. Appropriate replacement with blood bank products is important before surgical intervention. Leukopenia may also be seen but is a more difficult problem to manage. If surgery is performed electively, the timing can be coordinated with the anticipated cyclic effect of cytotoxic drugs.

Fluid and electrolyte levels also need to be increased because they are frequently in a state of imbalance. Postoperative prophylactic anticoagulation should be considered in all patients to reduce the risk of thrombophlebitis and pulmonary embolism.

In conclusion, the time spent in this detailed multisystem approach will pay off in diminished morbidity associated with surgical treatment of pathologic fractures.

References

1. Boring CC, Squires TS, Tong T: Cancer statistics, 1991. *CA* 1990; 41:19–36.

2. Yazawa Y, Frassica FJ, Chao EYS, et al: Metastatic bone disease: A study of the surgical treatment of 166 pathologic humeral and femoral fractures. *Clin Orthop* 1990;251:213–219.

3. Abrams HL, Spiro R, Goldstein N: Metastases in carcinoma: Analysis of 1000 autopsied cases. *Cancer* 1950;3:74–85.

4. Paget S: The distribution of secondary growths in cancer of the breast. *Lancet* 1889;1(3421):571–573.

5. Ewing J: *Neoplastic Diseases: A Treatise on Tumors*, ed 3. Philadelphia, WB Saunders, 1928, pp 77–89.

6. Batson OV: The function of the vertebral veins and their role in the spread of metastases. *Ann Surg* 1940;112:138–149.

7. Coman DR, deLong RP: The role of the vertebral venous system in the metastasis of cancer to the spinal column: Experiments with tumor-cell suspensions in rats and rabbits. *Cancer* 1951;4:610–618.

8. Galasko CSB: The pathological basis for skeletal scintigraphy. *J Bone Joint Surg* 1975;57B:353–359.

9. Galasko CSB: Mechanisms of bone destruction in the development of skeletal metastases. *Nature* 1976;263:507–508.

10. Dietrich JW, Goodson JM, Raisz LG: Stimulation of bone resorption by various prostaglandins in organ cultures. *Prostaglandins* 1975;10:231–240.

11. Klein DC, Raisz LG: Prostaglandins: Stimulation of bone resorption in culture. *Endocrinology* 1970;86:1436–1440.

12. Eilon G, Mundy GR: Direct resorption of bone by human breast cancer cells *in vitro*. *Nature* 1978;276:726–728.

13. Wahner HW, Brown ML: Role of bone scanning, in Sim FH (ed): *Diagnosis and Management of Metastatic Bone Disease: A Multidisciplinary Approach*. New York, Raven Press, 1988, pp 51–67.

14. Pugh J, Sherry HS, Futterman B, et al: Biomechanics of pathologic fractures. *Clin Orthop* 1982;169:109–114.

15. Mankin HJ, Lange TA, Spanier SS: The hazards of biopsy in patients with malignant primary bone and soft-tissue tumors. *J Bone Joint Surg* 1982;64A:1121–1127.

16. Simon MA, Karluk MB: Skeletal metastases of unknown origin: Diagnostic strategy for orthopedic surgeons. *Clin Orthop* 1982;166:96–103.

17. Chernow B, Wallner SF: Variables predictive of bone marrow metastasis. *Cancer* 1978;42:2373–2378.

18. Sim FH, Frassica FJ, Edmonson JH: Clinical and laboratory findings, in Sim FH (ed): *Diagnosis and Management of Metastatic Bone Disease: A Multidisciplinary Approach*. New York, Raven Press, 1988, pp 25–30.

19. Gitelis S: The treatment of pathological hip fractures. *Techniques Orthop (Rockville, MD)* 1989;4(2):73–80

20. Gitelis S, Sheinkop MB, Hammerberg K, et al: The role of prophylactic surgery in the management of metastatic hip disease. *Orthopedics* 1982;5:1004–1011.

21. Gitelis S, Sheinkop MB, Hammerberg K, et al: Pathological fractures of the upper end of the femur secondary to metastatic disease, in Tronzo RG (ed): *Surgery of the Hip Joint*, ed 2. New York, Springer-Verlag, 1987, vol 2, pp 339–349.

22. Hipp JA, McBroom RJ, Cheal EJ, et al: Structural consequences of endosteal metastatic lesions in long bones. *J Orthop Res* 1989;7:828–837.

23. Mirels H: Metastatic disease in long bones: A proposed scoring system for diagnosing impending pathologic fractures. *Clin Orthop* 1989;249:256–264.

24. deSantos LA, Murray JA, Ayala AG: The value of percutaneous needle biopsy in the management of primary bone tumors. *Cancer* 1979;43:735–744.

25. El-Khoury GY, Terepka RH, Mickelson MR, et al: Fine-needle aspiration biopsy of bone. *J Bone Joint Surg* 1983;65A:522–525.

26. Zimmer WD, Berquist TH, McLeod RA, et al: Bone tumors: Magnetic resonance imaging versus computed tomography. *Radiology* 1985;155:709–718.

27. Simon MA: Biopsy of musculoskeletal tumors. *J Bone Joint Surg* 1982;64A:1253–1257.

Differential Diagnosis and Surgical Treatment of Pathologic Spine Fractures

James N. Weinstein, DO

"The hopelessness associated with cancer is only partly related to the number of lives it claims. The most devastating aspect of neoplasia, however, is the spread from the primary site to distant organs, i.e. metastasis."[1]

The treatment of spinal column neoplasia continues to evolve rapidly. Improved systemic therapy and an aggressive surgical approach have improved both the short- and long-term outcomes. Unfortunately, there is currently no uniform approach to treatment of patients with spinal tumors and little uniformity in reporting outcome measures. Direct comparison of treatment protocols is difficult, and conclusions regarding definitive management are somewhat tenuous. However, in appropriately selected patients, surgical treatment now offers a reasonable likelihood of functional improvement, pain relief, and, in many cases, cure of the disease.

General Information

Neoplastic disease of the spine may arise from local lesions, which develop within or adjacent to the spinal column, or from distant malignancies, which spread to the spine or paraspinous tissues by hematogenous or lymphatic routes. Local involvement of the spine can result from primary tumors of bone, from primary lesions that arise in the spinal cord or its coverings, or from contiguous spread of tumors of the paraspinous soft tissues and lymphatics. Regional or distant spread of metastatic disease to the spine can occur with almost any malignancy.

History

By examining mummified human remains, researchers have traced metastatic bone disease back as far as 2,400 years. Pre-Columbian Incas and Egyptians of the 3rd and 5th Dynasties were found to have metastases.[2,3] In 1829 Joseph Claude Recamier[4] was the first to use the term "metastases." Many theories have been developed to explain metastatic spread. The "seed and soil" theory was advanced by Paget[5] in 1899. In 1928 James Ewing[6] proposed the "circulation theory" to explain the spread of tumor cells to various organs. Today, it is believed that tumor cells metastasize by complex mechanisms involving both systemic and mechanical factors.

Incidence

Both metastatic and primary tumors occur in all age groups and at all levels of the spinal column. However, metastatic tumors are far more common than primary lesions and account for skeletal disease in 40 times as many patients as do all other forms of bone cancer combined.[7] Between 50% and 70% of patients with carcinoma will develop skeletal metastases before they die, as will as many as 85% of women with breast carcinoma.[8] Primary tumors of the spine are very rare, and their relative incidence reflects that of skeletal tumors in general. Certain tumors, such as chordoma or osteoblastoma, do show a predilection for the spinal column, but they make up a very small proportion of all spinal tumors. Only about 5% of cases develop epidural metastases. Today, there are about 18,000 new cases of vertebral metastases per year.

Presentation

Tumors of the spinal column can remain asymptomatic for some time. Symptoms usually develop as a result of one or more of the following: (1) expansion of the cortex of the vertebral body by tumor mass, with fracture and invasion of paravertebral soft tissues; (2) compression or invasion of adjacent nerve roots; (3) pathologic fracture caused by vertebral destruction; (4) development of spinal instability; and/or (5) compression of the spinal cord.[9] Obviously, rapidly progressive symptoms of pain or neurologic compromise will be associated with the more malignant, rapidly destructive tumors, whereas patients whose symptoms have progressed slowly over the years will typically have slow-growing tumors and a better long-term prognosis.

Age

The relationship between age and metastatic disease is well known. Systemic diseases such as myeloma and lymphoma are also predominant after the fifth decade of life. Likewise, primary spinal neoplasms show a strong correlation between age and malignancy. In patients older than 21 years of age, more than 70% of primary tumors are malignant, while in those younger than 21, the majority of lesions are benign.[10]

Location

The location of the lesion within the vertebra also differs for benign and for malignant disease. The majority of malignant tumors, both primary and metastatic, originate anteriorly and involve the vertebral body and possibly one or both pedicles. Strictly posterior localization, even when more than one level is involved, is more typical of benign lesions.

Diagnosis

The clinical presentation usually provides clues that alert the physician to the presence of a spinal neoplasm.

Symptoms

The most consistent complaint is pain. The pain associated with neoplasia tends to be progressive and unrelenting, and it is not as closely associated with activity as is mechanical back pain. Night pain is particularly worrisome. Symptoms may localize to a specific spinal segment, and they may be reproduced by pressure or percussion over that segment. Radicular symptoms are less common but are still frequently observed in patients who have cervical or lumbar involvement. Radicular symptoms similar to those seen in herniated nucleus pulposus may lead to confusion in diagnosis and treatment. In 38 cases of bone tumors simulating lumbar disk herniation, Sim and associates[11] identified lumbar or sacral neoplasms in 23 patients, and they noted that the pain associated with these lesions was usually unremitting and progressive and was not relieved by rest or recumbency.

Spinal deformity, which can be associated with the onset of pain, usually results from paraspinous muscular spasm. Scoliosis, sometimes associated with osteoid osteoma or osteoblastoma, typically causes localized paravertebral pain and paravertebral muscle spasm and limits motion. The onset of such scoliosis may be rapid.[12] Although these deformities are usually correctable early in the process, curves neglected for prolonged periods may become structural.[13]

Neurologic deficit is common in patients with spinal tumors, but it is rarely the first symptom observed. Weakness, usually in the lower extremities, may not become apparent until months or years after the onset of back pain. Nonetheless, as many as 70% of patients will manifest clinical weakness by the time the correct diagnosis is made. This emphasizes the importance of a high index of suspicion in patients with persistent back or radicular pain, particularly those with a history of known systemic malignancies.[14–16]

Bowel and bladder dysfunction may develop before diagnosis in as many as half of patients with cord compression.[15] Rarely, patients with compression at the level of the conus medullaris may have isolated sphincter dysfunction.

Osteoporosis

Osteoporosis, or decreased bone mass, must also be differentiated from either primary or secondary tumors

in patients with vertebral fractures. Osteoporosis affects 15 to 20 million Americans, including one of every four women younger than 65 and one out of two older than 65, and causes 1.3 million fractures per year. In the spine, compression fractures can be associated with scoliosis and/or kyphosis. A spine survey of 2,000 women for vertebral compression fractures secondary to osteoporosis showed an incidence of 29% between the ages of 45 and 54; of 61% between 55 and 64; and 79% between the ages of 65 and 70. Absorptiometry and computed tomographic scan are the best early diagnostic tools. Surgery is rarely indicated for osteoporosis, prevention being the primary treatment.[17]

Imaging Techniques

Plain roentgenograms should be obtained in any case where a neoplasm is suspected. They can be used to identify some characteristic tumor types, but even when the specific tumor type remains unknown, the benign or malignant nature of the lesion can sometimes be deduced from the pattern of bony destruction. However, in its early stages, any lesion is difficult to detect, because radiographic evidence of bone destruction is not apparent until 30% to 50% of the trabecular bone has been destroyed.[18] The technetium Tc 99m bone scan can detect lesions as small as 2 mm, provided there is some osteoblastic response in the surrounding bone, but it cannot differentiate between fracture, infection, and neoplasm.

Osteoarthritis—the most common source of false-positive scans—is prevalent in the older population most at risk for metastatic disease.[19–21] Although bone scans lack specificity, patterns of uptake that show multiple areas of skeletal involvement are virtually diagnostic for metastatic disease in the patient with a known primary malignancy.

Computed tomography (CT) offers improved sensitivity in the detection of spinal neoplasms and alterations in bone mineralization. Lesions may be visualized at an earlier time in their development, before extensive bone destruction or intramedullary extension has occurred, and before cortical erosion has progressed to the point of impending fracture. Because it demonstrates neoplastic involvement far more reliably than plain radiographs, computed tomography is vital in planning surgical approaches and tumor resection.

Although myelography has long been used to evaluate epidural metastases and cord compression, there are a number of inherent risks involved in that test. Magnetic resonance imaging (MRI), which has proven useful in evaluating a variety of spinal diseases, is well tolerated, noninvasive, and safe. The superior soft-tissue contrast provided by magnetic resonance imaging and the ability to obtain multiplanar images enhance the diagnostic and treatment-planning capabilities of the surgeon considerably. Magnetic resonance imaging delineates soft-tissue tumor extension and adherence or invasion of paravertebral structures more clearly than does computed tomography. Direct sagittal and coronal images are superior to reconstructions available through computed tomography, and magnetic resonance imaging is able to depict the spinal cord directly, without the aid of intrathecal contrast material.[22]

Biopsy Techniques

Three forms of biopsy are available to the surgeon: excisional, incisional, and needle biopsy (aspiration). On occasion, a posterior lesion may prove suitable for an excisional biopsy, but most lesions of the spinal column will require either incisional or needle biopsy. Needle biopsies are subject to sampling errors and provide a small specimen for evaluation. The primary role of needle biopsy is confirmation—confirmation of metastatic disease, of recurrence of a known lesion, or of sarcomatous histology in an otherwise classic clinicoradiologic presentation of osteosarcoma.[23] When the differential is limited to lesions that are easily distinguished histologically, a needle biopsy may be ideal. In more complex lesions and in those with a more subtle differential, a specimen obtained by needle biopsy often proves inadequate.[24]

The incisional biopsy should be the last step in the staging of the patient and is performed just before the definitive surgical resection. The location of the biopsy incision should be chosen so that it will be excised with the tumor during the definitive procedure. Tissues should be handled carefully, and hemostasis should be meticulous. Bone should not be removed or windowed during biopsy unless absolutely necessary. All tissue contaminated during biopsy or by hematoma must be excised if surgical control is expected.[24] Once the tumor is exposed, an adequate sample of tissue must be obtained. The specimen should be large enough to allow histologic and ultrastructural analysis, as well as immunologic stains. The margin of the soft-tissue mass often provides the best information, because central portions can be necrotic. The surgeon should take care not to crush or distort the specimen so as to maintain its architecture.

Metastatic Tumors

Metastases are by far the most common skeletal tumors observed by the orthopaedist, and the spine is the most common site of skeletal involvement.[25] Skeletal metastases occur, most commonly, secondary to carcinoma of the breast, lung, or prostate; less frequently, they occur secondary to renal, thyroid, or gastrointestinal carcinoma (Table 1).

Table 1
Metastatic disease of bone: Location of primary neoplasms producing metastatic lesions of bone

Primary Site	No.	%
Breast	2,020	40
Lung	646	13
Prostate	296	6
Kidney	284	6
Gastrointestinal	255	5
Bladder	160	3
Thyroid	110	2
Miscellaneous	1,235	25
Total	5,006	

Reproduced with permission from McLain RF, Weinstein JN: Tumors of the spine. *Semin Spine Surg* 1990;2:157–180.

Table 2
Neoplasms producing spinal metasteses: Location of primary tumors producing metastatic disease of the spinal column

Primary Neoplasm	No.	%
Breast	576	21
Lung	377	14
Myeloma	245	9
Prostate	211	7.5
Lymphoma	180	6.5
Kidney	154	5.5
Gastrointestinal	134	5
Thyroid	73	2.5
Miscellaneous	798	29
Total	2,748	

Reproduced with permission from McLain RF, Weinstein JN: Tumors of the spine. *Semin Spin Surg* 1990;2:157–180.

Approximately 60% of spinal-column metastases arise from one of four primary tumor types: breast, lung, prostate, or lymphoreticular malignancies, including lymphoma and myeloma (Table 2). Although rarely mentioned in reviews of metastatic disease, tumors of the gastrointestinal system result in a considerable number of spinal metastases.

The clinical behavior of the primary tumor dictates the prevalence of its metastases and ultimately determines their clinical importance for each patient. Hence, patients with breast and prostate carcinoma have prolonged survivals and require treatment for their spinal metastases. Patients with pulmonary malignancies may succumb so rapidly that little more than supportive care can be offered. Those with gastrointestinal carcinoma, which tends to involve the liver and lungs long before it involves the spine, often die before their spinal lesions become apparent clinically.

In most patients, the primary cancer has been diagnosed months or years before symptoms of spinal involvement become apparent.[15,16,18–26] Regardless of how remote the history may be, metastatic disease must be suspected whenever symptoms develop in a patient with a previous malignancy.

Table 3
Survival in solitary plasmacytomas of the spine: Characteristics of patients with multiple myeloma, solitary plasmacytoma of bone, and solitary plasmacytoma of the spine

Tumor	5-Year Survival %	% Male	Age at Presentation		Disease-Free Interval (Months)	Overall Survival (Months)
			Male	Female		
Multiple myeloma	18	51	60	61	—	24
Solitary plasmacytoma of bone	35	68	50	55	78	86
Solitary plasmacytoma of the spine	60	74	51	57	76	92

Reproduced with permission from McLain, RF, Weinstein JN: Solitary plasmacytomas of the spine: A review of 84 cases. *J Spinal Disorders* 1989;2:69–74.

Patients with metastatic disease are, by definition, systemically ill. Those receiving chemotherapy may be immunosuppressed and thrombocytopenic. Preoperative renal function should be assessed and serum calcium and phosphorus followed serially to avoid the development of malignant hypercalcemia.[7] Whenever possible, hematologic abnormalities should be corrected and the patient's overall fitness maximized before surgery is attempted. In patients who remain severely compromised, the risk of surgical mortality must be weighed carefully against the risks of incapacitating pain, paralysis, and a shortened life expectancy if surgical treatment is withheld.

Probably the most important determinant of the course of metastatic disease is the tumor type. Although sex, age, location, and interval between diagnosis of disease and appearance of metastases have all been correlated with differences in outcome, none of these is independent of tumor type.

Although radiotherapy remains the most reasonable treatment option for many patients, significant differences in radiosensitivity exist between different tumor types and between different clones of the same tumor type. Prostatic and lymphoreticular tumors are usually quite radiosensitive, and excellent clinical results can be obtained in most patients.[27-29] Metastases from breast carcinoma are usually responsive to irradiation, but as many as 30% of these patients demonstrate no clinical response with irradiation alone.[29,30] Gastrointestinal and renal tumors often prove radioresistant. The neurologic status of the patient at the time of presentation dictates the likely outcome following radiotherapy. Although 70% of patients who are ambulatory will retain that function following radiotherapy, it is rare for patients who have lost this ability to regain it through irradiation alone.[29]

Surgical treatment of metastatic disease provides good to excellent pain relief in 80% to 95% of patients.[31,32] In selected cases, with appropriate decompressions, there is also a high likelihood of restoring neurologic function. In one series, 40% of patients treated with posterior decompression and 75% of those treated with anterior decompression had significant neurologic improvement.[32]

Malignant Multiple Myeloma and Solitary Plasmacytoma

Most investigators today would consider multiple myeloma and solitary plasmacytoma two manifestations in a continuum of B-cell lymphoproliferative diseases. Because the natural history of these two lesions differs so significantly, the clinical distinction between solitary plasmacytoma and multiple myeloma remains pertinent.

True solitary plasmacytoma is a rare entity comprising only 3% of all plasma cell neoplasms.[33] Though the course of multiple myeloma is usually rapidly progressive and lethal, patients with solitary plasmacytoma may have prolonged survival rates despite eventual progression.[34] Three quarters of patients with multiple myeloma involving the spinal column die within one year of their diagnosis, and most die within four years,[34] but the five-year survival rate in spinal solitary plasmacytoma is roughly 60% (Table 3). Survival periods of 20 years and more have been reported.[12,34,36]

The treatment of choice for solitary plasmacytoma and multiple myeloma is radiation. Because of the radiosensitivity of this tumor, surgical treatment has less influence in determining outcome than it does in other tumor types. We have not seen any case of onset or progression of neurologic deficit during radiotherapy and do not recommend surgical intervention unless cord compression or spinal instability is present. Dissemination of myeloma may occur after many years of disease-free survival, and routine follow-up is indicated for an indefinite period.

Lymphoma

Lymphoma can be a systemic disease with skeletal manifestations, or it can be an isolated bony tumor or reticulum cell sarcoma. Because some investigators consider the lesion a metastatic lesion, it is not consistently included in reviews of primary bone tumors. Whether considered primary or metastatic, lymphomas account for a large number of spinal neoplasms requiring treatment.

Children's Tumors

Tumors of the immature spine differ in type from those seen in adults, particularly in terms of the malignant lesions. Nearly 70% of the primary bone tumors observed in children are benign. Osteoid osteomas and osteoblastomas, osteochondromas, and aneurysmal bone cysts account for over 40% of all primary spinal lesions observed in children. Ewing's sarcoma is the most common primary malignancy, but it is more commonly a metastatic lesion (Table 4).[10] Metastatic or contiguous spread are most common from neuroblastoma, embryonal carcinoma, and sarcoma. Neuroblastoma alone accounts for between 20% and 30% of all pediatric spine tumors and for 51% of the metastases seen.[37-39] These are highly aggressive lesions and have a poor prognosis regardless of treatment.

Leukemia must also be considered in the differential of children's back pain and vertebral collapse.[40] Children with leukemia manifest a variety of nonspecific constitutional symptoms—lethargy, anemia, and fever—and the correct diagnosis is often difficult to make. Radiographs may be normal or they may show focal lytic lesions, occasional sclerotic lesions, or isolated periosteal reactions. Results of radionuclide scans are unreliable in patients with leukemia.[41]

Aside from the usual complexities of treating the neoplasm itself, the added dimension in the care of children's tumors is the management of spinal deformities that can develop as a result of treatment. Progressive deformity may occur for any of a number of reasons. As in adults, deformity can result from structural deficiencies caused by the erosion of bone, either by tumor or by aggressive surgical resection. However, these deformities may be more severe or progressive in children, particularly in postlaminectomy kyphosis and in the thoracic spine. The younger the child at the time of laminectomy, the more severe the eventual deformity is likely to be.[37] Irradiation and rib resection are well-known factors in the development of iatrogenic scoliosis. Deformity following congenital or acquired paraplegia is also common and tends to be more severe in children who have an earlier onset of paralysis and higher levels of cord injury. Surgical management of these patients must anticipate the later development of deformity and seek to minimize it. Patients in whom deformity is certain must be identified early on and treatment must be instituted to halt progression.

Spinal Cord Compression

Spinal cord compression, which occurs in 5% to 20% of patients who have widespread cancer,[42,43] results from one of four processes: (1) direct compression by an enlarging soft-tissue mass; (2) fracture and retropulsion of bony fragments into the canal; (3) severe

Table 4

Primary tumors of the pediatric spine: Primary bone tumors found in the spinal column in 31 patients younger than 18 years of age

Tumor	No.
Benign	
Osteoblastoma	4
Osteochondroma	4
Aneurysmal bone cyst	4
Giant cell tumor	3
Eosinophilic granuloma	2
Osteoid osteoma	2
Hemangioma	1
Angiolipoma	1
Malignant	
Ewing's sarcoma	3
Chordoma	1
Osteosarcoma	1
Malignant giant cell tumor	1
Chondrosarcoma	1
Others	3

Reproduced with permission from Weinstein JN, McLain RF: Primary tumors of the spine. *Spine* 1987;12:843–851.

kyphosis following vertebral collapse; or (4) intradural metastases.[44] The most common cause of cord compression is mechanical pressure, either from tumor tissue or from bone extruded from the collapsing vertebral body.[9] Because of the flexion moment acting on the vertebrae of the thoracic spine, erosion causes the vertebral body to collapse into kyphosis, extruding tumor tissue and the posterior vertebral cortex dorsally into the spinal canal. Direct compression of the cord may occur without vertebral erosion if the tumor extends directly into the canal.

Recognition of spinal cord compression is critical to providing early intervention and preventing progressive and permanent neurologic injury.[45] The most prominent symptoms are back pain, radicular or "girdle" pain, weakness in the lower limbs, sensory loss, and finally, loss of sphincter control. Although nearly all patients experience some localized back pain, patients with cervical and lumbosacral lesions are also likely to experience radicular pain.

The prognosis for neurologic outcome is determined by (1) tumor biology, (2) pretreatment neurologic status, and (3) the location of the tumor within the spinal canal.[43] The inherent nature of any neoplasm determines its biologic behavior, dictating which will have slow or rapid growth, which will be invasive, and which will produce metastases. Although metastatic lesions usually demonstrate behavior similar to their parent lesions, this is not always true; some metastases may be far more invasive or rapid-growing than the primary lesions from which they come. It is this biologic behavior that determines the likelihood of spinal cord compression; rapid expansion or vertebral erosion and fracture result in acute cord compression and a poorer prognosis.

Table 5
Neurologic recovery in cord decompression: Maintenance and recovery of neurologic function in patients treated surgically for cord compression due to metastatic or primary spinal tumor

Author	No. of Patients	% Improvement	% Satisfactory Outcome
Anterior decompression			
Manabe[48]	28	82	89
Harrington[46]	77	84	73
Kostuik[32]	70	73	84
Sundaresan[51]	160	80	78
Fidler[47]	17	73	78
Siegal[26]	75	80	80
Posterior decompression			
Kostuik[32]	30	36	37
Sherman[50]	149	27	48
Siegal[26]	25	39	39
Nather[49]	42	13	29
Gilbert[15]	65	45	46
White[52]	226	38	37
Hall[45]	123	30	29
Wright[53]	86	35	33

Reproduced with permission from McLain RF, Weinstein JN: Tumors of the spine. *Semin Spine Surg* 1990;2:157–180.

The pretreatment neurologic status clearly correlates with posttreatment outcome in terms of the likelihood and extent of recovery of ambulatory function and sphincter control. Between 60% and 95% of the patients still walking at the time of diagnosis will retain that ability following treatment, but only 35% to 65% of paraparetic patients and fewer than 30% of paraplegic patients will regain ambulation.[14,32,45–49] The rate of progression of the neurologic deficit also has prognostic significance. If a patient progresses from the earliest onset of symptoms to a major deficit in less than 24 hours, the prognosis for recovery is poor irrespective of treatment. Conversely, a lesion that has slowly evolved over a course of months has a far more favorable prognosis for recovery following treatment.[9]

The location of the neoplasm within the vertebral body or spinal canal determines the symptoms and signs produced, and dictates the surgical approach required for treatment. Cord compression occurs most commonly in the thoracic region of the spine, where the cord is relatively large with respect to the vertebral canal. As the mechanical demands on the vertebral elements differ from anterior to posterior, location also has value in predicting which lesions will lead to vertebral collapse and segmental instability. For both of these reasons, tumors of the anterior and middle columns are associated with more frequent and more profound neurologic injury.

Cord decompression can provide dramatic improvement in neurologic function even in advanced deficits, depending on the rate of progression, the interval from paralysis to treatment, and the surgical approach. Radiation therapy has been the traditional standard for treatment of metastatic cord impingement, with surgical decompression usually consisting of a laminectomy and removal of whatever tumor could be reached laterally or through the pedicle. Although laminectomy was sometimes combined with posterior stabilization, and frequently combined with radiotherapy, the results were no better than those from radiotherapy alone and often resulted in iatrogenic instability.[9,15,50] Constans and associates[42] reported that 46% of patients treated with laminectomy and radiotherapy showed improved neurologic function, compared with 49% of patients treated with radiotherapy alone. Still, fewer than half the patients treated by either method had a satisfactory result in terms of neurologic function. The results of surgical decompression through the anterior approach have been more favorable, and now offer a genuine improvement over treatment by radiotherapy alone. Table 5 shows the results of anterior and posterior decompressions documented in a number of studies.

Surgical Approaches and Treatment

General

Indications for surgical treatment have been outlined by a number of different investigators. Gilbert and associates[15] and Siegal and Siegal[54] suggested that decompressive laminectomy was indicated in metastatic disease when (1) the nature of the primary tumor was not known or the diagnosis was in doubt; (2) when tumor growth recurred following maximum radiotherapy to that segment; and (3) when symptoms progressed inexorably during radiotherapy treatments. With the acceptance of more aggressive surgical methods, these indications have been expanded; recently investigators have recommended surgical intervention in instances of (1) an isolated primary or metastatic lesion or a solitary site of relapse; (2) pathologic fracture or deformity producing neurologic symptoms or pain; (3) radioresistant tumors—metastatic or primary; and (4) segmental instability following radiotherapy.[9,10,32,43,48,51,55] All of these indications presume a patient who is healthy enough to survive surgery, but they are not incumbent on a long-term expected survival. Any patient with expectations of surviving six weeks or longer and who is not hopelessly bedridden should be considered for surgery.

There are a number of different surgical approaches available to the spine surgeon and variations of each have been described (Table 6). Choosing the correct approach for the given situation is, perhaps, the most important step in treating these conditions.

Resection

Although some investigators have advised that attempts at surgical extirpation are fruitless and should not be attempted,[56] it is clear from others[10,16,57,58] that

Table 6
Surgical approaches to spinal neoplasms

Level	Anterior	Posterior
Cervical		
C1-2	Transoral	Midline posterior
C1-T2	Anterolateral Transsternal	Posterolateral
Thoracic	Thoracotomy	Midline posterior Costotransversectomy
Thoracolumbar		
T11-L2	Thoracoabdominal 10th to 12th rib resection, detachment of diaphragm	Midline posterior Posterolateral
Lumbar	Retroperitoneal Transabdominal	Midline posterior

Reproduced with permission from McLain RF, Weinstein JN: Tumors of the spine. *Semin Spine Surg* 1990;2:157–180.

the ability to completely resect the primary tumor plays a role in overall patient survival and in recovery and maintenance of neurologic function. Although there are no true anatomic compartments in the spinal column, anatomic structures do provide natural planes for dissection and excision. The vertebral body, anterior and posterior longitudinal ligaments, the intervertebral disks, and the dura may all be resected to avoid leaving residual tumor behind. Neural, muscular, and vascular structures may all be sacrificed to obtain an adequate surgical margin. Such an aggressive approach is justified. As in extremity surgery, extirpation provides the best prognosis for local control and cure of the disease.

The vertebral body may be divided into four zones, I–IV. Tumor extension is designated as A,B,C for (A) intraosseous, (B) extraosseous, and (C) distant tumor spread (Fig. 1).[59] Zone IA includes the spinous process to the pars intraarticularis and the inferior facets. Zone IIA includes the superior articular facet, the transverse process, and the pedicle from the level of the pars to its junction with the vertebral body. Zone IIIA includes the anterior three fourths of the vertebral body, and zone IVA designates involvement of the posterior one fourth of the body, that segment immediately anterior to the cord. Zones IB to IVB are the extraosseous ex-

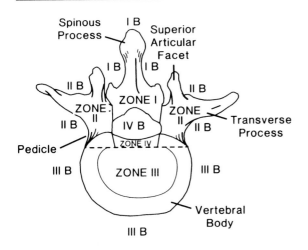

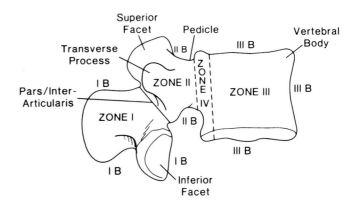

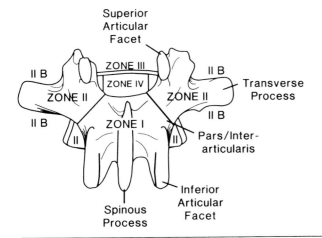

Fig. 1 **Top left,** Vertebral cross-section at the lumbar level depicting the borders of resection zone I A, II A, III A, and IV A. **Top right,** Lateral drawing. **Bottom,** Posterior drawing demonstrating anatomic depiction of zones I A through IV A. Tumors eroding through adjoining cortex should be classed according to their anatomic locations as stage B lesions. (Reproduced with permission from Weinstein JN: Spinal tumors, in Weinstein JN, Wiesel S (eds): *The Lumbar Spine.* Philadelphia, WB Saunders, 1990, pp 741–759.)

Table 7
Surgical approach by zone and potential margin of resection

Zone	Procedure for Excision	Potential Margin
IA* (B, C)	Posterior	Wide
IIA* (B, C)	Posterior	Wide/marginal
IIIA* (B, C)	Anterior	Wide/marginal
IVA* (B, C)	Anterior/posterior	Wide/intralesional

*The extent of extraosseous soft tissue (nerve, vessel, muscle) involvement may limit the potential margin of excision for zones I to IV, B and C lesions. (Reproduced with permission from McLain RF, Weinstein JN: Tumors of the spine. *Semin Spine Surg* 1990;2:157–180.)

tensions of tumor beyond the boundaries of the cortical bone, and zones IC to IVC designate associated regional or distant metastatic involvement. Surgical outcome is determined by the zone involved, by the extent of the local or distant tumor spread, by the type of tumor, and by its grade (Table 7).

Complete radiographic evaluation, including computed tomography and magnetic resonance imaging, allows accurate determination of the tumor location and extension and will allow a more informed prediction of the tumor's grade if not its actual tissue type.

It is important to determine accurately the most likely tumor type before undertaking surgery. Overtreatment of benign disease can be nearly as disastrous as undertreatment of malignancy. We have developed an algorithm for the evaluation of patients presenting for the first time with a spine lesion (Fig. 2).

In many locally aggressive or malignant tumors, it is essential to obtain the widest margin possible. An adequate margin can be extremely difficult to obtain in type B lesions. IB to IVB lesions of the lumbosacral or cervical regions may not be resectable without producing serious neurologic deficits. In these cases, surgery is marginal at best and usually intralesional. The decision to attempt a wide or radical resection in these cases must be weighed against the risk.

The surgical approach selected must provide sufficient access both for tumor excision and for stabilization of the spine thereafter. If both operations cannot be performed through the same incision, the surgeon must plan for a combined approach (Fig. 3). Zone I lesions are best approached posteriorly, and the extent of excision must be based on any soft-tissue extension seen on preoperative studies. Zone II lesions are also more easily excised through a posterior or posterolateral approach[60] and should be similarly stabilized.

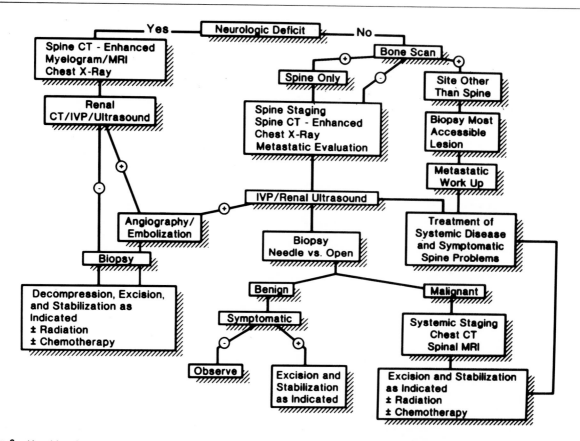

Fig. 2 Algorithm demonstrating a systematic approach to tumors of the spine. (Reproduced with permission from Weinstein JN: Spinal tumors, in Weinstein JN, Wiesel S (eds): *The Lumbar Spine*. Philadelphia, WB Saunders, 1990, pp 741–759.)

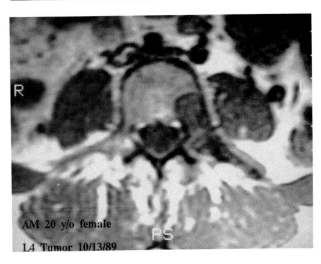
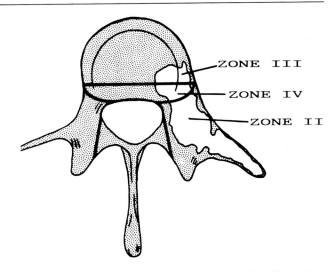

Fig. 3 **Left,** CT scan of an L3 aneurysmal bone cyst involving the vertebral body, pedicle, and transverse process. **Right,** Schematic demonstrating resection zones involved by this aneurysmal bone cyst showing involvement of zones II, III, and IV without soft-tissue extension. (Reproduced with permission from Weinstein JN: Spinal tumors, in Weinstein JN, Wiesel S (eds): *The Lumbar Spine*. Philadelphia, WB Saunders, 1990, pp 741–759.)

Once laminectomy and excision are performed, the resulting tensile loads are best minimized through posterior instrumentation of the surgeon's choice with autologous bone graft.

Lesions in zone III should be approached anteriorly. Adequate resection of type A lesions can usually be obtained throughout the spinal column, but type B lesions should be analyzed carefully before surgery to anticipate invasion or adherence to critical adjacent structures. Reconstruction can be performed with or without internal fixation, depending on the extent of the resection and the inherent stability of the residual elements.

Zone IV lesions require a combined anterior and posterior surgical approach. These lesions, which involve the most inaccessible region of the vertebral body, are the most difficult lesions to reconstruct. Zones I, II, and/or III must be crossed at some point to provide access to zone IV lesions, and frequently more than one zone may be involved with tumor. Complete excision can be obtained through vertebrectomy, essentially separating zone II from zone III through combined approaches. In such cases both anterior and posterior stabilization are necessary (Fig. 4).

Metastatic Lesions

In situations where conservative therapy of a metastatic focus is not feasible or has proven ineffective, surgical decompression is indicated. In lesions of the cervical spine above the level of C-3, a posterior approach is advocated. In all other regions laminectomy should be restricted to those cases where the site of compression has been shown to be strictly posterior.[47] An anterior approach with decompression and meth-

ylmethacrylate stabilization is generally recommended for metastatic lesions involving a single level or two, but Kostuik and associates[32,61] prefer a posterolateral approach to lesions involving multiple adjacent levels and perform a posterolateral decompression followed by segmental fixation and sublaminar wiring, with methylmethacrylate augmentation as needed. In contrast, Harrington[62] has reported good results with anterior stabilization using longitudinal rods and methylmethacrylate in lesions involving up to seven vertebral levels.

Renal tumors present a special challenge to the surgical oncologist; patients frequently present with osseous metastases at the time of initial diagnosis, and demonstrate a highly variable course in terms of survival (Fig. 5).[63,64] Sundaresan and associates[65] found that patients undergoing complete resection of tumor survived longer than those treated with radiotherapy alone. Significant neurologic improvement was seen in 70% of surgical patients compared to 45% of radiated patients.[64] Preoperative angiography and embolization may prove lifesaving in these patients, and two courses of embolization are sometimes necessary to identify all of the major vessels feeding the lesion.

Posterior Approach

Whether laminectomy provides patients who have cord compression with any significant benefit beyond that provided by radiotherapy is debatable.[15,16,66] Although Constans and associates[42] showed some improvement in results using laminectomy with radiotherapy, Gilbert and associates[15] showed very little difference between patients treated with radiotherapy alone and those treated with both laminectomy and

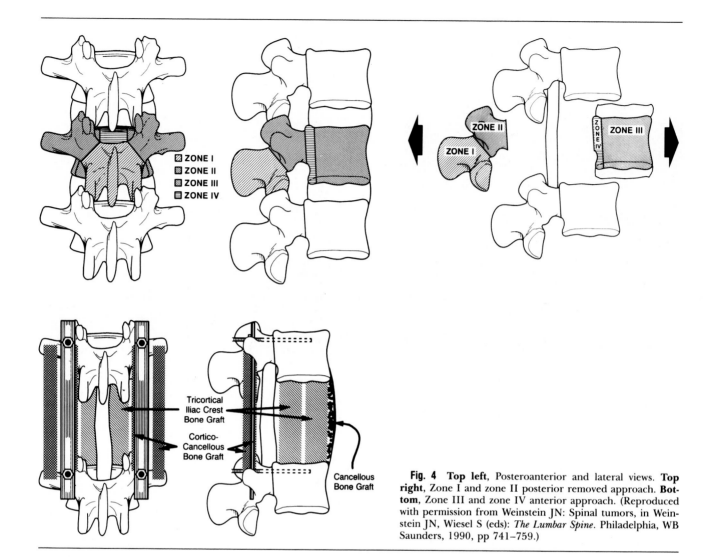

Tricortical
Iliac Crest
Bone Graft

Cortico-
Cancellous
Bone Graft

Cancellous
Bone Graft

ZONE I
ZONE II
ZONE III
ZONE IV

ZONE II
ZONE I
ZONE IV
ZONE III

Fig. 4   Top left, Posteroanterior and lateral views. **Top right,** Zone I and zone II posterior removed approach. **Bottom,** Zone III and zone IV anterior approach. (Reproduced with permission from Weinstein JN: Spinal tumors, in Weinstein JN, Wiesel S (eds): *The Lumbar Spine*. Philadelphia, WB Saunders, 1990, pp 741–759.)

radiation. The proportion of satisfactory outcomes was less than 50% in each case.

Although comparison of data for anterior and posterior approaches is made difficult by the lack of continuity in reported outcome measures, the trend seen in such a comparison is still quite clear (Table 5). Of 746 patients treated with posterior decompression only, 38% had a satisfactory neurologic outcome. In those with a severe deficit, results were even poorer. Although stabilization significantly improved the pain relief and maintenance of neurologic function relative to laminectomy alone, the overall results were still somewhat disappointing.[50]

Anterior Approach

Anterior decompression has been used successfully to treat cord compression caused by a variety of different lesions, including fracture, neoplasm, infection, and congenital deformity. Improvement in neurologic function has been most dramatic in those with acute compression, as seen in fracture, infection, and tumor.

Significant neurologic improvement was documented in 75% to 93% of patients decompressed anteriorly for metastatic disease.[47,62,67]

In one of the few prospective studies of surgical decompression of epidural tumors, Siegal and Siegal[54] chose an anterior approach and decompression for lesions located ventral to the cord and a posterior laminectomy for lesions located dorsally. Only 40% of patients treated with laminectomy retained or regained the ability to walk, as opposed to 80% of the vertebrectomy patients. Of 13 paraplegic patients treated by anterior decompression, all but one improved at least one grade in neurologic function, whereas five of 25 patients treated with laminectomy actually deteriorated as a result of treatment. The operative mortality was similar for both approaches, but postoperative complications were far more frequent in the laminectomy group, usually as a result of poor wound healing after operations performed through irradiated tissue.[54] In 427 cases of anterior decompression in which objective grading of neurologic recovery was reported,

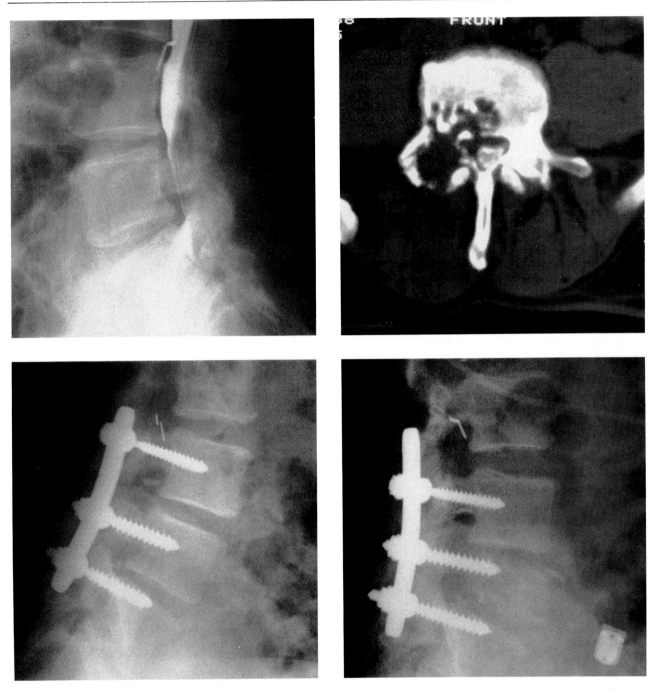

Fig. 5   Renal cell carcinoma of the L4 vertebral body. **Top left**, Lateral myelogram demonstrating cord compression secondary to soft-tissue mass. Vertebral destruction cannot be appreciated at this time. **Top right**, CT scan of the L4 vertebral body demonstrating lytic lesion involving the vertebral body, pedicle, and lamina and displacing the thecal sac. **Bottom left**, Patient underwent embolization, posterior decompression, and VSP plating. Neurologic symptoms improved significantly. **Bottom right**, Thirteen months postoperatively, the patient remains neurologically intact with some back pain. Lateral roentgenogram demonstrates extensive destruction of the vertebral body secondary to progression of the tumor. (Reproduced with permission from McLain RF, Weinstein JN: Tumors of spine. *Semin Spine Surg* 1990;2:157–180.

79% had a significant improvement in grade and 77% obtained a satisfactory outcome: independent ambulation and intact autonomic function. These results are significantly better than those seen with posterior decompression.

Harrington[46] reported an estimated blood loss of between 200 and 550 ml for anterior decompressions, depending on level. The mean estimated blood loss for combined anterior and posterior procedures was considerably greater, at 2,250 ml. Operative time for Harrington's patients was just less than 2.5 hours for cervical lesions and just under four hours for thoracic and thoracolumbar lesions.[46]

Reconstruction

Whether a tumor is resected posteriorly or anteriorly, posterior stabilization is frequently indicated to prevent early, progressive deformity and to allow incorporation of bone graft. A wide variety of instrumentation systems have been used successfully to provide posterior fixation, and the surgeon must choose his hardware to meet the challenges of each individual case.

Harrington distraction and compression rods have been used for many years to stabilize lesions of the thoracic and lumbar spine. Distraction rods are sufficient to stabilize the vertebral column following laminectomy or in cases of compression fracture. When both the anterior and middle columns are involved, as is seen in extensive vertebral fracture or erosion, the three point fixation of the Harrington system cannot counter the excessive bending and tension loads and is at risk for failure.[68-70] Although the Harrington system can restore proper alignment and in some cases restore appropriate vertebral heights to the spinal elements, retropulsed vertebral fragments responsible for cord impingement are not reduced. Even with an intact posterior longitudinal ligament, reduction of the fracture is associated with a 25% residual stenosis.[69]

Stabilization with Luque instrumentation and sublaminar wiring has been successful in cervical, thoracic, and lumbar segments. Although there are risks involved in passing sublaminar wires, this technique may provide better fixation than the Harrington system in soft bone.[71,72] Wires may be passed over the transverse processes or throughout the neural foramina at operated segments.[55]

Regardless of the technique used, posterior instrumentation alone cannot provide a stable construct in all cases. When the anterior and middle columns of the spine have already been compromised by extensive vertebral collapse,[72] laminectomy is likely to result in severe postoperative instability. These patients are placed at high risk for iatrogenic cord injury and paraplegia. Even when a solid fusion is obtained posteriorly, motion of the anterior elements may still occur without reconstruction of the anterior and middle columns (Fig. 6). Despite rigid fixation of the posterior elements there can be substantial motion anteriorly in response to physiologic compression and bending loads.[68] There is, furthermore, a higher complication rate when methylmethacrylate is used with posterior rather than anterior stabilization.[73] Of 24 complications reported by McAfee and associates,[74] only five occurred after anterior stabilization using methylmethacrylate.

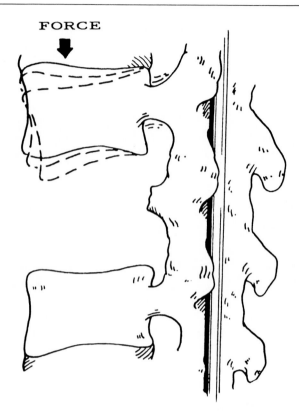

Fig. 6 Despite solid fixation or fusion of the posterior elements, significant motion of the anterior construct can occur if no anterior stabilization has been provided. Significant bending stresses applied anteriorly can result in failure of the posterior construct, fracture of the pedicle, or failure of an inadequate construct. (Reproduced with permission from McLain RF, Weinstein JN: Tumors of spine. *Semin Spine Surg* 1990;2:157–180.)

Because of the increased incidence of infection and wound breakdown associated with posterior instrumentation, Harrington[46] recommended posterior stabilization only when (1) combined anterior and posterior decompression is necessary; (2) lengthy anterior fixation is inadequate to restore stability; (3) posterior instability is produced by tumor lysis of posterior elements; and/or (4) the lesion is located distal to the L3 vertebral body.

A number of techniques of anterior stabilization have been developed. Some of these rely on methylmethacrylate or other synthetic spacers. Others use bone graft in anticipation of a solid arthrodesis. Bone grafting is clearly favored in the treatment of benign or slow-growing tumors, where patient survival is expected to be measured in years. In metastatic lesions, bone graft is commonly augmented by internal fixation and a methylmethacrylate construct (Fig. 7). Methylmethacrylate functions as an adjunct to stabilization, providing a temporary internal splint in anticipation of eventual bony arthrodesis. If arthrodesis is not obtained, it is only a matter of time before the methacrylate construct fails. Only patients with a very limited life expectancy

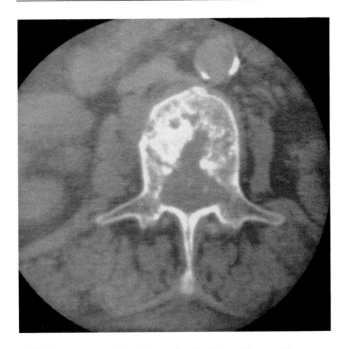

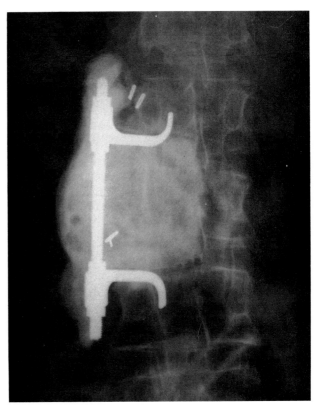

Fig. 7 Chordoma of the L2 vertebral body in a 77-year-old woman. **Left**, CT scan demonstrating erosion of the vertebral body with extension into the spinal canal. **Right**, Anteroposterior roentgenogram following hemivertebrectomy and anterior stabilization with polymethylmethacrylate augmentation. Patient was neurologically intact and pain free postoperatively. (Reproduced with permission from McLain RF, Weinstein JN: Tumors of spine. *Semin Spine Surg* 1990;2:157–180.)

are candidates for methacrylate fixation without bone grafting.[74]

Used in anterior reconstructions where, functioning as a spacer, it is primarily exposed to compressive loads, methylmethacrylate proves quite resilient and dependable.[68] Reinforcing methacrylate with wire or wire mesh increases its tensile strength and improves its ability to withstand bending loads, particularly when used in posterior stabilizations. Longitudinal Steinmann pins used anteriorly enhance both the bending resistance of the construct and its fixation to the adjacent vertebral bodies.[51] Seigal and associates[26] have advocated the use of Harrington distraction rods, and more recently, Moe sacral hooks and threaded rods to obtain anterior purchase. Harrington[9,62] has used Knodt rods for several years for the same purpose.

In reconstructing the vertebral body with methylmethacrylate, care must be taken to avoid contact of the cement with the dural sac posteriorly. Cement used in the dough phase allows better control of placement, and interposing a sheet of gelfoam anterior to the dural elements will further shield them.[75] During polymerization, a steady flow of saline irrigation will minimize the transmission of heat to surrounding tissues.

Because of problems with fixation and cord impingement, some authors have recommended against the use

of methylmethacrylate in patients whose life expectancy is greater than one year.[73] On the other hand, biomechanical studies in postmortem specimens have shown excellent stability in the cervical spine as long as seven years after fixation with methacrylate.[76] The key to longevity in methylmethacrylate fixation is adequate augmentation with bone graft.

Summary

The prognosis for survival has improved dramatically for cancer patients over the past three decades. Advances in systemic therapy have prolonged survival even in those who cannot be cured. The importance of managing spinal column disease and protecting the spinal cord has subsequently been amplified. Almost any patient presenting with detectable neurologic function and enough physical reserve to withstand an operation will benefit from a spinal stabilization, pain relief, and neural decompression; there are few exceptions.

Advances in surgical technique and biomaterials have not only improved survival and functional outcome, they have diminished many of the postoperative complications that plagued earlier treatment techniques. Methods of preventing or correcting iatrogenic deformity have improved outcome. Newer fixation techniques promise to eliminate many of the causes of hardware and fixation failure previously seen.

Improved medical management, antibiotics, and preoperative planning, along with techniques of preoperative embolization and early postoperative mobilization have made surgical management much less risky. Vertebrectomy, considered a last alternative in the past, is now coming to be seen as the conservative approach to tumor management in many situations.

Appropriate surgical treatment can have a dramatic impact on function and outcome in patients with tumors of the spinal column, and should never be dismissed as an option without serious consideration. Advances in fixation systems, local and systemic therapy, and in our understanding of the biology of cancer promise even greater improvements for the future.

References

1. Fidler I, Gersten D, Hart I: The biology of cancer invasion and metastasis. *Ad Cancer Res* 1978;28:149–250.
2. Urteage O, Pack GT: On the antiquity of melanoma. *Cancer* 1966;19:607–610
3. Wells C: Ancient Egyptian pathology. *J Laryngol Otol* 1963;77:261–265.
4. Recamier JCA: Recherches sur la traitment du cancer par la compression simple ou combine, cum l'historie generale de la meme maladie. Paris, Chez Gabon Libraire-Editeur, 1829.
5. Paget S: The distribution of secondary growths in cancer of the breast. *Lancet* 1889;1:571–573.
6. Ewing J: *Neoplastic Disease: A Treatise on Tumors*, ed 3. Philadelphia, WB Saunders, 1928.
7. Harrington KD: *Orthopaedic Management of Metastatic Bone Disease*. St. Louis, CV Mosby, 1988, pp 309–383.
8. Jaffe HL: *Tumors and Tumorous Conditions of the Bones and Joints.* Philadelphia, Lea & Febiger, 1958.
9. Harrington KD: Metastatic disease of the spine. *J Bone Joint Surg* 1986;68A:1110–1115.
10. Weinstein JN, McLain RF: Primary tumors of the spine. *Spine* 1987;12:843–851.
11. Sim FH, Dahlin DC, Stauffer RN, et al: Primary bone tumors simulating lumbar disc syndrome. *Spine* 1977;2:65–74.
12. Keim HA, Reina EG: Osteoid-osteoma as a cause of scoliosis. *J Bone Joint Surg* 1975;57A:159–163.
13. Pettine KA, Klassen RA: Osteoid-osteoma and osteoblastoma of the spine. *J Bone Joint Surg* 1986;68A:354–361.
14. Black P: Spinal metastasis: Current status and recommended guidelines for management. *Neurosurgery* 1979;5:726–746.
15. Gilbert RW, Kim JH, Posner JB: Epidural spinal cord compression from metastatic tumor: Diagnosis and treatment. *Ann Neurol* 1978;3:40–51.
16. Shives TC, Dahlin DC, Sim FH, et al: Osteosarcoma of the spine. *J Bone Joint Surg* 1986;68A:660–668.
17. National Institute of Arthritis, Musculoskeletal, and Skin Diseases: *Osteoporosis: Cause, Treatment, Prevention*. Bethesda, MD, National Institutes of Health, Rev. May 1986. NIH Publication No. 86-226.
18. Edelstyn GA, Gillespie PJ, Grebbell FS: The radiological demonstration of osseous metastases: Experimental observations. *Clin Radiol* 1967;18:158–162.
19. Corcoran RJ, Thrall JH, Kyle RW, et al: Solitary abnormalities in bone scans of patients with extraosseous malignancies. *Radiology* 1976;121:663–667.
20. Citrin DL, Bessent RG, Greig WR: A comparison of the sensitivity and accuracy of the 99TCm-phosphate bone scan and skeletal radiograph in the diagnosis of bone metastases. *Clin Radiol* 1977;28:107–117.
21. Waxman AD: In favor: Bone scans are of sufficient accuracy and sensitivity to be part of the routine workup prior to definitive surgical treatment of breast cancer, in Van Scoy-Mosher MB (ed): *Medical Oncology: Controversies in Cancer Treatment*. Boston, GK Hall, 1981, pp 69–76.
22. Godersky JC, Smoker WRK, Knutzon R: Use of magnetic resonance imaging in the evaluation of metastatic spinal disease. *Neurosurgery* 1987;21:676–680.
23. Mirra JM: *Bone Tumors: Clinical, Radiologic, and Pathologic Correlations*. Philadelphia, Lea & Febiger, 1989, pp 31–33.
24. Springfield DS, Enneking WF, Neff JR, et al: Principles of tumor management, in Murray JA (ed): American Academy of Orthopaedic Surgeons *Instructional Course Lectures, XXXIII*. St. Louis, CV Mosby, 1984, pp 1–25.
25. Dahlin DC: *Bone Tumors: General Aspects and Data on 6,221 Cases*, ed 3. Springfield, IL, Charles Thomas, 1978.
26. Siegal T, Tiqva P, Siegal T: Vertebral body resection for epidural compression by malignant tumors: Results of forty-seven consecutive operative procedures. *J Bone Joint Surg* 1985;67A:375–382.
27. Bruckman JE, Bloomer WD: Management of spinal cord compression. *Semin Oncol* 1978;5:135–140.
28. Millburn L, Hibbs GG, Hendrickson FR: Treatment of spinal cord compression from metastatic carcinoma: Review of literature and presentation of a new method of treatment. *Cancer* 1968;21:447–452.
29. Tomita T, Galicich JH, Sundaresan N: Radiation therapy for spinal epidural metastases with complete block. *Acta Radiol [Oncol]* 1983;22:135–143.
30. Greenberg HS, Kim JH, Posner JB: Epidural spinal cord compression from metastatic tumor: Results with a new treatment protocol. *Ann Neurol* 1980;8:361–366.
31. O'Neil J, Gardner V, Armstrong G: Treatment of tumors of the thoracic and lumbar spinal column. *Clin Orthop* 1988;227:103–112.
32. Kostuik JP, Errico TJ, Gleason TF, et al: Spinal stabilization of vertebral column tumors. *Spine* 1988;13:250–256.
33. Corwin J, Lindberg RD: Solitary plasmacytoma of bone vs. extramedullary plasmacytoma and their relationship to multiple myeloma. *Cancer* 1979;43:1007–1013.
34. McLain RF, Weinstein JN: Solitary plasmacytomas of the spine: A review of 84 cases. *J Spinal Disorders* 1989;2:69–74.
35. Valderrama JA, Bullough PG: Solitary myeloma of the spine. *J Bone Joint Surg* 1968;50B:82–90.
36. Schajowicz F: *Tumors and Tumorlike Lesions of Bone and Joints*. New York, Springer-Verlag, 1981, pp 281–302.
37. Fraser RD, Paterson DC, Simpson DA: Orthopaedic aspects of spinal tumors in children. *J Bone Joint Surg* 1977;59B:143–151.
38. Leeson MC, Makley JT, Carter JR: Metastatic skeletal disease in the pediatric population. *J Pediatr Orthop* 1985;5:261–267.
39. Tachdjian MO, Matson DD: Orthopaedic aspects of intraspinal tumors in infants and children. *J Bone Joint Surg* 1965;47A:223–248.
40. Rogalsky RJ, Black GB, Reed MH: Orthopaedic manifestations of leukemia in children. *J Bone Joint Surg* 1986;68A:494–501.
41. Clausen N, Gøtze H, Pedersen A, et al: Skeletal scintigraphy and radiography at onset of acute lymphocytic leukemia in children. *Med Pediatr Oncol* 1983;11:291–296.
42. Constans JP, deDivitiis E, Donzelli R, et al: Spinal metastases with neurological manifestations: Review of 600 cases. *J Neurosurg* 1983;59:111–118.
43. Siegal T, Siegal T: Current considerations in the management of neoplastic spinal cord compression. *Spine* 1989;14:223–228.
44. Boland PJ, Lane JM, Sundaresan N: Metastatic disease of the spine. *Clin Orthop* 1982;169:95–102.

45. Hall AJ, Mackay NNS: The results of laminectomy for compression of the cord or cauda equina by extradural malignant tumour. *J Bone Joint Surg* 1973;55B:497–505.

46. Harrington KD: Anterior decompression and stabilization of the spine as a treatment for vertebral collapse and spinal cord compression from metastatic malignancy. *Clin Orthop* 1988;233:177–197.

47. Fidler MW: Anterior decompression and stabilisation of metastatic spinal fractures. *J Bone Joint Surg* 1986;68B:83–90.

48. Manabe S, Tateishi A, Abe M, et al: Surgical treatment of metastatic tumors of the spine. *Spine* 1989;14:41–47.

49. Nather A, Bose K: The results of decompression of cord or cauda equina compression from metastatic extradural tumors. *Clin Orthop* 1982;169:103–108.

50. Sherman RMP, Waddell JP: Laminectomy for metastatic epidural spinal cord tumors: Posterior stabilization, radiotheraphy, and preoperative assessment. *Clin Orthop* 1986;207:55–63.

51. Sundaresan N, Galicich JH, Lane JM, et al: Treatment of neoplastic epidural cord compression by vertebral body resection and stabilization. *J Neurosurg* 1985;63:676–684.

52. White WA, Patterson RH Jr, Bergland RM: Role of surgery in the treatment of spinal cord compression by metastatic neoplasm. *Cancer* 1971;27:558–561.

53. Wright RL: Malignant tumors in the spinal extradural space: Results of surgical treatment. *Ann Surg* 1963;157:227–231.

54. Siegal T, Siegal T: Surgical decompression of anterior and posterior malignant epidural tumors compressing the spinal cord: A prospective study. *Neurosurgery* 1985;17:424–432.

55. Flatley TJ, Anderson MH, Anast GT: Spinal instability due to malignant disease: Treatment by segmental spinal stabilization. *J Bone Joint Surg* 1984;66A:47–52.

56. Bohlman HH, Sachs BL, Carter JR, et al: Primary neoplasms of the cervical spine: Diagnosis and treatment of twenty-three patients. *J Bone Joint Surg* 1986;68A:483–494.

57. Stener B: Total spondylectomy in chondrosarcoma arising from the seventh thoracic vertebra. *J Bone Joint Surg* 1971;53B:288–295.

58. Stener B, Johnsen OE: Complete removal of three vertebrae for giant-cell tumour. *J Bone Joint Surg* 1971;53B:278–287.

59. Weinstein JN: Surgical approach to spine tumors. *Orthopedics* 1989;12:897–905.

60. Lesoin F, Rousseaux M, Lozes G, et al: Posterolateral approach to tumours of the dorsolumbar spine. *Acta Neurochir* 1986;81:40–44.

61. Kostuik JP: Anterior spinal cord decompression for lesions of the thoracic and lumbar spine, techniques, new methods of internal fixation results. *Spine* 1983;8:512–531.

62. Harrington KD: The use of methylmethacrylate for vertebral-body replacement and anterior stabilization of pathologic fracture-dislocation of the spine due to metastatic malignant disease. *J Bone Joint Surg* 1981;63A:36–46.

63. Skinner DG, Colvin RB, Vermillion CD, et al: Diagnosis and management of renal cell carcinoma: A clinical and pathologic study of 309 cases. *Cancer* 1971;28:1165–1177.

64. Saitoh H, Hida M, Nakamura K, et al: Metastatic processes and a potential indication of treatment for metastatic lesions of renal adenocarcinoma. *J Urol* 1982;128:916–918.

65. Sundaresan N, Scher H, DiGiacinto GV, et al: Surgical treatment of spinal cord compression in kidney cancer. *J Clin Oncol* 1986;4:1851–1856.

66. Nicholls PJ, Jarecky TW: The value of posterior decompression by laminectomy for malignant tumors of the spine. *Clin Orthop* 1985;201:210–213.

67. Johnson JR, Leatherman KD, Holt RT: Anterior decompression of the spinal cord for neurological deficit. *Spine* 1983;8:396–405.

68. Gertzbein SD, Macmichael D, Tile M: Harrington instrumentation as a method of fixation in fractures of the spine. *J Bone Joint Surg* 1982;64B:526–529.

69. White AA III, Panjabi MM: *Clinical Biomechanics of the Spine.* Philadelphia, JB Lippincott, 1978, pp 423–431.

70. Willén J, Lindahl S, Irstam L, et al: Unstable thoracolumbar fractures: A study by CT and conventional roentgenology of the reduction effect of Harrington instrumentation. *Spine* 1984;9:214–219.

71. Cybulski GR, Von Roenn KA, D'Angelo CM, et al: Luque rod stabilization for metastatic disease of the spine. *Surg Neurol* 1987;28:277–283.

72. DeWald RL, Bridwell KH, Prodromas C, et al: Reconstructive spinal surgery as palliation for metastatic malignancies of the spine. *Spine* 1985;10:21–26.

73. Denis F: The three column spine and its significance in the classification of acute thoracolumbar spine injuries. *Spine* 1983;8:817–831.

74. McAfee PC, Bohlman HH, Ducker T, et al: Failure of stabilization of the spine with methylmethacrylate: A retrospective analysis of twenty-four cases. *J Bone Joint Surg* 1986;68A:1145–1157.

75. Clark CR, Keggi KJ, Panjabi MM: Methylmethacrylate stabilization of the cervical spine. *J Bone Joint Surg* 1984;66A:40–46.

76. Dolin MG: Acute massive dural compression secondary to methylmethacrylate replacement of a tumorous lumbar vertebral body. *Spine* 1989;14:108–110.

Metastatic Bone Disease of the Pelvis and Femur

Franklin H. Sim, MD

Improvements in the oncologic management of patients with disseminated cancer have resulted in increased survival.[1,2] Because of this, orthopaedic surgeons are being called on more frequently to manage patients who have metastatic bone disease. The pelvis and femur are common sites for metastatic involvement.[3] The pelvis is the second most frequent site for osseous metastasis (after vertebral column); 40% of osseous metastases occur in the pelvis. The femur has the third highest incidence of osseous metastases, accounting for 25%. Moreover, the femur accounts for two-thirds of all long-bone pathologic fractures; most involve the proximal femur because of the high stresses in that region. Pathologic fractures of the hip most frequently involve the femoral neck (approximately one half). Twenty percent occur in the intertrochanteric region, and the remainder are in the subtrochanteric region.

The development of a pathologic fracture of the hip or femur is a catastrophic event. The major goal in the management of the patient is to relieve pain and to restore function and ambulation. Recognition of the full therapeutic potential of each situation is essential. This usually requires a team effort, with close cooperation among multidisciplinary groups. Careful attention to the patient's general health and correction of nutritional and metabolic problems are essential. It is important to recognize and manage hematopoietic suppression, particularly in patients who are considered for surgical treatment. Moreover, aggressive systemic treatment to control the basic neoplastic process has resulted in increased survival. The prime treatment modality to achieve local control of the tumor is radiotherapy, which provides effective pain relief for up to one year in 80% of patients.[4] After fixation of pathologic fractures, the entire component and preferably the entire bone are treated because this may help decrease the risk of metastatic disease developing in the adjacent bone, resulting in loss of fixation or a second pathologic fracture.

Nonsurgical Management

There is little role for conservative management of pathologic fractures of the hip and femur. At times, terminally ill patients and, occasionally, nonambulatory patients who are comfortable are treated nonsurgically. In a terminal patient, treatment might include simple support with pillows, Buck's traction,[5] or skeletal traction.[6] However, effective prolonged fracture immobilization by bracing is rarely successful in the debilitated patient, and the only means of nonsurgical treatment is bedrest. Effective prolonged fracture immobilization in bed is difficult to achieve and relief of pain requires large doses of narcotic analgesics.

Unstable fractures typically require a plaster hip spica cast to immobilize the limb sufficiently to allow transfer of the patient to and from the radiotherapy unit. In this circumstance, the morbidity from radiation is increased and the skin-sparing effect is lost because an electron buildup occurs as the beam traverses the cast.[7] However, the most compelling argument against conservative treatment is the development of significant medical complications that accompany bedrest and immobilization. Deleterious effects include decubitus ulcers, pneumonia, and urinary tract infections, as well as difficulty in nursing care. Two complications peculiar to systemic malignancy and enforced immobilization are the development of disseminated intravascular coagulopathy and malignant hypercalcemia. Therefore, if conservative treatment is elected, care must be taken to avoid the secondary complications associated with prolonged recumbency.

Surgical Management

General Considerations

Because of the problems associated with nonsurgical treatment, pathologic fractures of a major weightbearing bone, such as the hip or the femur, have been managed primarily by surgical techniques whenever possible. However, careful preoperative assessment is necessary to determine whether the patient's general condition is good enough to withstand the operation. Because guidelines cannot reliably predict whether an individual patient will survive, we favor surgical treatment whenever the patient's condition permits surgery. As mentioned, careful medical management of these high-risk patients is mandatory. Moreover, careful consideration as to the extent of bone destruction at the site of fracture is helpful in planning the procedure. In planning surgery for a lesion of the proximal femur, careful assessment of associated acetabular disease is important because of the high incidence of involvement in this area. For the patient with a femoral fracture, it is necessary to obtain a radiograph of the entire femur, so that if there are other lesions within the femur, they can be prophylactically fixed at the time of surgery. Moreover, bilateral involvement of the hips in many patients makes surgical intervention to restore stability and function even more necessary.

Management of pathologic fractures must be individualized. Surgical techniques vary depending on the location of the fracture, extent of bone destruction, and general condition and expected length of survival of the patient. Previously, many surgical methods failed because of the extensive bone destruction adjacent to the fracture.[8-10] Thus, the goals of the surgery were not achieved because fixation was not secure. However, much progress has been made in surgical management of pathologic fractures. Recent advances in the management of traumatic fractures as well as in reconstructive orthopaedic surgery and joint replacement have been applied to metastatic bone disease. As a result, patients now predictably benefit from secure fixation of the fracture or from joint replacement with a stable prosthesis. Moreover, in patients with extensive destruction, the adjuvant use of methylmethacrylate has been shown to enhance the stability of fixation.[1,11,12] When methylmethacrylate is used with an intramedullary device, greater fixation is achieved and improvement is noted in bending strength and rotational stability. When used to augment a nail-plate apparatus, there is improved fixation of the screws in the weakened bone as well as greater resistance to torsional stress. One of the earliest reports on the adjuvant use of methylmethacrylate in 97 Mayo Clinic cases showed the potential benefits of this technique.[13] Gitelis and associates[11] showed that methylmethacrylate aided in fracture stabilization in 99 consecutive hip fractures. Habermann and associates[12] also reported improved functional results and fewer failures of fixation devices in their series of 114 patients with pathologic fractures of the hip. There is good evidence that radiotherapy is not adversely affected by the presence of acrylic cement.[1]

Prophylactic Fixation

The benefits of prophylactically fixing pathologic lesions in high-stress areas, such as the hip and femur, that are prone to spontaneous fracture have been well documented.[14-17] Such prophylactic fixation lessens the surgical morbidity and decreases the hospitalization time. Moreover, it enhances the ability to preserve function and restore the patient's activity status.

Extensive invasion of metastatic cells alters the inherent mechanical properties of the bone. Pugh and associates[18] described the biomechanical changes that greatly decrease the ability of involved bone to support functional stresses, which are extremely high in the femur. Radiographic criteria can predict the probability of fractures of a lytic metastatic lesion, and the indications for prophylactic fixation have become more

clearly defined. The size of the lesion is an important consideration.[19] High-risk lesions include those that are greater than 2.5 cm in diameter. Moreover, Fidler[16] demonstrated that, if not prophylactically reinforced, a long-bone lesion involving at least 50% of the cortex had at least a 50% chance of spontaneous fracture. The worrisome finding of avulsion of the lesser trochanter suggests an imminent pathologic fracture in this region. Moreover, the type of lesion is an important consideration, particularly when there is pure lytic destruction. Lesions such as those of the lung and kidney, which result in extensive permeative destruction, have a high risk of subsequent fracture.[20] It it important to consider the initial hyperemic response to radiotherapy, which increases the risk of spontaneous fracture. Because of the high stresses in the hip and femur, the prophylactic surgical procedure should be done before radiotherapy is begun. Once prophylactic fixation has been achieved, radiotherapy can be completed without the risk of fracture. There is good evidence that radiotherapy is not adversely affected by the presence of acrylic cement[1] nor does it interfere with the stability of fixation.[21]

Specific Pathologic Fractures

There are individual considerations pertinent to the management of pathologic fractures in the pelvis and femur. Various techniques can be used, depending on the location and on the extent of bone destruction. The surgeon must be thoroughly familiar with the device being used as well as with the associated technical problems. In general, instead of relying on one standard internal fixation device, the surgeon should, in each case, choose a device that will provide the best fracture stability, depending on the individual circumstances.

Femoral Neck Fracture

There is general consensus that replacement arthroplasty is the procedure of choice for lesions in the femoral head and neck. Internal fixation has not been effective because the high loads applied to the hip result in failure of the apparatus in tumor-destroyed bone. Moreover, pathologic fractures of the femor neck, even undisplaced ones, almost never heal.[22,23]

Replacement arthroplasty has become a reliable and predictable technique for the management of pathologic fractures of the femoral neck. Lane and associates[24] reported excellent pain relief, improvement in function, and restoration of ambulation in 167 consecutive patients treated by endoprosthetic replacement. Currently, my colleagues and I favor an articulated endoprosthesis of a bipolar design for routine use, except for patients with extensive acetabular involvement, in which case we use total hip arthroplasty. Habermann and associates[12] recommended routine use of total hip arthroplasty because of the high incidence of acetabular involvement in metastatic disease. This view, however, does not appear to be generally favored. Harrington[23] reported less than 1% complication of migration of an endoprosthesis because of a weakened periacetabular bone. He also felt, however, that a total hip replacement was necessary if the acetabulum was grossly involved. If there is no palpable structural weakness of the acetabular articular cartilage, a bipolar proximal femoral endoprosthesis is used.

Whether a total hip replacement, femoral endoprosthesis, or a bipolar femoral prosthesis is used, a long-stem femoral component is useful to prophylactically reinforce the remaining proximal femur, particularly if there is any evidence of weakening by lytic metastasis (Fig. 1). Moreover, restoration of femoral length is critical to minimize leg-length discrepancy and to ensure hip joint stability.

Peritrochanteric Fractures

Fractures in the intertrochanteric area may be difficult to manage. Neoplastic destruction weakens the cortex and results in instability of the fracture.

The surgical repair of pathologic peritrochanteric fractures is controversial. Some surgeons advocate internal stabilization of the fracture using a combination compression hip screw and intramedullary methylmethacrylate; others prefer to use a femoral prosthesis. Internal fixation with a hip compression screw device is most commonly advocated. This technique can be used to preserve the hip when the integrity of the head and neck fragment allows secure fixation. However, the success of this procedure requires restoration of stability by reconstructing the medial cortical continuity with methylmethacrylate. The cement provides increased resistance to compression loads, enhancing the strength of the compression screw and methacrylate composite.

Use of the sliding hip screw and side plate appears adequate for the majority of these fractures and is technically straightforward. The technique for internal fixation is similar to that used in conventional fixation of hip fracture. There are different opinions as to whether the compression screw should be inserted before or after injection of the bone cement. Some surgeons have chosen to hollow out the femoral head and neck by drilling up to the subchondral bone. Cement of liquid consistency is placed in the defect, and a compression screw is placed in the cement. Advocates argue that the screw is thus embedded in cement rather than in bone of questionable integrity, and that the combination of screw threads and cement gives a better surface area of contact for the fixation device in the femoral head, thus reducing the risk of the screw cutting out of the head. Critics, however, stated that drilling out the head can cause osteonecrosis of the head or microemboli of cement in the rich vascular plexus of the head of the

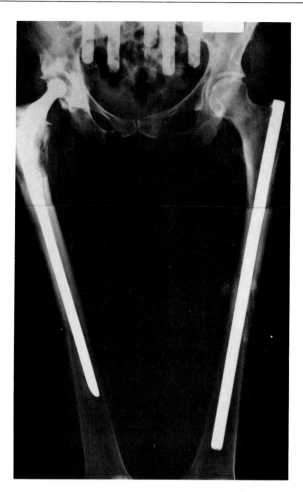

Fig. 1 Anteroposterior view of both femurs shows long-stem Charnley total hip arthroplasty in right femur and prophylactic intramedullary rod in left femur. (By permission of Mayo Foundation.)

femur.[23] I prefer to place the screws through partially hardened methylmethacrylate, although it is also effective to inject the cement into the tumor cavity after the device has been applied. Care must be taken to prevent extrusion of cement through the cortex, because extruded cement can interfere with periosteal bone formation and fracture healing.

Many surgeons advocate the use of a prosthesis because of the extent of proximal and distal destruction of cortical bone.[12,24,25] Currently, the availability of prosthetic implants of varying neck lengths and calcar replacement potential has extended the indications for replacement arthroplasty in the management of peritrochanteric fractures. This technique provides excellent pain relief and early weightbearing function. Replacement arthroplasty is usually necessary when the metastatic process extends into the proximal fragment and the remaining bone is insufficient to adequately secure a nail-plate apparatus. These advantages—early mobilization and immediate weightbearing—have led to an increase in the use of replacement arthroplasty for

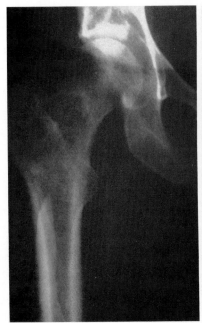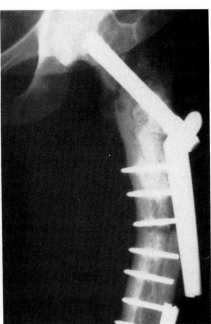

Fig. 2   Anteroposterior view of left proximal femur shows internal fixation of pathologic fracture with long nail-plate apparatus augmented with methylmethacrylate. Defect in medial cortex collapsed with failure of internal fixation. (By permission of Mayo Foundation.)

lesions in this region. However, we must consider that prosthetic replacement is a more extensive surgical procedure and has a potential for increased blood loss and surgical morbidity. In addition, the use of hip replacement arthroplasty introduces the problems of reattaching the trochanteric and abductor mechanism as well as dislocation.

The use of condylocephalic or Ender's nails[26] has been advocated for fixation of pathologic fractures in the intertrochanteric area, because fixation can be achieved without opening the fracture site. This method has fallen into disfavor because of the high rate of complications, including loss of reduction, caused primarily by malrotation, in addition to distal migration of the pins.[27] On occasion, fractures that appear to be primarily in the intertrochanteric region will extend into the subtrochanteric region where lytic metastasis is evident. Although a compression screw and a long reinforced side plate augmented by methylmethacrylate may be satisfactory, it may be best to internally fix such fractures with an intramedullary device such as a Zickel nail or Russell-Taylor reconstruction rod.

Subtrochanteric Fractures

Metastatic involvement in the subtrochanteric area is common and is prone to pathologic fracture because of the tremendous loads applied to this area. These fractures occur between the lesser trochanter and 5 cm distally.[28] This region consists primarily of cortical bone, and treatment is complicated by the loss of bone substance and strength associated with the metastatic disease. Because of these anatomic and mechanical considerations, a stable reduction is difficult to maintain

with a nail-plate apparatus. Even a small defect in the medial cortex leads to medial collapse and bending of the lateral plate. Therefore, when a nail-plate apparatus is used, methylmethacrylate is essential for reinforcement. However, there is still a high failure rate because of the high torque and shear stress on the plate (Fig. 2).

With the development of intramedullary devices, such as the Zickel nail or the Russell-Taylor reconstruction nail, major advances have been made in the management of pathologic fractures in this region. Biomechanically, the most practical position for a subtrochanteric fixation device is within the medullary canal at the femur. There is eccentric loading of the femur at the subtrochanteric level and the magnitude of forces is higher than at any other level. The medial cortex has been shown to be subjected to compressive forces in excess of 1,200 lb per sq. in. (psi), whereas the lateral cortex must resist tensile stresses exceeding 900 psi. Intramedullary devices compensate for these eccentric loads by affording balanced resistance midway between the cortices. Bending forces on intramedullary devices are much lower than on laterally located plates.

The Zickel nail is a device typically advocated for subtrochanteric pathologic fractures (Fig. 3). The large proximal portion of the Zickel nail provides improved proximal fragment fixation, and stability of fixation is achieved by the nail inserted into the head and neck fragment. This device is designed to tolerate the high stresses in this region, allowing early weightbearing to achieve impaction and restore the medial cortical bony buttress. In extensive lesions, intramedullary methylmethacrylate can be used after inserting the device to

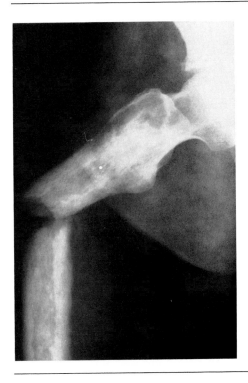

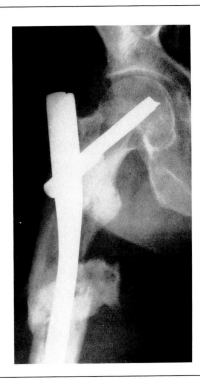

Fig. 3 **Left,** Anteroposterior view of right proximal femur shows pathologic subtrochanteric fracture secondary to prostate carcinoma. **Right,** After internal fixation with Zickel nail and methylmethacrylate. (By permission of Mayo Foundation.)

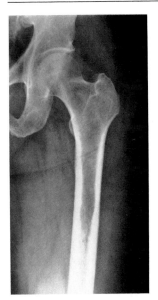

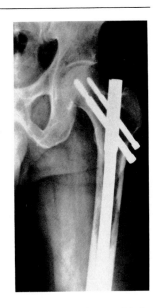

Fig. 4 **Left,** Anteroposterior view of left proximal femur with destruction secondary to metastatic breast carcinoma. **Right,** After prophylactic internal fixation with Russell-Taylor rod. (By permission of Mayo Foundation.)

prevent rotation of the distal shaft fragments, to reinforce fixation of the head, and to prevent shortening.[20] Another device that is gaining popularity in managing pathologic subtrochanteric fractures is the Russell-Taylor reconstruction rod. This device seems technically less demanding than the Zickel nail and recent experience has been excellent (Fig. 4).

The indications for prosthetic replacement are being extended for fractures in the subtrochanteric region. This technique is generally reserved for patients who have fractures in this region with extensive osseous involvement in which inadequate proximal fixation can be achieved by the internal fixation device (Fig. 5). In these instances, resection and proximal femoral replacement have been effective in achieving pain relief and allowing early progressive weightbearing. Moreover, this technique has proven particularly useful for salvaging internal fixation devices that have failed in patients with pathologic fractures in this region (Fig. 6). Although Khong and associates[29] reported excellent results in the Mayo Clinic series of 33 patients with metastatic disease who underwent proximal femoral replacement arthroplasty, it is a more extensive procedure with increased morbidity and complications. Moreover, the loss of the abductor mechanism compromises function and results in an abductor limp. In order to improve abductor function, a bioimplant has been advocated for the reconstruction when it is necessary to resect the proximal femur. With this technique, the allograft sleeve around the prosthesis provides a biologic structure for reattachment of the remaining functional muscles.[30] This technique, however, is a more extensive procedure, is still limited by its availability, and is associated with higher potential complications, such as infection and nonunion, particularly when radiotherapy and chemotherapy are used.[31] Fortunately, a great majority of patients with subtrochanteric lesions can be managed effectively by stan-

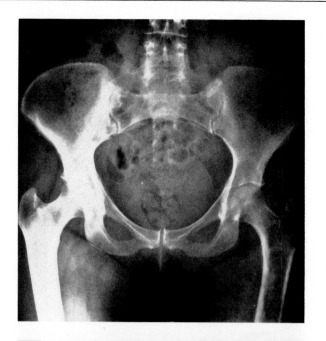

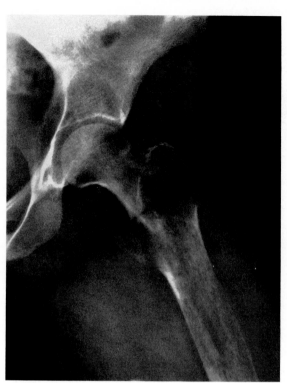

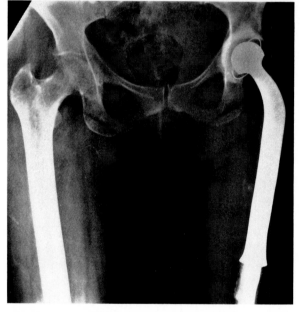

Fig. 5 **Top left**, Anteroposterior view of pelvis and proximal femur. **Top right**, Lateral view of left proximal femur shows extensive involvement of left proximal femur secondary to breast carcinoma. Lesion extends into femoral neck and trochanteric region, so adequate fixation cannot be achieved with Zickel nail. **Bottom left**, Anteroposterior view of proximal femur after resection and proximal femoral replacement. (By permission of Mayo Foundation.)

dard internal fixation devices such as a Zickel nail or a Russell-Taylor reconstruction nail.

Femoral Shaft

One-third of metastatic lesions involving the femur are located in the femoral shaft or supracondylar region. The patient with a pathologic fracture of the femur secondary to metastatic disease is a primary candidate for internal fixation because of the weightbearing function. Even though small painful lesions in this region may be treated with radiation therapy alone, the limb must be protected with partial weightbearing. For larger, more destructive lesions,

prophylactic fixation should be considered. Although biomechanical studies have shown that one or two large plates provide stronger fixation than intramedullary rods,[32,33] the latter is the preferred method of stabilization. When plates are used, there are additional concerns such as stress-shielding[20] or fractures through other areas in the femur from additional metastatic sites.[34]

Small femoral shaft lesions can be stabilized by closed femoral nailing. The technique is similar to that used in conventional traumatic fractures. A nail of the largest diameter possible should be used to provide maximal stability. Moreover, pre-bent intramedullary rods

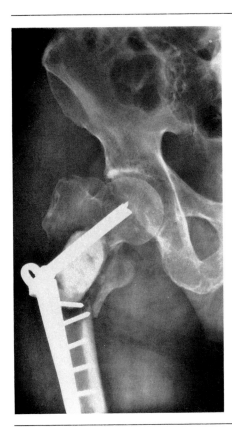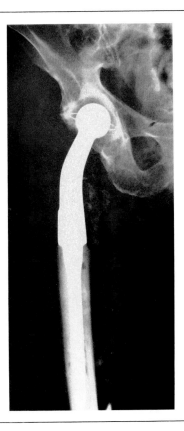

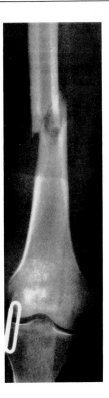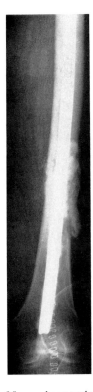

Fig. 6 **Left**, Anteroposterior view of right hip shows failure of internal fixation and pathologic fracture due to metastasis from carcinoma of breast. **Right**, After salvage by proximal femoral replacement. (By permission of Mayo Foundation.)

are preferred in order to prevent extrusion in the anterior femur. When there is a large amount of cortical destruction associated with the pathologic fracture (greater than 75% of the diameter), a more extensive procedure must be considered. In such circumstances, the addition of intramedullary methylmethacrylate is beneficial (Fig. 7). Interlocking medullary rods have been used extensively for comminuted or shortened fractures of the femur. I have found these rods to be effective in prophylactic placement of rods with proximal and distal interlocking screws. However, in extensive femoral lesions with bony destruction, collapse with excessive stresses on the interlocking screw areas may occur. Therefore, in fractures associated with extensive bone loss, methylmethacrylate should be used for added stability and to prevent collapse.

Supracondylar Fractures

Pathologic fractures involving the distal femur are challenging to treat because of comminution and poor bone stock. Surgical stabilization is simplified if the procedure is done prophylactically before fracture and comminution occur. Improvements in nail-plate and dynamic screw-plate devices of various lengths have provided improved fixation. Moreover, augmentation of the device with methylmethacrylate is important because the bone stock is usually poor. Healy and Lane[35] reported satisfactory results using a Zickel device designed for treatment of these fractures. Occasionally,

Fig. 7 **Left**, Anteroposterior view of femur shows pathologic fracture secondary to metastatic breast carcinoma. **Right**, After open reduction and internal fixation with medullary rod and methylmethacrylate.

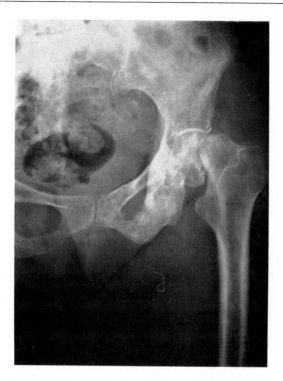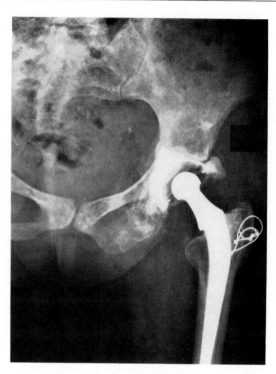

Fig. 8 **Left**, Anteroposterior view of left hip shows transcervical fracture. **Right**, After resection and total hip arthroplasty. (By permission of Mayo Foundation.)

the bone destruction is very extensive or the adjacent knee joint is compromised and, in these cases, a custom distal femoral replacement is warranted.

Lesions of the Pelvis

Metastatic involvement of the pelvis is a frequent clinical problem, resulting in pain and disability depending on the location and extent of the disease. Lesions involving the nonweightbearing portion of the pelvis may be managed effectively by radiotherapy and protected weightbearing.

Pathologic fractures involving the periacetabular region of the pelvis pose a difficult therapeutic problem. The degree of destruction has important implications for treatment. Previously, patients with massive involvement often became bedridden with incapacitating pain despite radiotherapy or a Girdlestone procedure. However, current advances in techniques of acetabular reconstruction have provided effective functional restoration in these patients.

Acetabular reconstruction using total hip arthroplasty must ensure that the acetabular component will remain securely positioned. This requires careful analysis of the extent of periacetabular bone destruction in order to determine which locations have sufficient strength to anchor the acetabular component. Moreover, the reconstruction must be able to transmit the weightbearing stresses in a manner that will prevent subsequent migration of the prosthesis. To accomplish

these aims, a classification system was formulated by Harrington.[36]

In class I, minor involvement, only a small region of the acetabulum is involved by tumor, and most of the acetabular globe remains intact. In these patients, with intact lateral cortices and superior medial parts of the acetabular globe, there is sufficient acetabular bone stock for conventional fixation of an acetabular component (Fig. 8).

In class II, there is major involvement of the acetabulum with deficiency of the medial wall as well as the superior part of the globe. However, the peripheral rim of the acetabulum remains intact. In these cases, a protrusio ring such as the Oh-Harris device transmits the stresses from the intact rim, avoiding stresses on the involved medial and superior aspects of the globe (Fig. 9).[12,37] In these patients, an acetabular mesh can be used to reinforce the medial wall and to prevent extrusion of cement. When the protrusio ring is used, it is important to ensure that the neck of the femoral component is long enough to avoid mechanical impingement against the ring, which could cause dislocation. Moreover, Levy and associates[37] cautioned that since the protrusio ring fits against the resected rim of the acetabulum in a more vertical manner, independent placement of the acetabular component in the correct position is essential to minimize the risk of dislocation.

Patients with class III, massive involvement of the acetabulum, have extensive bone loss. There is destruc-

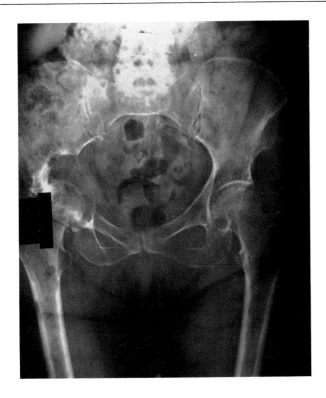
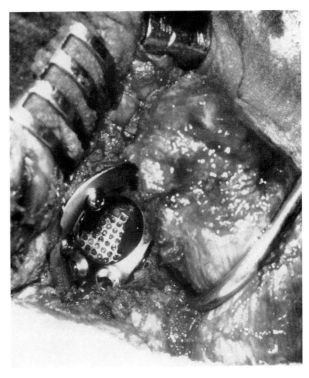
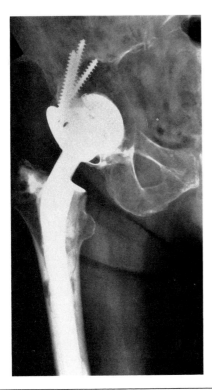
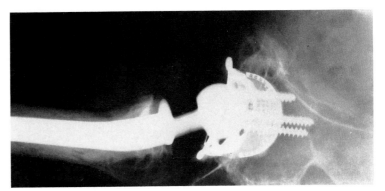

Fig. 9 **Top left**, Anteroposterior view of pelvis and right proximal femur shows extensive destruction of acetabulum by myeloma. **Top right**, Surgical view of acetabular reconstruction with wire mesh and screws. (By permission of Mayo Foundation.) **Bottom left**, Anteroposterior view of right hip after total hip replacement with acetabular reconstruction. **Bottom right**, Lateral view of right hip after total hip replacement with acetabular reconstruction. (By permission of Mayo Foundation.)

tion of the superior part of the acetabular wall in addition to destruction of the medial wall of the acetabulum and lateral rim. In such a situation, effective fixation of the acetabular prosthetic component in its normal location would be impossible even if the Oh-

Harris protrusio ring was used. In these cases, special techniques have been developed[36] to transmit stresses away from the acetabulum, which has been destroyed by tumor, and into the superior part of the ilium and sacrum. This procedure involves removal of gross tu-

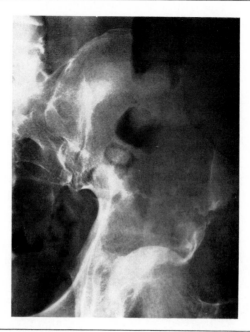
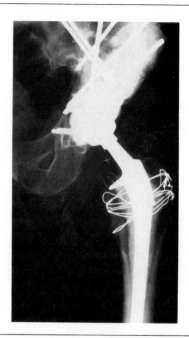

Fig. 10   **Left**, Anteroposterior view of left hemipelvis with extensive destruction from metastatic hypernephroma. This massive acetabular involvement corresponds to a Harrington class III defect. **Right**, After acetabular reconstruction utilizing Steinmann pins, methylmethacrylate, and an acetabular protrusio ring. (By permission of Mayo Foundation.)

mor tissue and bone fragments until solid bone can be palpated superiorly. Flexible Steinmann pins are placed in the remaining superior ilium and across the sacroiliac joint of the sacrum to transmit the weightbearing stresses to the structurally intact area. After placement of the threaded pins, the defect is packed with methylmethacrylate before the protrusio ring is inserted. The presence of the pins allows the stresses from the ring to be transferred superiorly to the intact bone (Fig. 10).

Because of the extensive nature of the surgery in patients with class III acetabular involvement, these patients should have the potential for prolonged survival, such as one anticipates in patients with carcinoma of the breast or prostate. Another important consideration is the vascularity of the lesion. If the preoperative assessment suggests a highly vascular lesion, angiography with selective embolization of the arterial trunk has proved beneficial. The experience at the Mayo Clinic[13,25] and that of Levy and associates[37] have shown gratifying results in patients undergoing acetabular reconstruction for metastatic disease. In Harrington's series[36] of 58 patients with reconstruction for periacetabular metastatic disease, only 5 had loosening of the acetabular component with loss of fixation. Moreover, in patients with class III or extensive involvement, none had loosening. In that series, two-thirds of the patients had satisfactory pain relief, and approximately half of the patients remained ambulatory at two years. The mean survival was 19 months.

Summary

Metastatic bone disease involving the pelvis and femur is a common clinical occurrence. A pathologic frac-

ture in this region is a catastrophic event that results in significant pain and loss of function. Recent advances in surgical management of pathologic fractures, resulting in secure fracture stability or stable joint replacement, have allowed these patients to resume their pre-fracture level of activity and ambulation. The surgeon must be familiar with the various devices available, because the choice of surgical procedure depends on the location of the tumor. In selected patients with extensive destruction, methylmethacrylate can be used to enhance the security of fixation and stability. Moreover, a more aggressive approach to prophylactic fixation before a catastrophic fracture develops has distinct advantages.

References

1. Harrington KD, Sim FH, Enis JE, et al: Methylmethacrylate as an adjunct in internal fixation of pathological fractures: Experience with three hundred and seventy-five cases. *J Bone Joint Surg* 1976;58A:1047–1055.

2. McKenna RJ: Bone metastases: Rehabilitation. Presented at the Bone Metastases Workshop, University of Southern California Comprehensive Cancer Center, Sept. 21, 1979.

3. Clain A: Secondary malignant disease of bone. *Br J Cancer* 1965; 19:15–29.

4. Schray MF, Gunderson LL: Principles of radiation-therapy, in Sim FH (ed): *Diagnosis and Management of Metastatic Bone Disease: A Multidisciplinary Approach*. New York, Raven Press, 1988, pp 141–146.

5. Cleveland M, Bosworth DM, Thompson FR: Management of the trochanteric fracture of the femur. *JAMA* 1948;137:1186–1190.

6. Aufranc OE, Jones WN, Turner RH: Severely comminuted intertrochanteric hip fracture. *JAMA* 1967;199:994–997.

7. Perez CA, Bradfield JS, Morgan HC: Management of pathologic fractures. *Cancer* 1972;29:684–693.

8. Francis KC, Higinbotham NL, Carroll RE, et al: The treatment

of pathological fractures of the femoral neck by resection. *J Trauma* 1962;2:465–473.

9. Koskinen EV, Nieminen RA: Surgical treatment of metastatic pathological fracture of major long bones. *Acta Orthop Scand* 1973;44:539–549.

10. McLaughlin HL: Intramedullary fixation of pathologic fractures. *Clin Orthop* 1953;2:108–114.

11. Gitelis S, Sheinkop MB, Hammerberg K: The treatment of metastatic foci of the proximal femur: A retrospective review (abstract). *Orthop Trans* 1981;5:428.

12. Habermann ET, Sachs R, Stern RE, et al: The pathology and treatment of metastatic disease of the femur. *Clin Orthop* 1982; 169:70–82.

13. Sim FH, Daugherty TW, Ivins JC: The adjunctive use of methylmethacrylate in fixation of pathological fractures. *J Bone Joint Surg* 1974;56A:40–48.

14. Beals RK, Lawton GD, Snell WE: Prophylactic internal fixation of the femur in metastatic breast cancer. *Cancer* 1971;28:1350–1354.

15. Coran AG, Banks HH, Aliapoulios MA, et al: The management of pathologic fractures in patients with metastatic carcinoma of the breast. *Surg Gynecol Obstet* 1968;127:1225–1230.

16. Fidler M: Prophylactic internal fixation of secondary neoplastic deposits in long bones. *Br Med J* 1973;1:341–343.

17. Parrish FF, Murray JA: Surgical treatment for secondary neoplastic fractures: A retrospective study of ninety-six patients. *J Bone Joint Surg* 1970;52A:665–686.

18. Pugh J, Sherry HS, Futterman B, et al: Biomechanics of pathologic fractures. *Clin Orthop* 1982;169:109–114.

19. Chao EYS, Sim FH, Shives TC, et al: Management of pathologic fracture: Biomechanical considerations, in Sim FH (ed): *Diagnosis and Management of Metastatic Bone Disease: A Multidisciplinary Approach.* New York, Raven Press, 1988, pp 171–181.

20. Zickel RE, Mouradian WH: Intramedullary fixation of pathological fractures and lesions of the subtrochanteric region of the femur. *J Bone Joint Surg* 1976;58A:1061–1066.

21. Bartucci EJ, Gonzalez MH, Cooperman DR, et al: The effect of adjunctive methylmethacrylate on failures of fixation and function in patients with intertrochanteric fractures and osteoporosis. *J Bone Joint Surg* 1985;67A:1094–1107.

22. Graham WD: Pathological fractures due to metastatic cancer (abstract). *J Bone Joint Surg* 1963;45B:617.

23. Harrington KD: New trends in the management of lower extremity metastases. *Clin Orthop* 1982;169:53–61.

24. Lane JM, Sculco TP, Zolan S: Treatment of pathological fractures of the hip by endoprosthetic replacement. *J Bone Joint Surg* 1980; 62A:954–959.

25. Sim FH, Hartz CR, Chao EYS: Total hip arthroplasty for tumors of the hip. *Hip* 1976;4:246–259.

26. Pankovich AM, Tarabishy IE: Ender nailing of intertrochanteric and subtrochanteric fractures of the femur. Complications, failures, and errors. *J Bone Joint Surg* 1980;62A:635–645.

27. Levy RN, Siegel M, Sedlin ED, et al: Complications of Ender-pin fixation in basicervical, intertrochanteric, and subtrochanteric fractures of the hip. *J Bone Joint Surg* 1983;65A:66–69.

28. Fielding JW, Magliato HJ: Subtrochanteric fractures. *Surg Gynecol Obstet* 1966;122:555–560.

29. Khong K-S, Chao EYS, Sim FH: Long-term performance of custom prosthetic replacement for neoplastic disease of the proximal femur, in Yamamuro T (ed): *New Developments for Limb Salvage in Musculoskeletal Tumors.* Berlin, Springer-Verlag, 1989, pp 403–411.

30. Woo SL-Y, Akeson WH, Coutts RD, et al: A comparison of cortical bone atrophy secondary to fixation with plates with large differences in bending stiffness. *J Bone Joint Surg* 1976;58A:190–195.

31. Czitrom AA, Gross AE, Langer F, et al: Bone banks and allografts in community practice, in Bassett FH III (ed): American Academy of Orthopaedic Surgeons *Instructional Course Lectures, XXXVII.* Park Ridge, IL, American Academy of Orthopaedic Surgeons, 1988, pp 13–24.

32. Anderson JT, Erickson JM, Thompson RC Jr, et al: Pathologic femoral shaft fractures comparing fixation techniques using cement. *Clin Orthop* 1978;131:273–278.

33. Mensch JS, Markolf KL, Roberts SB, et al: Experimental stabilization of segmental defects in the human femur: A torsional study. *J Bone Joint Surg* 1976;58A:185–190.

34. Albright JA, Gillespie TE, Butaud TR: Treatment of bone metastases. *Semin Oncol* 1980;7:418–434.

35. Healy JH, Lane JM: Treatment of pathologic fractures of the distal femur with the Zickel supracondylar nail. *Clin Orthop* 1990; 250:216–220.

36. Harrington KD: The management of acetabular insufficiency secondary to metastatic malignant disease. *J Bone Joint Surg* 1981; 63A:653–664.

37. Levy RN, Sherry HS, Siffert RS: Surgical management of metastatic disease of bone at the hip. *Clin Orthop* 1982;169:62–69.

Metastatic Lesions of the Humerus and the Upper Extremity

Michael G. Rock, MD

Introduction

Metastases are much less likely to occur in the upper extremity than in the spine, pelvis, and lower extremity. In extensive postmortem examinations of patients who died of cancer, Jaffe[1] found 85% overall had osseous metastases. Of these, 69% were in the vertebrae, 41% in the pelvis, 25% in the femur, and 25% in the ribs. Considerably fewer than 20% were in the upper extremity. Similar findings were recorded by Clain.[2] Of upper extremity lesions, the humerus is by far the most common site, accounting for approximately 50% of cases. The remaining lesions are equally distributed between the scapula and the clavicle. Lesions below the elbow are extremely rare and account for less than 1% of osseous metastases. The two most common histologic types to metastasize to forearm, hand, and wrist are lung and renal cell carcinoma.

Upper extremity involvement markedly interferes with patients' ability to feed themselves and perform routine hygiene and perineal care. It is also detrimental psychologically and can render bed-to-chair transfers and the use of external aids for lower extremity, pelvic, or spinal involvement impossible. Therefore, prophylactic fixation of impending pathologic fractures assumes significance in the upper extremity just as it does in the lower extremity.

Most patients with upper extremity metastases have a pathologic fracture or pain, prompting imaging of the area. It is not entirely unusual, however, to have patients appear with large destructive lesions of the upper extremity that are asymptomatic and are detected by routine bone scintigraphy or skeletal surveys. Treatment of upper extremity lesions is done prophylactically in patients who are experiencing significant pain, who are in need of a stable upper extremity to allow use of external aids, or who are at risk of fracture. Those with pathologic fractures are treated surgically, to relieve pain and restore function, because a flail upper extremity is painful and nonfunctional, and conservative management of a pathologic fracture will not promote healing. It is necessary to consider curative resection of upper extremity lesions only in rare cases that occur with unifocal thyroid or renal carcinoma, both of which have a predilection for upper humerus involvement. The use of radical procedures for metastasis is recommended only after thorough restaging of the primary and possible other metastatic sites and thorough discussions among the patient, medical oncologists, and surgeons.

Treatment Options

Treatment options include nonsurgical medical management, palliative surgical stabilization, and surgical cure.[3-8] Factors affecting this determination include the anticipated longevity of the patient, as determined by overall tumor load; the patient's medical status and ability to withstand a major surgical procedure; the extent of upper extremity involvement; the necessity for using external aids to ambulate; and the histogenesis of the tumor involved.

Nonsurgical management is usually reserved for small symptomatic lesions that are not at risk of fracture, for patients who are not currently using or who do not anticipate using external aids for ambulation, for extensive upper extremity involvement precluding adequate stabilization, and for patients with limited longevity (less than 3 months). These patients may be treated with radiation therapy,[9] chemical or hormonal treatment, and dynamic splinting of the upper extremity to minimize fracture translation and pain.[10]

Preoperative considerations in those selected for surgical stabilization include the extent of involvement of the principal lesion, additional areas of involvement in the same bone, additional areas of involvement remote from the principal lesion but within the same upper extremity, existence of an impending or actual pathologic fracture, and histogenesis of the primary tumor. Thorough imaging of the involved upper extremity should be performed. If the primary site is unknown, abdominal ultrasonography and serum electrophoresis should be performed to rule out the two pathologic processes, namely renal cell carcinoma and myeloma, that are known to be extremely vascular and would benefit from embolization of the lesion before surgical intervention. Additionally, several alternative forms of reconstruction must be considered and should be available at operation. With impending pathologic fractures, it is important to position and prepare the patient to minimize the risk of creating a pathologic fracture; at the same time the chosen positioning should allow for various alternative procedures, if necessary, at the time of exposure.

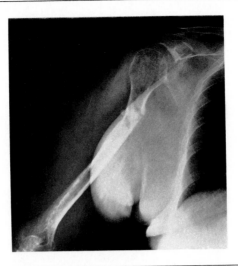
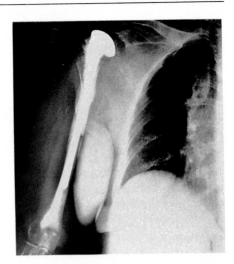

Fig. 1 **Left**, A 63-year-old woman with extensive metastatic breast carcinoma involving the humeral head and neck with an associated pathologic fracture of proximal shaft. **Right**, Treatment consisted of humeral head replacement with the stem of the implant serving as an intramedullary nail supporting the fracture.

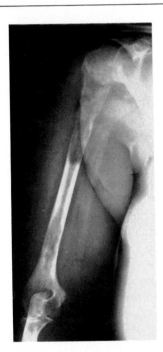
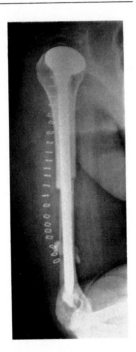

Fig. 2 **Left**, A 59-year-old man with extensive solitary myeloma of proximal right humerus. **Right**, Extent of tumor involvement precluded stable fixation. En bloc resection was performed. Reconstruction was performed with allograft custom long-stem Cofield prosthesis. The patient is alive 2 years postoperatively with good stable shoulder function.

Humerus

Humeral Head and Neck

The most frequently involved area in the upper extremity is the humerus, which can be considered as three separate anatomic regions. Proximal head and neck involvement is best treated with unipolar humeral replacement. Because intra-articular, and specifically

glenoid, involvement is rare, conversion to total shoulder replacement is usually not necessary. The approach is through a typical deltopectoral incision that exposes the shoulder joint. After the tumor has been removed, it may be necessary to cement the implant proud and to advance the rotator cuff into the remaining viable proximal humeral shaft (Fig. 1). If involvement includes the upper shaft of the humerus, additional alternative reconstructions are available. These include custom proximal humeral replacements, conventional shoulder replacement humeral components with intramedullary nails that extend into the remaining uninvolved humerus, or allograft prosthetic composites or osteoarticular allografts.[11] Allograft reconstructions are recommended for individuals whose anticipated life span exceeds one year, because they allow a more functional and stable shoulder. Large custom humeral implants have no provision for allowing rotator cuff advancement and, thus, are less stable. If an allograft is chosen for these reasons, the fixation device used should span the full length of the allograft, and cement should be applied in the intramedullary portion of the allograft to increase fixation strength (Fig. 2).

Humeral Shaft

The most frequently involved anatomic area in the upper extremity is probably the humeral shaft. Risk factors that apply to lower extremity shaft lesions—pain after radiation, 50% or more of cortical destruction, and lesions 2 cm or more in size—may not apply to upper extremities, specifically humeral lesions.[5] These determinations assume weightbearing demands that are not present with upper extremity lesions. A more applicable and universal risk-for-fracture scheme has been proposed based on such variables as anatomic location, pain, size, and radiographic appearance. Each of four variables is scored one, two, or three, and the likelihood of fracture increases dramatically with a score of 8 or

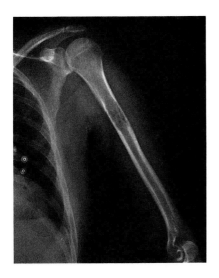
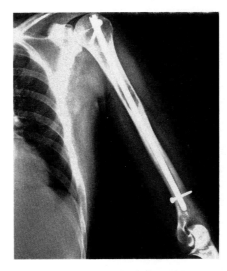

Fig. 3 **Left**, Metastatic renal cell carcinoma in 59-year-old man. **Right**, Locked intramedullary nail for impending fracture.

Table 1
Risk of fracture

Variable	Score		
	1	2	3
Site	Upper limb	Lower limb	Peritrochanter
Pain	Mild	Moderate	Functional
Lesion	Blastic	Mixed	Lytic
Size (diameter)	<1/3	1/3 to 2/3	>2/3

(Reproduced with permission from Mirels H: Metastatic disease in long bones: A proposed scoring system for diagnosing impending pathologic fractures. *Clin Orthop* 1989;249:256–264.)

more points out of the possible total of 12 (Table 1).[12] Although not absolute, these factors can help the surgeon decide if surgical stabilization is advisable.

The nature of the involvement of the humeral shaft can dictate whether treatment should be by an open or a closed procedure. Impending pathologic fractures of the shaft of the humerus can be treated effectively with either anterograde or retrograde closed intramedullary nailing performed under fluoroscopic control.[13] The intramedullary device can be introduced proximally, at the tuberosity, or distally, above the olecranon fossa. The type of implant used usually reflects the surgeon's preference. Rush rods, Ender's nails, or Hackenthall nails are more flexible and are not quite as rigid as the Richard or Seidel locked humeral nails. Furthermore, the locked intramedullary nails prevent the migration that can be a problem with Rush rods and Ender's nails (Fig. 3). Actual pathologic fractures of the humerus warrant open reduction, removal of tumor, and augmentation of the selected fixation device with methylmethacrylate. Additional options for humeral shaft fractures include resection and shortening, for lesions less than 4 cm in size with no obvious evidence of additional involvement in the proximal or dis-

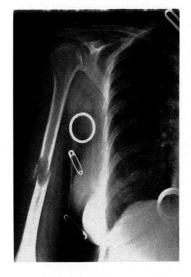
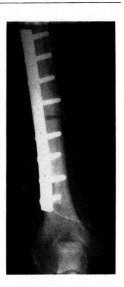

Fig. 4 **Left**, Metastatic breast carcinoma with pathologic fracture in 57-year-old woman. **Right**, Treatment consisted of excision, shortening, plating, and reinforcement with intramedullary methylmethacrylate.

tal segment (Fig. 4), or resection and replacement by an intercalary prosthesis cemented into the proximal and distal remaining segments (Fig. 5).[14] It is generally best to obtain fixation with intramedullary devices rather than with plate and screws, because future bone involvement above or below the plate can put this type of reconstruction at risk for failure.

Distal Humerus

Distal humeral involvement at or slightly above the condyles is best treated with crossed Rush rods introduced from the medial and lateral epicondyles (Fig. 6). This area can be exposed with the patient prone,

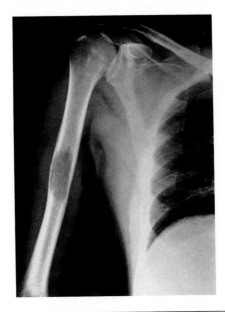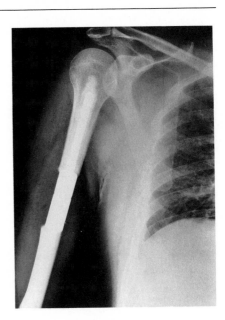

Fig. 5 Left, Midshaft impending pathologic fracture of right humerus in 67-year-old man with known renal cell carcinoma. **Right**, Because of the vascularity of renal cell metastases, the area involved was removed en bloc and reconstructed with an intercalary metal spacer cemented into proximal and distal humeral canals.

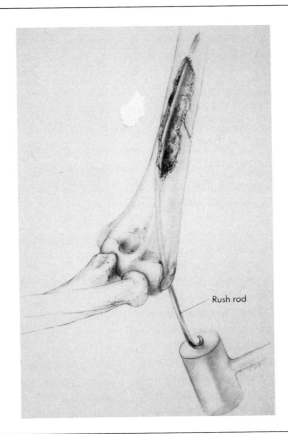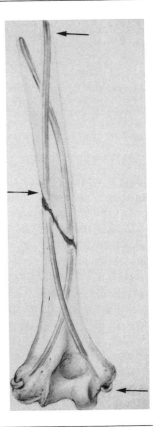

Rush rod

Fig. 6 Left, Rush rod introduced into lateral epicondyle. **Right**, Crossed Rush rods with three-point fixation (**arrows**) stabilizing distal humerus fracture. (Reproduced with permission from Harrington KD: *Orthopaedic Management of Metastatic Bone Disease*. St. Louis, CV Mosby, 1988, pp 255–281.)

through a posterior incision, by elevating the triceps off the proximal ulna as recommended in the Morrey-Bryant approach for total elbow replacement. This approach allows visualization of the entire distal shaft of the humerus. It may be necessary to isolate and possibly even transpose the ulnar nerve to avoid injury to this structure. An alternate approach splits the triceps and gives access to the tumor in the condylar or distal shaft segment. Other reconstructive options in this area include pelvic reconstruction plates on both the medial and lateral columns reinforced with methylmethacrylate. This assumes no evidence of tumor proximal to the distal segment of the humerus. Additionally, if the tumor is extensive in this area, resection and replacement with total elbow arthroplasty is a reasonable alternative.

Scapula

Other areas of involvement in the upper extremity are rare. Scapular involvement tends to be in the periglenoid region, specifically the neck. Fortunately, this rarely involves the articular surface. Apart from allowing some local collapse of the neck, the overall shoulder joint is usually not transgressed. Similarly, body involvement of the scapula does not interfere with contiguous joint function. These patients are best treated nonsurgically with appropriate medical management that allows shoulder immobilization for pain control while radiotherapy and medical management are being administered. Once the patient is more comfortable, therapeutic endeavors should be initiated to obtain glenohumeral motion and avoid shoulder ankylosis.

Similarly, clavicular lesions rarely, if ever, require surgical stabilization. Lesions in the outer third of the clavicle can be successfully treated with resection, but midshaft or medial lesions rarely need stabilization with plate and screws augmented with methylmethacrylate. Because of the propensity for migration, intramedullary Kirschner wires should be avoided in this region.

Forearm

Involvement below the elbow, although extremely uncommon, should raise concern, because most of these are renal cell carcinomas with some contribution from lung. Careful preoperative determination of the underlying histogenesis is important to minimize the risk of excessive blood loss. Fortunately, in this anatomic area, a tourniquet can be applied to the upper arm, making the procedure safe to perform.

In summary, the indications and requisites for surgical stabilization of upper extremity metastatic deposits have been discussed, as have preoperative planning and the various surgical options currently available. The reconstruction must be biomechanically sound to withstand the stresses being applied through this area for the remaining life of the patient. Because fractures will not heal in the presence of radiation therapy or tumor, conventional fixation techniques may be inappropriate or unsatisfactory for this patient population.

References

1. Jaffe HL: *Tumors and Tumorous Conditions of the Bones and Joints.* Philadelphia, Lea & Febiger, 1958.
2. Clain A: Secondary malignant disease of bone. *Br J Cancer* 1965; 19:15–29.
3. Coran AG, Banks HH, Aliapoulios MA, et al: The management of pathologic fractures in patients with metastatic carcinoma of the breast. *Surg Gynecol Obstet* 1968;127:1225–1230.
4. Douglass HO Jr, Shukla SK, Mindell E: Treatment of pathological fractures of long bones excluding those due to breast cancer. *J Bone Joint Surg* 1976;58A:1055–1061.
5. Harrington KD, Sim FH, Enis JE, et al: Methylmethacrylate as an adjunct in internal fixation of pathological fractures: Experience with three hundred and seventy-five cases. *J Bone Joint Surg* 1976;58A:1047–1055.
6. Lewallen RP, Pritchard DJ, Sim FH: Treatment of pathologic fractures or impending fractures of the humerus with Rush rods and methylmethacrylate: Experience with 55 cases in 54 patients, 1968–1977. *Clin Orthop* 1982;166:193–198.
7. Parrish FF, Murray JA: Surgical treatment for secondary neoplastic fractures: A retrospective study of ninety-six patients. *J Bone Joint Surg* 1970;52A:665–686.
8. Sim FH, Daugherty TW, Ivins JC: The adjunctive use of methylmethacrylate in fixation of pathological fractures. *J Bone Joint Surg* 1974;56A:40–48.
9. Blake DD: Radiation treatment of metastatic bone disease. *Clin Orthop* 1970;73:89–100.
10. Sarmiento A, Kinman PB, Galvin EG, et al: Functional bracing of fractures of the shaft of the humerus. *J Bone Joint Surg* 1977; 59A:596–601.
11. Rock MG: Intercalary allograft and custom Neer prosthesis after en bloc resection of the proximal humerus, in Enneking WF (ed): *Limb Salvage in Musculoskeletal Oncology.* New York, Churchill Livingstone, 1987, pp 586–597.
12. Mirels H: Metastatic disease in long bones: A proposed scoring system for diagnosing impending pathologic fractures. *Clin Orthop* 1989;249:256–264.
13. Stern PJ, Mattingly DA, Pomeroy DL, et al: Intramedullary fixation of humeral shaft fractures. *J Bone Joint Surg* 1984;66A: 639–646.
14. Chin HC, Frassica FJ, Hein TJ, et al: Metastatic diaphyseal fractures of the shaft of the humerus: The structural strength evaluation of a new method of treatment with a segmental defect prosthesis. *Clin Orthop* 1989;248:231–239.

Serious Fractures and Joint Injuries in Children

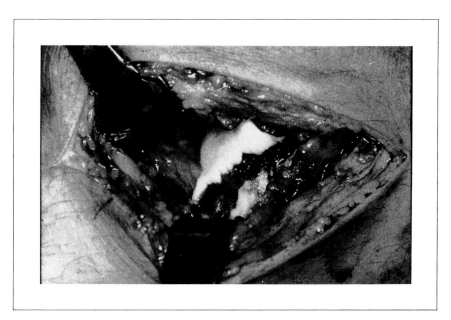

CHAPTER 35

General Features of Fractures in Children

Colin F. Moseley, MD

Children differ qualitatively and quantitatively from adults, and some of these differences have a direct bearing on the occurrence and treatment of fractures. This chapter deals with certain general principles of fractures in children. The consideration of specific fractures will be covered elsewhere.

Growth

The most obvious difference between children and adults is that children are growing and adults are not, and future growth frequently must be considered in deciding how to manage fractures in children. Growth can be helpful or harmful, sometimes contributing to problems and complications and at other times tending to resolve them.

Growth Arrest

In the Salter-Harris type V epiphyseal plate injury, cells of the growth plate are injured by compression, but there is no actual disruption or fracture of the plate. Therefore, by definition, radiographs taken after the injury are normal, and the diagnosis of a type V fracture can only be made in retrospect. The cells at the tips of the cell columns produce growth in the growth plate, and their blood supply comes from the epiphyseal side and passes through the small cell layer of the growth plate to ramify at the tips of the columns. The existence of a type V fracture assumes that this blood supply can be interrupted by compression or microfracture without gross disruption of the plate. Some people doubt that such fractures exist, preferring to believe instead that an initial disruption was present, which might have been seen had other radiographs been taken.

Figure 1 shows a radiograph of a boy's wrist one year after a hyperextension injury. No radiographs were taken at the time of the injury. The result has been premature closure of the distal radial epiphyseal plate with radial deviation of the wrist. It is likely that the growth plate was injured originally, possibly in a type V injury.

Figure 2 provides more convincing evidence that the type V fracture exists. The anteroposterior and lateral views shown are among a number of views taken after the patient stepped on the foot of another player during a basketball game and suffered a twisting injury. None of the radiographs showed a fracture or disrup-

tion of the growth plate. One year later, however, the girl had developed premature closure of the medial aspect of her distal tibial epiphyseal plate with an 18-degree angular deformity.

Bony Bridge

Certain fractures are particularly susceptible to the formation of bony bridges, which tether the bone of the epiphysis to that of the metaphysis and prevent further growth. Figure 3 shows a diagram of such a fracture and illustrates how the bone of the epiphysis of the displaced fracture fragment can come to lie in apposition to the bone of the metaphysis. It is clear that healing in this area will tether the epiphysis to the metaphysis and prevent further longitudinal growth. The type IV fracture as it occurs in the ankle is a particularly good example.

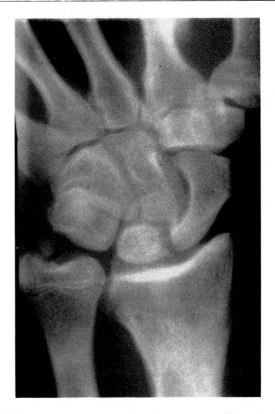

Fig. 1 This boy suffered a hyperextension injury of his wrist playing football. It was treated as a sprain and no radiographs were taken at the time. One year later he was found to have premature closure of the distal radial physis. His original injury may have been a type V injury of the growth plate.

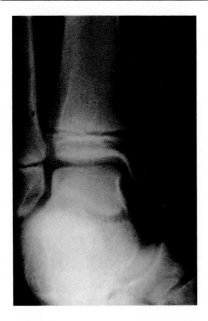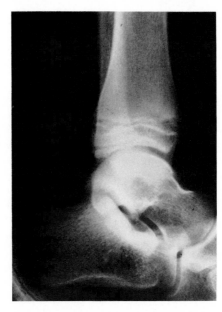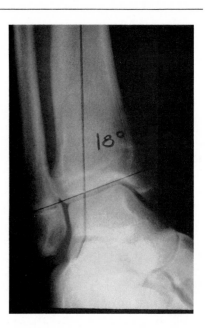

Fig. 2 **Left** and **center**, These are anteroposterior and lateral radiographs of the ankle of a 12-year-old girl who twisted her ankle playing basketball. Other views were also taken and no view showed any evidence of fracture. **Right**, Fifteen months later she had developed an 18-degree tilt of her ankle joint caused by asymmetrical growth of the distal tibial physis. This is convincing evidence of a type V injury.

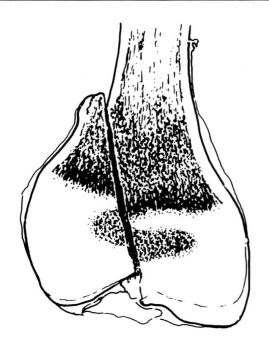

Fig. 3 A diagrammatic section of a type IV fracture showing how the epiphyseal bone of the displaced fragment comes to lie in apposition to the bone of the metaphysis. It is clear that the healing at this location will tether the epiphysis to the metaphysis and will prevent future growth.

It is worth noting that certain type IV fractures, such as those about the elbow, are avulsion fractures with separation of the fragments. They are prone to nonunion rather than bridge formation.

Even minimally displaced type IV fractures can suffer this complication. Figure 4 shows a bimalleolar fracture in a 10-year-old boy with a type IV fracture of the medial malleolus and a type II fracture of the distal fibula. This fracture is minimally displaced and was treated without reduction in a plaster cast. Eleven months later, a radiograph of the ankle showed deformity of the epiphysis and joint surface and the suggestion of a medial bony bridge. These findings were confirmed by tomogram. This boy underwent successful surgical excision of the bony bridge, but early accurate reduction of the fracture with internal fixation could have avoided this complication.

Growth Stimulation

It is common knowledge that fractures of the femur have a tendency to overgrow in children, possibly because the hypervascularity of the healing fracture also affects the neighboring growth plates. A particularly interesting example of overgrowth, however, is that of the valgus deformity, which tends to occur following fractures of the proximal tibial metaphysis. This deformity may represent a malunion, but in most cases results from a growth disturbance. Its genesis and treatment are covered in detail elsewhere.

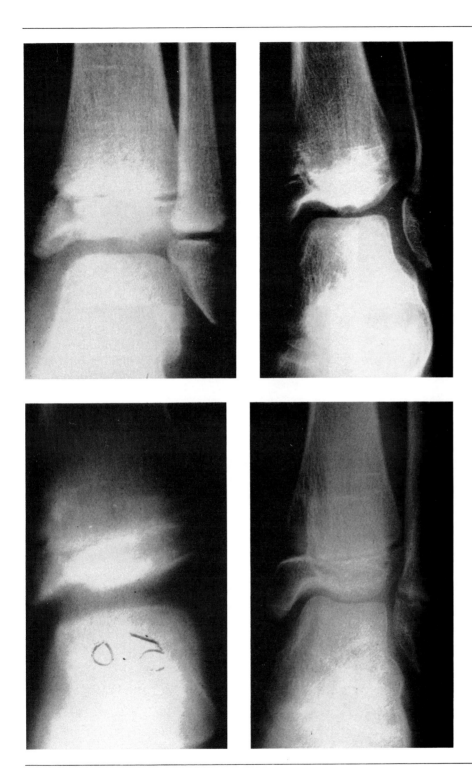

Fig. 4 **Top left,** This 10-year-old boy suffered a bimalleolar fracture of his ankle. The radiograph shows a type II injury of the distal fibula, and a type IV injury of the distal tibia. The displacement was thought to be minimal, and he was treated in a cast without reduction. **Top right,** Eleven months after the injury, he complained of pain and a radiograph showed deformity of the physis and suggested formation of a physeal bridge. **Bottom left,** The presence of a small peripheral bridge was confirmed by computed tomography. **Bottom right,** The bridge was excised, and 18 months later he was seen to be growing relatively normally although there was persistent deformity of the epiphysis.

Healing

There is no question that the rate of healing of a fracture slows with age. A femoral fracture takes one week to heal in the newborn, four weeks in the 5-year-old, eight weeks in the 10-year-old, three months in the adolescent, and four months or longer in the adult.

There are instances, however, when the difference in healing ability is more than quantitative; where the quantitative difference can result in a qualitatively different treatment approach.

Figure 5 shows an example. In this case, a 6-year-old girl suffered proximal fractures of both the radius and ulna. A closed reduction achieved a satisfactory but not

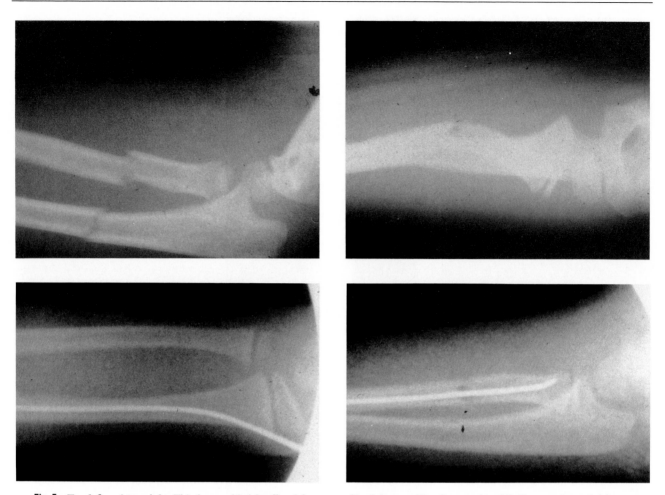

Fig. 5   **Top left** and **top right**, This 6-year-old girl suffered fractures of both bones of her forearm in a fall. Because the radial fracture is particularly proximal, plating of both bones would run the risk of cross-union. **Bottom left** and **bottom right**, Because of the superior healing ability of children, less-than-rigid fixation with a intramedullary Kirschner wire maintained alignment, allowing healing, and minimized the intervention. Bending the tip of the wire slightly aids in directing the wire across the fracture.

perfect reduction, but a radiograph taken four days later showed that the reduction had been lost and that the deformity had recurred.

Suitable treatment in an adult would have involved plating both bones, which would have been difficult with such proximal fractures. In the child, however, with the ability to heal rapidly, it was possible to treat this problem with minimal intervention. A flexible intramedullary Kirschner-wire was introduced into the radius to maintain alignment. Because of the child's superior healing abilities, it was not necessary to provide rigid internal fixation, and the simple maintenance of alignment allowed this fracture to go on to heal in excellent position without rigid internal fixation.

Remodeling

There are two methods of remodeling. One, described by Wolff in the late 19th century, involves the

laying down of new bone where it is needed and the removal of bone where it is not. In angulated fractures, for example, bone is laid down in the concavity and is removed from the convexity, with the result that the bone tends to become straight. This kind of remodeling does take place in adults, but in children the process is more efficient.

A second form of remodeling occurs in accordance with the Heuter-Volkman law, which states that the growth plate tends to align itself perpendicular to the resultant force acting across it. This means that asymmetrical growth of the physis can actually change the orientation of the joint at the end of the bone. This mechanism occurs in children but is obviously impossible in adults, who lack growth plates. Adults, therefore, cannot realign their joints through remodeling, but children can.

Figure 6 shows an example of remodeling by Wolff's law. Although the bone was regaining its straight configuration, it had not regained its normal strength and

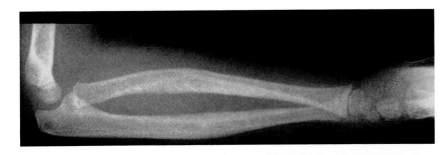

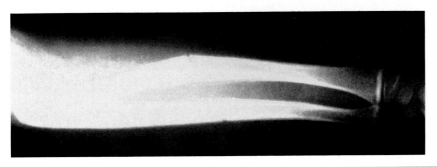

Fig. 6 Top, This radiograph shows the result of remodeling by Wolff's Law. New bone has been added in the concavity and the convexity has been rounded off with the result that the bone is regaining its normal shape. **Bottom,** Unfortunately the new bone has substance but not architecture and is prone to refracture.

this patient suffered a refracture through the bone, which had not yet gained a strong architecture. Figure 7 shows anteroposterior and lateral radiographs of a completely displaced supracondylar fracture in a 5-year-old girl who was not brought in for medical care until two weeks after her injury. Some subperiosteal new bone is already visible. The decision was made to allow this fracture to heal and trust that remodeling would achieve a satisfactory outcome. With the passage of time, the anterior spike of bone slowly disappeared through remodeling and presented less obstruction to elbow flexion. In addition, the growth of the elbow joint away from the site of the fracture and the humeral spike also contributed to the recovery of motion. Final radiographs, taken 1.5 years after the injury, show excellent reconstitution of the configuration of the humerus. At that time the child had regained full flexion of the elbow.

The ability of a fracture to remodel is greater if it is near the growth plate, if the child has significant growth remaining, and if the plane of deformity of the fracture is in the major plane of motion of the adjacent joint.

Mechanical Properties

The mechanical properties of musculoskeletal tissues change constantly during life, and there are significant differences between children and adults. These changes are present in the material properties of bone as a tissue and the physical properties of bones as structures.

Structural Properties

The major feature of children's bones as structures is the presence of the growth plate, which is a region of relative weakness. In the face of trauma, the growth plate is usually, but not always, disrupted before the ligaments of the adjacent joint. This might be considered an advantage for children, because epiphyseal plate fractures usually go on to 100% recovery, and ligamentous disruptions usually do not. This difference is shown diagrammatically in Figure 8 with respect to the knee. The diagnosis can usually be made clinically, before any radiographs have been taken, by palpating the epiphyseal plate while performing a stress test. This is not as painful as it might sound, because the soft tissues are completely disrupted and are not placed into tension.

The distal tibial growth plate has a distinctive pattern of closure, which relates to certain fractures in children. It closes first on the medial side and the closure progresses gradually towards the lateral. This means that there is a period of time during which the medial side is closed and the lateral side is not.

The Tillaux fracture (Fig. 9) results from an external rotation injury in which the anterolateral part of the distal tibial epiphysis is avulsed by the anterior tibial fibular ligament. The fracture through the plate occurs only through the part of the plate that is still open, and not through the part that has closed, which is the reason why this fracture happens in children who are within two years of the end of growth. This fracture demands anatomic reduction for the sake of the articular surface. The growth plate is not an important consideration, because growth is effectively complete.

The triplane fracture of the distal tibia (Fig. 10) occurs in the same place as the Tillaux fracture and at the same age. The triplane fracture occurs in the coronal plane in the metaphysis, the horizontal plane

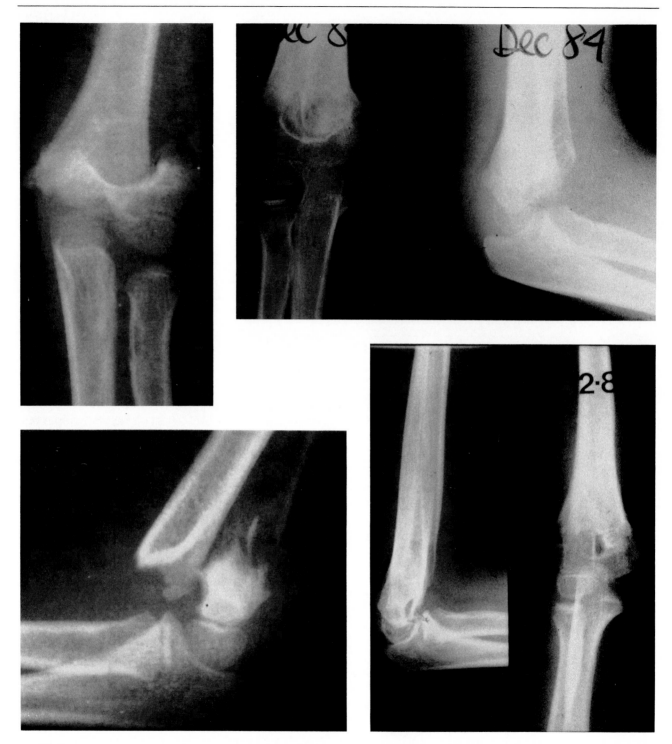

Fig. 7 Top left and **bottom left**, This 6-year-old girl suffered a completely displaced supracondylar fracture. For the first two weeks she was treated at home with compresses and herbal medicines. These radiographs at two weeks show that subperiosteal bone was already beginning to form. It was decided to allow the fracture to heal in this position and allow natural remodeling. **Top right**, Five months later the space beneath the stripped periosteum had filled in with new bone, the joint was growing away from the fracture, and remodeling had begun. **Bottom right**, At 18 months she had regained full elbow flexion, had normal alignment, and the humerus showed excellent remodeling.

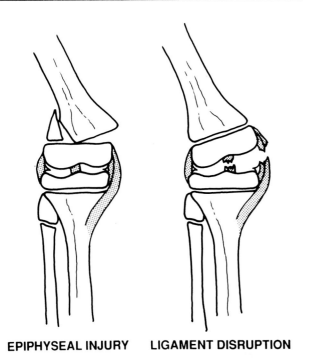

EPIPHYSEAL INJURY   LIGAMENT DISRUPTION

Fig. 8 A diagrammatic representation of the typical injuries suffered by the knees of children and adults when subjected to valgus trauma. The injuries are different by virtue of the presence of the epiphyseal plate, which tends to fail before the ligaments of the adjacent joint.

through part of the physis, and a complex, curved, partially sagittal plane through the epiphysis. In this fracture, like the Tillaux fracture, the joint surface requires

anatomic reduction, probably with internal fixation, but the growth plate, as important as it is for the genesis of the fracture, is relatively unimportant in prognosis because growth is virtually finished.

Material Properties

Bone, as a tissue, is not the same in children as it is in adults. While adult bone is brittle and breaks without bending, children's bone has the ability to undergo plastic deformation and it can bend without breaking or it can break partially. The greenstick fracture begins on the tension side of the bone and continues toward the compression side, but it leaves a part of the cortex on the compression side that is plastically deformed, but not fractured.

The most commonly bent bones are in the forearm, usually as a result of falls. The curvature of bent bones will slowly remodel with growth, and the question of whether or not a reduction is necessary usually depends on the direction of the curvature and the clinical finding of whether or not pronation and supination of the forearm are significantly reduced. If a reduction is necessary, it is sometimes possible to bend the bones back into proper alignment without breaking them. This procedure involves a significant risk of fracture, but the fracture, if it occurs, is easily treated.

The term "greenstick fracture," which is somewhat loosely applied to children, is sometimes used to include all minimally displaced fractures of the forearm. In this context, however, it is best to use the term to describe only those fractures in which part of the circumference of the bone is fractured and part is plastically deformed. It is usually impossible to reduce these fractures to their

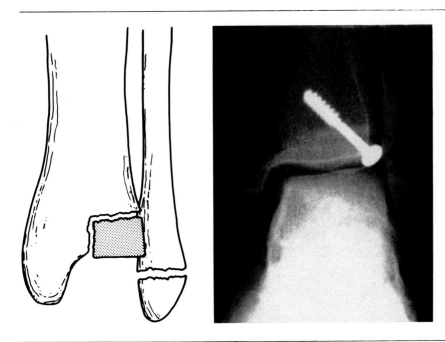

Fig. 9 Left, A diagrammatic representation of a Tillaux fracture. This fracture results from forced external rotation of the ankle. Tension in the anterior tibio-fibular ligament avulses that part of the distal tibial epiphysis where the growth plate has not yet closed. **Right,** This fracture requires anatomic reduction for the sake of the articular surface. Screw fixation that crosses the physis is of no concern, because this fracture only happens when the plate is closing.

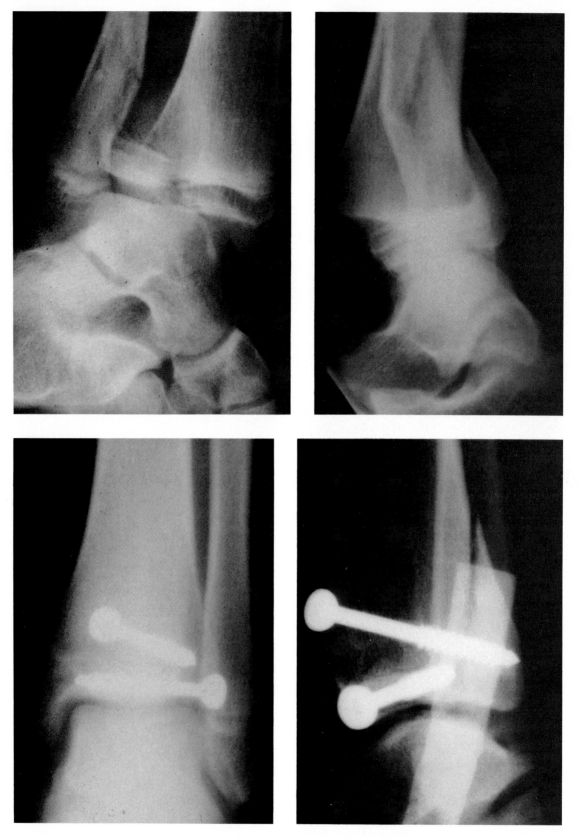

Fig. 10 Top left and **top right**, These radiographs show a triplane fracture. The fracture components through the three planes of the metaphysis, physis, and epiphysis are evident. **Bottom left** and **bottom right**, The most important part of the treatment is the reduction and fixation of the articular surface, which can usually be accomplished by a single screw. The reduction of the epiphysis to the metaphysis is less important and sometimes can be achieved by a lag screw from the anterolateral incision. Sometimes direct visualization, through a second posterolateral incision, is necessary.

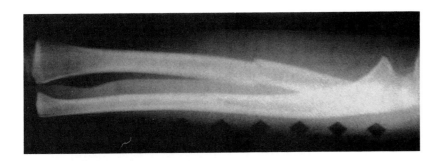

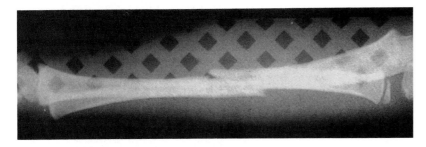

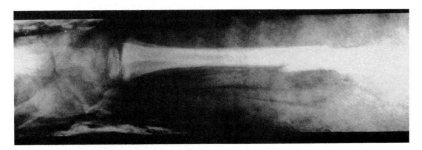

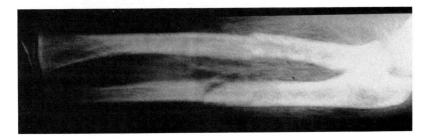

Fig. 11 **Top** and **top center**, This boy fractured both forearm bones in a fall from a tree. The wound was recognized to be open by virtue of a pinhole laceration over the sharp end of the ulnar fragment and was irrigated but not debrided. This radiograph was taken nine hours after the reduction because the patient was complaining of pain. Lucent lines are present in the soft tissue planes of the forearm. **Bottom center** and **bottom**, A radiograph taken 29 hours after the fracture and after transporting the child to a major medical center showed gas in all compartments of the forearm and extending in the common extensor compartment above the elbow. The boy was very sick but recovered following elbow disarticulation and administration of antibiotics and hyperbaric oxygen.

anatomic position by manipulation, because it is impossible to reverse the deformity during the manipulation. For the deformity to be corrected, the fracture may have to be completed.

There is one other area in which the material properties of children's bone have a bearing on treatment, and that is in the femoral neck. Children, unlike older adults, have very solid bone in the femoral neck, and it is often possible to apply internal fixation into the neck without extending across the epiphyseal plate into the epiphysis.

Pitfalls

Child Abuse

The orthopaedic surgeon treating children's fractures must constantly be on the lookout for child abuse. This diagnosis is only made if clinical suspicion exists and problems beyond the fracture itself are considered. There is an extraordinarily high incidence of child abuse in long bone fractures in very young children, and it may be that as many as 50% of the long bone fractures seen in children under the age of one year, and 80% under the age of six months, result from child abuse. The hallmark of child abuse is multiple fractures in different stages of healing, but the astute orthopaedic surgeon will recognize discrepancies between the pattern of the fracture and the history. If a suspicion of child abuse exists, there is a legal and moral obligation to protect the child, and the child should be kept in the hospital until the question can be resolved.

Open Fractures

This particular pitfall is much the same in children as it is in adults. Open fractures should be treated with great care, because of the risks involved. In particular, small pinhole fractures, which are caused by the sharp ends of fractured bones, should not be considered any cleaner or less risky than fractures compounded from without.

Figure 11 shows anteroposterior and lateral views of a forearm fracture, which was recognized to be compounded by the sharp end of the ulnar fragment. The fracture was not opened or debrided, and the boy experienced severe pain and developed gas shadows in the soft tissues of his arm. Ultimately, this patient required an elbow disarticulation as a life-saving measure. All compound fractures should be explored, and the laceration should be widened, if necessary. The bone ends should be exposed, foreign materials and dead tissue debrided, and thorough irrigation carried out. It is best to leave the wound open to undergo secondary closure later, either in the operating room or by gradual closure with adhesive tape.

Conclusion

The orthopaedic surgeon treating fractures in children must embrace a set of principles different from those used in treating fractures in adults. The general principles presented above will be repeated elsewhere as they apply to specific fractures.

Initial Management of the Multiply Injured Child: The ABC's

Peter F. Armstrong, MD, FRCSC, FACS

Introduction

The leading cause of death in childhood is blunt trauma. Falls and motor vehicle accidents (including pedestrian, passenger, bicycle, etc.) account for at least 80% of these deaths. Many of the deaths occur because the injuries are so serious that even prompt, thorough resuscitation and treatment are inadequate to sustain life. This is particularly true of serious head injuries. Unfortunately, other deaths occur that could have been prevented with proper medical attention. The real tragedy is when the patient makes it to the hospital with treatable injuries but dies there as a result of errors in management. The most common errors involve the management of problems of hypoxia or hypovolemia or the failure to detect hidden, serious injuries.

Care of the injured child requires a systematic, multidisciplinary, predetermined approach that will ensure the thorough evaluation of all organ systems and the implementation of prompt, appropriate therapy. The processes of evaluation and treatment are carried out simultaneously. Care of the injured child also requires a high index of suspicion and frequent, repeated examinations to insure that no injuries are missed. Ignorance of these principles is no excuse. In my opinion, any surgeon involved in the management of acute trauma should be well trained in the principles of initial resuscitation and stabilization. Excellent courses, such as the Advanced Trauma Life Support course provided by the American College of Surgeons, are available to provide this training.[1] Part of this course deals specifically with the pediatric trauma patient.

Patterns of Injury

The patterns of injury in the child differ from those in the adult. Because the child is smaller, the force per unit area may be significantly higher than for the adult. Because the force is being applied to someone with less subcutaneous fat, less elastic connective tissue, and closer proximity of multiple organs, there is a high incidence of multisystem injury. Head injuries occur in over 80% of severely injured children. Abdominal injuries are also more frequent because the abdominal muscles are not sufficiently developed to protect the abdominal viscera. Because of the elasticity of the thoracic cage, fractures of the ribs and sternum are unusual. Nevertheless, severe parenchymal damage to the lungs and heart can occur with little external evidence of injury. Greater mediastinal flexibility allows a more significant lateral shift in instances of tension pneumothorax and can lead to compromised cardiac filling and ventilation of the opposite lung.

Physiologic Response to Injury

The physiologic response of a child to trauma also differs in some respects from that of an adult. Some of these differences are beneficial to the patient. Usually the child does not have any preexisting disease that affects the major organs. There are usually larger cardiac and pulmonary reserves. The child can withstand longer periods of hypoxia than the adult. The neurologic system shows a phenomenal capacity for recovery following severe injury.

The fact that the vascular system is able to maintain the systolic pressure in the normal range despite the existence of significant hypovolemia can give a false sense of security and lead to a delay in proper volume replacement. If hypovolemia continues, eventually the pressure can no longer be maintained and will start to drop, often quite rapidly. Tachycardia does occur early in hypovolemia and should be looked for carefully.

Because of the high ratio of surface area to weight, the child is very prone to develop hypothermia. This causes muscle shivering and peripheral vasoconstriction leading to lactic acidemia. This can adversely affect the response to the treatment of shock.

Primary Survey and Resuscitation

Attention must obviously be directed first to any situation that threatens the life of the patient. Attention must be paid to the well known ABC's of trauma management—Airway, Breathing, and Circulation.

History

Obviously a brief history is necessary. The mnemonic, AMPLE, is a reminder that this should include information regarding: Allergies, Medications, Past medical history, Last meal, and Events (details of the accident and any management already received). This information can be gathered as the primary survey and resuscitation proceed.

Airway and Breathing Management

Cervical Spine Control

Although the incidence of cervical-spine injury in children is quite low, nevertheless, it is recommended that all multiply injured children be treated as though they have a cervical-spine injury until this possibility has been ruled out clinically and radiographically. Immobilization is most frequently accomplished with sandbags and taping. In many cases, a rigid collar will already have been applied by the ambulance personnel. Because a child has a relatively large occiput, a regular spine board will flex the cervical spine. For this reason, special pediatric spine boards have been designed that have a depression in which the head rests.

Clearing and Maintaining the Airway

Obvious foreign material, as well as blood, mucus, and vomit, are removed from the mouth and oropharynx. Remember that, in infants, it is important to ensure that the nostrils are clear as well. The jaw thrust or lift will help maintain a clear airway. Insertion of an oral airway in a patient with an intact gag reflex is not recommended, because to do so can precipitate choking, laryngospasm, or vomiting. In the unconscious child, the airway is best controlled by the insertion of an uncuffed orotracheal tube, as described below.

If these methods fail, direct access to the trachea is best achieved by needle cricothyroidectomy. Needle jet insufflation can then be used. This emergency measure is temporary and is used only until a more definitive way of securing an airway, such as intubation or, in rare circumstances, a tracheostomy, can be carried out. If a tracheostomy is required, it should be performed by someone experienced with the technique and is done in a controlled environment, such as an operating room.

Tracheal Intubation

Obviously, this is the most reliable way to gain control of an airway in a child with ventilatory compromise. For patients that require intubation, the orotracheal route is recommended. As a rough guide, the tube used should have about the same external diameter as the child's external nares or baby finger. Uncuffed tubes are generally used for all children up to the time of puberty. There should always be a small leak of gas around the tube during inflation. Always check carefully for endobronchial intubation by listening in the axillae for air entry into each lung. The air entry must be reassessed frequently in order to detect an evolving ventilatory disfunction.

Gastric Decompression

Almost all infants and children swallow air, often in large quantities, when they are stressed. The gastric dilatation this creates can produce vomiting, with the

Table 1
Normal values for pediatric vital signs in non-crying patients

Age	Pulse (rate/min)	Blood Pressure (mm Hg)	Respirations (rate/min)
Less than 1 year	120 to 140	70 to 90	30 to 40
2 to 5 years	100 to 120	80 to 90	20 to 30
5 to 12 years	80 to 100	90 to 110	15 to 20

Formula to estimate a child's systolic blood pressure: [(Age in years × 2) + 80].

risk of aspiration. It can also cause splinting of the diaphragm and interfere with ventilation. The vena cava can be compressed, resulting in decreased venous return and causing or aggravating hypotension. A nasogastric tube should be used for decompression if there are no contraindications, such as facial fractures with damage to the cribriform plate.

Circulation (Shock)

Diagnosis

Significant blood loss is common in an injured child. The child, as mentioned previously, has a tremendous physiologic reserve. The relevance of this to management is that, despite significant hypovolemia, the child is able to maintain reasonably normal vital signs. There is a limit to this reserve, however, and when it is exceeded the vital signs can deteriorate rapidly.

The first sign of hypovolemia is tachycardia. Because hypovolemia is obviously not the only cause of tachycardia, it is also necessary to monitor the other systems. The normal circulating blood volume in a child is 80 ml/kg. A child's vital signs are age dependent. It is, therefore, very important to know the normal values for the various age groups in order to be able to detect when they are abnormal (Table 1). Close monitoring of the functions of the heart, kidneys, central nervous system, and skin makes diagnosis fairly easy and allows the physician to assess the severity of the hypovolemia and to follow the patient's response to treatment. Table 2 shows the changes seen in the functions of these four organ systems with increasing degrees of blood loss.

Venous Access

Early access to the cardiovascular system should be established. In general, this is best accomplished by a percutaneous route and, failing that, by a cutdown, or venostomy. The common sites for a cutdown are: (1) Greater saphenous at the ankle, (2) Median cephalic at the elbow, (3) Main cephalic higher in the arm, (4) External jugular, and (5) Long-bone marrow (intraosseous infusion).

The percutaneous route can be difficult to achieve in hypovolemic, younger children, and intraosseous infusion provides quick, convenient access to the venous

Table 2
Systemic responses to blood loss in the pediatric patient

System	Blood Volume Loss		
	Early (Less than 25%)	Prehypotensive (25%)	Hypotensive (40%)
Cardiac	Weak, thready pulse, increased heart rate	+ Tilt test, increased heart rate	Frank hypotension, tachycardia to bradycardia
Central Nervous System	Lethargic, irritable, confused, combative	Changes in level of consciousness, dulled response to pain	Comatose
Skin	Cool, clammy	Cyanotic, decreased capillary refill, cold extremities	Pale, cold
Kidneys	Decreased urinary output; increased specific gravity	Increased BUN	No urinary output

circulation. The recommended site is the anterior tibial metaphysis, 2 to 3 cm below the tibial tuberosity. An alternate location is the distal, anterolateral femoral metaphysis, approximately 3 cm above the lateral femoral condyle. For obvious reasons, the cannula should not be introduced below the site of a fracture. A 16- to 18-gauge needle with trocar is introduced at a right angle or up to 60 degrees caudad with the bevel up. If marrow is aspirated, the needle is in the correct place. Infusion is carried out at the same rate as for the intravenous route.

Fluid Resuscitation

The principles governing fluid resuscitation in the child are virtually the same as those that are applied to the adult. Because the manifestations of clinical shock indicate a blood loss of 25% or more, the initial fluid management is to give a bolus of crystalloid equal to approximately one fourth of the circulating blood volume (20 ml/kg). By the "3 for 1 rule," which applies in children as well as adults, it would take three such boluses to replace a 25% loss in circulating blood volume. If there is no response to the first bolus, a second is started and preparations are made to start administering blood. A surgical opinion is very important at this stage.

Blood Replacement

If the child fails to respond to a second crystalloid bolus, blood infusion should be started. If fully cross-matched or type-specific blood is not yet available, O Rh-negative blood may be given. Packed cells are usually reconstituted with plasma and given as a bolus of 10 mg/kg. If the child does not respond to this bolus, then surgery is probably indicated, depending on the probable site of the ongoing blood loss.

Chest Trauma

The flexibility and pliancy of the pediatric chest wall has already been mentioned. Its significance is that a child can sustain major intrathoracic injury with very little external evidence of this injury. The problems of tension pneumothorax and hemopneumothorax are poorly tolerated by the child because of the mobility of the mediastinal structures. When these problems occur, they must be recognized promptly and managed in exactly the same manner as they would be in the adult. The chest must be reevaluated both clinically and radiographically from time to time to avoid overlooking a serious pulmonary contusion that becomes more manifest with time.

Abdominal Trauma

Blunt trauma to the abdomen, which is very common in the multiply injured child, can occur in the unrestrained passenger in a car, as well as in a child restrained by a lap belt. The abdomen is examined clinically for tenderness, guarding, bowel sounds, etc. The peritoneal lavage is rarely used to evaluate the presence of intraperitoneal bleeding. Instead, the child is usually assessed by abdominal computed tomographic scan and frequent clinical reevaluations. The frequency of gastric distension caused by air swallowing has been mentioned. Such distension is best managed by the insertion of a nasogastric tube.

Head Injury

Head injuries in children are often devastating and are the largest, single cause of nonpreventable death. Some head injuries, however, are potentially survivable but become fatal because of inadequate treatment of hypoxia and/or hypovolemia. Respiratory insufficiency and shock must be treated quickly and effectively. Fluid restriction, to avoid exacerbating cerebral edema, has no place in the management of the injured child in shock.

Conclusion

Although the approach to the seriously injured child is no different from the ABC approach to the seriously injured adult, there are certain anatomic and physiologic differences that must be familiar to those who may find themselves managing one of these children. Use of the systematic, multidisciplinary, predetermined approach outlined above should eliminate the tragedy of a preventable death.

References

1. Pediatric trauma, in *Advanced Trauma Life Support Course for Physicians Instructors Manual*. Chicago, American College of Surgeons, 1988, pp 215–233.

Injuries of the Epiphyseal Plate

Robert B. Salter, OC, MD, FRCSC

Injuries of the epiphyseal plate present special problems in both diagnosis and management. The dread complication of significant disturbance of growth is usually predictable and can often be prevented. Thus, knowledge of the prognosis for a given injury to the epiphyseal plate in a particular child is of considerable importance to the orthopaedic surgeon, who has the dual responsibility of treating the child and advising the parents.

Applied Histology

A knowledge of the microscopic features of the normal epiphyseal plate is pivotal in understanding the problems associated with the various types of injuries to which it may be subjected. When seen in longitudinal section, four distinct layers can be identified in the normal epiphyseal plate; the layer of resting cells, the layer of proliferating cells, the layer of hypertrophying cells, and the layer of endochondral ossification. The space between the cells is filled with cartilage matrix or intercellular substance. It is this intercellular substance, and not the cells, that provides the strength of the epiphyseal plate, particularly its resistance to shear. The intercellular substance of cartilage is made up of collagen fibers embedded in an amorphous cement substance. Because the refractive indexes of these two components are the same, the collagen fibers cannot be identified in ordinary preparations, but they can be seen by special techniques, for instance, phase-contrast microscopy.

These collagen fibers in the matrix of the epiphyseal plate are arranged longitudinally and no doubt play a role similar to that of the steel rods in reinforced concrete. In the first two layers of the plate the matrix is abundant, and here the plate is strong.

In the third layer the matrix is scanty, and here the plate is weak. On the metaphyseal side of this layer, however, the matrix is calcified, forming the so-called zone of provisional calcification. The addition of calcification seems to reinforce this part of the third layer, because the plane of cleavage after separation lies in the third layer at approximately the junction of the calcified and uncalcified parts. It seems logical, then, that the constancy of the plane of cleavage is the direct result of the structural details of the normal plate. The significance of the constant location of the plane of cleavage after complete epiphyseal separation is that the growing cells remain attached to the epiphysis. Thus, if the nutrition of these cells is not damaged by the separation, there is no reason why growth should not continue in a normal fashion.

Mechanism of Nutrition

Two separate systems of blood vessels provide nutrition to the epiphyseal plate. The epiphyseal system arises from vessels in the epiphysis that penetrate the bone plate of the epiphysis. These vessels end in capillary tufts or loops in the layer of resting cells of the plate. These vessels are essential to the viability of the chondrocytes of the epiphyseal plate. The metaphyseal system arises in the marrow of the shaft and ends in vascular loops in the layer of endochondral ossification.

Dale and Harris[1] have demonstrated that the nutrient vessels of the epiphysis (from which the terminal vascular loops to the epiphyseal side of the plate are derived) enter in one of two ways. The first, and more common, of these ways occurs when the sides of the epiphysis are covered with periosteum, as is the case in the distal femoral and proximal tibial epiphyses, in which the nutrient vessels penetrate the side of the epiphysis at a point remote from the epiphyseal plate. The second, and decidedly less common, mode of entrance occurs when the entire epiphysis is intra-articular and, hence, is covered with articular cartilage. The upper femoral epiphysis is the main example of this type; the upper radial epiphysis probably belongs to this group as well. In epiphyses of this type, the nutrient vessels enter the epiphysis by traversing the rim of the epiphyseal plate. It is easy to see that the vessels of this type are in danger in the event of epiphyseal separation and might easily be ruptured.

Relative Strength

The cartilaginous epiphyseal plate is obviously less strong than bone, and yet fractures through bone are much more common in children than are epiphyseal separations. The probable explanation for this apparent paradox is that only shearing and avulsion forces are capable of separating an epiphysis.

In adolescents, the epiphyseal plate is also less strong than normal tendons and ligaments. For this reason, injuries that may result in complete tear of a major ligament in the adult actually produce a separation of the epiphysis in the adolescent. For example, an abduction injury of an adolescent's knee will result in epiphyseal separation rather than a rupture of the medial collateral ligament of the knee. Thus, tears or ruptures of major ligaments are very uncommon in adolescence, and every adolescent suspected of having torn a major ligament should have a radiographic examination to study the epiphyses of the area. By the same token, the epiphyseal plate is not as strong as the fibrous joint capsule, and traumatic dislocations of major joints, such as the knee, during adolescence are thus decidedly less common than epiphyseal separations. Stress radiographs are useful in differentiating between epiphyseal plate separations and other injuries in the area.

Relative Growth at the Ends of Long Bones

In the lower extremity, more longitudinal growth occurs in the region of the knee than in the regions of the hip or ankle. In the femur, 70% of growth occurs in the distal end and 30% occurs in the proximal end. In the tibia, 55% of growth occurs in the proximal end and 45% occurs in the distal end.

Diagnosis

Clinical Diagnosis

Although the accurate diagnosis of epiphyseal plate injuries depends on radiographic examination, the surgeon must suspect such an injury in any child or adolescent who exhibits evidence of a fracture near the end of a long bone, a dislocation, ligamentous rupture, or even a severe sprain of a joint. Remember that an epiphysis may be displaced at the moment of injury and then return to its normal position, in which case clinical examination is likely to be of considerable importance in recognizing the nature of the injury. The history of the mechanism of injury, although often inadequate, may arouse suspicion of a crushing type of epiphyseal plate injury, which is difficult to detect radiographically.

Radiographic Diagnosis

Accurate interpretation of the radiographs of adolescent bones and joints requires a knowledge of the normal appearance of epiphyses and epiphyseal plates at various ages. Two views at right angles to each other are essential, and often two additional oblique views are required. If in doubt, it may be helpful to obtain comparable views of the opposite uninjured extremity.

When the clinical examination suggests an epiphyseal plate injury but the radiographs do not reveal such an injury, stress radiographs taken while the patient is under general anesthesia frequently reveal that a sepa-

ration through the epiphyseal plate has, in fact, occurred and that in the initial radiographs the epiphysis had returned to its normal position.

Late radiographic diagnosis of an undisplaced epiphyseal separation can be made by demonstrating subperiosteal new bone formation in the metaphyseal region ten days or more after injury.

Injuries of Epiphyseal Plates

Of all injuries to the long bones during childhood, approximately 15% involve the epiphyseal plate.[2,3]

Age and Sex Incidence

Although injuries to the epiphyseal plates can occur at any age during childhood, they are somewhat more common during periods of rapid skeletal growth—in the first year and during the prepuberty growth spurt. These injuries—and others—are more frequent in boys than in girls, presumably because, in general, boys are more active physically.

Site

In general, epiphyseal plates that provide the most growth are the ones most commonly separated by injury. This is not true, however, of two types of epiphyseal injury—fractures that cross or crush the epiphyseal plate.

The lower radial epiphyseal plate is by far the one most frequently separated by injury; indeed, injuries to this epiphyseal plate are nearly as frequent as all other injuries to the epiphyseal plates combined.[4] In order of decreasing frequently, separations of other epiphyses are found in the lower ulnar, lower humeral (lateral condyle), upper radial (head), lower tibial, lower femoral, upper humeral, upper femoral (head), upper tibial and phalangeal epiphyseal plates.

Possible Effects of Epiphyseal Injuries

Fortunately, most epiphyseal plate injuries are not associated with any disturbance of growth. After separation of an epiphysis through its epiphyseal plate there may be a slight and transient acceleration of growth, in which case no significant deformity ensues.

The clinical problem associated with premature cessation of growth depends on several factors, including the bone involved, the extent of involvement of the epiphyseal plate, and the amount of remaining growth normally expected in the involved epiphyseal plate.

If the entire epiphyseal plate ceases to grow, the result is progressive shortening without angulation. However, if the involved bone is one of a parallel pair (such as tibia and fibula or radius and ulna), progressive shortening of the one bone will produce progressive angulatory deformity in the neighboring joint. If

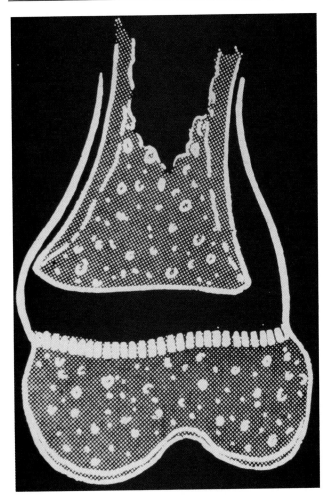

Fig. 1 Type I epiphyseal plate injury. Separation of the epiphysis.

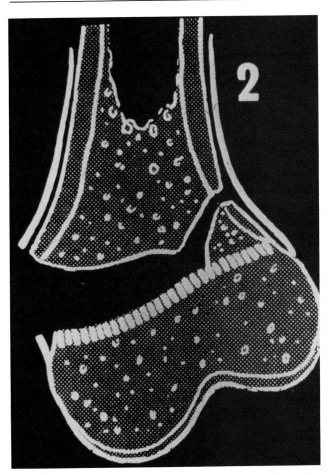

Fig. 2 Type II epiphyseal plate injury. Fracture-separation of the epiphysis.

growth in one part of the epiphyseal plate ceases but continues in the rest of the plate, progressive angulatory deformity occurs.

Cessation of growth does not necessarily occur immediately after injury to the epiphyseal plate, and, indeed, growth arrest can be delayed for six months or even longer. Furthermore, there may be a period of growth retardation before growth ceases completely.

Classification of Epiphyseal Injuries

The following classification, developed by Salter and Harris, is based on the mechanism of injury and the relationship of the fracture line to the growing cells of the epiphyseal plate. This classification scheme is also correlated with the method of treatment and the prognosis for growth disturbance.[5-8]

Type I In a type I epiphyseal plate injury (Fig. 1) there is a complete separation of the epiphysis from the metaphysis without any bony fracture. The growing cells

of the epiphyseal plate remain with the epiphysis. This type of injury, which is caused by a shearing or avulsion force, is more common in birth injuries and during early childhood, when the epiphyseal plate is relatively thick. It is also seen in pathologic separations of the epiphysis associated with scurvy, rickets, osteomyelitis, and endocrine imbalance. Wide displacement is uncommon because the periosteal attachment is usually intact. Reduction is not difficult, and the prognosis for future growth is excellent unless the epiphysis involved is entirely covered by cartilage (eg, upper end of the femur), in which case the blood supply is frequently damaged with resultant premature closure of the epiphyseal plate.

Type II In a type II epiphyseal plate injury (Fig. 2), which is the most common type, the line of separation extends along the epiphyseal plate for a variable distance and then moves out through a portion of the metaphysis, providing the familiar triangular metaphyseal fragment sometimes referred to as Thurston Holland's sign. This type of injury, which usually occurs in children older than 10 years of age, is the result of

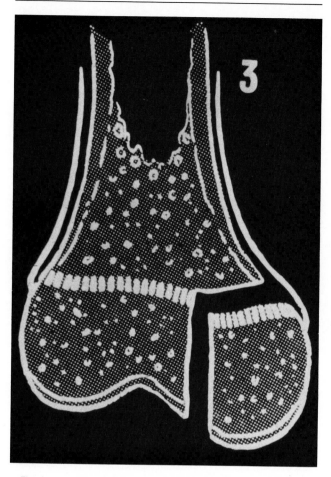

Fig. 3 Type III epiphyseal plate injury. Fracture of part of the epiphysis.

shearing injury or an avulsion force. The periosteum is torn on the convex side of the angulation, but is intact on the concave side, that is, the side on which the metaphyseal fragment is seen. Reduction is relatively easy to obtain and to maintain; because of the intact periosteal hinge and the metaphyseal fragment, over-reduction cannot occur. The growing cartilage cells of the epiphyseal plate remain with the epiphysis, and thus the prognosis for growth is excellent, provided the circulation to the epiphysis is intact (it nearly always is).

Type III In a type III epiphyseal injury (Fig. 3) the fracture, which is intra-articular, extends from the joint surface to the weak zone of the epiphyseal plate and then along the plate to its periphery. This type of injury is uncommon, but when it does occur it usually happens near the end of skeletal growth, most often in the upper or lower tibial epiphyses, and it is caused by an intra-articular shearing force. Accurate reduction is essential, not so much for the sake of the epiphyseal plate as for the restoration of a smooth joint surface; surgery may be necessary to obtain such reduction. As in types I and II injuries, the prognosis is good, provided the blood supply to the separated portion of the epiphysis is intact.

Type IV In a type IV epiphyseal injury (Fig. 4) the fracture, which is intra-articular, extends from the joint surface through the epiphysis, across the full thickness of the epiphyseal plate, and through a portion of the metaphysis, thereby producing a complete split. Perfect reduction of a type IV epiphyseal plate injury is essential, not only for the sake of the epiphyseal plate but also for the restoration of a smooth joint surface. Unless the fracture is undisplaced, open reduction is al-

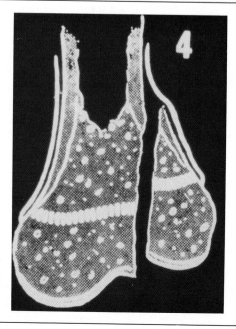
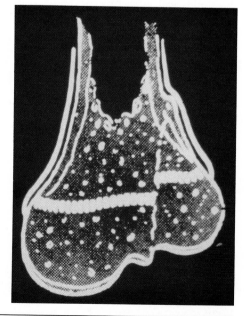

Fig. 4 Type IV epiphyseal plate injury: **Left,** Fracture of the epiphysis and epiphyseal plate. **Right,** Bony union across epiphyseal plate at fracture site.

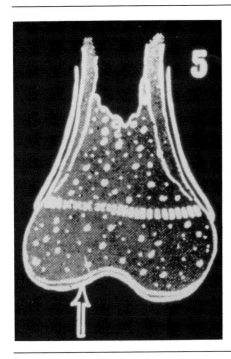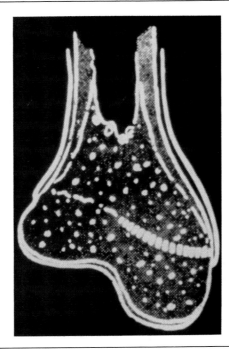

Fig. 5 Type V epiphyseal plate injury. **Left,** Crushing of the epiphyseal plate. **Right,** Premature closure of the epiphyseal plate.

ways necessary. The epiphyseal plate must be accurately realigned in order to prevent bony union across the plate with resultant local premature cessation of growth. If metal fixation is required to obtain stability, it is preferable to place it across the metaphysis, although fine, smooth Kirschner wires left to traverse the plate for a few weeks will not interfere with subsequent growth.

Type V The type V epiphyseal injury (Fig. 5), a relatively uncommon type of injury, results from a severe crushing force applied through the epiphysis to one area of the epiphyseal plate. It occurs in joints that move in one plane only, such as the ankle or the knee. A severe abduction or adduction injury to a joint that normally only flexes or extends is likely to produce crushing of the epiphyseal plate. Displacement of the epiphysis under these circumstances is unusual, and the initial radiograph gives little indication of the serious nature of the injury; indeed, the injury may be dismissed as a sprain. Suspect crushing of the epiphyseal plate under such circumstances, and prevent weight bearing for three weeks in the hope of preventing the almost inevitable premature cessation of growth. The prognosis in type V epiphyseal plate injuries is decidedly poor.

Type VI To this five-type classification, a sixth type has been added by Rang.[9] This type consists of an injury to the perichondrial ring of the epiphyseal plate. If the perichondrial ring is either removed by a sharp object in an open injury or is avulsed by an injury to a ligament attached to it, bone will grow across the epiphyseal plate from epiphysis to metaphysis, thereby producing a bony

bridge and a resultant progressive angulatory deformity.

Other Classifications

Epiphyseal injuries have also been classified by Poland,[10] Aitken and Magill,[11] and, more recently, by Ogden[12] but the Salter-Harris classification is probably the one most widely used. At the distal end of the tibia near the end of skeletal growth, closure of the epiphyseal plate begins medially and proceeds laterally. While this closure is in progress an injury may produce a "triplane fracture," which combines a type II injury with either a type III or even a type IV injury as described by Cooperman and associates.[13] In the triplane fracture, there may be either two or three fragments. Radiographic examination may be difficult to interpret, and a computed tomographic scan is indicated to determine the nature of the fracture as well as the precise position of the fragments. The type III and type IV components of the triplane fracture require accurate reduction and maintenance of such reduction; this may necessitate open reduction and internal fixation.

Factors in Estimating the Prognosis Regarding Growth Disturbance

Significant growth disturbance follows approximately 10% of epiphyseal plate injuries, although minor disturbances are seen in a higher percentage of patients. Although it is not possible in a given patient with a given epiphyseal plate injury to predict the prognosis with absolute accuracy, several factors help considerably in estimating prognosis.

Type of Injury

The anatomic type of injury, described above, is important from the prognostic point of view. In general, types I, II, and III injuries have a good prognosis for growth, provided the blood supply of the epiphysis is intact and the injury has not been severe, such as an automobile accident or a fall from a great height. The prognosis for type IV epiphyseal injuries is bad, unless the fracture across the epiphyseal plate is completely reduced. Type V injuries associated with actual crushing of the cartilaginous plate have the worst prognosis.

Age at the Time of Injury

The age of the patient makes it possible to predict the amount of growth normally expected in the particular epiphyseal plate during the remaining years of growth. Obviously, the younger the patient at the time of injury, the more serious any growth disturbance will be. On the other hand, even a serious injury incurred during the last year of growth will not produce a significant deformity, because so little normal growth potential remains.

Blood Supply to the Epiphysis

The epiphyseal plate is nourished by blood vessels of the epiphysis. If this blood supply is destroyed, the epiphyseal plate degenerates and growth ceases. Thus, interference with the blood supply to the epiphysis (a common complication of epiphyseal injuries of the femoral and radial heads) is associated with a poor prognosis. Fortunately, in other regions, the blood vessels enter the epiphyses directly and, here, separation of these epiphyses does not usually disturb the blood supply.

Severity of the Injury (Velocity and Force)

When a given type of injury occurs in an epiphyseal plate as the result of a violent injury, such as an automobile accident or a fall from a great height, there may be some crushing of the plate even in a type I, II, or III injury. The prognosis for subsequent growth may thus be poor, even though with a less severe injury the prognosis might have been good.

Method of Reduction

Unduly forceful manipulation of an epiphysis can injure the epiphyseal plate; this is particularly true if the manipulation is carried out past the tenth day after injury. Likewise, instruments used to pry on an epiphyseal plate during surgical reduction can crush the plate. Screw nails or threaded wires that traverse the epiphyseal plate also increase the risk of premature cessation of growth. Excessive soft-tissue stripping of an epiphysis at the time of open reduction can lead to avascular necrosis of that epiphysis and the underlying epiphyseal plate with resultant premature cessation of growth.

Closed or Open Injury

Open (formerly called "compound") injuries of the epiphyseal plate are uncommon. However, they have a poorer prognosis than do closed injuries because of the added factor of contamination and possible infection. If infection develops at the site of an epiphyseal plate injury, the cartilaginous epiphyseal plate is usually destroyed by the process of chondrolysis, and the prognosis is therefore very poor indeed.

General Principles of Treatment

Gentleness in Reduction

In types I, II, and III epiphyseal plate injuries, in contrast to fractures through bone, one of the fracture surfaces is composed of delicate, vulnerable cartilage of the epiphyseal plate. Consequently, in order to prevent damage to the plate, the surgeon must avoid unduly forceful manipulation of such an injury. This principle also applies to surgical methods of reducing a displaced epiphysis. No instrument should be used to pry a displaced epiphysis back into place.

Time of Reduction

The best time to reduce an epiphyseal plate injury is on the day of the injury, because reduction becomes progressively more difficult with each passing day. Indeed, after about 10 days the fragments, particularly in types I and II injuries, are difficult to shift without using excessive force. Under these circumstances, forceful manipulation may further damage the cartilaginous plate and should be avoided; at this stage it is wiser to accept an imperfect reduction than to risk either forceful manipulation or open operation. Perform a corrective osteotomy later if necessary. In types III and IV injuries, however, delayed reduction, although not desirable, is preferable to leaving the intraarticular fragment displaced.

Method of Reduction

The vast majority of types I and II epiphyseal plate injuries are readily reduced by closed means, and furthermore the reduction is easily maintained. Type III injuries sometimes require open reduction to obtain a smooth joint surface, and displaced type IV injuries nearly always require open reduction. When internal fixation is deemed necessary, it is preferable to place such fixation through the metaphysis rather than through the epiphysis. Never insert screw nails or threaded wires across the epiphyseal plate; fine smooth Kirschner wires that cross the plate at right angles may be used with impunity but should be removed when the injury is healed. Take great care to avoid damage to the blood supply of the epiphysis.

The contour of the epiphyseal plate is such that perfect reduction of types I and II injuries is usually possible. If, however, there is residual moderate displacement (anterior, posterior, medial, or lateral) or slight angulation, repeat manipulation is not necessary, because remodeling of the bone from the periosteum is adequate. The criteria for acceptable position are less rigid in the region of a multiplane joint, such as the shoulder, than in the region of a single-plane joint, such as the knee. Types III and IV injuries must be perfectly reduced, as explained previously.

Period of Immobilization

Types I, II, and III injuries unite in approximately half the time required for union of a fracture through the metaphysis of the same bone in the same age group; therefore, the period of immobilization may be correspondingly reduced. Type IV injuries, because of their location, require the same period for union as metaphyseal fractures do.

Estimation and Discussion of Prognosis

In a given epiphyseal plate injury, consider the prognosis for growth disturbance at least in the general terms described above. Part of the surgeon's responsibility in the treatment of these injuries is to provide the parents with some indication of the prognosis without causing them undue anxiety. Stress the importance of follow-up examination.

Period of Follow-up Observation

The need for regular follow-up observation of epiphyseal plate injuries is obvious; it is not always obvious just how long a period of observation is required. Because growth disturbance can be delayed, at least in its manifestations, for up to one year, a one-year period of observation is the minimum. Six months after injury examine the full length of the injured bone and its opposite number in the healthy extremity with x-rays. If little growth has occurred in the uninjured bone during this six-month period, six more months of observation will be needed before a definitive prognosis can be made.

Complications of Epiphyseal Injuries

Failure of Early Diagnosis

The clinical and radiographic diagnosis of epiphyseal plate injuries, discussed above, merits emphasis in order to avoid failure of early diagnosis. Failure of diagnosis of a type I injury is difficult to avoid in infants when the involved epiphysis is not yet ossified, for example, in a birth injury that produces a fracture-separation of the unossified proximal femoral epiphysis. Initially, this injury is difficult to differentiate radiographically from congenital or traumatic dislocation of the hip in the newborn, unless an arthrogram is performed. Within one week, however, periosteal new bone formation along the neck of the femur provides

a clue. Fracture-separation of the entire unossified distal humeral epiphysis in an infant presents the same problems in diagnosis.

Failure to diagnose an epiphyseal plate injury early means that appropriate treatment is delayed. This delay can be particularly serious with an unstable type IV injury of the lateral condyle of the humerus, which, if untreated, can go on to a nonunion. Failure to recognize a type IV injury in the knee or ankle can result in a malunion that will in turn lead to premature cessation of growth in the involved epiphyseal plate.

Malunion

When a type I or II epiphyseal plate injury has healed in an unsatisfactory position, there may be some spontaneous correction of the deformity, provided that the epiphyseal plate continues to grow, the child is young, and the deformity is in the plane of motion of the nearest joint, for example, posterior or anterior angulation in the femur at the site of a distal femoral epiphyseal separation. If the deformity does not, or is unlikely to, correct spontaneously, a corrective osteotomy is required. Malunion of a type III injury of the distal tibial epiphyseal plate can lead to post-traumatic degenerative arthritis unless the incongruity of the joint surface is corrected surgically. Malunion of a type IV injury of, for example, the distal tibial epiphyseal plate inevitably leads to a premature cessation of growth.

Nonunion

The most common site of nonunion after an epiphyseal plate injury is the type IV fracture-separation of the lateral condyle of the humerus, a complication that in turn leads to additional complications of lateral instability of the elbow joint and, eventually, a tardy ulnar nerve palsy. Displaced type IV injuries of the lateral condyle of the humerus represent an absolute indication for accurate open reduction and internal fixation in order to prevent malunion or nonunion.

Osteomyelitis

An open injury of an epiphyseal plate carries the same risk of osteomyelitis as any open fracture. Osteomyelitis in the region of the epiphyseal plate, however, especially if caused by *Staphylococcus aureus*, can result in chondrolysis of the cartilaginous plate and can lead to premature cessation of growth. Therefore, such injuries must be treated with meticulous debridement and prophylactic antibiotics; they should be left open initially, with a delayed skin closure.

Neurological Complications

An unreduced type II injury of the distal radial epiphysis with residual anterior angulation (dorsal tilt of the epiphysis) can cause compression of the median nerve, which is a form of carpal tunnel compression syndrome.

Hyperextension injuries in the region of the knee

(type I or II injuries of either the distal femoral or proximal tibial epiphyseal plates) are associated with a risk of serious injury to the medial popliteal nerve, usually of the traction type. Careful neurological examination and documentation before treatment are essential to differentiate between neurologic damage caused by the injury and that caused by the treatment.

Vascular Complications

Vascular injuries are seldom associated with epiphyseal plate injuries except in the region of the knee, where the popliteal artery is at risk along with the medial popliteal nerve for the same types of injuries mentioned above. Indeed, unrecognized intimal tears or disruptions of the popliteal artery secondary to hypertension may even lead to gangrene and can necessitate amputation.

Avascular Necrosis of the Epiphyses

The blood supply to the epiphysis has been discussed above. It is apparent that completely displaced type I injuries of the proximal femoral and proximal radial epiphyses carry a high risk of avascular necrosis of the epiphysis and, even more important, of the related epiphyseal plates. When an epiphyseal plate loses its blood supply, the chondrocytes of the plate die and are replaced by fibrocytes, with resultant cessation of epiphyseal plate growth.

Avascular necrosis of the proximal femoral epiphysis at an early age is therefore associated with failure of the femoral neck to grow in length, with continued poor growth of the greater trochanter, and with a functional coxa vara, which may necessitate a distal and lateral transfer of the greater trochanter to overcome the associated Trendelenburg limp.

Premature Cessation of Growth and its Management

After an epiphyseal plate injury, local growth may either cease immediately or it may continue at a retarded rate for a variable period of time before complete cessation. Furthermore, the growth disturbance may involve the entire epiphyseal plate or only one part of it. The resultant deformity progresses until the end of the growing period. Thus, the gravity of the clinical problem depends on several factors—the site of the growth disturbance, the extent of involvement of the epiphyseal plate, and the expected amount of growth remaining in the involved plate. The main types of deformity that can develop are progressive angulation, progressive shortening, or a combination. Considerable judgment is required to plan the most effective management of these progressive deformities.

Retardation or cessation of growth in one area of the epiphyseal plate with continuation of growth in the remainder produces a gradually progressive angulation. Under these circumstances, growth in the remainder of the plate eventually ceases prematurely, and

shortening becomes superimposed upon angulation. It is usually preferable to deal with progressive angulation by an open wedge type of osteotomy in order to preserve the growing potential of the undamaged portion of the epiphyseal plate and to gain some length in the extremity. Unless the entire epiphyseal plate has ceased growing, the osteotomy should overcorrect the deformity to delay its inevitable recurrence. When progressive angulation exists in a child, it may become necessary to repeat the osteotomy more than once. Epiphyseal arrest by stapling may help to correct a progressive angulation, but only if the damaged area of the epiphyseal plate is still growing. This method has the disadvantage, however, of further shortening the involved extremity.

Excision of a post-traumatic bony bridge that crosses the epiphyseal plate and insertion of a free fat graft, as developed by Langenskiöld,[14,15] offers hope of preventing a progressive angulatory deformity and even of restoring symmetric longitudinal growth, provided that the bony bridge does not exceed one third of the epiphyseal plate. Using Silastic inserts rather than free-fat grafts, Bright[16] has also had encouraging results.

If one of two paired bones (eg, radius or ulna, tibia or fibula) is the site of premature cessation of growth, the resultant discrepancy in length between the two bones will produce a progressive deformity (varus or valgus) of the nearest joint. For example, premature cessation of growth at the lower radial epiphyseal plate in the presence of continued growth at the lower ulnar epiphysis will produce a progressive valgus or radial deviation of the hand. To overcome this problem it may be necessary to lengthen the shorter bone or shorten the longer bone. At the same time, an epiphyseal arrest of the growing epiphysis will prevent a recurrence of the deformity.

When a single bone (femur or humerus) develops progressive shortening, the resultant problem is one of limb-length discrepancy, which is only significant in the lower extremity. An actual or predicted lower-limb discrepancy of more than 3 cm usually merits either surgical lengthening of the involved bone or epiphyseal arrest or surgical shortening of the opposite limb in accordance with the principles of leg-length equalization.

References

1. Dale GG, Harris WR: Prognosis of epiphyseal separation: An experimental study. *J Bone Joint Surg* 1958;40B:116–122.
2. Bisgard JD, Martenson L: Fractures in children. *Surg Gynecol Obstet* 1937;65:464–474.
3. Compere EL: Growth arrest in long bones as a result of fractures that include the epiphysis. *JAMA* 1935;105:2140–2146.
4. Eliason EL, Ferguson LK: Epiphyseal separation of the long bones. *Surg Gynecol Obstet* 1934;58:85–99.
5. Salter RB, Harris WR: Injuries involving the epiphyseal plate. *J Bone Joint Surg* 1963;45A:587–622.

6. Salter RB: Injuries of the ankle in children. *Orthop Clin North Am* 1974;5:147–152.

7. Salter RB: Epiphyseal injuries in the adolescent knee, in Kennedy JC (ed): *The Injured Adolescent Knee.* Baltimore, Williams & Wilkins, 1979, chap 3, pp 77–101.

8. Czitrom AA, Salter RB, Willis RB: Fractures involving the distal femoral epiphyseal plate of the femur. *Int Orthop* 1981;4:269–277.

9. Rang M: *Children's Fractures*, ed 2. Philadelphia, Lippincott, 1983, pp 23 & 315.

10. Poland J: *Traumatic separation of the epiphyses.* London, Smith, Elder & Co., 1898.

11. Aitken AP, Magill HK: Fractures involving the distal femoral epiphyseal cartilage. *J Bone Joint Surg* 1952;34A:96.

12. Ogden JA: *Skeletal Injury in the Child.* Philadelphia, Lea & Febiger, 1982.

13. Cooperman DR, Spiegel PG, Laros GS: Tibial fractures involving the ankle in children: The so-called triplane epiphyseal fracture. *J Bone Joint Surg* 1978;60A:1040–1046.

14. Langenskiöld A: An operation for partial closure of an epiphyseal plate in children, and its experimental basis. *J Bone Joint Surg* 1975;57B:325–330.

15. Langenskiöld A: Surgical treatment of partial closure of the growth plate. *J Pediatr Orthop* 1981;1:3–12.

16. Bright RW: Operative correction of partial epiphyseal plate closure by osseous-bridge resection and silicone rubber implant. *J Bone Joint Surg* 1974;56A:655–664.

Occult Fractures

Colin F. Moseley, MD

Occult fractures are fractures in children that occur partly or completely through the cartilage parts of immature bones. Because the part of the fracture that occurs through cartilage is not fully defined by plain radiographs, there is a risk of the fracture being misdiagnosed or missed completely. The orthopaedic surgeon treating fractures near the joints of young children must have a high index of suspicion and must take whatever measures are necessary to completely define the fracture before undertaking treatment.

Occult Fractures About the Hip

Occult fractures about the hip usually occur in relation to dislocation and involve chondral or osteo-chondral fractures of the femoral head or the margins of the acetabulum. The hip radiograph in Figure 1 was taken eight months after a closed reduction for traumatic dislocation. The reduction is clearly not concentric. An arthrogram shows separation of the joint surfaces, and computed tomography shows a fragment within the joint that was not visible on the plain radiographs. The radiograph of the fragment makes it clear that the large bulk of the fragment is cartilaginous. Because only a small part is bone, it was not evident on the radiograph of the hip.

The cartilaginous rim of the acetabulum, the labrum, can obstruct reduction if it is torn or infolded. Figure 2 shows a boy who dislocated his hip in a fall from a bicycle, and who had a nonconcentric closed reduction. The radiographs shown were taken nine months after

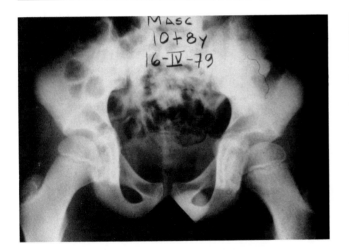

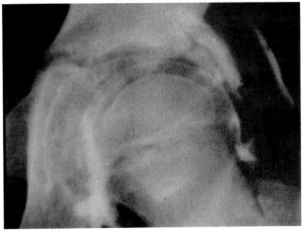

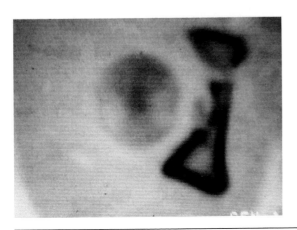

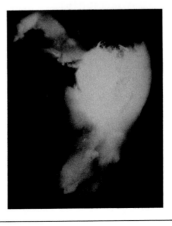

Fig. 1 Top left, A post-reduction film of a 10-year-old who suffered dislocation of the hip. The hip is not concentrically reduced, and there is widening of the medial joint space. **Top right,** Arthrogram shows separation of the joint surfaces. **Bottom left,** CT scan shows a fragment in the joint. **Bottom right,** A radiograph of the fragment removed by arthrotomy shows that it is largely cartilage, explaining why it did not show on plain radiographs.

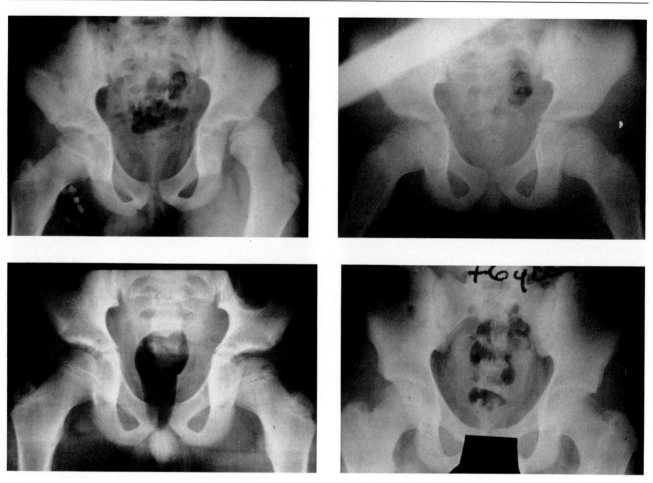

Fig. 2 **Top left**, A dislocation of the hip in a 10-year-old who fell from a bicycle. **Top right**, A closed reduction produced a nonconcentric reduction. **Bottom left**, Open reduction was carried out with repositioning of an infolded interposed labrum. **Bottom right**, The hip appeared normal six years later.

the injury. Exploration of his hip joint disclosed a torn labrum, a flap of which was interposed into the joint. Excision of the flap was required to achieve a concentric reduction. Figure 3 shows a nonconcentric reduction of the hip of a girl at the age of 7 and also at the age of 15 when she was seen because of hip pain. Computed tomography showed a bony fragment in the fovea of the acetabulum. In this case, because of the long delay in diagnosis, the dome of the acetabulum had actually remodeled to the new, slightly lateralized, position of the femoral head.

Open reduction of the dislocated hip is not required as often in children as it is in adults partly because the rim of the acetabulum is somewhat flexible, and also because the incidence of small bony chips in the acetabulum is much lower in children. The orthopaedic surgeon should examine post-reduction films very carefully for concentricity and should perform an open reduction in any case of nonconcentric reduction.

Occult Fractures About the Knee

Occult fractures about the knee, like those about the hip, are usually related to dislocation, in this case of the patellofemoral joint. Bony fragments can be knocked off the patella or the lateral femoral condyle at the time of dislocation and, if the bony component of the fragment is relatively small, can be invisible on a radiograph. Figure 4 shows a radiograph and an intraoperative photograph of the knee of a 15-year-old girl who dislocated her patella with a resulting acute hemarthrosis. In this case, because there was a significant bony component, the radiograph shows the fragment lying behind the femoral condyle. The fragment was large enough to be reduced and fixed internally.

Figure 5 shows a patient who injured his knee during a football game. The injury occurred between plays as he stooped down with a twisting motion to pick up the football. He felt a pop in his knee and developed an acute hemarthrosis. In this case, radiographs of the

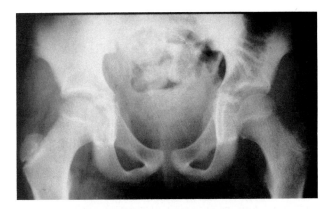

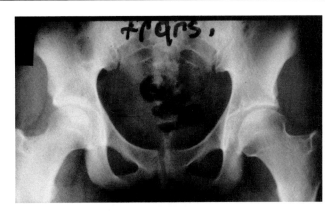

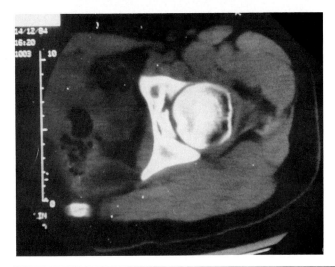

Fig. 3 **Top left**, Post-reduction film of a 7-year-old girl who had suffered a traumatic dislocation of the hip. The radiograph was read as normal, but, in retrospect, showed a nonconcentric reduction. **Top right**, Eight years later she complained of mild pain in the hip. The medial joint space is still wide, but the weightbearing dome has remodeled to the altered position of the femoral head and the joint is congruent. **Bottom**, CT shows a bone fragment in the fovea of the acetabulum.

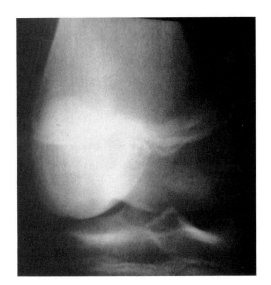

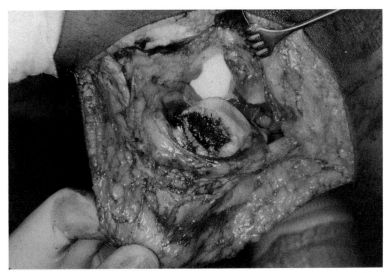

Fig. 4 **Left**, This 15-year-old girl suffered a traumatic dislocation of her patella. The radiograph shows a bone fragment overlying the femoral condyle. **Right**, At exploration the fragment was found to be larger than expected because of its large cartilaginous component.

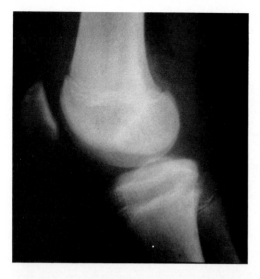

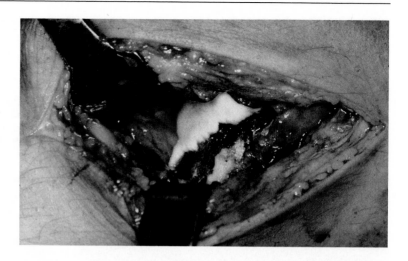

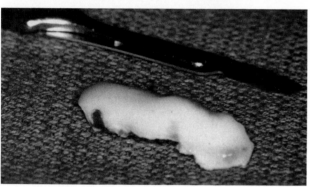

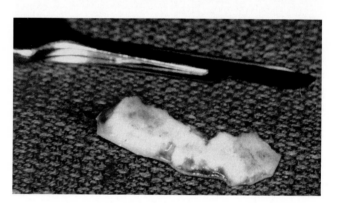

Fig. 5   Top left, This boy felt a pop as he stooped to pick up a football. Radiographs showed no evidence of fracture. **Top right** and **bottom left**, At exploration he was found to have peeled off a part of the articular cartilage from his femoral condyle. **Bottom right**, The fragment, which was composed almost entirely of cartilage, was not evident on the radiograph. Upon close examination of the fracture surface of the side of the fragment one can almost see Beninghoff's arcades and the tangential orientation of the surface collagen.

knee were completely normal, but arthroscopy and subsequent open arthrotomy showed that a large piece of articular cartilage had been torn off his femoral condyle, much like the peel from an orange. The photograph of the fragment shows that there is almost no bony component, which explains why this fracture was occult and not visible on the radiograph.

Tibial spine fractures can also be occult in young children, whose tibial spines are largely cartilaginous. There is always an occult component to tibial spine fractures, which may have very large cartilaginous flaps. The meniscus may be incarcerated beneath these flaps, which would not appear on the radiograph.

Occult Fractures Around the Elbow

Occult fractures around the elbow present the gravest risks and have the most serious implications for the orthopaedic surgeon. The variety of such fractures is numerous and their diagnosis is particularly difficult.

There are several specific types of radiograph that can be misinterpreted.

Dislocation Versus Type I Fracture

Children in the first 2 or 3 years of life can have a swollen and painful elbow following an injury. At that age, because very little ossification has occurred and no ossification centers may be present, radiographs may only disclose that the relationship of the forearm bones to the humerus is abnormal. This abnormal relationship may be caused by a type I fracture through the distal humerus or a dislocation of the elbow. In such cases, it is also conceivable that the injury could be a condylar fracture.

In these very young children, the incidence of dislocation is extremely low, and almost all such injuries are type I fractures of the distal humerus. However, to avoid treating the child merely on the basis of these odds, it is imperative that the surgeon determine the exact nature of the fracture. This is best done by arthrogram. In Figure 6, which shows just such an injury,

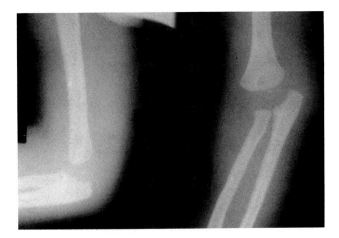 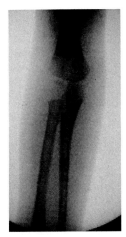 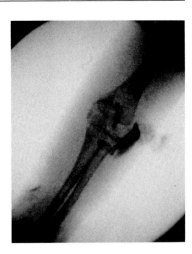

Fig. 6 **Left**, A 1-year-old child with a painful swollen elbow. To the astute observer the radiograph reveals a disturbed relationship between the forearm bones and the humerus, but does not disclose the nature of the injury. **Center**, The initial view on the image intensifier shows no abnormality. **Right**, The appearance of the arthrogram is altogether different. The outlines of the olecranon, radial head, and femoral condyles are clearly seen. Upon manipulation of the elbow, dye is seen to enter the growth plate but not between the condyles, indicating that the injury is a type I physeal injury. A condylar fracture can be confidently ruled out.

the plain films showed only an abnormal relationship between the forearm bones and the humerus, but an arthrogram outlined all of the cartilaginous components of the elbow. The arthrogram showed that there was no dislocation, that there was no dye intruding between the medial and lateral condyles, and that dye flowed into the fractured epiphyseal plate with manipulation of the elbow. Having established the exact nature of the injury, it was possible to proceed to definitive and correct treatment.

Growth Plate Fracture Versus Medial Condyle Fracture

For many children who have a swollen painful elbow following trauma, a radiograph shows only a flake of bone fractured from the lateral humeral metaphysis. Although this is almost always a type IV fracture of the lateral condyle, extending toward and perhaps into the elbow joint, it might also represent, instead, a type II fracture of the epiphyseal plate that does not involve the joint. These fractures are usually displaced type IV condylar fractures, which require open reduction and fixation. In case of a type II fracture, surgery is unnecessary. If there is any doubt, an arthrogram will determine the true nature of the injury.

In some cases, the metaphyseal fragments can be so small as to be invisible on plain films and the fracture can be completely missed. Figure 7 shows just such a case. The partial fracture of the olecranon was recognized, but the slight shift in position and contour of the ossification center of the capitellum was not. After the fracture had been treated on the basis of the incomplete diagnosis, subsequent radiographs showed further evidence that this was in fact a condylar fracture. This fracture went on to nonunion and significant disruption of the elbow. Figure 7 also shows the elbow

of a 28-year-old man who suffered a similar injury as a child and emphasizes the importance of treating these fractures appropriately in the initial stage.

Condylar Fracture Versus Epicondylar Fracture

Almost all fractures on the medial side of the elbow are epicondylar fractures, and almost all those on the lateral side are condylar fractures, but it is not very helpful to know this in the treatment of an individual case. Medial condylar fractures do exist, and, at certain ages, these fractures can be occult and not evident on plain radiographs.

Figure 8 shows anteroposterior and lateral views of a 6-year-old child with a swollen, painful elbow. Because the plain radiographs disclosed only a significant displacement of the ossification center of the medial epicondyle, it would have been very easy to treat this injury as an epicondylar fracture, which might or might not require open reduction. The child was taken to the operating room, however, where an arthrogram outlined the fracture fragment and showed quite clearly that the displaced ossification center was only a small part of a very large medial condyle fragment. Medial condyle fractures, like lateral condylar fractures, require open reduction and fixation. The arthrogram led to appropriate treatment.

Principles of Treatment of Occult Fractures

Orthopaedic surgeons treating children's fractures must repeatedly remind themselves about occult fractures, because only a high index of clinical suspicion will avoid the pitfalls mentioned above. Although a knowledge of the incidence and pathogenesis of frac-

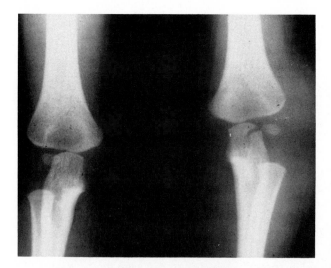
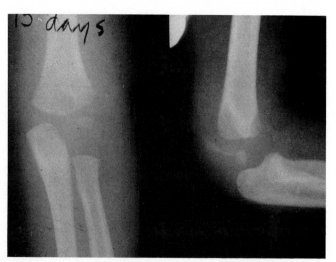
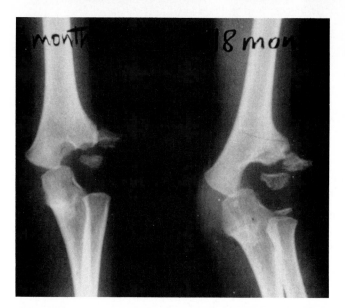
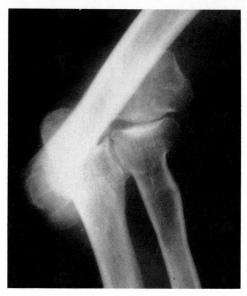

Fig. 7 **Top left**, This child had a painful swollen elbow after a fall. The fracture of the olecranon was recognized, but the slight changes in shape and position of the ossification center of the capitellum were not. **Top right** and **bottom left**, Films taken later revealed that the fracture was in reality a lateral condyle fracture that is ununited. **Bottom right**, The elbow of a 28-year-old man who had suffered a similar injury at the age of four. He has a severely disorganized elbow and significant disability.

tures is helpful, such knowledge is not sufficient to ensure proper treatment of these fractures. It behooves the treating surgeon to appreciate fully the nature of the injury and to make a complete and correct diagnosis before attempting treatment. One must treat the child for the injury that exists, not for the injury that most likely exists.

Further investigation should be performed whenever necessary to determine the exact nature of the injury. Computed tomographic scans are not helpful because the cartilage cannot be distinguished from articular fluid and, therefore, computed tomography cannot define intra-articular fractures through cartilage. Mag-

netic resonance imaging can make this distinction, but its resolution is not always sufficient to be confident about the nature of the fracture. In addition, obtaining a magnetic resonance image, which usually involves waiting hours or even days, delays treatment.

The arthrogram, unlike these modalities, can be performed quickly and easily in the operating room by the operating surgeon and, therefore, entails no delay in treatment. Many of these children will require open reduction and fixation in any case, so it is reasonable to bring them to the operating room to perform the arthrogram under general anesthesia. Having outlined the fracture fragments, one can then proceed to ap-

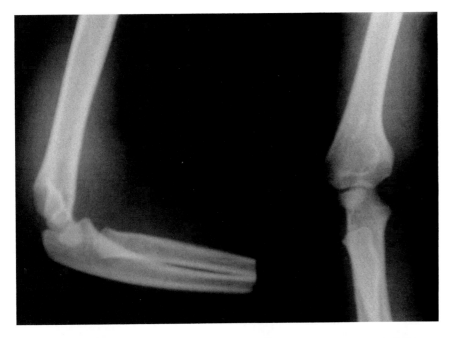

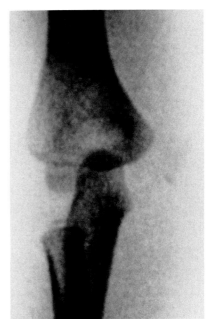

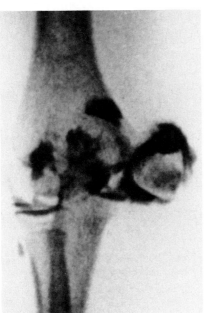

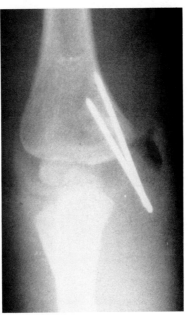

Fig. 8   Top left, This little girl presented with a painful, swollen elbow, mainly on the medial side. A radiograph showed a displaced ossification center of the medial epicondyle, such as would occur with a medial epicondyle avulsion fracture. **Top right**, The image intensifier shows only the displaced epicondylar ossification center. **Bottom left**, The arthrogram makes it evident that the fracture involves the condyle and not just the epicondyle. **Bottom right**, This fracture requires open reduction and internal fixation, which might not have been done had the orthopaedic surgeon assumed the most likely diagnosis, that of epicondyle fracture.

propriate treatment. The arthrogram is indicated in most elbow fractures when the patient is younger than three years of age and in many cases when the patient is younger than six.

Occult fractures can trap the unwary, but they represent an avoidable pitfall to the suspicious orthopaedic surgeon who is careful to take appropriate measures to reach a complete definitive diagnosis.

Fractures of the Proximal Humerus and Shaft in Children

James H. Beaty, MD

Proximal Humeral Fractures

Fractures of the proximal humeral physis account for approximately 3% of all physeal fractures.[1] Because the proximal humeral physis contributes 80% of the longitudinal growth of the humerus,[1-2] these injuries can have serious consequences. Proximal humeral fractures in children fall roughly into two groups: Salter-Harris type I fractures occur most frequently in children between birth and 5 years of age, and Salter-Harris type II fractures occur in children between 5 and 14 years of age. Salter-Harris types III and IV fractures of the proximal humerus are rare in children.[2] During infancy, the fracture may be caused by a fall, by catching the arm in a crib, or by child abuse. In later childhood, the most common mechanism is a fall.

In infants and young children, the physis is more transverse than conical, but with growth it becomes more "cone-shaped"[3] and more susceptible to Salter-Harris type II rather than type I injuries. The fracture

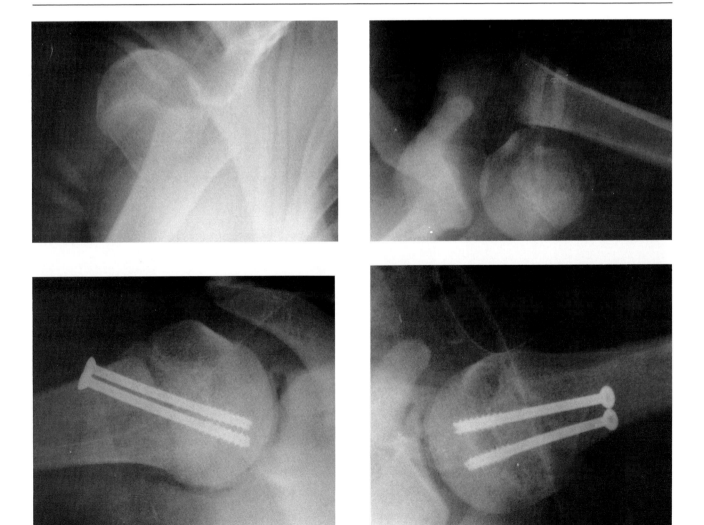

Fig. 1 **Top left** and **right,** Completely displaced, irreducible, Salter-Harris type II proximal humeral epiphyseal fracture in a 14-year-old girl. **Bottom left** and **right,** After open reduction and internal fixation.

369

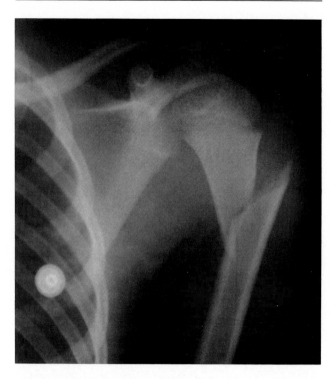

Fig. 2 Metaphyseal fracture of proximal humerus in 8-year-old boy, who was injured while playing football.

begins in the lateral aspect of the physis and continues medially into the metaphysis, leaving a metaphyseal fragment of variable size.[4] With severe injury, the distal fragment usually is displaced anterolaterally beneath the deltoid.[2] Periosteal stripping of the lateral metaphysis is frequent, and entrapment of the biceps between the fracture fragments can hinder reduction.

Diagnosis is made by roentgenogram because physical findings vary, depending on displacement. Swelling and localized tenderness around the shoulder joint usually are present, and ecchymosis may appear two to three days after injury.

Treatment, which depends primarily on the age of the patient and the degree of displacement, can be divided into four general categories: neonates, 1 to 5 years of age, 5 to 12 years of age, and 12 years and older. The younger the child, the more potential there is for physeal remodeling.[1,2] Most proximal humeral fractures in children can be treated with closed methods. Minimal attempts at reduction are indicated, and most authors report good results in very young children even with significant displacement.[1,2,5,6] Even in older children and adolescents, slight overriding of the fragments or mild varus usually is remodeled with growth. As a general guideline the following are acceptable positions for fracture alignment: (1) in children younger than 5 years, 70 degrees of angulation and total displacement; (2) in children between 5 and 12 years of

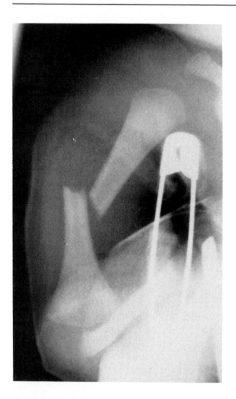
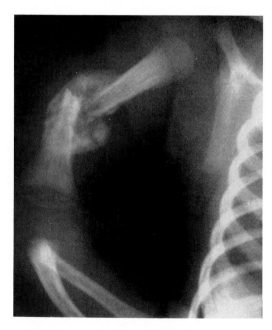
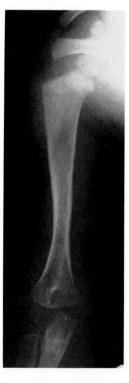

Fig. 3 **Left,** Fracture, shaft of the humerus in newborn. **Center,** Four weeks later, large mass of callus, varus angulation of 45 degrees. **Right,** At age 14 months, fracture remodeled to normal alignment.

age, 40 to 70 degrees of angulation; and (3) in children older than 12 years, 40 degrees of angulation and 50% apposition. As the teenager approaches the final years of growth, minimal angulation and displacement are acceptable.

Closed treatment methods include a collar-and-cuff, a shoulder spica cast, an abduction brace, or a hanging arm cast. Collar-and-cuff immobilization for two to three weeks usually is sufficient for fractures in infants and children up to 5 years of age or for minimally displaced fractures in older children. A hanging arm cast infrequently may be used in children between the ages of 5 and 12 years in whom fracture alignment is unsatisfactory or in whom shortening is more than 2 cm.

Surgical options include "blind" percutaneous pinning and open reduction and internal fixation. Blind percutaneous pinning generally is reserved for adolescents with completely displaced fractures and an unacceptable position. Open reduction and internal fixation rarely are indicated for proximal humeral fractures. Children with multiple injuries may require open reduction and internal fixation for stabilization of the fracture or of soft tissues (such as periosteum or the deltoid or biceps tendon), which can be entrapped between the fragments and prevent reduction. In children aged 12 years and older with completely displaced fracture, if open reduction and internal fixation are indicated, fixation may be with two removable, smooth Kirschner wires through a deltopectoral surgical approach. For teenagers approaching skeletal maturity, internal fixation by minifragment screws may be used as in adults (Fig. 1).

Complications after these fractures in children are rare.[7] The two most common are loss of motion after open reduction and varus deformity. Both, however, generally are well-tolerated because of the mobility of the shoulder joint. Rarely, physeal growth arrest causes limb length inequality extensive enough to be a cosmetic problem, but it rarely causes functional problems.

Special types of proximal humeral fractures include stress fractures, reported in young baseball players,[8,9] and fractures caused by birth trauma or child abuse.

Humeral Shaft Fractures

Humeral shaft fractures are less common in children than in adults. Metaphyseal fractures (Fig. 2) occur most frequently in children between the ages of 4 and 12 years. The diaphyseal area is more frequently fractured in children younger than 3 years of age or older than 12 years.[10] Most humeral shaft fractures are caused by indirect trauma, such as twisting, rather than by direct trauma. Humeral shaft fractures also occur in children with multiple trauma, as can result from

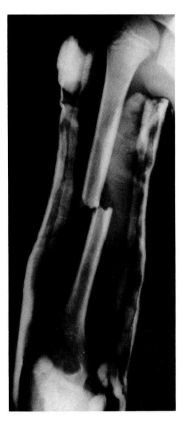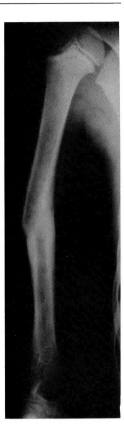

Fig. 4 Left, Diaphyseal humeral shaft fracture in 12-year-old boy treated in coaptation splint. **Right**, Union at 2 months with mild varus angulation.

motor vehicle accidents. Humeral shaft fractures can be transverse with part of the periosteum left intact, transverse with complete tear of the periosteum, oblique, or spiral.

Regardless of type, most humeral shaft fractures in children should be treated with closed methods. Anteroposterior and lateral roentgenograms should confirm satisfactory position after treatment. Overriding of 1 to 2 cm will be compensated by overgrowth of the humerus. For fracture of the middle or distal thirds, angulation of 15 degrees is acceptable, and in infants up to 45 degrees of angulation will remodel satisfactorily (Fig. 3). In more proximal fractures, angulation of 25 degrees usually will be corrected with growth and remodeling.[4] Immobilization may be by a collar and cuff, with or without a coaptation splint (Fig. 4), or rarely, by a hanging arm cast for severe shortening.

Because of its proximity to the humeral shaft, the radial nerve is vulnerable to injury;[10] however, radial nerve injuries in humeral shaft fractures in children are less common than in adult fractures with the classic Holstein configuration. They occur most frequently with fractures of the middle or distal third of the shaft. In general, the prognosis for radial nerve recovery is excellent, usually within eight to 12 weeks.[10] If the nerve is intact initially, but function decreases after any type of manipulation or cast immobilization, the radial nerve should be surgically explored.

For children with severe soft-tissue injuries, other types of treatment used include external fixation or overhead olecranon traction. Skeletally mature teenagers with polytrauma occasionally require open reduction and internal fixation of the humeral shaft fracture.

References

1. Neer CS II, Horowitz BS: Fractures of the humeral epiphysial plate. *Clin Orthop* 1965;41:24–31.
2. Dameron TB Jr, Reibel DB: Fractures involving the proximal humeral epiphyseal plate. *J Bone Joint Surg* 1969;51A:289–297.
3. Ogden JA, Murphy MJ, Southwick WO, et al: Radiology of postnatal skeletal development: XIII. C1-C2 interrelationships. *Skeletal Radiol* 1986;15:433–438.
4. Ogden JA: *Skeletal Injuries in the Child,* ed 2. Philadelphia, WB Saunders, 1990, pp 357–359.
5. Lentz W, Meuser P: The treatment of fractures of the proximal humerus. *Arch Orthop Trauma Surg* 1980;96:283–285.
6. Sherk HH, Probst C: Fractures of the proximal humeral epiphysis. *Orthop Clin North Am* 1975;6:401–413.
7. Baxter MP, Wiley JJ: Fractures of the proximal humeral epiphysis: Their influence on humeral growth. *J Bone Joint Surg* 1986;68B:570–573.
8. Barnett LS: Little league shoulder syndrome: Proximal humeral epiphysiolysis in adolescent baseball pitchers: A case report. *J Bone Joint Surg* 1986;67A:495–496.
9. Cahill BR, Tullos HS, Fain RH: Little league shoulder: Lesions of the proximal humeral epiphyseal plate. *J Sports Med* 1974;2:150–153.
10. Dameron TB Jr, Rockwood CA Jr: Fractures and dislocations of the shoulder, in Rockwood CA Jr, Wilkins KE, King RE (eds): *Fractures in Children.* Philadelphia, JB Lippincott, 1991, pp 577–682.

CHAPTER 40

Fractures and Dislocations About the Elbow in Children

James H. Beaty, MD

Fractures of the Lateral Humeral Condyle

Fractures of the lateral condyle account for 10% to 15% of elbow fractures in children.[1-6] Most occur in children around six years of age. Classification is based on the amount of displacement (Fig. 1): stage I is nondisplaced (1 to 2 mm of displacement); stage II is moderately displaced (2 to 4 mm of displacement; and stage III is completely displaced.[5] Treatment also depends on displacement. Stage I fractures generally can be treated with cast immobilization until union is seen on roentgenographs; however, serial roentgenographic evaluation should be carried out to detect any late displacement. Stage II and III fractures are best treated by open reduction and internal fixation.

Although type I fractures appear innocuous (Fig. 2), late displacement (Fig. 3) or late nonunion has been reported in as many as 10% of such injuries.[2,7-12] Varus stress views may be used to determine fracture stability and the presence or absence of a cartilaginous hinge. Arthrography also has been used in treating type I fractures to detect intra-articular displacement that requires surgical fixation.[1,12,13]

Open reduction is performed through a straight lateral approach, and the fragment is replaced and fixed with two smooth Kirschner wires (K-wires) (Fig. 4). The posterior soft tissues are left attached to the lateral condyle to protect its blood supply. The pins are removed at three to six weeks, as soon as satisfactory healing has occurred.

The most common complications after lateral condylar fractures are nonunion and progressive cubitus valgus deformity. These usually occur because the initial injury was unrecognized and untreated. In carefully selected patients, late open reduction and internal fixation may be performed.[9,14] The criteria for late treatment, as outlined by Flynn and associates,[9] are a large metaphyseal fragment, displacement less than 1 cm from the joint, and an open physis. Extra-articular late open reduction and internal fixation, which often requires bone grafting and screw fixation, can result in loss of range of motion (Fig. 5).

The natural history of nonunion of the lateral humeral condyle is progressive cubitus valgus with a high risk of tardy ulnar nerve palsy.[15] Children and adults with established nonunions are best treated by "benign neglect," with early transposition of the ulnar nerve when symptoms appear (Fig. 6).

Fractures of the Medial Epicondyle

About 40% of all medial epicondylar fractures in children occur with elbow dislocations.[16,17] Most occur in children between the ages of nine and 12 years.

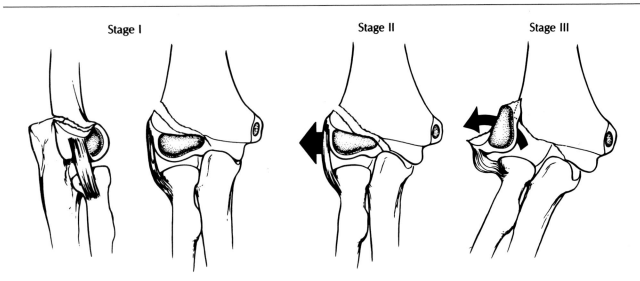

Fig. 1 Classification of fractures of lateral condyle: stage I nondisplaced, stage II moderately displaced, and stage III completely displaced. (Reproduced with permission from Wilkins KE: Fractures and dislocations of the elbow region, in Rockwood CA Jr, Wilkins KE, King RE (eds): *Fractures in Children*, ed 2. Philadelphia, JB Lippincott, 1991, vol 3, p 628.)

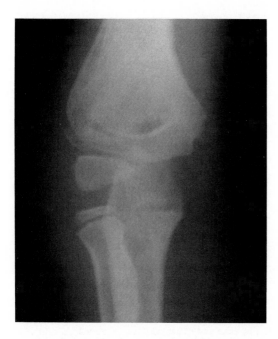

Fig. 2 Stage I fracture of lateral condyle. Note small metaphyseal fragment with 2 mm of displacement.

The medial epicondyle is a traction apophysis. In the early stages of ossification, it is part of the distal humeral epiphysis, but with growth it becomes separated by metaphyseal bone. Ossification of the apophysis begins at from 4 to 6 years of age, and fusion occurs at approximately 15 years. Irregularities of ossification may be misinterpreted as a fracture.[18]

Three mechanisms of medial epicondylar fractures have been proposed: a direct blow, pure muscle avulsion, and in association with an elbow dislocation. Direct trauma as a source of these injuries seems rare. Muscle avulsion injuries occur during a fall on an outstretched arm with the elbow in extension and the wrist and fingers hyperextended. The forearm flexor muscles place a tension force on the epicondyle and cause the avulsion.[19]

Fractures of the medial epicondyle are classified by the amount of displacement: type I is nondisplaced; type II is moderately displaced (less than 1 cm); and in type III there is intra-articular entrapment. Types I and II fractures can be treated with cast immobilization for three to four weeks. Occasionally, a type II injury with gross medial instability will require open reduction and internal fixation.[20] Open reduction and internal fixation are indicated for type III fractures if the medial epicondyle cannot be extracted from the joint by manipulation (valgus positioning, supination of the forearm, and dorsiflexion of the wrist) in a sedated patient. Open reduction and internal fixation are required if the fracture fragment is trapped within the joint (Fig. 7).[21] At one time, ulnar nerve dysfunction was an in-

dication for open reduction, and some authors recommended transposition of the nerve at the time of reduction. Bernstein and associates,[16] however, found that all patients with initial ulnar neuritis did well without surgery, and most authors now do not recommend nerve transposition. Delayed ulnar nerve symptoms are rare. Woods and Tullos[22] recommend that if gravity valgus stress testing shows significant instability, surgery is indicated, especially in athletes.

T-Condylar Fractures

T-condylar fractures are uncommon in young children and occur more frequently in older adolescents and teenagers.[23-25] These fractures represent type IV physeal injuries of each of the distal columns of the humerus. Occasionally the fracture is minimally displaced, but most are displaced with instability of all fragments. T-condylar fractures may be confused clinically with extension-type supracondylar fractures. In older children, a T-condylar fracture should be differentiated from a comminuted supracondylar fracture. Treatment depends on the extent of soft-tissue and bone injury. If swelling or comminution is severe, olecranon traction for two to three weeks may be required for reduction. If the fracture fragments are large and displaced, open reduction and internal fixation are indicated. Extensive dissection should be avoided to prevent osteonecrosis of the articular cartilage. K-wires, screws, or screw-reconstruction plate combinations may be used for fixation depending on the age of the child and the severity of the comminution (Fig. 8). The triceps splitting or "tongue" approach may be used, and olecranon osteotomy may be required to correct severe intra-articular comminution.

Monteggia Fracture-Dislocations

The Monteggia fracture-dislocation is a pronation injury consisting of fracture of the ulna with dislocation of the radial head (Fig. 9). Most of these injuries are caused by falls, and associated wrist injuries are common.[26-30] These injuries were classified by Bado[31] according to the direction of displacement of the radial head: in type I the displacement is anterior; in type II it is posterior; in type III it is lateral; and in type IV it is anterior with fracture of the ulna and radius. Anterior and lateral displacement of the radial head are the most common. The radial head dislocation may not be apparent on roentgenograms, because the elbow often is not included in the initial evaluation of forearm injuries. Roentgenograms of ulnar or radial fractures should include the elbow and wrist joints and should show the radial head in line with the middle of the

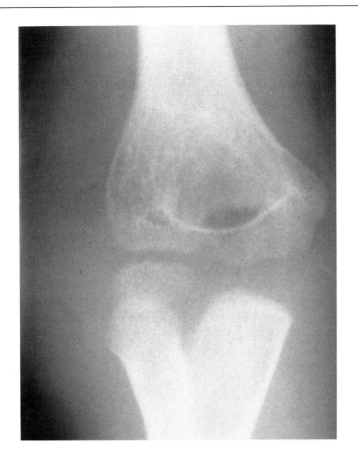

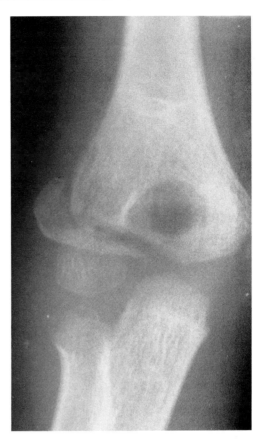

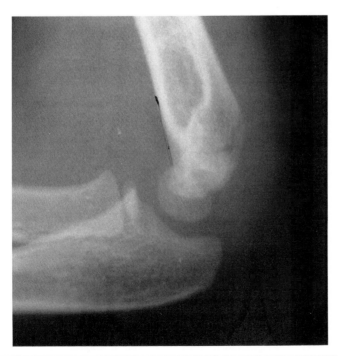

Fig. 3 Stage I fracture of lateral condyle with late displacement. **Top left**, Fracture is not visible on anteroposterior view. **Bottom left**, Displacement of 1 mm is seen on lateral view. **Top right**, Three weeks after injury, late displacement is obvious.

capitellum on all views, especially the lateral. This can be confirmed by drawing a straight line through the radial head and neck; in any position, this line should pass through the central portion of the capitellum.

For most Monteggia fracture-dislocations in children, closed manipulation can be used to reduce the ulnar fracture and the radial head dislocation.[32,33] A cast is applied with the arm in a stable position

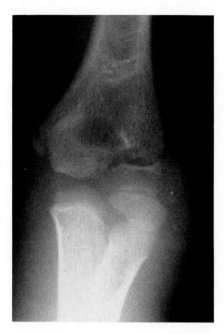
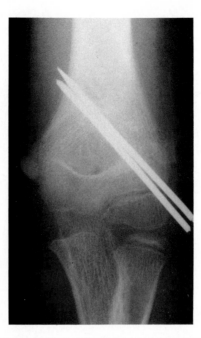

Fig. 4 **Left**, Completely displaced fracture of lateral condyle in 8-year-old. **Right**, After open reduction and internal fixation with two smooth 5/64-inch K-wires.

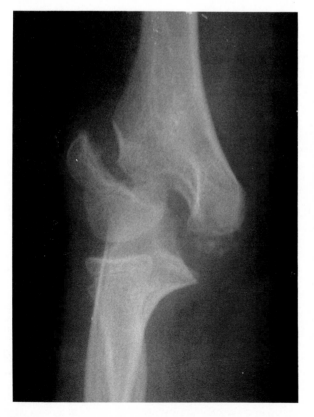
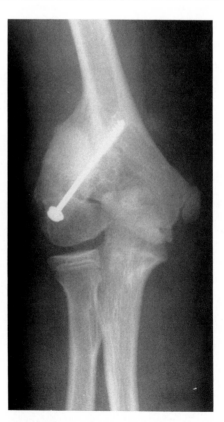

Fig. 5 **Left**, Nonunion two years after lateral condyle fracture with large metaphyseal fragment. **Right**, After open reduction, internal fixation, and iliac crest bone graft, metaphyseal fragment has united, and patient has good clinical range of motion.

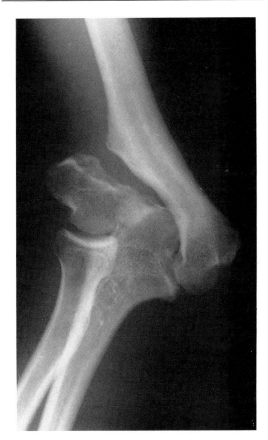
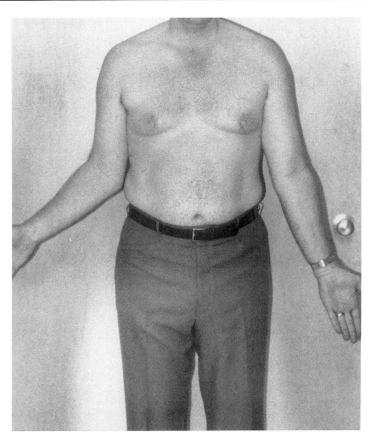

Fig. 6 **Left**, Established nonunion in 30-year-old man after untreated fracture of lateral humeral condyle. **Right**, Clinical appearance with cubitus valgus and mild elbow flexion contracture.

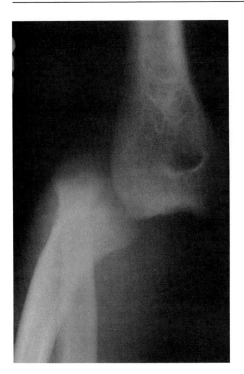
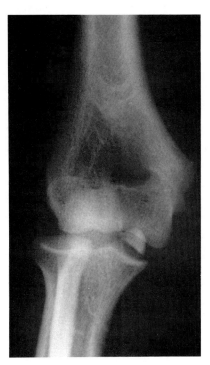
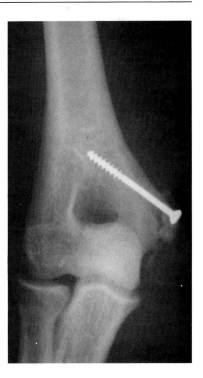

Fig. 7 **Left** and **center**, 15-year-old boy with posterolateral elbow dislocation and fracture of medial epicondyle, which was trapped in joint following reduction. **Right**, After open reduction and internal fixation with small fragment screw.

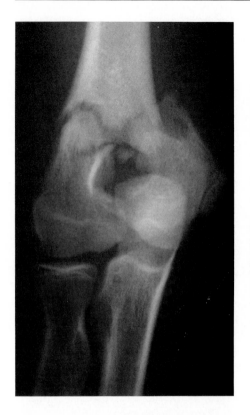

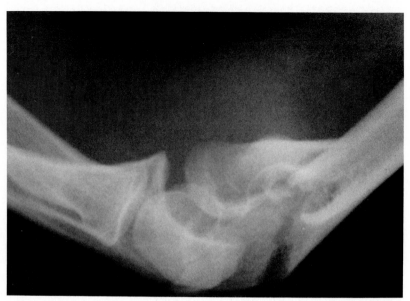

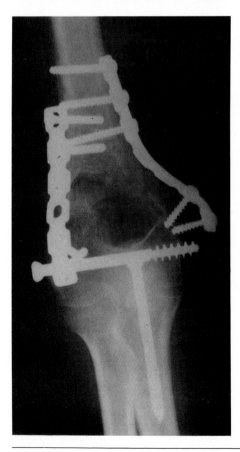

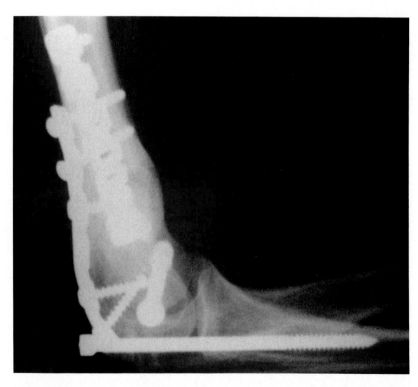

Fig. 8   **Top left** and **top right**, T-condylar fracture in 14-year-old girl. **Bottom left** and **bottom right**, After olecranon osteotomy, open reduction, and internal fixation with acetabular reconstruction plates and screws.

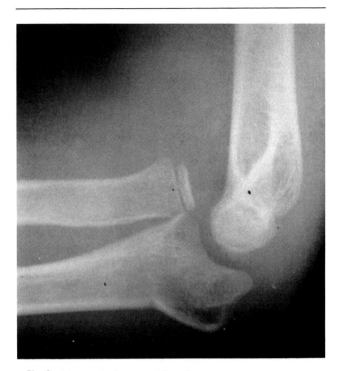

Fig. 9 Monteggia fracture-dislocation.

(flexion or extension) and remains in place for six to eight weeks. After closed reduction the position of the radial head relative to the capitellum should be confirmed by roentgenograms. Open reduction and internal fixation may be required if soft tissue interposition makes closed reduction of the radial head impossible. In younger children and adolescents, open reduction may be required for acute, irreducible injuries. If reduction of the ulnar fracture fails, soft tissue interposition (such as the annular ligament, capsule, or anconeus muscle) must be surgically corrected to obtain reduction of the radial head. The older the child, the more likely that ulnar fixation will be required. Intramedullary fixation or compression plating of the ulna, as in adults, may be performed depending on the age of the child and the level of the ulnar fracture (Fig. 10).

The treatment of undetected, untreated Monteggia lesions is controversial.[34-36] Historically, radial head resection after skeletal maturity has been recommended for symptomatic untreated Monteggia fracture-dislocations. Recent reports indicate that the radial head may be satisfactorily reduced as late as 24 months after dislocation. Late treatment may require reconstruction of the annular ligament, as well as a reduction of the radial head (Bell-Tawse proce-

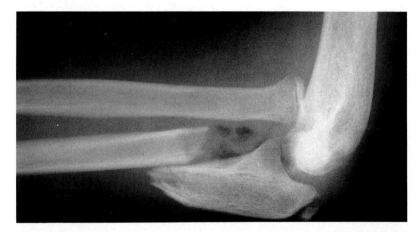

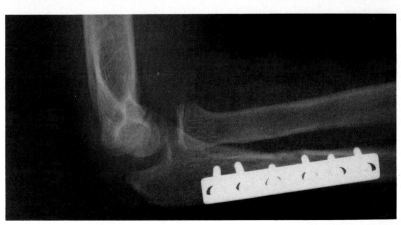

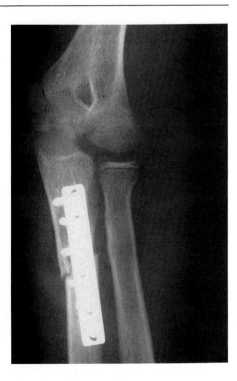

Fig. 10 Top left, A 13-year-old boy with anterior Monteggia fracture-dislocation, open Type I ulnar fracture. **Right** and **bottom left,** Postoperative irrigation and debridement ulnar fracture, compression plate fixation, reduction of radial head.

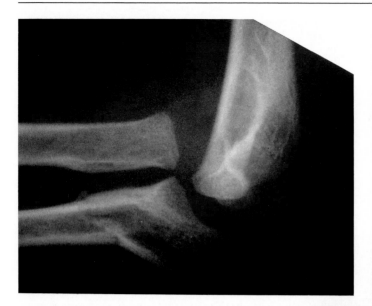

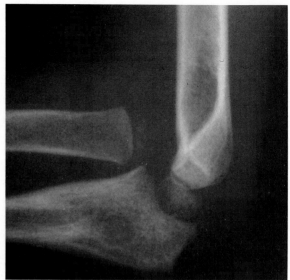

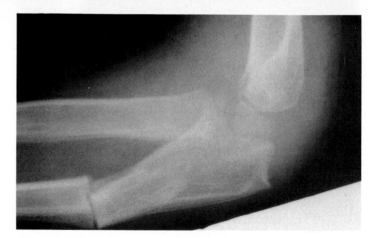

Fig. 11   Top left, A 5-year-old boy with acute anterior Monteggia lesion. **Top right,** Three months later, ulna healed, radial head dislocation undetected. **Bottom right,** Postoperative lengthening. Angulation osteotomy of ulna, annular ligament reconstruction, reduction of radial head.

dure).[37] Angulation-lengthening osteotomy of the ulna may be necessary to allow stable radial head reduction (Fig. 11).

Posterior interosseous nerve palsy is not infrequent with this injury, but most patients recover spontaneously.[34] Migration and breakage of transcapitellar pins also have been reported. Compartment syndrome, myositis, and synostosis of the proximal radius and ulna are infrequent complications.[38]

Fractures of the Olecranon

Fractures of the olecranon are infrequent in children, constituting only 5% of all elbow fractures.[39-41] These fractures generally result from a fall in which the child lands directly on the elbow. Olecranon fractures are of two types: physeal separation and metaphyseal fracture. They are classified by the mechanism of injury: flexion, extension, valgus, varus, or shear. If the fracture is displaced less than 5 mm, it should be immobilized in the most stable position, usually 45 degrees of elbow flexion, for three to six weeks. Open reduction and internal fixation using AO technique are indicated for unstable fractures. Olecranon fractures frequently occur in association with fractures of the radial head and neck, and these should be sought on initial roentgenograms. A "simple" olecranon fracture may be part of a Monteggia lesion, so radial head position should be evaluated carefully.

Fractures of the Radial Head and Neck

Fractures of the radial head and neck also are rare in children, and most occur in children between 4 and 14 years of age. The radial neck is fractured

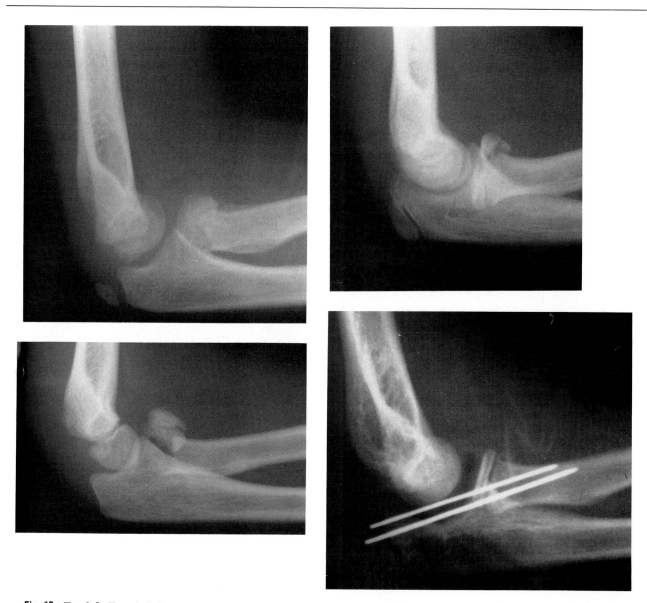

Fig. 12 **Top left,** Type A (Salter-Harris type II) fracture of radial neck. **Top right,** Type B (Salter-Harris type IV) fracture of radial head. **Bottom left,** Type C (completely displaced) fracture of radial neck with anterior displacement of proximal fragment. **Bottom right,** After open reduction and internal fixation with two small, oblique K-wires.

more frequently than the radial head, and most radial neck fractures occur through the metaphysis. The most common mechanism of injury is a fall.[42-47] These fractures are generally classified as a valgus fracture (type I) or a fracture with an elbow dislocation (type II). Wilkins[48] divided valgus injuries into three categories: type A, Salter-Harris types I and II fractures (Fig. 12, *top left*); type B, Salter-Harris type IV fractures (Fig. 12, *top right*); and, type C, fractures of only the proximal metaphysis. Displacement is characterized as degrees of angulation, percentage of translocation, or total displacement (Fig. 12, *bottom left* and *bottom right*).

Treatment should be by closed methods if possible. Satisfactory results can be obtained with angulation of 25 to 50 degrees and displacement or translation of less than 50%. If manipulation is required for reduction, traction should be used with a varus force and direct pressure applied to the radial head. Percutaneous manipulation with image intensification has been reported,[49] but long-term results are not yet available. Open reduction through a lateral approach is indicated when angulation is more than 60 degrees or displacement is more than 50%.[50-52] Fixation should be with small oblique K-wires, which are removed early, at three weeks if possible. Complica-

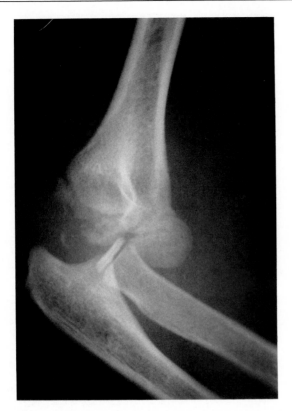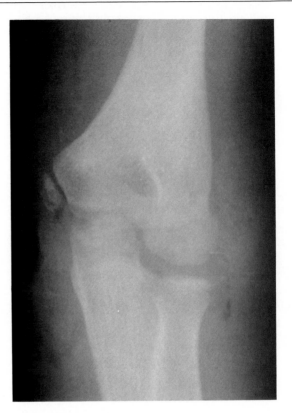

Fig. 13 Posterior elbow dislocation (**left**) that after reduction showed no associated fracture (**right**).

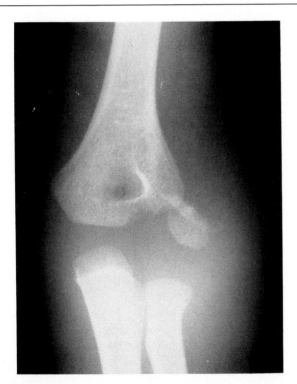

Fig. 14 Displaced fracture of lateral humeral condyle after posterior dislocation of elbow in 5-year-old boy.

tions include osteonecrosis, which appears to remodel somewhat with growth, and synostosis, which may occur after severe injury and surgical treatment.

Elbow Dislocations

Elbow dislocations, which account for approximately 6% of all elbow injuries, occur most frequently in males (70%). Generally elbow dislocations are classified as having the proximal radioulnar joint intact or divergent. Dislocations with intact joints (Fig. 13) may be posterior, anterior, medial, or lateral; most are posterior.[53] Dislocations with divergence of the joint may be anteroposterior or transverse; these are rare.[54]

Most posterior elbow dislocations can be treated with closed reduction by the use of traction and the application of pressure on the olecranon.[55] The elbow is immobilized for 10 to 14 days. Open reduction rarely is indicated for an irreducible dislocation, an open injury, or a dislocation associated with intraarticular fractures of the same elbow. There is a high incidence of associated fractures with elbow dislocations (as frequent as 50% in children), especially fractures of the radial head and neck (Fig. 14), the lateral condyle, and the medial epicondyle. Vascular injury is rare,[56] but should be suspected in open dislocations.[57] Nerve injuries occur in approximately 10% of patients, but most recover spontaneously. Rarely, the median nerve or brachial artery is entrapped after reduction and requires surgical correction.[56-63] Recurrent elbow dislocations have been reported occasionally, and these require special treatment.[64,65]

References

1. Akbarnia BA, Silberstein MJ, Rende RJ, et al: Arthrography in the diagnosis of fractures of the distal end of the humerus in infants. *J Bone Joint Surg* 1986;68A:599–602.
2. Badelon O, Bensahel H, Mazda K, et al: Lateral humeral condylar fractures in children: A report of 47 cases. *J Pediatr Orthop* 1988;8:31–34.
3. Foster DE, Sullivan JA, Gross RH: Lateral humeral condylar fractures in children. *J Pediatr Orthop* 1985;5:16–22.
4. Rutherford A: Fractures of the lateral humeral condyle in children. *J Bone Joint Surg* 1985;67A:851–856.
5. Jakob R, Fowles JV, Rang M, et al: Observations concerning fractures of the lateral humeral condyles in children. *J Bone Joint Surg* 1975;57B:430–436.
6. Wadsworth TG: Injuries of the capitular (lateral humeral condylar) epiphysis. *Clin Orthop* 1972;85:127–142.
7. Flynn JC, Richards JF Jr: Nonunion of minimally displaced fractures of the lateral condyle of humerus in children. *J Bone Joint Surg* 1971;53A:1096–1101.
8. Wood AB, Beaty JH: Fractures of the lateral humeral condyle in children. Presented at the 52nd Annual Meeting of the American Academy of Orthopaedic Surgeons, Las Vegas, NV, Jan 26, 1985.
9. Flynn JC, Richard JF Jr, Saltzman RI: Prevention and treatment of non-union of slightly displaced fractures of the lateral humeral condyle in children: An end-result study. *J Bone Joint Surg* 1975;57A:1087–1092.
10. Fowles JV, Kassab MT: Displaced fractures of the medial humeral condyle in children. *J Bone Joint Surg* 1980;62A:1159–1163.
11. Josefsson PO, Danielsson LG: Epicondylar elbow fracture in children: 35-year follow-up of 56 unreduced cases. *Acta Orthop Scand* 1986;57:313–315.
12. Herring JA, Fitch RD: Lateral condylar fracture of the elbow. *J Pediatr Orthop* 1986;6:724–727.
13. Yates C, Sullivan JA: Arthrographic diagnosis of elbow injuries in children. *J Pediatr Orthop* 1987;7:54–60.
14. Masada K, Kawai H, Kawabata H, et al: Osteosynthesis for old, established non-union of the lateral condyle of the humerus. *J Bone Joint Surg* 1990;72A:32–40.
15. Hardacre JA, Nahigian SH, Froimson AI, et al: Fractures of the lateral condyle of the humerus in children. *J Bone Joint Surg* 1971;53A:1083–1095.
16. Bernstein SM, King JD, Sanderson RA: Fractures of the medial epicondyle of the humerus. *Contemp Orthop* 1981;3:637–641.
17. Papavasiliou V, Nenopoulos S, Venturis T: Fractures of the medial condyle of the humerus in childhood. *J Pediatr Orthop* 1987;7:421–423.
18. Silberstein MJ, Brodeur AE, Graviss ER, et al: Some vagaries of the medial epicondyle. *J Bone Joint Surg* 1981;63A:524–528.
19. Fowles JV, Slimane N, Kassab MT: Elbow dislocation with avulsion of the medial humeral epicondyle. *J Bone Joint Surg* 1990;72B:102–104.
20. Hines RF, Herndon WA, Evans JP: Operative treatment of medial epicondyle fractures in children. *Clin Orthop* 1987;223:170–174.
21. Fowles JV, Kassab MT, Moula T: Untreated intra-articular entrapment of the medial humeral epicondyle. *J Bone Joint Surg* 1984;66B:562–565.
22. Woods GW, Tullos HS: Elbow instability and medial epicondyle fracture. *Am J Sports Med* 1977;5:23–30.
23. Beghin JL, Bucholz RW, Wenger DR: Intercondylar fractures of the humerus in young children: A report of two cases. *J Bone Joint Surg* 1982;64A:1083–1087.
24. Jarvis JG, D'Astous JL: Pediatric T-supracondylar fracture. *J Pediatr Orthop* 1984;4:697–699.
25. Peterson HA: Triplane fracture of the distal humeral epiphysis. *J Pediatr Orthop* 1983;3:81–84.
26. Letts M, Locht R, Wiens J: Monteggia fracture-dislocations in children. *J Bone Joint Surg* 1985;67B:724–727.
27. Lloyd-Roberts GC, Bucknill TM: Anterior dislocation of the radial head in children. *J Bone Joint Surg* 1977;59B:402–407.
28. Olney BW, Menelaus MB: Monteggia and equivalent lesions in childhood. *J Pediatr Orthop* 1989;9:219–223.
29. Wiley JJ, Galey JP: Monteggia injuries in children. *J Bone Joint Surg* 1985;67B:728–731.
30. Ovesen O, Brok KE, Arreskv J, et al: Monteggia lesions in children and adults: An analysis of etiology and long-term results of treatment. *Orthopedics* 1990;13:529–534.
31. Bado JL: The Monteggia lesion. *Clin Orthop* 1967;50:71–86.
32. Speed HS, Boyd HB: Treatment of fractures of ulna with dislocation of head of radius. *JAMA* 1940;115:1699–1705.
33. Boyd HB, Boals JC: The Monteggia lesion: A review of 159 cases. *Clin Orthop* 1969;66:94–100.
34. Holst-Nielsen F, Jensen V: Tardy posterior interosseous nerve palsy as a result of an unreduced radial head dislocation in Monteggia fractures: A report of two cases. *J Hand Surg* 1984;9A:572–575.
35. Hurst LC, Dubrow EN: Surgical treatment of symptomatic chronic radial head dislocation: A neglected Monteggia fracture. *J Pediatr Orthop* 1983;3:227–230.
36. Kalamchi A: Monteggia fracture-dislocation in children. Late treatment in two cases. *J Bone Joint Surg* 1986;68A:615–619.
37. Bell Tawse AJS: The treatment of malunited anterior Monteggia fractures in children. *J Bone Joint Surg* 1965;47B:718–723.
38. Fowles JV, Sliman N, Kassab MT: The Monteggia lesion in children. Fracture of the ulna and dislocation of the radial head. *J Bone Joint Surg* 1983;65A:1276–1283.
39. Dormans JP, Rang M: Fractures of the olecranon and radial neck in children. *Orthop Clin North Am* 1990;21:257–268.
40. Matthews JG: Fractures of the olecranon in children. *Injury* 1980;12:207–212.
41. Papavasiliou VA, Beslikas TA, Nenopoulos S: Isolated fractures of the olecranon in children. *Injury* 1987;18:100–102.
42. Fowles JV, Kassab MT: Observations concerning radial neck fractures in children. *J Pediatr Orthop* 1986;6:51–57.
43. Jeffrey CC: Fractures of the head of the radius in children. *J Bone Joint Surg* 1950;32B:314–324.
44. Landin LA, Danielsson LG: Elbow fractures in children: An epidemiological analysis of 589 cases. *Acta Orthop Scand* 1986;57:309–312.
45. Steinberg EL, Golomb D, Salama R, et al: Radial head and neck fractures in children. *J Pediatr Orthop* 1988;8:35–40.
46. Tibone JE, Stoltz M: Fracture of the radial head and neck in children. *J Bone Joint Surg* 1981;63A:100–106.
47. Vahvanen V, Gripenberg L: Fracture of the radial neck in children: A long-term follow-up study of 43 cases. *Acta Orthop Scand* 1978;49:32–38.
48. Wilkins KE: Fractures and dislocations of the elbow region, in Rockwood CA Jr, Wilkins KE, King RE (eds): *Fractures in Children*. Philadelphia, JB Lippincott, 1984, pp 501–529.
49. Wilkins KE: Fractures and dislocations of the elbow region, in Rockwood CA Jr, Wilkins KE, King RE (eds): *Fractures in Children*. ed 2. Philadelphia, JB Lippincott, 1991, pp 509–828.
50. Jones ERL, Esah M: Displaced fractures of the neck of the radius in children. *J Bone Joint Surg* 1971;53B:429–439.
51. Scullion JE, Miller JH: Fracture of the neck of the radius in

children. Prognostic factors and recommendations for management. *J Bone Joint Surg* 1985;67B:491.

52. Wedge JH, Robertson DE: Displaced fractures of the neck of the radius in children. *J Bone Joint Surg* 1982;64B:256.

53. Carlioz H, Abols Y: Posterior dislocation of the elbow in a child. *J Pediatr Orthop* 1984;4:8–12.

54. DeLee JC: Transverse divergent dislocation of the elbow in a child. *J Bone Joint Surg* 1981;63A:322–323.

55. Borris LC, Lassen MR, Christensen CS: Elbow dislocation in children and adults: A long-term follow-up of conservatively treated patients. *Acta Orthop Scand* 1987;58:649–651.

56. Hofammann KE III, Moneim MS, Omer GE, et al: Brachial artery disruption following closed posterior elbow dislocation in a child: Assessment with intravenous digital angiography: A case report with review of the literature. *Clin Orthop* 1984;184:145–149.

57. Rubens MK, Aulicino PL: Open elbow dislocation with brachial artery disruption. Case report and review of the literature. *Orthopedics* 1986;9:539–542.

58. Green NE: Entrapment of the median nerve following elbow dislocation. *J Pediatr Orthop* 1983;3:384–386.

59. Hallett J: Entrapment of the median nerve after dislocation of the elbow: A case report. *J Bone Joint Surg* 1981;63B:408–412.

60. Holmes JC, Hall JE: Tardy ulnar nerve palsy in children. *Clin Orthop* 1978;135:128–131.

61. Matev I: A radiological sign of entrapment of the median nerve in the elbow joint after posterior dislocation: A report of two cases. *J Bone Joint Surg* 1976:58B:353–355.

62. Pritchard DJ, Linscheid RL, Svien HJ: Intra-articular median nerve entrapment with dislocation of the elbow. *Clin Orthop* 1973;90:100–103.

63. Pritchett JW: Entrapment of the median nerve after dislocation of the elbow. *J Pediatr Orthop* 1984;4:752–753.

64. Trias A, Comeau Y: Recurrent dislocation of the elbow in children. *Clin Orthop* 1974;100:74–77.

65. Beaty JH, Donati N: Recurrent dislocation of the elbow in children. *J Pediatr Orthop* 1991;11:392–396.

Percutaneous Pinning of Supracondylar Fractures of the Humerus

James R. Kasser, MD

Introduction

Supracondylar fractures of the humerus (Fig. 1) are common in children. These fractures generally occur as a result of a fall on an outstretched hand, and their peak incidence is at approximately age five. The injury is notorious for associated neurovascular complications as well as residual deformity. The characteristic displacement of the distal humeral fragment, in extension-type injuries, is posteromedial in 90% of the cases and posterolateral in 10%. The flexion-type supracondylar fracture is a rare injury. This discussion deals with indications and technique for treatment by percutaneous pinning of the type III extension-type supracondylar fracture.

Percutaneous pinning of supracondylar fractures is certainly not a new technique. Miller[1] reported the technique of blind pinning in 1939. In 1948 Swenson[2] described ten cases treated successfully with crossed Kirschner wiring. In 1967 Jones[3] described blind pinning in 19 supracondylar fractures with no infection and no neurologic damage.

Physeal arrest was not seen. The statement was made that "an adequate surgeon will experience no difficulty in avoiding neuromuscular structures using this technique." Subsequently, Flynn and associates[4] and Pirone and associates[5] have reported excellent results with percutaneous pinning with a very low rate of malunion and no physeal arrest. Problems with vascular compromise, compartment syndromes, and Volkman's ischemic contracture have been greatly reduced with this technique.

Cubitus Varus Deformity

The deformity of cubitus varus is common after supracondylar fractures in nearly all series.[6] The incidence has been reported as high as 58%. The deformity is caused by medial displacement, internal rotation, and extension of the distal fragment on the proximal. The obliquity of the fracture line, together with internal rotation, converts pure rotation into angular deformity. Although in its mild forms cubitus varus deformity produces little functional problem, the appearance is disturbing. In some cases, it requires corrective osteotomy. Prevention is the optimal therapy. Malreduction accounts for the vast majority of cases of cubitus varus. Kirschner wire (K-wire) stabilization after reduction appears to be the best method to hold this fracture. A

growth abnormality with osteonecrosis of the trochlea can occur following a supracondylar fracture, with overgrowth of the lateral side of the distal humeral epiphysis leading to progressive cubitus varus (Fig. 2). These rare cases of progressive growth abnormality cannot be prevented by stabilization of the distal fragment.

Initial Evaluation

When presented with a child with a supracondylar fracture, the surgeon must document the neurovascular status before initiating therapy. The nerves most commonly injured in supracondylar fractures are the radial nerve and the median nerve.[5,7,8] In a series of supracondylar fractures, median nerve injuries greatly outnumbered radial nerve injuries, but this varies from series to series. The most common median nerve injury involves the anterior interosseous branch of the median nerve, which provides motor innervation to the flexor

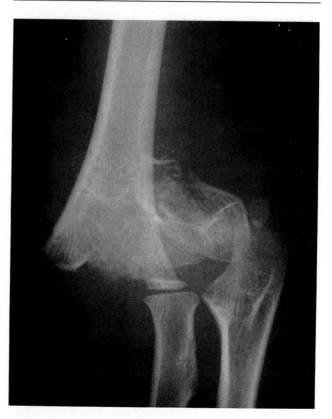

Fig. 1 The distal humeral fragment is displaced posteriorly and medially, with the typical anteroposterior appearance of a type III supracondylar fracture.

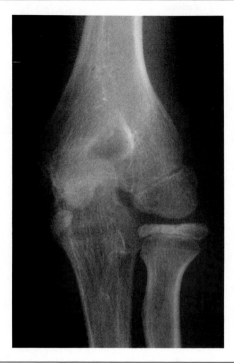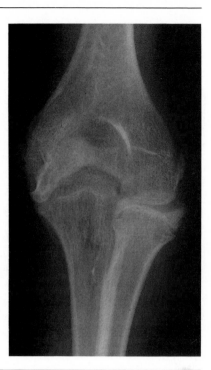

Fig. 2 Left, This patient had a supracondylar fracture at age 5. At age 8 he had a mildly progressive varus deformity with avascular necrosis of the trochlear. **Right**, Demonstrates further mild increase in varus deformity as physeal closure is approaching.

pollicis longus and the flexor digitorum longus to the index finger. These specific muscles should be tested in all cases of supracondylar fracture. Sensation in the discrete areas for median, ulnar, and radial nerve should always be tested. Passive extension and flexion of the fingers should be tested, because pain with this test can be a sign of compartment syndrome. The radial and ulnar pulses should be documented at the time of presentation. The unreduced fracture should be splinted acutely in about 30 degrees of flexion to avoid stretching the brachial artery over the proximal humeral fragment. Type I, type II, and type III extension supracondylar fractures refer to minimally displaced, periosteal hinged, and totally displaced fractures, respectively.[9]

Closed Reduction

The accurate closed reduction of a supracondylar fracture must precede stabilization (Fig. 3). To reduce the fracture, apply traction to disengage the proximal fragment from the brachialis muscle. Centralize the distal fragment medial to lateral in proper alignment with the shaft. In general, this requires lateral displacement of the distal fragment, because most fractures are posteromedially displaced. Correct the internal rotation deformity. Next, with the thumb over the olecranon, push the distal humeral fragment forward, flex the elbow to 120 degrees, and pronate the wrist to tighten the periosteal hinge. In the posterolateral fracture, supinate to tighten the lateral periosteal hinge. Check the anteroposterior and lateral position with the fluoroscopy (C-arm) unit. Generally, because the fracture is

stable in external rotation, a lateral view can be taken without moving the radiographic unit simply by externally rotating the shoulder 90 degrees. If closed reduction and casting were chosen, the cast should be applied at this point with the elbow with at least 120 degrees of flexion.[10] Because casting in this position creates some risk of vascular compromise, percutaneous pinning is the treatment of choice for a displaced type III supracondylar fracture and for most type II fractures.

Percutaneous Pinning

The C-arm provides the surface on which to operate and should be sterilely draped. Because the distal fragment is usually quite stable in 120 degrees of flexion in pronation, the arm can be moved from neutral to external rotation so that anteroposterior and lateral radiographs can be taken. An image taken in slight internal and external rotation will confirm that the medial and lateral columns are anatomically reduced. The procedure should be done as follows (Fig. 4).

With the arm flexed 120 degrees and the elbow resting on the screen of the C-arm, a .062- or .078-in K-wire is inserted laterally through the lateral condyle, crossing just lateral to the olecranon fossa and engaging the medial cortex. This wire passes through the capitellum and distal humeral growth plate. Anatomic reduction must precede pin placement, because stabilization is never a substitute for reduction. The position of the first pin should be checked in both anteroposterior and lateral views. For the lateral view, externally rotate the arm at the shoulder while maintaining the

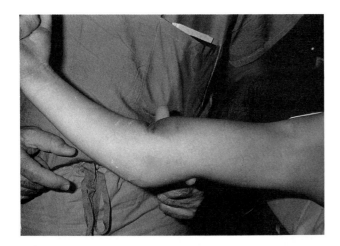

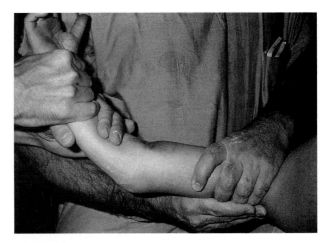

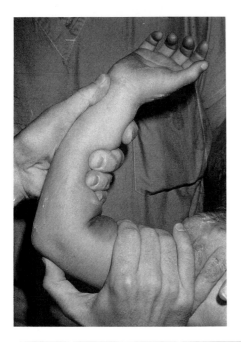

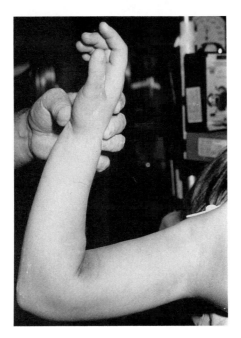

Fig. 3 Closed reduction of a supracondylar fracture. **Top left,** The distal fragment is posterior. **Top right,** Apply traction to disengage the proximal fragment from the brachialis and correct internal rotation. **Bottom left,** Centralize the distal fragment and flex with pressure over the olecranon. **Bottom right,** Pronate to tighten the periosteal hinge.

elbow flexed and the forearm pronated. A small medial incision is made over the medial epicondyle and the position of the K-wire on the medial epicondyle is checked by radiograph. A snap is used to spread down to the medial epicondyle to be sure the ulnar nerve is not injured. A small tissue protector can be used to protect the soft tissues adjacent to the medial epicondyle. A medial wire is then driven up the medial column of the distal humerus so that it crosses the lateral wire just proximal to the olecranon fossa. The pin should cross well above the fracture site to provide maximal stability. The elbow can then be extended and an anteroposterior image obtained on the C-arm to ensure proper alignment according to the Baumann angle. A lateral image can be obtained. Pins are bent over and left protruding through the skin to allow easy removal. Smooth pins are always used. When bending the pins,

secure the base of the pin with a pliers to avoid displacing the fracture while torquing the pins. The patient is splinted in 60 to 90 degrees of elbow flexion with the wrist in neutral. The pulse can be palpated and the hand left free for careful examination. A circular cast is not applied at this time. The patient is admitted to the hospital for observation of neurovascular status following this procedure.

After pinning, the optimal radiologic appearance should reveal an anatomic reduction with a wire up each column crossing above the fracture (Fig. 5).

Complications

The principal risks of percutaneous pinning are infection and nerve damage. In one series of supracon-

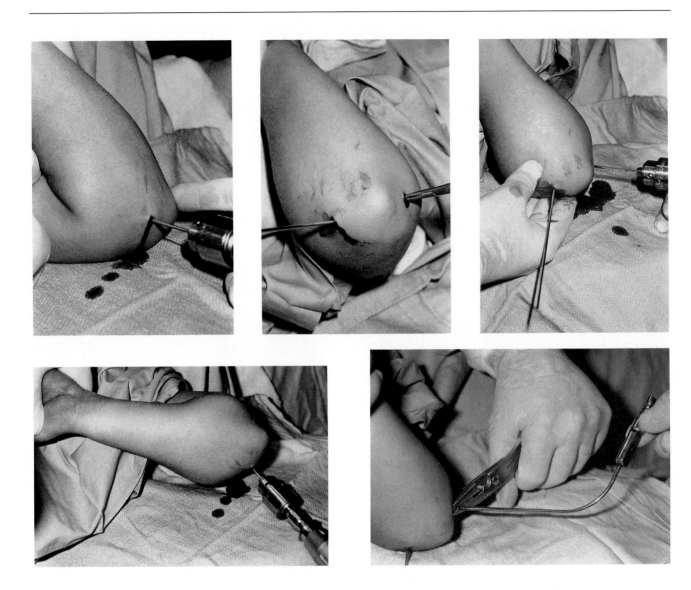

Fig. 4 After anatomic reduction is achieved, percutaneous pinning should be done using the sterilely draped C-arm as an operating surface. **Top left,** The lateral pin is placed first through a stab incision and an anteroposterior radiograph taken. **Bottom left,** The flexed pronated arm is externally rotated to obtain a lateral radiograph. **Top center,** A hemostat is used to spread soft tissue to the medial epicondyle. **Top right,** The medial pin is inserted with only 90 degrees of elbow flexion placing less tension on the ulnar nerve. **Bottom right,** Pins are bent and left protruding through the skin.

dylar fractures, incidence of nerve damage was approximately 3%.[7] Two cases occurred late, while the patient was in a cast, and were presumed to be secondary to the stretch of the ulnar nerve over the medial pin in a flexed position. In response to this, if the distal humeral fracture is very stable, two lateral pins are used, instead of cross K-wires, to stabilize the fracture. Another variation uses a single medial pin and two lateral pins arranged in such a way that, if there is any ulnar nerve dysfunction postoperatively, the medial pin can easily be removed without loss of fracture fixation. Acute nerve injuries at the time of surgery involved the ulnar and radial nerves. When such an injury occurs, the wire should be removed and consideration given to

exploring the nerve. Infection of a pin site can be managed with skin release and oral antibiotics. Deep infection of bone or joint is very rare and will require joint aspiration, pin removal, and parenteral antibiotics.

Vascular Insufficiency

When supracondylar fractures occur with vascular insufficiency the treatment of choice is rapid reduction and percutaneous pinning. Of 17 cases with vascular compromise on initial examination, four had a persistent absence of the pulse after reduction in a series at Children's Hospital in Boston.[8] Our indications for ex-

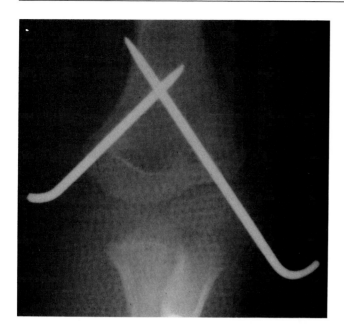
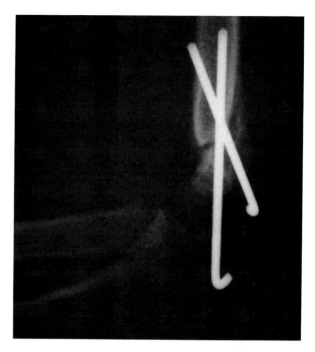

Fig. 5 Pins should cross above the fracture site (**left**) and engage the proximal cortex to insure maximal stability (**right**).

ploration of the artery were an absent pulse with signs of vascular compromise, specifically decreased capillary refill, suggestion of a compartment syndrome after reduction and pinning of the fracture, or the absence of pulse by Doppler. The presence of a totally normal hand with an absent pulse was not an indication for exploration in our series. One patient with an absent pulse, but normal hand, was watched, and pulse returned in four days. Three patients with abnormal vascular examination and absent pulse were explored with the findings of an intimal tear in two cases and a tethered artery in one. The two cases of intimal tear required vein graft. The one case of arterial entrapment simply required freeing the entrapped artery. Figure 6 demonstrates the findings at exploration of an injured brachial artery. Brachial artery injury generally occurs adjacent to the supracondylar fracture just proximal to the supratrochlear artery. The external appearance of the artery in this typical location is diagnostic of such an arterial injury.

Contraindications

Contraindications to percutaneous pinning include (1) massive swelling, (2) inability to obtain satisfactory closed reduction, (3) comminution in the supracondylar area extensive enough to render the medial column unstable, and (4) open fracture. Open fractures should be fully debrided and irrigated rather than undergoing closed reduction. Open supracondylar fractures can then be stabilized with percutaneous K-wire.

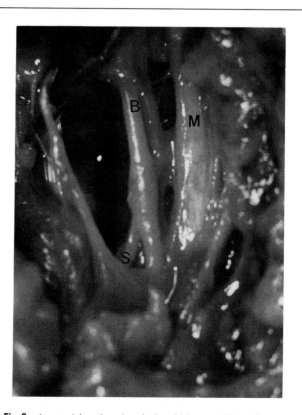

Fig. 6 At arterial exploration the brachial artery (B), median nerve (M), and supratrochlear branch of the brachial artery(s) are seen. The injured arterial segment is the swollen area just proximal to the supratrochlear artery.

Summary

Percutaneous pinning following closed reduction of supracondylar fractures is a preferred technique for management of type III injuries. If there is no pulse, rapid closed reduction with percutaneous fixation should be done. No arteriogram is indicated before treatment. Nerve damage is not a contraindication to this procedure but should be documented prior to surgery. The duration of immobilization is three to four weeks, with pins left protruding through the skin, to be removed in the office. Complications of vascular insufficiency and cubitus varus can be avoided with this technique.

References

1. Miller OL: Blind nailing of T fracture of the lower end of the humerus which involves the joint. *J Bone Joint Surg* 1939;21A: 933–938.

2. Swenson AL: The treatment of supracondylar fractures of the humerus by Kirschner-wire transfixation. *J Bone Joint Surg* 1948; 30A:993–997.

3. Jones KG: Percutaneous pin fixation of fractures of the lower end of the humerus. *Clin Orthop* 1967;50:53–69.

4. Flynn JC, Matthews JG, Price CT: Percutaneous pinning of the supracondylar fracture of the humerus: An overview of 26 years experience with long term follow up. *Orthop Trans* 1986;10:474–475.

5. Pirone AM, Graham HK, Krajbich JI: Management of displaced extension-type supracondylar fractures of the humerus in children. *J Bone Joint Surg* 1988;70A:641–650.

6. Smith L: Deformity following supracondylar fractures of the humerus. *J Bone Joint Surg* 1960;42A:235–252.

7. Royce RO, Dutkowsky JP, Kasser JR, et al: Neurologic complications after K-wire fixation of supracondylar humerus fractures in children. *J Pediatr Orthop* 1991;11:191–194.

8. Shaw BA, Kasser JR: Management of vascular injuries in displaced supracondylar humeral fractures without arteriography. *J Orthop Trauma* 1990;4:25–29.

9. Wilkins KE: Fractures and dislocations of the elbow region, in Rockwood CA Jr, Wilkins KE, King RE (eds): *Fractures in Children.* Philadelphia, JB Lippincott, 1984, vol 3.

10. Millis MB, Singer IJ, Hall JE, et al: Supracondylar fractures of the humerus in children: Further experience with a study in orthopaedic decision-making. *Clin Orthop* 1984;188:90–97.

Forearm Fractures

James R. Kasser, MD

Forearm fractures represent 55% of all children's fractures.[1] Of forearm fractures, 75% occur in the distal third of the radius. The usual mechanism of injury is a fall on the outstretched hand. Because this is the same mechanism of injury that results in supracondylar fractures, it is not surprising that these two injuries frequently occur simultaneously. The cause of the injury is almost always accidental trauma.

Normal forearm mechanics involve the rotation of a complex bowed radius about a straight fixed ulna. The anatomy of the radius (Fig. 1) is such that as the forearm is moved from the position of supination into pronation an intimate relationship between the volar flat surface of the radius and the ulna is established in the proximal forearm. The acceptable range of angulation, therefore, is much different in the proximal compared to the distal forearm. The question is frequently asked, "What is acceptable deformity?" Based on the bench studies of Tarr and associates[2] and Matthews and associates,[3] the clinical study of forearm remodeling of Friberg,[4,5] and the review of malunion in forearm fractures by Price and associates,[6] the acceptable limit in the distal radius is 20 degrees of angulation and no more than 20 degrees of malrotation. Malrotation results in motion loss in a one-to-one ratio, but little effect on motion occurs with less than 20 degrees of angulation. If the fracture is in a young child, up to 30 degrees of angulation is probably acceptable. The amount of angulation acceptable is related to the age of the patient, the proximity to the growth plate, and the degree of difficulty in correcting the deformity. It has been suggested that radial deviation is more of a problem than volar/dorsal angulation in terms of subsequent motion loss.[7,8] Bayonet apposition is acceptable up to age eight in the mid and distal radius. In children older than 8, no more than 10 degrees of angulation

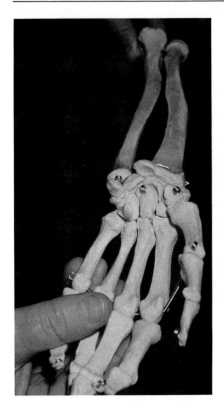 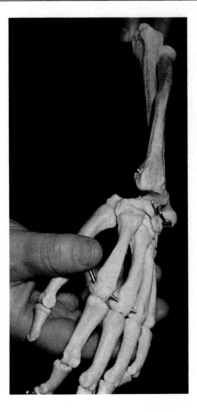 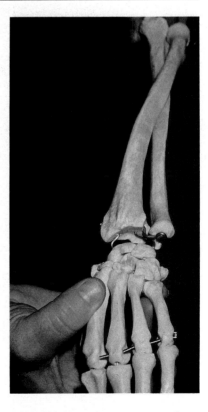

Fig. 1 **Left,** In supination there is a broad interosseous space in the forearm. **Center,** In neutral position the radius crosses over the ulna. Angular deformity in the proximal and midshaft of the radius will have a greater effect on rotation. **Right,** In full pronation the flat volar surface of the radius intimately apposes the ulna.

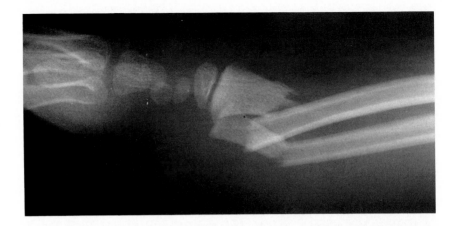

Fig. 2   The distal one-third radius fracture requires hyperextension for reduction and is held in a long arm cast with a volar mold. The rotational position of immobilization is controversial.

is acceptable in the proximal diaphyseal radius, and bayonet apposition is unacceptable.

Types of Fractures

Distal One-Third of the Radius

In the common distal one-third of the radius fracture (Fig. 2) the distal fragment is usually displaced dorsally relative to the proximal and is supinated. This is the most common upper extremity fracture in children. The periosteal hinge remains intact dorsally. Muscle spasm and shortening can make reduction difficult, at times requiring general anesthesia. With simple reductions not requiring much manipulation, sedation or the use of self-administered nitrous oxide may be of value.[9] Hematoma block and axillary block are useful. If shortening is greater than 1 cm or if the patient is very muscular, I'd favor general anesthesia.

The reduction maneuver is usually done by increasing the supination and dorsiflexion of the distal fragment. With the surgeon's dominant thumb, the distal fragment is usually pushed forward as it is hyperextended, clicking the distal fragment over the proximal. At this point the fragment is palmar flexed and secured in position. The distal one-third of the radius fracture is often very stable (Fig. 3), allowing immobilization in pronation, supination, or a neutral position. There are advocates of each position. In a study at our hospital we had a nearly constant rate of 15% repeat reduction of these fractures regardless of position. I advocate immobilization in 30 degrees of supination for this particular fracture if it is rotationally stable, because this position can decrease the degree of volar angulation, is a more stable position for the radial ulnar joint, and is generally a comfortable position for the patient. Finally, if motion is compromised in any way, pronation can be compensated for by shoulder abduction, whereas supination cannot be compensated. This fracture is generally immobilized in a long arm cast for

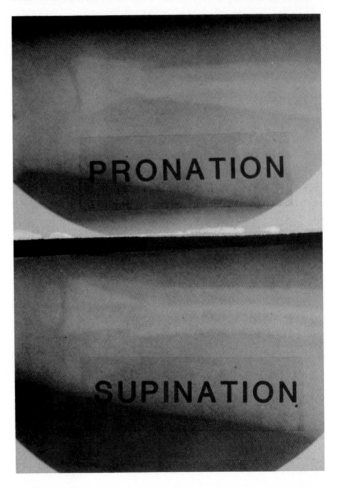

Fig. 3   After reduction, the rotationally stable distal one-third radius fracture may be immobilized in pronation, neutral, or supination. Check for stability at various rotations. The fracture shown above is stable in pronation and supination as shown.

four weeks and then converted to a short arm cast until healing is documented. Occasionally the distal one-third of the radius fracture occurs in isolation, pre-

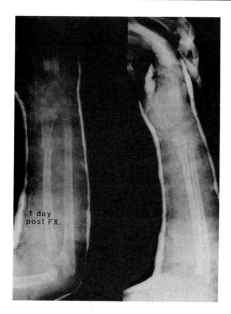
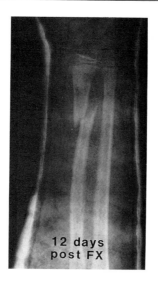
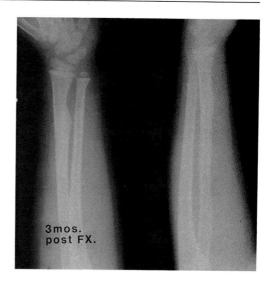

Fig. 4 **Left**, The "isolated" distal radius fracture is sometimes equivalent to the adult Galeazzi fracture. If possible, it should be casted in supination after reduction to treat the distal radial ulnar joint injury. **Center**, If significant radial shortening occurs with an intact ulna, skeletal fixation to reestablish radial length may be indicated. **Right**, Pins and plaster were used to restore radial length in this case.

sumably in association with a distal radial ulnar joint injury (Fig. 4).[10] In such cases, closed reduction and immobilization in supination can be tried, but, if radial shortening occurs, length should be maintained by internal or external skeletal fixation or repeat closed reduction. The adult Galeazzi-type fracture does occur in children but is quite rare.

The Greenstick Fracture

Greenstick fractures, which are peculiar to young children, occur because at that age individuals have a relatively thick periosteum and their bone has a long plastic range of deformation before it fails. The greenstick fracture generally occurs in the midshaft of the radius and ulna. The fracture in general is a rotational and angular injury without translation. In the volar apex fracture, there is generally a supination deformity of the distal fragment relative to the proximal. In the dorsal apex fracture, there is generally a pronation deformity of the distal fragment relative to the proximal.

Greenstick fractures may be reduced by correcting the primary rotational abnormality in aligning the bones or by breaking the remaining cortex and casting the fracture in neutral. My preference for reduction of greenstick fractures is a rotational reduction. In this way, the rotational deformity is corrected first, and, if no deformity remains, the opposite cortex is not broken. This method of reduction works quite satisfactorily. In doing it we use "the rule of thumb."

Figure 5, *left*, shows a typical greenstick fracture. Although it is difficult to see in radiographs, there is a supination deformity of the distal fragment. The reduction is done by pronating the distal fragment or rotating the thumb toward the volar apex, hence the name, "the rule of thumb." In doing this technique sedation is all that is required. The forearm is pronated to correct the radial deformity. If ulnar angular deformity remains, gentle pressure is applied over the ulnar apex. Figure 5, *right*, shows radiographs after a simple pronation reduction. Similarly, a dorsal angulated fracture with a pronation deformity can be reduced by rotating the thumb toward the dorsal apex or, simply stated, supinating the distal fragment to reduce the deformity. Patients should be casted in 45 degrees of pronation or supination and not in a more extreme position.

An occasional greenstick fracture occurs that has no rotational deformity, only simple angular deformity with plastic deformation of the remaining cortex. In this case, break the opposite cortex and cast the fracture in neutral as is traditionally recommended for greenstick fractures.

Although the fracture method can be used for all greenstick fractures, it does risk converting a stable greenstick fracture to an unstable diaphyseal fracture. I recommend trying the rule of thumb or rotational method of reduction on the next greenstick fracture encountered, because it works splendidly and involves little discomfort for the patient.

Diaphyseal Fractures

Diaphyseal fractures of the forearm should be treated closed in most growing children. To do this, the

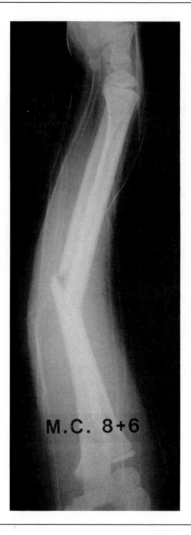

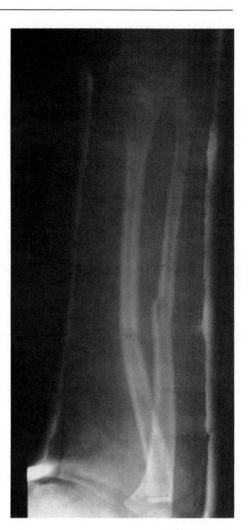

Fig. 5 **Left**, This greenstick fracture has a supination deformity of the distal fragment. **Right**, Reduction may be accomplished with pronation and pressure on the volar ulnar apex if angular deformity remains.

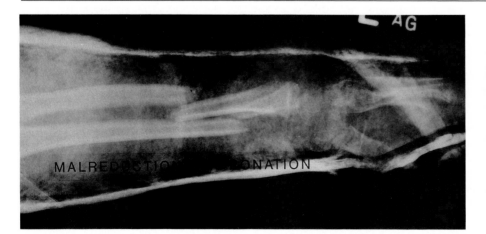

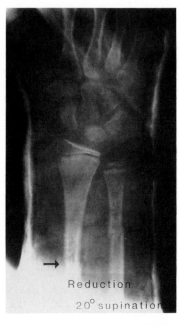

Fig. 6 **Left**, Unstable fractures require reduction by aligning the distal with the proximal fragment. Severe malrotation is obvious in this case. **Right**, Proper alignment was achieved in mild supination using fluoroscopy to check cortical alignment, as well as the position of the bicipital tuberosity.

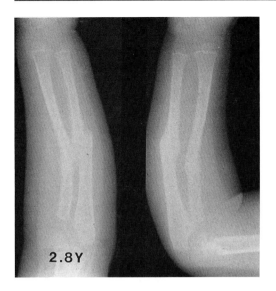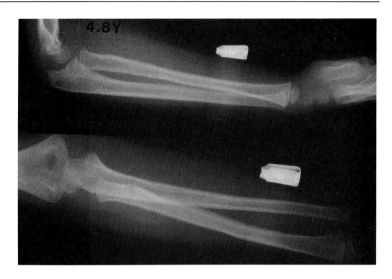

Fig. 7 **Left**, This deformity after fracture in a 2-year-old child remodels completely. **Right**, In older children, this does not occur to this extent.

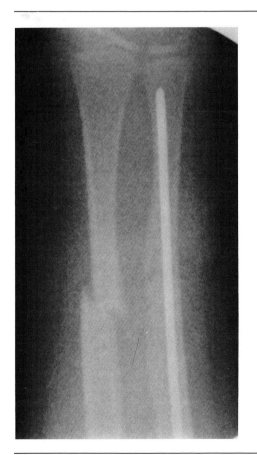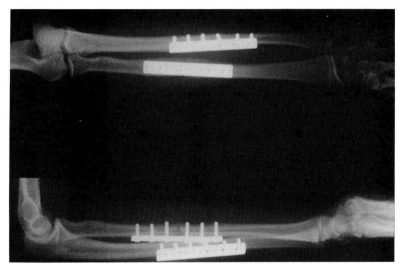

Fig. 8 Internal fixation should be done with either intramedullar rodding (**left**) or plate fixation (**right**). If a radial rod is required, a thin flexible rod should be threaded retrograde via the radial metaphysis.

distal fragment must be brought into proper alignment with the proximal fragment and immobilized in this position. Greenstick fractures and fractures of the distal one-third of the radius do not necessarily require

this treatment. The C-arm is often helpful in obtaining proper alignment of a totally displaced forearm fracture. Figure 6 shows a distal radius and ulnar fracture that was initially reduced in pronation and clearly is significantly malrotated. Using the C-arm, together with a knowledge of the position of the bicipital tuberosity and the relationship between the radial styloid and the bicipital tuberosity,[11] an adequate reduction is obtained in 20 degrees of supination. Greater than 50% apposition of the bones, as well as less than 20 degrees of angular deformity, is obtained. This patient went on to heal with satisfactory outcome after long arm cast immobilization for six weeks followed by short arm cast immobilization. Radiologic documentation as well as clinical lack of tenderness is necessary to judge duration of immobilization. The position of immobilization must correspond to the position of the proximal fragment and the position of best reduction.

In very young children, massive degrees of deformity can be tolerated (Fig. 7) with a satisfactory outcome. Deformity up to 30 degrees can be accepted, but the goal at the time of reduction remains 20 degrees. In children younger than eight years of age, bayonet apposition is entirely acceptable, as long as there is not impingement on the interosseous space with risk of cross union.

In boys older than 12 years of age or girls older than 10 years of age, bayonet apposition is not acceptable. If the fracture is unstable, and angulation less than 20 degrees cannot be maintained, open reduction and internal fixation is indicated.[12] This can be done either with intramedullary rodding[13,14] or plate fixation (Fig. 8).[8,15]

Price has found, contrary to recent publications, that even in the teenager[1] return to full motion is possible, despite significant deformity. I would suggest that any angulation in the proximal radius will impair motion, but up to 20 degrees is tolerated in the distal radius.

The methods of fixation appropriate for children's forearm fractures include oblique Kirschner wire fixation, intramedullary rod fixation, AO plate fixation, and external fixation devices. In general, the indications for skeletal fixation are: (1) open fracture with severe soft tissue injury; (2) an irreducible fracture; and (3) an unstable fracture in a child older than 10 years of age.

Open Fractures

Open fractures in children require irrigation and debridement of the fracture site in all cases. This includes grade I injuries. It is a serious error to allow the puncture wound in the emergency room to be treated with superficial wash with betadine, antibiotics, and splinting. All open fractures should be opened, irrigated, and debrided. Most children's open forearm fractures can then be treated with partial closure of the wound (leaving the initial wound wide open), a short course of antibiotics, and cast immobilization without external

fixation. Arms with severe soft-tissue injury can be treated with an external fixture to stabilize the bones while soft tissue is being treated. As is true in adults, the open forearm fracture in childhood is not a contraindication to internal fixation.[8]

Conclusion

Forearm fractures in children are managed somewhat differently from those in adults, because a thick periosteum renders the fracture quite stable and growth leads to significant remodeling. Keeping the principles described in this paper in mind will allow proper treatment of forearm fractures in children.

References

1. Mann DC, Rajmaira S: Distribution of physeal and nonphyseal fractures in 2,650 long-bone fractures in children aged 0–16 years. *J Pediatr Orthop* 1990;10:713–716.
2. Tarr RR, Garfinkel AI, Sarmiento A: The effects of angular and rotational deformities of both bones of the forearm: An in vitro study. *J Bone Joint Surg* 1984;66A:65–70.
3. Matthews LS, Kaufer H, Garver DF, et al: The effect on supination-pronation of angular malalignment of fractures of both bones of the forearm. *J Bone Joint Surg* 1982;64A:14–17.
4. Friberg KS: Part I: Remodeling after distal forearm fractures in children. The effect of residual angulation on the spatial orientation of the epiphyseal plates. *Acta Orthop Scand* 1979;50:537–546.
5. Friberg KS: Part II: Remodeling after distal forearm fractures in children. The final orientation of the distal and proximal epiphyseal plates of the radius. Part III: Remodeling after distal forearm fractures in children. Correction of residual angulation in fractures of the radius. *Acta Orthop Scand* 1979;50:731–749.
6. Price CT, Scott DS, Kurzner ME, et al: Malunited forearm fractures in children. *J Pediatr Orthop* 1990;10:705–712.
7. Fuller DJ, McCullough CJ: Malunited fractures of the forearm in children. *J Bone Joint Surg* 1982;64B:364–367.
8. Moed BR, Kellam JF, Foster RJ: Immediate internal fixation of open forearm fractures of the diaphysis of the forearm. *J Bone Joint Surg* 1986;68A:1008–1017.
9. Wattenmaker I, Kasser JR, McGarvey A: Self administered nitrous oxide for fracture reduction in the E.W. setting. *J Orthop Trauma* 1990;4:35–38.
10. Walsh HP, McLaren CA, Owen R: Galeazzi fractures in children. *J Bone Joint Surg* 1987;69B:730–733.
11. Evans EM: Fractures of the radius and ulna. *J Bone Joint Surg* 1951;33B:548–561.
12. Kay S, Smith C, Oppenheim WL: Both-bone midshaft forearm fractures in children. *J Pediatr Orthop* 1986;6:306–310.
13. Amit Y, Salai M, Chechik A, et al: Closing intramedullary nailing for the treatment of diaphyseal forearm fractures in adolescence: A preliminary report. *J Pediatr Orthop* 1985;5:143–146.
14. Verstreken L, Delronge G, Lamoureux J: Shaft forearm fractures in children: Intramedullary nailing with immediate motion: A preliminary report. *J Pediatr Orthop* 1988;8:450–453.
15. Anderson LD, Sisk TD, Tooms RE, et al: Compression-plate fixation in acute diaphyseal fractures of the radius and ulna. *J Bone Joint Surg* 1975;57A:287–297.

Fractures and Dislocations of the Hip

Colin F. Moseley, MD

Fractures and traumatic dislocations of the hip are not common injuries in children. A review of 10 years experience of a hospital seeing more than 20,000 children a year in its Emergency Department revealed fewer than 100 dislocations and fewer than 50 fractures.

Dislocations of the Hip

The causes of dislocations of the hip are shown in Table 1. Falls are the single most common cause. The dislocations are best classified on an anatomic basis. The acetabulum has three bony ridges running away from it, and the femoral head, when it dislocates, falls into one of the three valleys between these ridges. In anterior dislocations, the femoral head lies between the ilium and the pubis, in posterior dislocations between the ilium and the ischium, and in obturator dislocations between the pubis and ischium in the obturator foramen.

For the most common dislocation, the posterior, the mechanism is usually a blow on the knee when the hip is flexed, as can happen to a child who is riding unrestrained in a car and strikes one knee again the dashboard. A similar mechanism occurred in one child who was struck on the back by a falling object while crawling on all fours. Anterior dislocations are usually caused by excessive external rotation but can result from a direct blow to the greater trochanter with the hip externally rotated. Obturator dislocations are rare and are usually caused by forced abduction.

It is important to keep in mind that there are important soft tissues around the hip, which may be damaged at the time of a hip dislocation. The capsule and Y-ligament can be stretched or torn. The head can buttonhole through a rent in the capsule, and the damage to the capsule can predispose to recurrent dislocation. The ligamentum teres can be torn, which is of little significance, but it can also avulse a fragment from the femoral head, which can then be an obstruction to concentric reduction. The sciatic nerve lies directly behind the head and, therefore, can be contused or torn in a posterior dislocation. The blood supply of the femoral head is in close proximity to the capsule and can be injured with capsular injury. Some authors believe that femoral head necrosis can result from the pressure of an intracapsular hematoma in those cases where the capsule is not torn. The cartilaginous labrum of the acetabulum is an important structure in the child and can be damaged in dislocation. It can be torn or infolded and obstruct reduction.

Of particular concern is the possibility of associated fractures. The appearance of the dislocation is usually so striking on the initial radiographs that attention may be diverted from the possibility of associated fractures, which can involve either the femoral head and neck, the femoral shaft, the acetabulum and pelvis, or, in cases in which the knee has struck the dashboard, the patella. Figure 1 shows a patient with a dislocated hip and an associated fracture through the proximal femoral physis. The fracture through the physis was not immediately obvious, was not detected, and an attempted reduction resulted in a reduction of the neck but not of the head. The appropriate approach to this kind of injury involves open reduction of the epiphysis into the acetabulum, reduction of the neck onto the epiphysis, and pin fixation.

The major complications of dislocations of the hip are nonconcentric reduction, avascular necrosis, recurrent dislocation, and heterotopic ossification.

Nonconcentric Reduction

Nonconcentric reductions usually result from a chondral or osteochondral fracture with the fracture fragment intruding into the acetabulum. A torn ligamentum teres or labrum can also become interposed between the head and the acetabulum during reduction. Figure 2 shows a dislocated hip in an 11-year-old boy who fell while skiing. A closed reduction, which resulted in a nonconcentric reduction, was followed by an open reduction to excise an osteochondral fragment.

Osteonecrosis is rare if the hip is reduced within 6 to 8 hours after dislocation and is unusual even if the interval to reduction extends towards 24 hours. Osteonecrosis can result from one or all of a number of

Table 1
Pathogenesis of dislocations of the hip in children*

Mechanism of Injuries	%
Falls	50
Motor vehicle accidents	30
Sports and recreation	18
Other	2

*52 children, The Hospital for Sick Children, Toronto, Canada

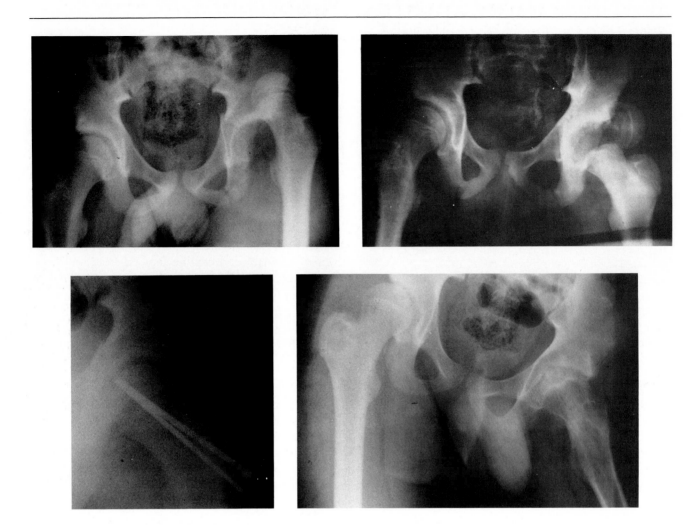

Fig. 1   **Top left**, Dislocation of the left hip. Widening of the epiphyseal plate is visible, but was undetected at the time. **Top right**, An attempt at closed reduction succeeded in reducing the neck into the acetabulum, leaving the head behind. **Bottom left**, An open reduction of the head into the acetabulum followed by reduction of the neck onto the head and pin fixation. **Bottom right**, Osteonecrosis, an almost universal complication with fractures through the physis, occurred.

factors, including direct damage to the blood vessels that surround the hip and supply the head and pressure from the intracapsular hematoma that accumulates if the capsule is not disrupted.

Recurrent Dislocation

Recurrent dislocation is unusual because muscle tension is usually enough to keep the head reduced. In cases where there is a fracture of the acetabular lip or a tearing of the capsule, particularly the posterior capsule, redislocation is more likely. In such cases, if any sense of instability exists at the time of reduction, postoperative immobilization is indicated during the period of soft-tissue healing.

Principles of Treatment

The essential elements of the treatment of a dislocated hip in the child are to rule out any associated injuries, to perform a closed reduction of the hip on an urgent basis as long as associated injuries permit it, to accept only a perfectly concentric reduction with an open reduction in the cases of nonconcentric reductions, and immobilization in traction or a spica if the associated soft-tissue damage impairs stability.

Fractures of the Femoral Neck

The incidence of fractures of the femoral neck is fairly even across the years, but boys are injured twice as frequently as girls.

Characteristics of Pediatric Hip Fractures

The major feature that differentiates femoral neck fractures in children from those in adults derives from the fact that children have strong bone in their femoral necks. This means that there has to be fairly severe trauma to cause such a fracture, or that the bone must

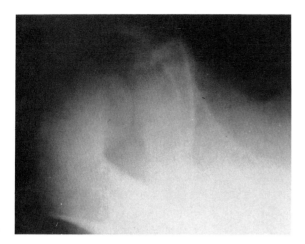

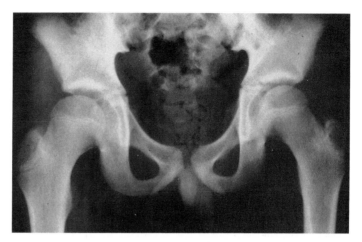

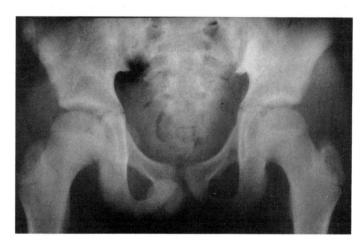

Fig. 2   Top left, Dislocation of the right hip in an 11-year-old boy suffered in a fall while skiing. **Top right**, Following closed reduction, the radiograph showed that the reduction was not concentric. **Bottom right**, Following open reduction to remove an interposed fragment, the reduction was concentric.

be somehow abnormal to predispose to it. In children, there is usually a distinct fracture line with two discrete fragments and without the comminution and crushing that occurs in adults. In addition, the strong bone allows internal fixation to be placed into the neck only, without extending across the physis into the epiphysis, and be quite secure.

Because children have much stronger periosteum than adults, it is possible for the femoral neck to crack without much displacement, leaving much of the periosteum intact. Such fractures will be significantly more stable than similar fractures in adults. There is, however, a very strong tendency for femoral neck fractures to drift into varus even if the initial displacement is minimal.

Pathologic Fractures

This is the single most common group of femoral neck fractures in children and involves fractures through tumors, such as unicameral bone cysts and fibrous dysplasia, and fractures through bone weakened by such diseases as osteogenesis imperfecta and metabolic bone disease. Figure 3 shows a fracture through a unicameral bone cyst of the proximal femur.

Classification

Fractures of the femoral neck are usually classified along anatomic grounds. Although systems classifying types of fractures by number have been described by various authors, these classification systems are not consistent, and it is better to refer to the fractures by their anatomic location. The three major categories are physeal fractures, which are true fractures and distinct from slipped epiphyses; fractures of the neck, which can be subclassified into subcapital fractures and fractures of the base of the neck; and trochanteric fractures. The trochanteric fractures are extracapsular and, because of this, the risk of circulatory disturbance is much less. Figure 4 shows a fracture through the physis and a fracture through the base of the neck.

Complications of Hip Fractures

Hip fractures are serious fractures and the risk of complications is high. The major complications are osteonecrosis and malunion.

The incidence of osteonecrosis is directly related to the location of the fracture. The incidence in fractures through the physis is greater than 80%, and the inci-

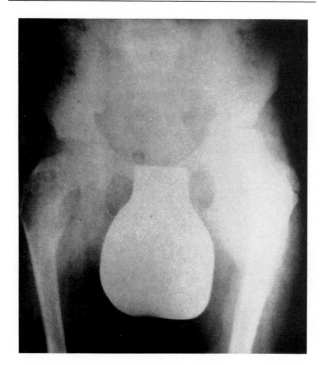

Fig. 3 A pathologic fracture through a unicameral bone cyst of the proximal femur.

dence decreases to about 20% in fractures of the base of the neck and to 0% in trochanteric fractures.

The pattern of involvement of osteonecrosis is particularly interesting because it can involve not only the physis, but the epiphysis and the proximal fragment of the neck as well. If the proximal neck fragment becomes avascular, then revascularization can be slow, and secondary fractures through this part of the neck have been reported. Osteonecrosis can affect growth either by a complete arrest and premature closure of the epiphyseal plate, resulting in leg length discrepancy, or by a differential involvement of the growth plate, leading to asymmetrical growth and angular deformity, usually coxa vara. The avascularity can also contribute to delayed union or nonunion, in which case the outcome is almost always poor. These fractures can heal, even in the face of osteonecrosis of the proximal neck fragment, from the distal side of the fracture.

There is a very marked tendency for these fractures to develop varus malunion with components of retroversion (external rotation) and extension. About 40% of cases of coxa vara are caused by poor reduction or lost position, and the other 60% result from osteonecrosis and growth disturbance.

Principles of Treatment

Almost all intracapsular fractures of the femoral neck are treated by closed or, possibly, open reduction fol-

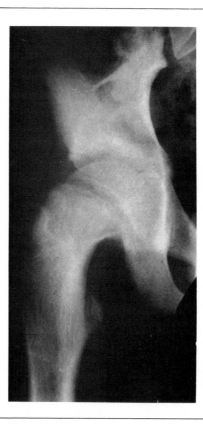
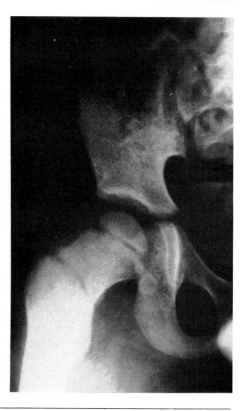

Fig. 4 Left, An acute fracture through the physis. There is a suggestion of remodeling of the femoral neck, which indicates that there may have been a preexisting chronic slip even though there were no prodromal symptoms. **Right**, A fracture through the base of the neck. This fracture may be part intracapsular and part extracapsular.

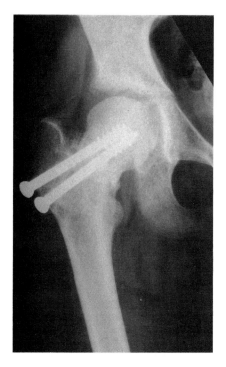 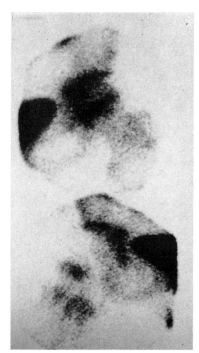 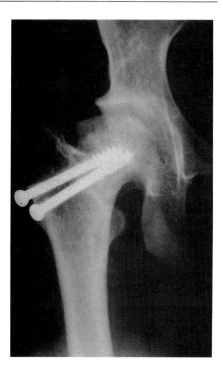

Fig. 5 **Left**, This radiograph shows a fracture through the base of the femoral neck fixed with two screws. **Center**, A bone scan at the time showed a "cold" femoral epiphysis. **Right**, The femoral head became necrotic.

lowed by internal fixation. The value of aspiration of the intracapsular hematoma is questionable and, although rational, it is not commonly performed. The best kind of fixation is with cancellous screws extending into the proximal part of the neck but not across the epiphyseal plate (Fig. 5).

Undisplaced fractures can be treated observantly with hip spica immobilization, but, because there is a tendency for these fractures to drift into varus, it is mandatory that the position be checked every few days by radiograph for the first few weeks. If a change in position is seen, reduction and internal fixation should be carried out.

Extracapsular fractures have a much lower risk of complications and, in particular, do not have the same risk of drifting into varus. Although many of these fractures can be treated without surgery, by immobilization in hip spica, they are frequently treated with reduction and internal fixation for the same reasons that apply to intracapsular fractures.

Conclusion

Because fractures and dislocations of the hip are not common injuries of children, no orthopaedic surgeon treats many of them. It is necessary to remain aware of the potential complications and how to avoid them.

CHAPTER 44

Femur Fractures in Children

James R. Kasser, MD

Femur fractures in children are quite common. In children younger than 4 years of age, 8.5% of femur fractures occur from violent trauma, 12.5% are pathologic fractures, 30% are abuse related, and 49% are the results of normal trauma to normal children. In children younger than 1 year of age, 70% of femur fractures are abuse related. Abuse should be suspected if there is: (1) unreasonable history; (2) inappropriate delay in coming to the hospital; (3) previous history of abuse; (4) evidence of other fractures in various stages of healing; (5) multiple acute fractures; and, (6) characteristic fracture patterns.[1] Figure 1 demonstrates characteristic fracture patterns diagnostic of abuse, with symmetrical epiphyseal separations in the proximal tibia and posterior rib fractures.[2] The most common abuse-related fractures are diaphyseal transverse or short oblique injuries, which look the same as other fractures. Fracture pattern alone does not rule out abuse.

Pathologic fractures occur in the femur quite commonly secondary to osteogenesis imperfecta, rickets, disuse osteopenia in neurologic disorders, or pathologic lesions of bone. At times osteogenesis imperfecta is easy to recognize, but it can be much more subtle as seen in Figure 2. When repeated long bone fractures occur in childhood, one has to have the abuse team assess the patient, but it is also necessary to consider the possibility of osteogenesis imperfecta in its mild forms. Pathologic fractures through bone cysts in the proximal femur occur frequently and are easily diagnosed on radiograph.

Treatment

In the child from 0 to 6 years of age, immediate spica[3,4] is the treatment of choice. Indications for this

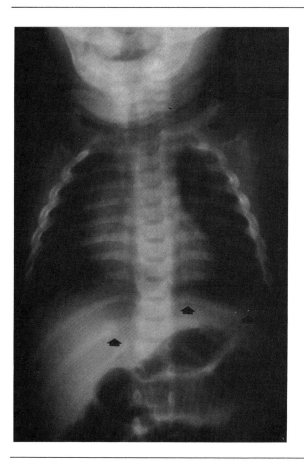

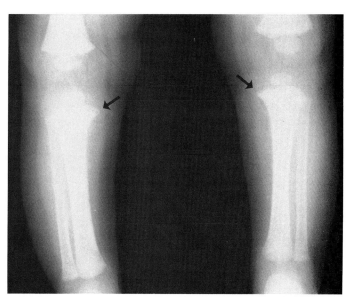

Fig. 1 Posterior rib fractures (**left**) and symmetrical epiphyseal separations (**right**) are fractures that are diagnostic of abuse.

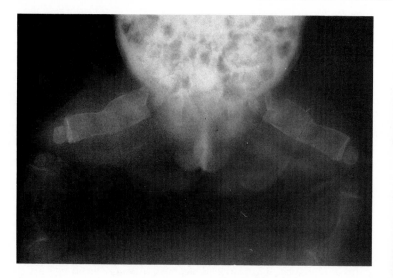
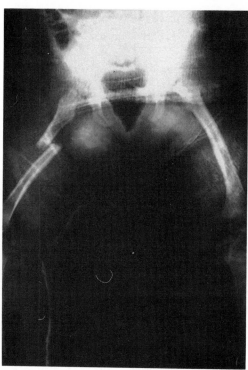

Fig. 2   Left, Osteogenesis imperfecta may present radiologically with thin cortices, marked osteopenia, and multiple fractures. **Right**, It may also present as multiple fractures with a nearly normal roentgenographic appearance.

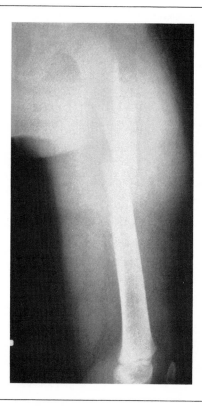
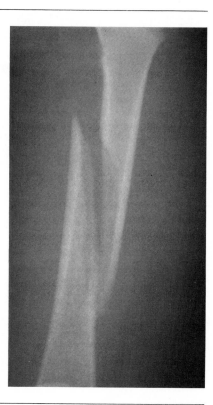

Fig. 3   An immediate spica can be used in most femur fractures regardless of fracture type in children less than 6 years of age, if there is less than 2.5 cm of shortening on initial radiographs. The transverse fracture (**left**) and the long oblique fracture (**right**) are common fracture patterns that are well treated with this technique.

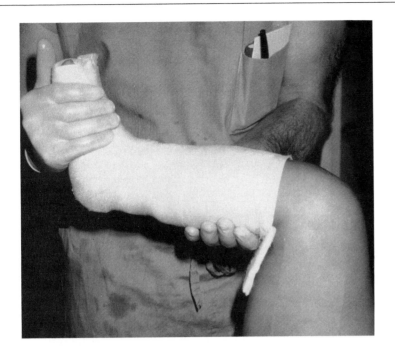

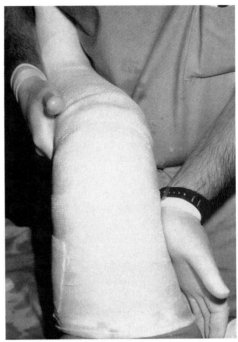

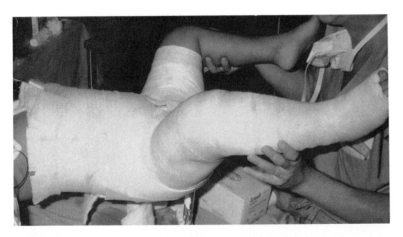

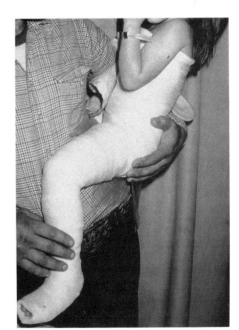

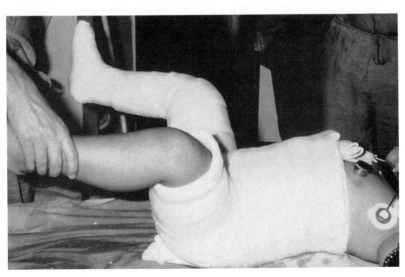

Fig. 4 In making an immediate spica, a 90-90 position (sitting) is used for most femur fractures. **Top left,** Make a short leg cast with a pad in the popliteal fossa on the involved leg. **Top right,** Extend this to a long leg cast with the knee flexed 90 degrees and a valgus mold over the fracture site. **Center left,** Place the child on a spica table with appropriate padding. **Bottom left,** A 1.5 spica is constructed using fiberglass. **Bottom right,** Fiberglass is strong enough to allow construction without a bar between the legs allowing greater ease in handling and toileting.

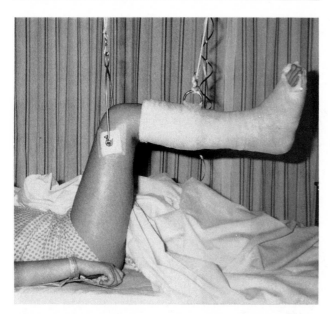

Fig. 5 Skeletal 90-90 traction is best accomplished with a distal femoral threaded pin, and a cast, splint, or sling over the lower leg.

technique are (1) fracture with less than 2.5 cm of initial shortening, (2) no history of any abuse, and (3) intact soft tissue without evidence of compartment syndrome.

The fracture may be a short oblique or transverse fracture as seen in Figure 3. The immediate spica I find most beneficial for all fractures regardless of location in the femur is a 90, 90 spica, also called a sitting spica. It is applied as shown in Figure 4. A valgus mold over the femur fracture is mandatory. I prefer the distal to proximal technique of making this cast, because it ensures the ability to hold the fracture in a valgus position. Malreduction from femur fractures is almost always seen with the fracture fragments falling into a varus position. The 90, 90 position of casting is chosen because it simplifies patient care. The child can be sat on a toilet or held on the parent's hip, which makes management much easier. When loss of reduction does occur in an immediate spica cast (this should be relatively rare), reduction can be salvaged by closed manipulation and casting, or by returning the child to traction. Weekly radiologic follow-up is indicated for the first three weeks to ensure satisfactory alignment. The limits of acceptability at the time of casting are 5 degrees of varus, 10 degrees of valgus, 20 degrees of anterior bow, and 10 degrees of posterior bow. If immediate casting is not appropriate, traction (either skin or skeletal) is used until the fracture is stable.

In the child from 6 to 12 years of age, the traditional treatment is traction followed by casting. The traction can be skeletal as in 90, 90 (Fig. 5) or skin traction with the leg resting on a Thomas splint. The benefit of 90

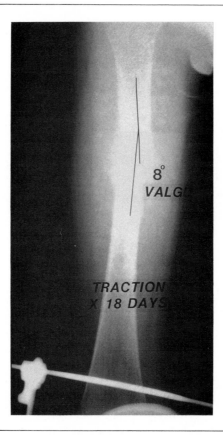

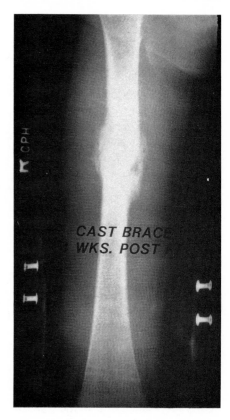

Fig. 6 Left, Alignment in traction should be in a few degrees of valgus, because the fracture will usually settle into varus (**right**) in a cast brace or spica.

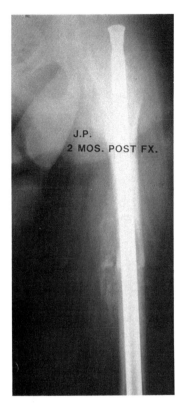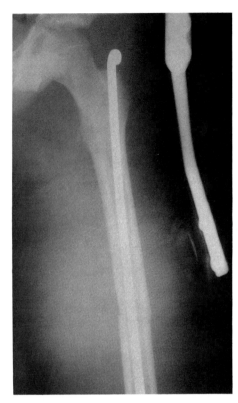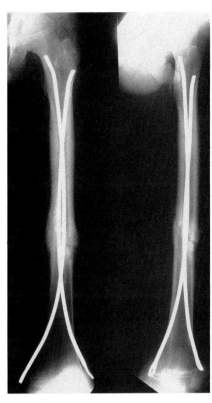

Fig. 7 Intramedullary rodding for femur fractures in children may use a reamed rod in the teenager (**left**), an antegrade rush rod (**center**), often requiring external supplementation with a long leg brace and pelvic band, or retrograde rodding with an Ender rod (**right**).

degrees-90 degrees traction is ease in patient management. Tibial pin traction should be avoided[5] because of the possibility of injury to the proximal tibial physis and the risk of growth arrest after diaphyseal fracture. After three weeks of traction, when the callus has begun to mature, the child can be placed in a cast, a brace, or a spica cast. Figure 6 documents the use of traction followed by casting. The femur should be placed in a few degrees of valgus while in traction, because it will generally fall back to a straight position as it heals. Varus in the early cast brace or spica period tends to increase during the period of fracture healing. If this does occur and is mild it can be corrected by manipulation and spica casting. If the varus angulation is associated with significant shortening, rodding may be necessary to correct this problem in the older child. In the child between 2 and 10 years of age, the desirable position in traction is 0.5 to 1.5 cm short to allow for overgrowth.[6,7]

Areas of controversy in the age group from 6 to 12 include the use of intramedullary fixation or the use of external skeletal fixation devices. Both techniques have been used, and series are being reported in these techniques. The child between 6 and 10 or 11 years of age is at considerable risk of overgrowth. The risk of overgrowth with the use of internal fixation is not yet

entirely clear. The standard treatment in this age group is traction followed by casting. In a child over 100 lbs, with multiple fractures or head trauma, or with an open fracture, skeletal stabilization is indicated.

Femur fractures in children over 12 should probably be treated with intramedullary fixation when appropriate. There still may be a role for traction followed by cast bracing. Series on traction and cast bracing in this age group document a significant incidence of shortening and varus deformity, which has not occurred in the femoral rod group. The series of traction-treated femoral fractures by Kirby and associates,[8] Humberger and Eyring,[9] Gross and associates,[10] and Scott and associates[11] all document significant problems in the larger child with diaphyseal femur fractures resulting in angular deformity and shortening. Just as the femoral rod has become standard treatment in the adult, it is rapidly becoming a standard treatment in the child over 12 years of age (Fig. 7). A straightforward transverse fracture could be treated either with a reamed femoral rod, ensuring good stability, or a non-reamed rod with external supplementation and use of a cast brace if necessary. Retrograde Ender rodding is gaining popularity and offers greater stability than a single Rush rod (Fig. 7). Either of these techniques will shorten hospitalization and ensure satisfactory alignment. The use of locked rods for unstable fractures is also excellent treatment in the teenager. Greater trochanteric growth after about the ages of 8 to 10 is minimal with appositional growth predominating. Growth across the superior aspect of the femoral neck does occur and may be compromised by standard femoral rodding techniques. Early rodding may lead to growth alterations of the proximal femur with coxa valga and neck hypoplasia. The technique of rodding femur fractures that seems best in younger children (aged 6 to 12) is retrograde metaphyseal insertion of flexible nails, because it offers similar benefit with less risk. Studies are underway to analyze this but I don't think its use is generally acceptable in a child who can be treated easily with traction and casting.

Conclusion

The appropriate management of femoral fractures in children includes the immediate spica as the primary treatment for children 0 to 6 years of age. Traction followed by cast, brace, or a spica is indicated in a child between 6 and 12 years of age. Flexible nonreamed rodding may have a role in this age group. In children older than 12 years of age, femoral rodding is the treatment of choice. For the future, more aggressive methods of fracture fixation in the 6- to 12-year-old child may be indicated. In the child with multiple fractures or head injury there is a need for early fracture stabilization at all ages.

References

1. Beals RK, Tufts E: Fractured femur in infancy: The role of child abuse. *J Pediatr Orthop* 1983;3:583–586.
2. Akbarnia B, Torg JS, Kirkpatrick J, et al: Manifestations of battered-child syndrome. *J Bone Joint Surg* 1974;56A:1159–1166.
3. Irani RN, Nicholson JT, Chung SMK: Long-term results in the treatment of femoral-shaft fractures in young children by immediate spica immobilization. *j Bone Joint Surg* 1976;58A:945–951.
4. Staheli LT, Sheridan GW: Early spica cast management of femoral shaft fractures in young children. *Clin Orthop* 1977;126:162–166.
5. Miller PR, Welch MC: The hazards of tibial pin replacement in 90–90 skeletal traction. *Clin Orthop* 1978;135:97–100.
6. Griffin PP: Fractures of the femoral diaphysis in children. *Orthop Clin North Am* 1976;7:633–638.
7. Shapiro F: Fractures of the femoral shaft in children: The overgrowth phenomenon. *Acta Orthop Scand* 1981;52:649–655.
8. Kirby RM, Winquist RA, Hansen ST Jr: Femoral shaft fractures in adolescents: A comparison between traction plus cast treatment and closed intramedullary nailing. *J Pediatr Orthop* 1981;1:193–197.
9. Humberger FW, Eyring EJ: Proximal tibial 90–90 traction in treatment of children with femoral-shaft fractures. *J Bone Joint Surg* 1969;151A:499–504.
10. Gross RH, Davidson R, Sullivan JA, et al: Cast brace management of the femoral shaft fracture in children and young adults. *J Pediatr Orthop* 1983;3:572–582.
11. Scott J, Wardlaw D, McLauchlin J: Cast bracing of femoral shaft fractures in children: A preliminary report. *J Pediatr Orthop* 1981;1:199–201.

Pathogenesis of Progressive Valgus Deformity Following Fractures of the Proximal Metaphyseal Region of the Tibia in Young Children

Robert B. Salter, OC, MD, FRCSC

Trevor N. Best, FRACS

Introduction

An incomplete fracture of the proximal metaphyseal region of the tibia in young children may appear to be an insignificant bony injury, but it has the potential to produce a progressive valgus deformity of the involved lower limb during the ensuing year and a half. The first orthopaedic surgeon to recognize and report this curious phenomenon was Cozen in 1953.[1] Since then, it has been reported by Jackson and Cozen,[2] Salter and Best,[3] and Rooker and Salter.[4]

This chapter reports on a clinical investigation of the pathogenesis of such progressive valgus deformity following incomplete fractures of the proximal metaphysis of the tibia in young children.

The Problem

The typical fracture is of the greenstick type: it is transverse or oblique, involves the medial, but not the lateral, cortex of the proximal metaphysis, and may or may not be associated with an undisplaced fracture of the neck of the fibula. The fracture site is usually open on the medial side (Fig. 1). The potential for progressive deformity following this completely innocuous-looking fracture is usually not appreciated. Consequently, it is often treated by simple immobilization of the involved lower limb with the knee in 90 degrees of flexion (a position that cannot control valgus or varus malalignment). Over the next 18 months, however, the child's lower limb can develop a progressive valgus deformity that is obvious both clinically and radiographically (Fig. 2). Understandably, the unexpected deformity is disturbing to the concerned parents as well as to the perplexed surgeon and can even lead to litigation.

Clinical Investigation

Methods

The clinical investigation, which was entirely retrospective, included clinical assessment of the valgus deformity and photographic documentation of the full length of both lower limbs. The radiographic assessment of the lower limbs included measurement of the valgus deformity at the fracture site, total valgus deformity of the entire limb, and measurement of the lengths of both tibias and both fibulas.

Mechanism of Injury

In all of the children, the recorded mechanism of injury was a valgus or abduction injury with the knee extended.

Clinical Material

The clinical investigation included 21 children, 16 boys and five girls. Their ages at the time of injury ranged from 2 to 8 years. All of the children had a preexistent bilateral genu valgum of the physiologic type.

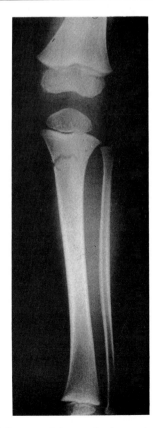

Fig. 1 Medial fracture of the proximal metaphyseal region of the tibia.

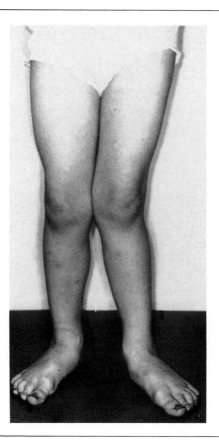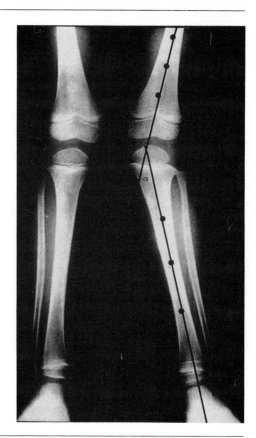

Fig. 2 Left, Photograph. **Right**, Radiograph showing valgus deformity.

Results

Of the 21 children, 13 (62%) exhibited a significant valgus deformity (more than 10 degrees greater than the valgus configuration of the opposite lower limb). The range of excessive valgus was from 13 degrees to 25 degrees (mean, 19.3).

The valgus deformity proved to be a combination of the following factors: (a) Excessive valgus deformity at the fracture site (malunion); (b) Transient acceleration of proximal tibial epiphyseal growth on the medial side; and (c) Tethering effect of the fibula in the presence of overgrowth of the fractured tibia (range, 0.3 to 1.0 cm; mean, 0.6 cm).

In addition, the relative overgrowth of the tibia produced a valgus deformity at the ankle secondary to elevation of the distal end of the fibula (range, 0 to 0.6 cm; mean, 0.3 cm).

Initial Treatment

In 12 of the 13 children who developed a valgus deformity, the initial treatment had consisted of immobilization of the involved lower limb in a long leg plaster cast with the knee at approximately 90 degrees of flexion. No attempt had been made to reduce the valgus deformity at the fracture site. In the remaining one of the 13 children, an attempt at reduction had been performed and the lower limb had been immobilized in a plaster cast with the knee extended.

Possible Prevention of the Valgus Deformity

Theoretically, if children with this fracture had been treated by closed reduction of the gap on the medial side of the tibia, and immobilization of the lower limb in a long leg, nonwalking cast with the knee in extension, the malunion component of the valgus deformity could have been eliminated or at least minimized. Furthermore, this might hasten the healing time and decrease the amount of overgrowth of the medial part of the proximal tibial epiphyseal plate. In this way, at least two of the aforementioned factors in the pathogenesis of progressive valgus deformity following fracture of the proximal metaphyseal region of the tibia in these children could be decreased.

Possible Spontaneous Correction of the Valgus Deformity

MacEwen and associates[5] reported that "adequate clinical correction (of the valgus deformity) occurred spontaneously in six of the seven patients" in their series. However, this group of patients had a less severe deformity than the patients in our clinical investigation. Furthermore, the mean amount of correction was only 4 degrees. Nevertheless, MacEwen has quite rightly recommended delaying surgical correction as long as possible to determine how much spontaneous correction might occur.

Surgical Correction of Severe Residual Valgus Deformity

From our experience with correction of severe residual valgus deformity as a complication of an incomplete fracture in the proximal tibia of young children, we learned that the optimum surgical treatment (to avoid recurrence of the deformity) includes shortening of the tibia approximately 0.5 cm in excess of the radiographically measured tibial overgrowth; osteotomy of the fibula, overcorrection of the tibial valgus de-

formity by a few degrees; and internal fixation of the osteotomy site by means of staples.

References

1. Cozen L: Fracture of the proximal portion of the tibia in children followed by valgus deformity. *Surg Gynecol Obstet* 1953;97:183–188.
2. Jackson DW, Cozen L: Genu valgum as a complication of proximal tibial metaphyseal fractures in children. *J Bone Joint Surg* 1971;53A:1571–1578.
3. Salter RB, Best T: Pathogenesis and prevention of valgus deformity following fractures of the proximal metaphyseal region of the tibia in children. *J Bone Joint Surg* 1972;54B:767.
4. Rooker GD, Salter RB: Prevention of valgus deformity following fracture of the proximal metaphysis of the tibia in children. *J Bone Joint Surg* 1980;62B:527.
5. Zionts LE, Sharps C, MacEwen GD: Spontaneous improvement of post-traumatic tibia valga. Presented at the 53rd Annual Meeting of the American Academy of Orthopaedic Surgeons, New Orleans, LA, Feb 20–25, 1986.

CHAPTER 46

Serious Fractures and Joint Injuries Involving the Foot and Ankle

Peter F. Armstrong, MD, FRCSC, FACS

Fractures involving the distal tibial epiphysis, such as Tillaux and triplane fractures, and the type III/IV fracture of the medial malleolus are serious injuries that have the potential for significant complications if they are not treated appropriately. Although serious fractures of the talus and calcaneus (os calcis) are uncommon in children, certain guidelines are important to remember in managing these injuries when they do occur.

Fractures Involving the Distal Tibial Epiphysis

The distal tibial physis fuses first centrally, then medially, and, finally, laterally. The closure seems to begin posteriorly rather than anteriorly. The process takes approximately 18 months.[1] If, during this period of varying degrees of incomplete physeal fusion, the ankle is subjected to angular and torsional forces, a peculiar pattern of injury occurs. The injury involves the sagittal, transverse, and coronal planes.[1-6] There may be two, three, or four fragments. The fracture enters the ankle joint and also crosses the physis. The latter two characteristics obviously indicate that this is a fracture that requires anatomic reduction. Two types of fractures occur during this transitional period from immaturity to maturity, the triplane fracture, which tends to occur in the earlier part of this period, and the Tillaux, which occurs, more commonly, in the latter part.[7]

Tillaux Fractures

The Tillaux fracture is a Salter-Harris type III injury that involves the anterolateral aspect of the distal tibial physis.[1] It occurs as a result of an external rotation injury when the central and medial regions of the physis have closed. The anterior tibiofibular ligament attaches to the distal tibial epiphysis at this point. The inherent strength of the ligament and its attachment to bone is greater than that of the attachment of the epiphysis to the rest of the tibia. The cleavage plane passes along the physis until it reaches the fused part of the plate. At this point the direction is changed to cross the epiphysis and enter the joint.[4,5]

Radiographs of the ankle (three views) should easily demonstrate the injury (Fig. 1). Letts[8] stressed the need to take mortise views of the ankle, because small Tillaux fractures tend not to be obvious on the standard anteroposterior radiograph of the ankle. The lateral view should be carefully reviewed to make sure that the injury is not, in fact, a triplane fracture.[4]

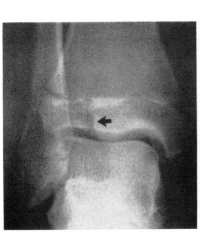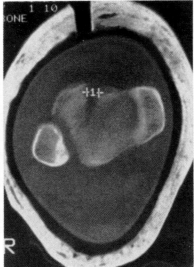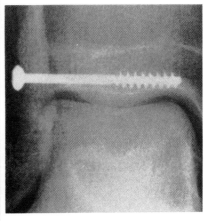

Fig. 1 Juvenile Tillaux fracture. **Left,** Pre-reduction. **Center,** After attempted closed reduction (1 cm gap). **Right,** Following open reduction and internal fixation. (Reproduced with permission from Herzenberg J: Computed tomography of paediatric distal tibial growth plate fractures: Practical guide. *Techniques Orthop* 1989;4:56–61.)

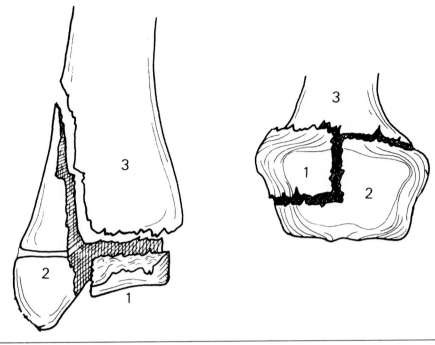

Fig. 2 Typical pattern of a three-part triplane fracture. (Reproduced with permission from Dias LS: Fractures of the tibia and fibula. Part II: Fractures of the distal tibial and fibular physes, in Rockwood CA Jr, Wilkins KE, King RE (eds): *Fractures in Children*. Philadelphia, JB Lippincott, 1984, vol 3, pp 1014–1042.)

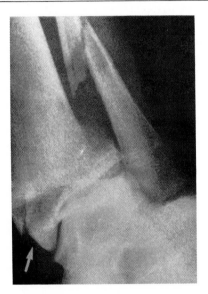 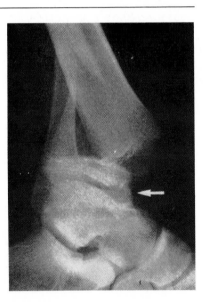

Fig. 3 Severely displaced triplane fracture. **Left,** Note medial malleolar fragment (arrow). **Right,** Lateral view shows large posterior metaphyseal spike.

The goal in the management of this injury is to restore the articular congruity of the joint. Because the majority of the distal tibial epiphysis is already fused, there is no concern about the development of a growth arrest.

It is generally agreed that 2 mm or more of intra-articular transverse displacement and any amount of vertical displacement is unacceptable and must be corrected.[2-4,7,9,10] In many cases, correction can be accomplished by closed reduction, usually under general anesthetic. Because the force that created the injury was an external rotation force, reduction is carried out by applying an internal rotation force. Direct pressure over the fragment can help push it back into place. The ankle is then dorsiflexed to ensure correct vertical alignment of the fragment. The limb is placed in a long leg cast with the knee flexed and the foot held in an internally rotated inverted position with the ankle at 90 degrees. The quality of reduction is best evaluated either by tomograms or by a computed tomographic scan.[4,5,11] This cast is maintained for three weeks and is then usually changed to a below-knee walking cast for

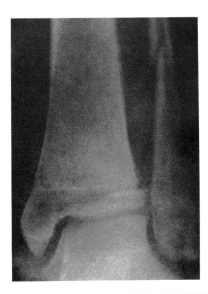
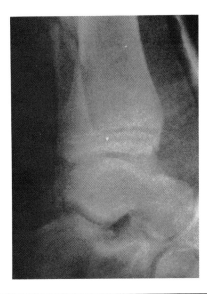

Fig. 4 Following closed reduction the plain films look quite acceptable.

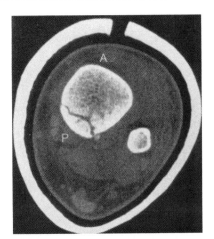
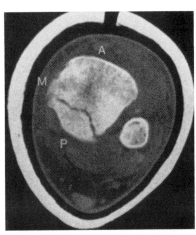
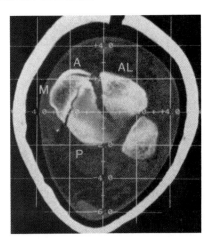

Fig. 5 **Left**, Proximal computed tomographic slice shows the posterior (P) and the anterior (A) fragments. **Center**, The distal cut through the distal metaphysis and the physis shows both the posterior (P) and anterior (A) fragments to be larger. The proximal tip of the medial malleolar fragment (M) is seen. **Right**, The cut through the epiphysis shows the posterior (P) fragment, the remaining small portion of the anterior (A) fragment, the medial malleolar (M) fragment, and the anterolateral (AL) fragment. This is an example of a 4-part fracture. The anterior gap is 5 mm and therefore unacceptable.

a further three weeks. The maintenance of reduction must be checked, by radiograph, weekly for the first three weeks to ensure that reduction has not been lost.

If satisfactory reduction is not achieved, an open reduction with internal fixation of the fragment must be performed. The fragment is approached through an anterolateral incision. Obviously, care must be taken not to denude the fragment of its soft-tissue attachments. Any impediments to reduction are removed, and the reduction is carried out. The reduction is fixed with a cancellous lag screw. The screw can cross the physis because little growth potential remains.

One other method of reduction can be attempted.

Using the image intensifier, a Kirschner wire can be inserted into the displaced fragment. The Kirschner wire is then used to manipulate the fragment into a reduced position. If the reduction is acceptable on the image, and is confirmed with proper plain films, the wire can then be driven across into the tibia. A small-fragment cannulated screw is used to achieve compression across the fracture (J Wedge, personal communication, 1988). Continuous passive motion (CPM) is used for three or four days following surgery and can be continued at home if the equipment is available. Weightbearing is not permitted for the first three weeks. Gradual progression to full weightbearing oc-

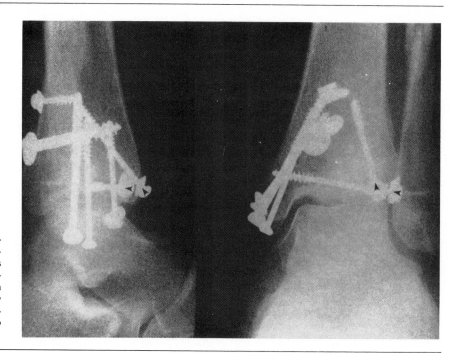

Fig. 6 On the basis of the computed tomographic scan, an open reduction and internal fixation of this four-part fracture was performed using a medial and an anterolateral incision. (Reproduced with permission from Herzenberg J: Computed tomography of paediatric distal tibial growth plate fractures: Practical guide. *Techniques Orthop* 1989;4:56–61.)

curs over the next three weeks. Removal of the screw is at the discretion of the surgeon.

Triplane Fractures

Triplane fractures are much more extensive than Tillaux fractures. The injury can produce from two to four fragments (Fig. 2). Often the plain films are insufficient to determine the morphology of the fracture. The computed tomographic scan, particularly with three-dimensional reconstruction, has proven to be invaluable in determining the number and displacement of the fracture fragments.[2–6,9,11,12] This information is critical in order to plan the most appropriate treatment. In cases of the two-fragment type, the principal displaced fragment may be either medial or lateral.[5] Two-fragment fractures can often be treated successfully by closed reduction. The quality of reduction must be determined accurately, and a computed tomographic scan offers the best method for doing this.[11] Again, a gap greater than 2 mm or any vertical displacement is unacceptable.[2–4,7,9,10] If an acceptable reduction has been achieved, the fracture is treated with a long leg cast as described for the Tillaux fracture. Three- and four-part fractures are more likely to require open reduction and internal fixation, but, even in these cases, a closed reduction may be attempted first. In these cases, the computed tomographic scan made before surgery is used to determine the number and location of incisions necessary to achieve an anatomic reduction (Figs. 3–6).[11] In younger patients, it is recommended that the fixation not cross the physis, because there is still significant growth remaining.

Salter Type III/IV Fractures of the Medial Malleolus

This fracture is not confined to the transition period of adolescence. The mechanism of injury is forced inversion of the ankle. These injuries must be treated with respect because of the significant potential for growth disturbance, particularly if the fracture is improperly managed. The fracture is an intra-articular physeal injury, which requires anatomic reduction and, in most cases, stable, internal fixation.[13,14] It is important to realize that even with anatomic reduction the risk of partial growth arrest is significant, probably because of some crushing of the physis that also occurred at the time of injury.[4,5,15–17]

Careful review of the plain films of what seems to be a type III fracture may, in fact, reveal a very small metaphyseal flake of bone attached to the displaced fragment. The radiograph may fail to reveal the full extent of the cartilage injury, which can extend beyond the visible bony injury.[5]

Unless the fracture is completely undisplaced, an open reduction must be performed. Anatomic reduction of the articular surface and the physis must be achieved. It is frequently helpful to excise the small metaphyseal flake to improve visualization of the physis. Transepiphyseal fixation, using Kirschner wires, threaded pins, or small fragment screws, is preferred. If there is a large metaphyseal piece, transmetaphyseal fixation can be used. Transphyseal fixation should be avoided, if possible (Fig. 7).

These fractures need to be followed every six months for at least two years in order to watch for the development of a partial growth arrest.[2,4,5,14,16] The Harris

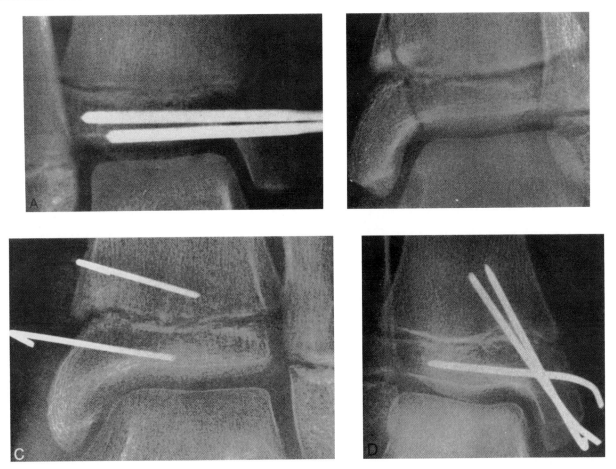

Fig. 7 Fixation of type IV medial malleolar injury. **Top left,** Transepiphyseal pins. **Top right,** Acute injury. **Bottom left,** Transmetaphyseal and transepiphyseal pins. **Bottom right,** Transepiphyseal and transphyseal pins (least recommended). (Reproduced with permission from Ogden JA: Tibia and fibula (Distal Epiphyseal and Physeal Injuries), in Ogden JA (ed): *Skeletal Injury in the Child*, ed 2. Philadelphia, WB Saunders, 1990, pp 832–863.)

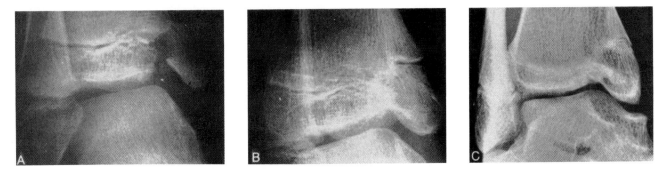

Fig. 8 Type III medial malleolar fracture. **Left,** Prereduction, treated by closed reduction. **Center,** Formation of osseus bridge 8 months later. **Right,** Two years following injury. (Reproduced with permission from Ogden JA: Tibia and fibula (Distal Epiphyseal and Physeal Injuries), in Ogden JA (ed): *Skeletal Injury in the Child*, ed 2. Philadelphia, WB Saunders, 1990, pp 832–863.)

growth arrest lines provide a convenient way of monitoring for a developing bar. This line will converge with the physis on the medial side if a growth arrest is developing. Even if there is no evidence of growth disturbance, follow-up should continue annually until maturity. Premature distal tibial physeal closure has been reported following this injury.[2,4,7] Obviously, a partial arrest will lead to the progressive development of a

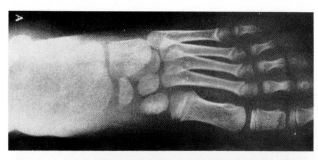

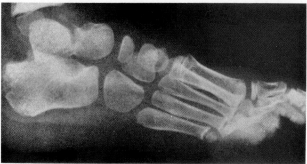

Fig. 9   Displaced fracture of the talar neck in a 7.2-year-old boy.

varus deformity at the ankle (Fig. 8). The general principles of the management of bony bridges should be applied. The bar may be resected with appropriate interposition material, so long as the fused portion of the plate does not exceed 40% of the total. If the fused portion exceeds 50%, the remaining distal tibial plate and the distal fibular plate should be fused by epiph-

ysiodesis. If a significant angular deformity has developed, it may be necessary to perform a distal tibial medial opening wedge osteotomy.

Fractures Involving the Foot

Fractures of the Talus

Fractures of the talus are rare in childhood.[18-21] This may be because a large portion of the talus in children is cartilage and is less likely to be injured by bending and axial loading. Nevertheless, these fractures do occur and can lead to osteonecrosis of the body of the talus. The most common mechanism of injury is forced dorsiflexion of the ankle, with impingement of the neck of the talus on the anterior aspect of the tibial plafond. The displacement is often minimal, and these fractures frequently are missed.[20] Despite the minimal displacement, osteonecrosis can occur. Letts and Gibeault[18] reviewed 12 patients ranging in age from 2 to 14 years of age. Although none had significant displacement, three of the 12 (25%) developed osteonecrosis of the body of the talus.

The initial management of this injury usually involves rest and elevation until the swelling subsides. If the fracture is either undisplaced or minimally displaced, the injury can be managed by immobilization in a non-weightbearing cast with the ankle in some equinus for six to eight weeks.[20,21]

If the fracture is displaced, a closed reduction is performed under general anesthetic, and the extremity is immobilized as above. If the reduction is unstable, percutaneous pinning may be required.[20,21]

In the event that an acceptable closed reduction is

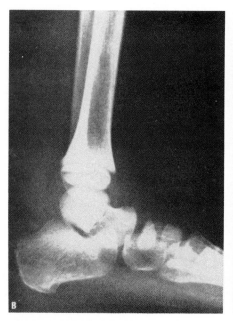

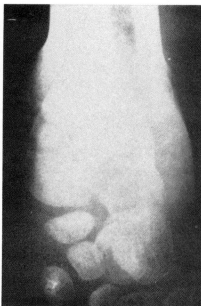

Fig. 10   Position after closed reduction by plantar flexion of the foot.

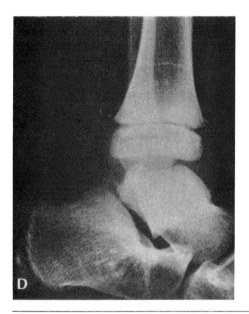

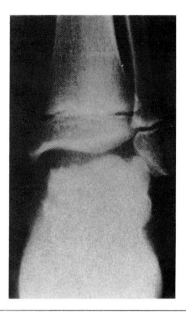

Fig. 11 Obvious avascular necrosis with secondary collapse (30 months after injury). (Reproduced with permission from Gross RH: Fractures and dislocation of the foot, in Rockwood CA Jr, Wilkins KE, King RE (eds): *Fractures in Children*. Philadelphia, JB Lippincott, 1984, vol 3, pp 1043–1103.)

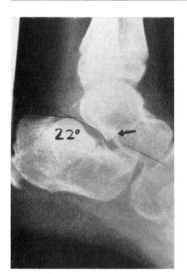

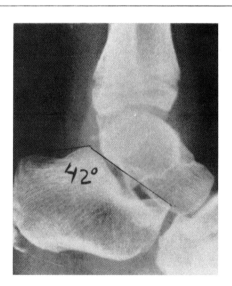

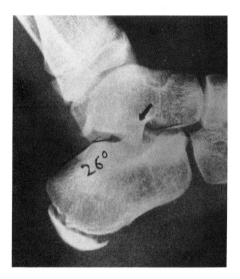

Fig. 12 **Left**, Fractures of the calcaneus in an 11.3-year-old boy. Joint depression type, Bohler's angle is 22 degrees. **Center**, Normal foot of the same boy with Bohler's angle of 42 degrees. **Right**, Fracture is healed 3 months later. Bohler's angle is still flattened, but the lateral process has enlarged and remodeled to accommodate the joint depression. (Reproduced with permission from Gross RH: Fractures and dislocation of the foot, in Rockwood CA Jr, Wilkins KE, King RE (eds): *Fractures in Children*. Philadelphia, JB Lippincott, 1984, vol 3, pp 1043–1103.)

not achieved, an open reduction may be necessary. The lateral approach is preferred, because it is less likely to cause further damage to the blood supply.[20]

Osteonecrosis is more likely to develop in children who have displaced fractures of the neck, crush injuries, or talar dislocation. Osteonecrosis can also be produced iatrogenically after open reduction. It may take as long as six months for evidence of osteonecrosis to appear, and, therefore, the child must be followed closely during this period of time (Figs. 9–11).[21] Hawk-

ins sign is unreliable in children under the age of 10 years.[20] A technetium bone scan may be helpful in making the diagnosis.[18,20,21] The recommended treatment for osteonecrosis is prolonged nonweightbearing until revascularization and reossification have occurred.[18,20]

Fractures of the Calcaneus

Fractures of the calcaneus are the most common tarsal injuries in children.[20-24] In the younger child, they may be caused by rather trivial trauma.[20] The possibility of this injury should, however, be considered in any child who has developed a limp.[20,25] The most common mechanism is a fall or jump from a height,[26] but more serious injuries can occur as a result of motor vehicle and lawn mower accidents. Schmidt and Weiner[24] reported that associated fractures, such as spinal fractures, were found in 20% of children younger than 12 years of age, compared with 50% of children of 13 years of age or older.

It is often extremely difficult to diagnose these injuries on radiographs. Technetium scanning has been used if there is some suspicion of a calcaneal fracture.[20,25] Because of the normal developmental anatomy of the child's calcaneus, Bohler's angle, used as an indicator of calcaneal injury in the adult, is not reliable in children.[20] The fractures are generally classified as extra-articular or intra-articular, and extra-articular fractures are more common in the younger child.[20,25] In more comminuted fractures, a computed tomographic scan can be very useful in delineating the morphology of the fracture fragments.[20,27]

For talar fractures, the initial management consists of rest and elevation to allow the swelling to subside. Often, no reduction is necessary. After three to four days, a below-knee cast is applied with the foot in a neutral position. The cast is usually maintained for six weeks and weightbearing is further protected for an additional four to six weeks. In the child younger than 10 years of age, remodeling takes place, and even displaced intra-articular fractures do well after closed reduction (Fig. 12).[24,26] Open reduction is more frequently required in children older than 10 years of age, who have displaced intra-articular fractures. Very few significant complications are reported as a result of this injury in children. In children with depressed intra-articular fractures, the subtalar joint is frequently stiff, but the children are pain-free.

References

1. Kleiger B, Mankin HJ: Fracture of the lateral portion of the distal tibial epiphysis. *J Bone Joint Surg* 1964;46A:25–32.
2. Dias LS: Fractures of the tibia and fibula. Part II: Fractures of the distal tibial and fibular physes, in Rockwood CA Jr, Wilkins KE, King RE (eds): *Fractures in Children*. Philadelphia, JB Lippincott, 1984, vol 3, pp 1014–1042.
3. Cooperman DR, Spiegel PG, Laros GS: Tibial fractures involving the ankle in children. The so-called triplane epiphyseal fracture. *J Bone Joint Surg* 1978;60A:1040–1046.
4. Mosca V: The management of displaced distal tibial injuries involving the physis. *Techniques Orthop* 1989;4:65–73.
5. Ogden JA: Tibia and fibula (Distal Epiphyseal and Physeal Injuries), in Ogden JA (ed): *Skeletal Injury in the Child*, ed 2. Philadelphia, WB Saunders, 1990, pp 832–863.
6. Dias LS, Giegerich CR: Fractures of the distal tibial epiphysis in adolescence. *J Bone Joint Surg* 1983;65A:438–444.
7. Spiegel PG, Cooperman DR, Laros GS: Epiphyseal fractures of the distal ends of the tibia and fibula: A retrospective study of two hundred and thirty-seven cases in children. *J Bone Joint Surg* 1978;60A:1046–1050.
8. Letts RM: The hidden adolescent ankle fracture. *J Pediatr Orthop* 1982;2:161–164.
9. Kärrholm J, Hansson LI, Laurin S: Computed tomography of intraarticular supination-eversion fractures of the ankle in adolescents. *J Pediatr Orthop* 1981;1:181–187.
10. Spiegel PG, Mast JW, Cooperman DR: Triplane fractures of the distal tibial epiphysis. *Clin Orthop* 1984;188:74–89.
11. Herzenberg J: Computed tomography of paediatric distal tibial growth plate fractures: Practical guide. *Techniques Orthop* 1989; 4:53–64.
12. Von Laer L: Classification, diagnosis, and treatment of transitional fractures of the distal part of the tibia. *J Bone Joint Surg* 1985;67A:687–698.
13. Dias LS, Tachdjian MO: Physeal injuries of the ankle in children: Classification. *Clin Orthop* 1978;136:230–233.
14. Salter RB, Harris WR: Injuries involving the epiphyseal plate. *J Bone Joint Surg* 1963;45A:587–622.
15. Aitken AP: The end results of the fractured distal tibial epiphysis. *J Bone Joint Surg* 1936;18A:685–691.
16. Kling TF Jr, Bright RW, Hensinger RN: Distal tibial physeal fractures in children that may require open reduction. *J Bone Joint Surg* 1984;66A:647–657.
17. Weber BG, Süssenbach F: Malleolar fractures, in Weber B, Brunner C, Freuler F (eds): *Treatment of Fractures in Children and Adolescents*. Berlin, Springer-Verlag, 1980, pp 350–372.
18. Letts R, Gibeault D: Fractures of the neck of the talus in children. *Foot Ankle* 1980;1:74–77.
19. Canale ST, Kelly FB Jr: Fractures of the neck of the talus: Long-term evaluation of seventy-one cases. *J Bone Joint Surg* 1980;60A: 143–156.
20. Ogden JA: Foot, in Ogden JA (ed): *Skeletal Injury in the Child*, ed 2. Philadelphia, WB Saunders, 1990, pp 865–906.
21. Gross RH: Fractures and dislocation of the foot, in Rockwood CA Jr, Wilkins KE, King RE (eds): *Fractures in Children*. Philadelphia, JB Lippincott, 1984, vol 3, pp 1043–1103.
22. Schantz K, Rasmussen F: Calcaneus fracture in the child. *Acta Orthop Scand* 1987;58:507–509.
23. Marti R: Fractures of the talus and calcaneus, in Weber B, Brunner C, Freuler F (eds): *Treatment of Fractures in Children and Adolescents*. Berlin, Springer-Verlag, 1980, pp 373–384.
24. Schmidt TL, Weiner DS: Calcaneal fractures in children: An evaluation of the nature of the injury in 56 children. *Clin Orthop* 1982;171:150–155.
25. Starshak RJ, Simons GW, Sty JR: Occult fracture of the calcaneus—Another toddler's fracture. *Pediatr Radiol* 1984;14:37.
26. Wiley JJ, Profitt A: Fractures of the os calcis in children. *Clin Orthop* 1984;188:131–138.
27. Pablot SM, Daneman A, Stringer DA, et al: The value of computed tomography in the early assessment of comminuted fractures of the calcaneus: A review of three patients. *J Pediatr Orthop* 1985;5:435–438.

Lower Extremity Growth Disturbances

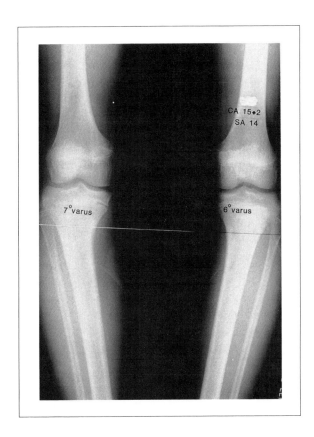

Current Trends in the Treatment of Simple and Complex Bone Deformities Using the Ilizarov Method

Maurizio A. Catagni, MD

Introduction

The introduction of the Ilizarov method in Italy in 1981 opened new horizons in the treatment of long bone and joint deformities, both congenital and post-traumatic.

Using compression and distraction to alter the shape and dimensions of bones, treatment of angular deformities with external fixation has progressed from applications limited to the stabilization of open fractures or osteotomies to correction of complex deformities using only limited open surgical techniques. By the unique application of hinges, Ilizarov has converted the simple fixator into a versatile apparatus for the reconstruction and correction of limb deformities.

Simple Correction of Axial Deformities

A simple angular deformity is one in which the anatomic axes of the bone segments intersect at the apex of the deformity without concurrent rotatory deformity. Figure 1-A demonstrates correction of angular deformity in a long bone with congenital or acquired abnormality of the anatomic axis. For this simple correction, an apparatus is put in place that

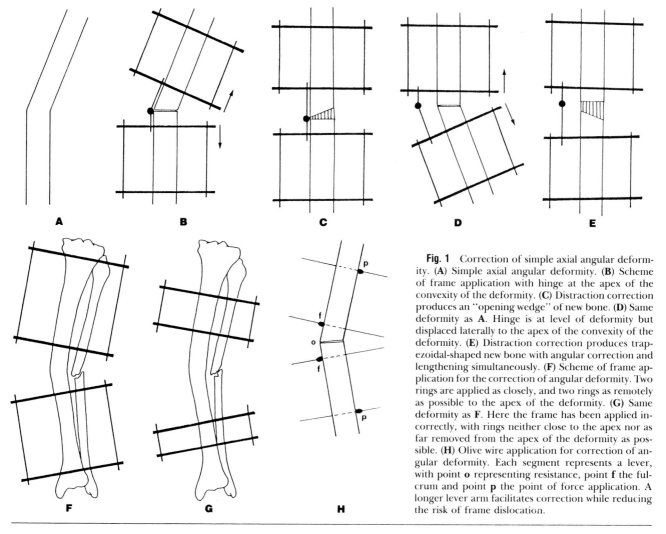

Fig. 1 Correction of simple axial angular deformity. (**A**) Simple axial angular deformity. (**B**) Scheme of frame application with hinge at the apex of the convexity of the deformity. (**C**) Distraction correction produces an "opening wedge" of new bone. (**D**) Same deformity as **A**. Hinge is at level of deformity but displaced laterally to the apex of the convexity of the deformity. (**E**) Distraction correction produces trapezoidal-shaped new bone with angular correction and lengthening simultaneously. (**F**) Scheme of frame application for the correction of angular deformity. Two rings are applied as closely, and two rings as remotely as possible to the apex of the deformity. (**G**) Same deformity as **F**. Here the frame has been applied incorrectly, with rings neither close to the apex nor as far removed from the apex of the deformity as possible. (**H**) Olive wire application for correction of angular deformity. Each segment represents a lever, with point **o** representing resistance, point **f** the fulcrum and point **p** the point of force application. A longer lever arm facilitates correction while reducing the risk of frame dislocation.

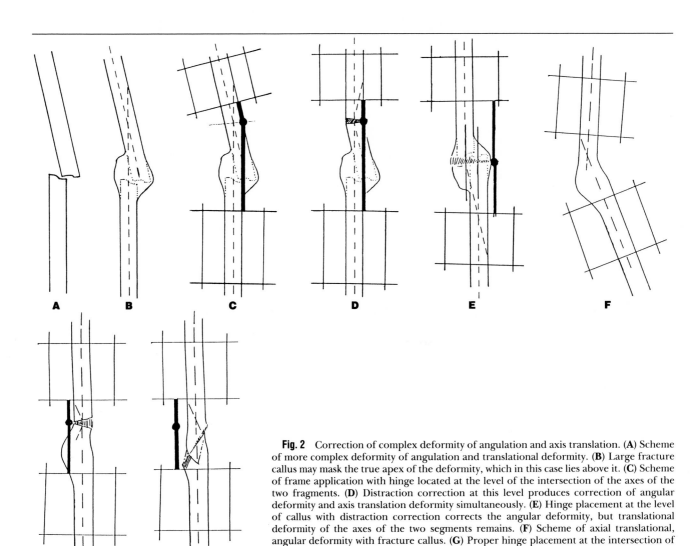

Fig. 2 Correction of complex deformity of angulation and axis translation. (**A**) Scheme of more complex deformity of angulation and translational deformity. (**B**) Large fracture callus may mask the true apex of the deformity, which in this case lies above it. (**C**) Scheme of frame application with hinge located at the level of the intersection of the axes of the two fragments. (**D**) Distraction correction at this level produces correction of angular deformity and axis translation deformity simultaneously. (**E**) Hinge placement at the level of callus with distraction correction corrects the angular deformity, but translational deformity of the axes of the two segments remains. (**F**) Scheme of axial translational, angular deformity with fracture callus. (**G**) Proper hinge placement at the intersection of the axes results in correction, but fracture callus may leave unsightly bump. (**H**) Proper hinge placement for the same deformity but with corticotomy through the callus, which may improve cosmesis while allowing correction of the deformity.

has two rings above the apex and two rings below the apex of the deformity. A corticotomy is then performed at the apex of the deformity, using the method described by Ilizarov. The hinges are placed at the apex of the deformity. It is essential that the axis of the hinges be perpendicular to the plane of deformity (Fig. 1-B).

A distraction force is applied opposite the apex of the deformity at a rate that will separate the bone ends at the concavity by 0.25 mm every six hours. This procedure causes an opening wedge of new bone to be produced (Fig. 1-C).

Using the same frame, lengthening of the bone, in addition to angular correction, may be obtained by moving the hinges away from the axis of the deformity in the direction of the convexity. In the previous example (Fig. 1-A), moving the hinges away from the apex (Fig. 1-D) will create new bone formation in the shape of a trapezoid (Fig. 1-E), thus lengthening the bone while correcting the deformity.

A stable construct requires two long lever arms. Each lever arm or segment is fixed with one ring placed as near and one ring placed as far as possible from the corticotomy site. Figures 1-F and 1-G demonstrate the correct and incorrect methods of application of this principle.

In order to keep the bone from moving along the wire and to increase stability of the frame, Ilizarov introduced the use of stop wires, commonly called olive wires. In angular corrections these wires are applied in the following manner. On the two rings adjacent to the corticotomy, olive wires are inserted with the stopper on the convexity. On the two rings farthest from the corticotomy, olive wires are placed on the concavity. Mechanical considerations are demonstrated in Figure 1-H. Each segment represents a lever, with point **o** representing resistance, point **f** the fulcrum, and point **p** the point of force application. A longer lever arm facilitates correction while reducing the risk of frame dislocation.

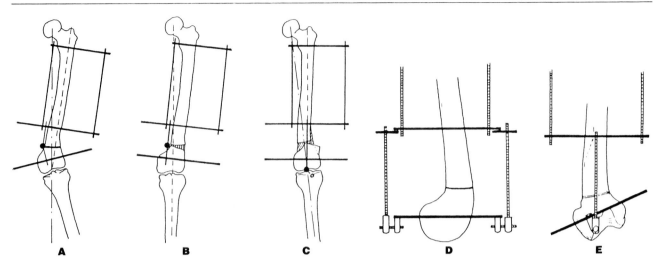

Fig. 3 Correction of angular deformity of the distal femur. (**A**) Scheme of frame application for correction of distal femoral valgus deformity with distal femoral corticotomy and hinge application at the level of the corticotomy. (**B**) Simple distraction correction corrects the angular deformity but axial translation deformity remains, producing a new deformity resembling a golf club. This occurs because the mechanical and anatomic axes of the leg intersect at the level of the knee. This example is directly analogous to angular and axial translational deformity correction. (**C**) Correct application of the hinges at the level of the intersection of the anatomic and mechanical axes, with simultaneous correction of angular deformity and axial translational deformity. (**D**) Lateral and (**E**) anteroposterior view of construction of hinges to allow correction as illustrated in **C**.

Correction of Axial Deviation With Translation

In many cases of angular deformity, especially those resulting from posttraumatic malunions and nonunions, a translational deformity coexists with the angular deformity. Figure 2-A shows a case in which a malunion is present with translation. It is important to note that the anatomic axes do not intersect at the apex within the hypertrophic callous (Fig. 2-B). The hinges must be applied at the intersection of the anatomic axes in order to achieve translational and anatomic correction (Figs. 2-C and 2-D). If the hinges were applied at the level of the deformity, the mechanical axis would be correct but a translation deformity would remain (Fig. 2-E).

When correcting deformities involving both translation and axial deviation, primary consideration must be given to placement of the hinges. The level of the corticotomy may be altered to improve cosmesis if hinge placement remains unchanged. Figure 2-F demonstrates a combined deformity with significant hypertrophic callous. If the corticotomy is performed at the level shown, an unacceptable cosmetic deformity will result (Fig. 2-G). This is especially important in the tibia where only minimal soft-tissue coverage exists. Performing a corticotomy through the hypertrophic callous can achieve correction and improve cosmesis at the same time (Fig. 2-H).

When the anatomic axis corresponds to the mechanical axis of the bone the application of the apparatus is relatively simple. When the anatomic axis and the mechanical axis differ, as in the femur, correction is more complex.

Distal Femoral Correction

In many cases, including congenital hemimelia and acquired or posttraumatic deformities, the surgeon must correct the axis of the distal femur. In such situations, the simple application of the device as described above will not suffice, because during correction of one deformity, a second, equally serious deformity can be created. Figure 3-A demonstrates the schema of a simple hinged apparatus used, with the hinges placed at the level of corticotomy, to correct a valgus deformity of the distal femur. Figure 3-B shows how the resultant restoration of the mechanical axis has resulted in simultaneous medial translation of the distal femoral segment, leading to an S-shaped deformity (usually called golf club deformity). This abnormality occurs when correction of the mechanical axis is carried out without respect for the anatomic axis. Because the point of intersection of the anatomic and the mechanical axes is the center of the knee, correction of an angular deformity, with or without lengthening, should be performed with the hinges at the level of the knee joint. In the example in Figure 3-A the hinges should be placed distal to the distal ring (Figs. 3-D and 3-E), resulting in the correction shown in Figure 3-C. With this technique it is possible to correct not only angular deviation but also translation. To determine the exact

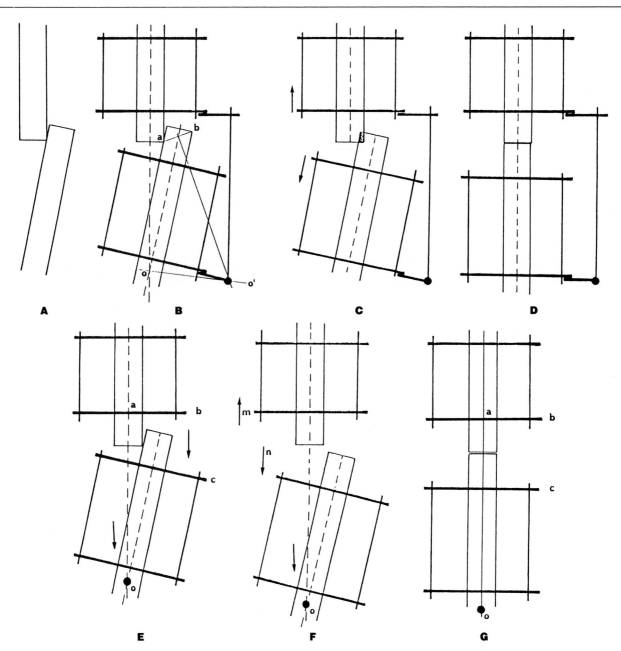

Fig. 4 Complex deformity with overlap of segments. (**A**) Scheme of angular and axis translational deformity of bone segments with overlap of segments. (**B**) Determination of intersection of axes and translation allows the determination of the point of deformity correction (hinge application), as explained in the text. (**C**) Correction occurs with distraction in the concavity of the deformity but requires overlap of the segments (shaded area). (**D**) Completion of deformity correction with simultaneous correction of overlap, angular, and axial translational deformity. (**E**) Same deformity and frame scheme as for (A,B,C,D) but with hinge application at the intersection of the axes of the bone segments. Overlap deformity is corrected initially by simultaneous distraction between points **a** and **o**, and points **b** and **c**. (**F**) After overlap deformity has been corrected, distraction between points **m** and **n** corrects angular and axial translational deformities through hinge at point **o**. (**G**) At the end of treatment, angular, axial, translational, and overlap deformities have been corrected without bone impingement.

point of hinge application preoperatively, tracings or templates should be made. A corticotomy can then be simulated, and the optimal position of the center of rotation determined.

Distractions With Complex Deformity Correction

This technique, which is generally required for post-traumatic deformities with shortening, also has appli-

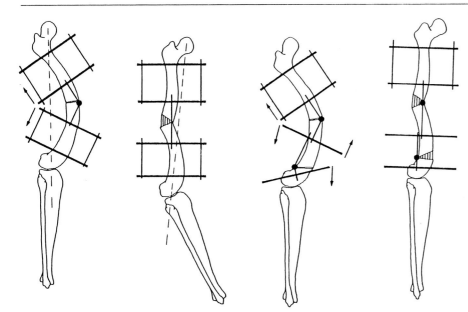

Fig. 5 Correction of severe angular deformity with periarticular deformity. **Left,** Severe procurvatum of the femur with recurvatum of the knee. **Left center,** Simple angular correction of the procurvatum aggravates the knee recurvatum. **Right center,** Scheme of two-level correction of both procurvatum of femur and recurvatum of the knee by opening wedge osteotomy. **Right,** Resultant correction of angulatory deformity as well as recurvatum of the knee by double-level corticotomy.

cations in congenital pseudarthrosis. Angular deformity may occur with concomitant bayonet apposition as seen in Figure 4-A. In theory both deformities can be corrected simultaneously with one motor force. The position of the hinge and motor would be calculated as shown in Figure 4-B. The intersection of the anatomic axis of the two segments is determined (point **o**). The angle formed by the axes is then bisected by the line **o-o'**. A perpendicular to the line connecting the bone ends (points **a** and **b**) is constructed. The intersection of the above perpendicular with line **o-o'** is the point of placement of the hinges. A distraction force is then applied opposite the apex as demonstrated by the arrows on Figure 4-C. The complete correction of angulation, translation, and lengthening is shown in Figure 4-D. In practice, however, simultaneous correction is not possible because of impingement of the bone ends. Therefore, apparatus construction differs as shown in Figure 4-E. Two rings are applied to each segment as previously described. Hinges are applied at point **o** anteriorly and posteriorly. Distraction is then applied equally between points **a** and **o** and points **b** and **c** until the overlap is eliminated. At this time distraction between the fragments is stopped and angular correction is accomplished by distraction between points **m** and **n** (Fig. 4-F). Completion of correction is demonstrated in Figure 4-G. Throughout treatment the basic frame is unchanged. All that is required is the exchange of the pushing mechanism at the completion of lengthening to achieve angular correction.

Several other methods of achieving the same correction are available. However, frequently many additional maneuvers are required, including insertion of olive wires. The method described above is by far the most appropriate, both theoretically and clinically.

Multiple Level Correction

In many pathologic conditions, long-bone deformities cannot be corrected with a single angular correction. In these cases restoration of the mechanical and anatomic axes requires two or more corticotomies and the construction of an apparatus that can produce correction at multiple levels.

The application of a simple frame to a complex deformity may produce an undesirable deformity. Figure 5, *left* shows how an attempt to correct procurvatum of the femur can result in recurvatum of the knee (Fig. 5, *left center*). In such cases, it is always necessary to prepare a careful tracing of the proposed correction. Such a tracing can demonstrate the need to perform a second correction in the opposite direction. In this example, a flexion osteotomy of the distal femur not only restores the anatomic axis but also maintains the integrity of the knee joint (Fig. 5, *right center* and *right*).

Similarly, if a marked procurvatum in the middle third of the tibia is corrected with a single osteotomy (Fig. 6, *left*), a seemingly acceptable reconstruction of the anatomic axis results in a residual abnormal angulation of the tibiotalar joint (Fig. 6, *center*). A double corticotomy with two levels of correction will avoid this problem. Figure 6, *right*, demonstrates the proper application of the apparatus to restore normal ankle alignment. When correction is performed in the lower limb, it is important to consider the alignment of the ankle

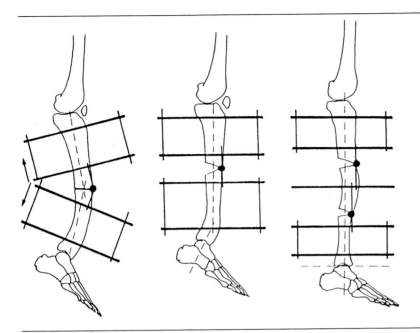

Fig. 6 Scheme of correction of tibia recurvatum with distal tibial deformity. **Left,** Severe procurvatum of tibia. Scheme of single level correction. **Center,** After single-level corticotomy, distal tibial angular deformity remains. **Right,** After double-level corticotomy, axis of tibia and ankle deformity have been corrected.

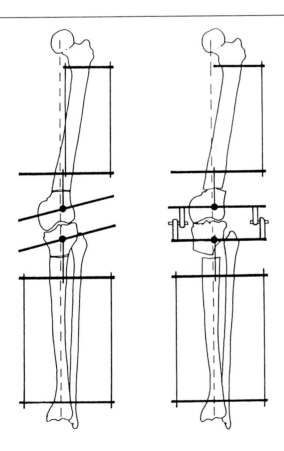

Fig. 7 Correction of joint obliquity with normal mechanical axis. **Left,** Limb with normal mechanical axis but oblique joint surface. Scheme of frame application. **Right,** Using hinge principles described previously, mechanical axis preserved while joint obliquity is corrected. Distal femoral and proximal tibial rings may be hinged to allow joint range of motion during the treatment period.

and knee joints because they are weightbearing and subject to increased forces; alignment is relatively less important in the upper extremity.

Abnormal obliquity in joint alignment may coexist with a normal mechanical axis. Although both mechanical and anatomic axes about the limb are normal, shear forces across the joint are increased. Figure 7, *left* illustrates such a deformity about the knee. In such cases, it is necessary to perform a double correction consisting of varus realignment of the distal femur and valgus of the proximal tibia.

The end result of correction would demonstrate normal axial and joint alignment (Fig. 7, *right*). To achieve correction of joint obliquity, hinges must be placed at the center of rotation of the knee joint, between the femoral and tibial frames. Joint obliquity is often accompanied by other deformities, most commonly leglength discrepancy. As with any lengthening, muscle tension can create abnormal compressive forces on articular cartilage; a small amount of distraction through the hinges across the knee joint preserves the joint surface, maintains motion, and prevents joint dislocation.

Correction of Residual Translational Malalignment

Residual translational malalignment may exist after angular correction. It is imperative that the surgeon know techniques that can correct this deformity. One technique involves the use of olive wires to apply traction in opposing directions on the bone segments (Fig. 8, *left* and *left center*). A noninvasive alternative method, perimounting, involves the modification of or addition

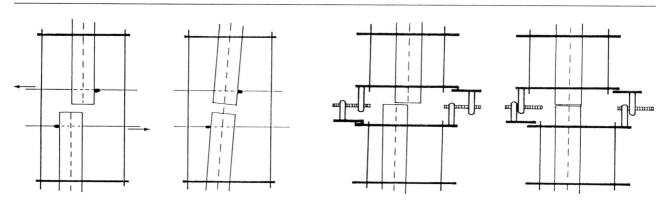

Fig. 8 Correction of translational deformity. **Left**, Olive wires may be placed with olive on the cortex away from the direction of translation required. **Left center**, With either acute or gradual tensioning of the olive wire, the bone is translated laterally. **Right center**, Scheme of frame perimounting to correct angular deformity. Posts from rings closest to the corticotomy are connected transversely by threaded rods. **Right**, By turning the threaded rods appropriately, one segment can be translated laterally on the other.

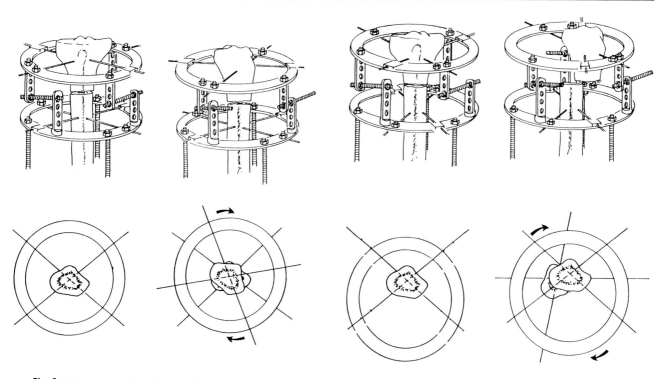

Fig. 9 Correction of rotational deformity. **Left** and **left center**, Rings closest to corticotomy are connected by posts and threaded rods, usually at three locations. By compressing the points together, one segment is rotated on the other. If both segments are located in the middle of the apparatus, no transational deformity results from this procedure. **Right** and **right center**, Frame scheme as for **left**. However, the bone is eccentrically located within the frame. Thus, with rotation correction located on the rings, one segment translates laterally on the other. May be secondarily corrected by the technique described for translational deformity.

to an existing frame. In translational perimounting, posts are attached to the closest ring of each segment and are then connected by threaded rod so that the posts can be moved along the rod to correct the translational deformity (Fig. 8, *right center* and *right*).

Rotational Correction

A small degree of rotational correction may be performed acutely during corticotomy, but corrections of more than 20 degrees require the construction of a device capable of progressive rotational correction. This construct consists of a basic frame with the rings adjacent to the corticotomy site connected by a series of posts and threaded rods (Fig. 9, *left* and *left center*). The nuts on the connecting rods are rotated at the rate of 2 to 4 mm per day.

When the axis of the bone corresponds to the center of rotation, only rotational movement is needed. When the center of the bone is not at the center of rotation, translation must accompany rotation (Fig. 9, *right center* and *right*).

Once rotational correction has been achieved, it will be possible to eliminate undesired translation by the method described above for translational deformities.

Management of Fibular Hemimelia Using the Ilizarov Method

Maurizio A. Catagni, MD

Introduction

The introduction of Ilizarov's methodology and external fixation device to Italy in 1981 has greatly changed the management of fibular hemimelia in our country. This applies particularly to the more severe forms of this congenital anomaly. In Italy, parents as a rule will not accept the traditional North American approach to the more severe forms, Syme's amputation. The purpose of this chapter is to present a functional classification of this disorder and to describe various ways of using the Ilizarov method to treat the different forms.

Classification and Management

The condition of fibular hemimelia is often associated with anomalies in the involved limb as well as other extremities. Foot, ankle, knee, and femoral deformities in the involved limb are frequent with the more severe forms of fibular hemimelia. We make a distinction between this deformity and others where fibular hemimelia, although present, is not the major or overriding deformity. Proximal femoral focal deficiency with associated fibular hemimelia is an example of the latter situation, and disorders of this type are not the subject of this chapter.

Grade I Fibular Hemimelia

Grade I fibular hemimelia is the mildest form of fibular hemimelia and is characterized by mild shortening of the fibula with associated shortening of the tibia. As a rule, there is no significant associated angular deformity of the tibia, femur, or foot, nor is knee or ankle instability present. Shortening of the lower leg is variable but averages 3 to 5 cm by the end of growth. The ankle may be ball-and-socket shaped but is stable. A lateral ray may be absent, but this is not functionally significant (Fig. 1, *left*).

This form of fibular hemimelia can be treated by simple lengthening of the leg at the appropriate stage for the patient. As a rule, it is not necessary to include the foot in the frame, because there is no significant ankle instability or foot deformity. Thus, the treating surgeon can use the external fixator of his choice for the lengthening. We prefer to use the Ilizarov frame because of the great flexibility of the device, the high patient tolerance for wire fixation, and the ability to extend the frame to the foot, if necessary.

The ideal time for lengthening is at or near the end of growth. At this point, the degree of functional shortening is readily apparent, and the patient is young enough that a relatively uneventful course can be expected.

Grade II Fibular Hemimelia

This lesion is more severe, consisting of severe shortening of the fibular, with no functional lateral malleolus (Fig. 1, *center*). The degree of ankle deformity varies with the degree of lateral malleolar hypoplasia (Fig. 2). Ankle instability can occur with the more severe deformity during lengthening or deformity correction. Lengthening procedures must incorporate the foot to prevent dislocation. Furthermore, the foot is often deformed, with equinovalgus of the ankle, pronation of the foot, and, frequently, absence of one or two lateral rays. The tibia, in addition to more severe shortening than is seen in grade I, may have associated valgus and procurvatum (anterior bow) angular deformity. In such cases, the first tibial frame must address and correct these deformities. The femur may be involved with

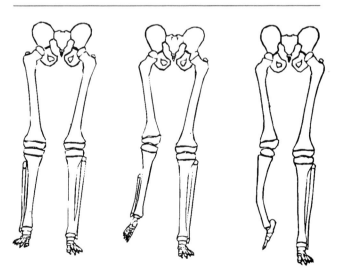

Fig. 1 Left, Grade I fibular hemimelia. **Center,** Grade II fibular hemimelia. **Right,** Grade III fibular hemimelia.

431

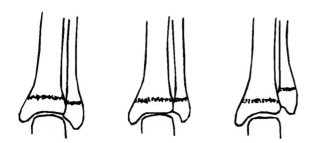

Fig. 2 Types of ankle deformity that can be associated with grade II fibular hemimelia. **Left,** Ball-and-socket ankle with fibula present. Ankle is usually stable in this configuration. **Center,** Hypoplastic fibula with intact mortise. **Right,** Severely hypoplastic or aplastic fibula. Talus usually unstable in the mortise, and may dislocate during lengthening or marked angular deformity correction.

shortening and/or hypoplasia of the lateral condyle (causing valgus of the knee and possible knee instability).

In this more severe disorder, we recommend the Ilizarov apparatus not only for the reasons mentioned above, but also because it has the ability to stabilize the ankle and the knee as necessary during the deformity correction.

Our program for these patients involves the following steps. First, patients who are old enough to walk are fitted with orthoses, as necessary. Second, at 10 to 12 years of age, patients undergo tibial angular correction (if it is needed), ankle stabilization, and the first tibial lengthening (Fig. 3). The ankle is stabilized by pulling the calcaneus into varus (either acutely or gradually) with olive wires, and by drawing the fibular remnant distally through the epiphysis. An alternative procedure involves a metaphyseal corticotomy with an anteroposterior wire, independent of the tibia (Fig. 4). The tibial portion of the frame is applied to allow gradual deformity correction and lengthening of the tibia as desired and tolerated. The more severe the initial foot deformity, the less the amount of lengthening that should be attempted at this stage.

The third stage involves a second lengthening and/or axial deformity correction of femur, tibia, or both and can be done at or near skeletal maturity. The extent or even the need for this stage depends on the degree of deformity and response to the previous treatment; it is usually not necessary. If repeat tibial lengthening is combined with femoral lengthening and axial deformity correction, we use the femoral-tibial frame described below in the section on grade III deformities. Again, if the tibia is lengthened or corrected, the foot must be included in the frame.

Grade III Fibular Hemimelia

This is the most severe form of fibular hemimelia, with functionally absent fibula, severe tibial deformity

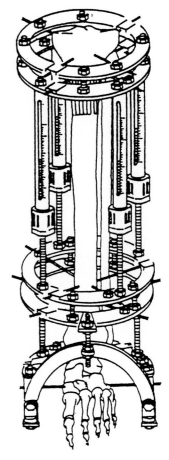

Fig. 3 Scheme of frame application for simple lengthening of the tibia, with stabilization of the foot within the frame to prevent dislocation.

and shortening, equinovalgus foot deformity or ankle dislocation, and femoral involvement (Fig. 1, *right*). The femoral involvement includes a variable amount of shortening, hypoplasia of the lateral condyle with valgus and instability of the knee, external rotation of the leg, and femoral neck deformity. Because of the absence of the fibula and the more severe degree of shortening and foot deformity, treatment is more extensive than for grade II cases.

Our treatment program includes the following steps. At 3 to 6 months of age, a soft-tissue release of the ankle is done to bring the foot into a plantigrade position. This is followed by orthoses for walking until the next stage.

At 5 to 6 years of age, the first tibial angular deformity correction is carried out. The foot is always incorporated in the frame, as for treatment of grade II lesions (Fig. 5). The extent of tibial lengthening to be undertaken at this stage is determined by the degree of pre-existing equinovalgus deformity of the ankle. The more severe the deformity, the less one should try to lengthen at this stage, concentrating rather on dealing with the foot and ankle deformity.

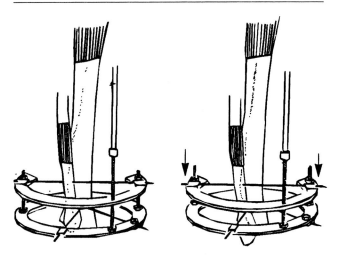

Fig. 4 Lateral malleolus hypoplasia correction. **Left,** At the distal end of the leg, the tibia and fibula are secured to separate rings. **Right,** The ring secured to the distal fibula is transported more distally than the tibia, functionally lengthening the fibula, and restoring a more competent lateral malleolus.

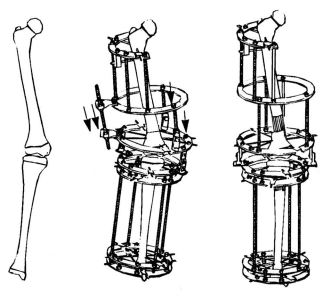

Fig. 6 **Left,** Scheme of simultaneous correction of femoral and tibial deformities, with lengthening. Grade III hemimelia with associated femoral shortening, valgus deformity. **Center,** Scheme of frame application for simultaneous angular correction of the femur and tibia. **Right,** After angular deformity correction, lengthening of the femur, tibia, or both may be carried out as necessary.

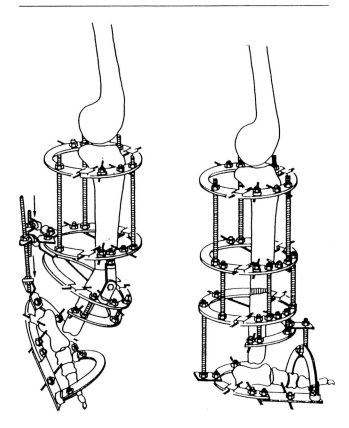

Fig. 5 **Left,** Scheme of apparatus for correction of tibia angular deformity and simultaneous correction of foot equinus. **Right,** Opening wedge correction of the tibia angular deformity. The amount of lengthening to be undertaken varies inversely with the severity of angular and foot deformities.

At 8 to 10 years of age, the second tibial lengthening is done, in conjunction with the first femoral lengthening and angular deformity correction. The frame thus extends the length of the leg, from upper femur to the foot. Again, because of the need to stabilize ankle and knee, we recommend using the Ilizarov device. We use the Lecco modification for the femoral frame, with 5-mm (4-mm in the very small femur) conical pins proximally, and full rings and wires distally. This frame must correct the valgus deformity of the femur gradually. The femoral frame is connected to a standard tibial lengthening frame, thus stabilizing the knee. The tibia and femur are lengthened simultaneously (Fig. 6). Again, the foot is also incorporated in the frame to prevent ankle equinus and valgus.

This procedure is repeated as needed to correct the extent of shortening involved. Usually, two further sessions are required, one at age 12 to 13, and another at skeletal maturity. Thus, for patients with grade III fibular hemimelia, five treatment sessions (at 3 to 6 months of age, 5 to 6 years of age, 8 to 10 years of age, 12 to 13 years of age, and at skeletal maturity) including four tibial lengthenings with the foot incorporated in the frame, are planned. Not all patients require all stages, nor does each session necessarily require both femoral and tibial lengthenings; however, with each tibial lengthening, the ankle is stabilized in the frame. Before the final session, if pain or instability dictate, an arthrodesis of the tibiotalar joint may be done. This of course can also be done at any time during adult life if necessary to treat ankle pain.

Patients Presenting Late With Grade II or III Fibular Hemimelia

Occasionally, a patient is seen with an untreated grade II or III fibular hemimelia. A program as described above may be instituted in these cases. The first step, however, is always to bring the foot into a plantigrade position, followed by correction of the tibial angular deformity. These steps can be followed by staged tibial and femoral lengthenings. The older the patient, the more severe the foot and ankle deformity, and the more significant the shortening of the extremity overall, the more difficult a total correction program will be. We think that if a patient is older than 15 years of age and has greater than 20% total shortening together with severe equinovalgus foot deformity, such as dislocation of the foot, it is wiser not to attempt a total correction. Rather, we prefer to straighten the femoral valgus deformity and bring the foot into a good position for an extension orthosis. In Italy, a Syme's amputation is usually not done even in these cases because of patient refusal.

Results

A total of 29 patients with grade I, 24 patients with grade II, and 18 patients with grade III fibular hemimelia have been treated thus far. A total of 94 segments have been lengthened, including 73 tibias and 21 femurs. The total limb lengthening ranged from 4 to 37 cm.

At this time, all of the grade I patients have completed treatment. In all patients leg-length discrepancy was corrected to within 1 to 2 cm. There were no significant complications that affected the final result. Joint function was satisfactory in all cases and patients were satisfied with the functional and cosmetic results.

Of the 24 grade II patients, seven have completed treatment. Two patients required reconstruction in two stages. Six patients underwent correction of ankle/foot deformity and instability by independent lengthening of the fibula, and one underwent foot correction by distal tibial osteotomy. The complications in this group

included one posterior subluxation of the knee during leg lengthening, one residual knee stiffness (flexion limited to 90 degrees one year after frame removal), one supracondylar fracture during lengthening, and two significant knee-flexion contractures, corrected by extension of the apparatus above the knee. Overall, the goals of treatment have been met in all patients who have completed treatment.

Four grade III patients have completed treatment. Five of the eighteen patients in this group have undergone two-stage correction, and one has undergone three-stage correction. Two have undergone foot correction by distal tibial osteotomy, and two have undergone ankle arthrodesis at the conclusion of treatment. Two patients underwent quadricepsplasty for extension contracture after lengthening.

Complications in this groups included two significant knee-flexion contractures requiring extension of the apparatus across the knee, one residual knee-extension contracture (flexion limited to 45 degrees), four foot deformity relapses, two fractures through regenerate bone treated with the apparatus, and one stiff edema of the leg.

Conclusions

The treatment of fibular hemimelia traditionally involves the use of orthotics for mild deformities; leg lengthening, epiphysiodesis, or both for mild to moderate leg-length discrepancy; and Syme amputation for patients with moderate to severe deformities and length discrepancies. In Italy, the management of fibular hemimelia has long been influenced by patient refusal of amputation. More recently, experience with techniques of limb lengthening and deformity correction introduced by Ilizarov have been applied to the spectrum of deformities associated with fibular hemimelia. The application of these techniques has significantly facilitated our management of these difficult cases.

Our functional classification and treatment plan addresses the leg-length discrepancy, angular deformity, and foot deformity, and treats them in single or staged procedures. It will be many years before enough patients treated in this manner will have reached skeletal maturity to make possible a full accounting of our management. Our preliminary results are encouraging in that treatment goals have been met in most cases.

Symes Amputation for Fibular Hemimelia: A Second Look in the Ilizarov Era

John A. Herring, MD

In 1986, Bill Barnhill, Carol Gafney, and I published a study of 21 patients who had undergone Symes amputations, in most cases because of fibular hemimelia.[1] The study showed that these children and adolescents were able to function almost normally. We were aware at the outset that they did well, but we were surprised at the high level of function they achieved. Based on that experience, we recommended Symes amputation as the treatment of choice for children with complete fibular hemimelia. Although that recommendation was valid for its time, we are now in the Ilizarov era and things have changed. Using Ilizarov techniques, the concomitant possibilities of lengthening and angular correction are astonishing. This chapter seeks to place in perspective our previous experience with Symes amputation as it now relates to this exciting new technology.

In our review of patients with Symes amputations, we found that two thirds of the patients of high-school age participated in varsity athletics. We presumed that this was at or even above the norm for children of that age. We also observed that some of these young people were among the best performers on their teams. In Texas, athletics means football, baseball, and basketball. Two boys in the study were outstanding football players. Their quadriceps function, as measured on the Cybex, exceeded that of their peers. One boy with bilateral Symes amputations was an excellent basketball player and also had a black belt in karate. We went along with his request to have his prostheses lengthened so that he could go from 5 feet 10 inches in height as a sophomore to 6 feet 2 inches as a junior, but denied his later request to add another 9 inches. Other athletes in the study included a competition skate-boarder (Fig. 1), a cycling expert, and a number of outstanding skiers. In short, these young people could participate in almost any sport, and, given the proper determination and native abilities, could compete at the highest levels without being limited by their prostheses.

These anecdotes are nice, but the real purpose of our review was to quantitate function. Evaluating physical function was easy. Their times for the fifty-yard dash ranged between the 4th and 67th percentiles of their age groups. Quadriceps power ranged from 50% to 105% of normal with a mean of 76.4%. Hamstring power ranged from 53% to 130% of normal and averaged 81.8%.

Results of psychological testing were more difficult to interpret. Family stress correlated most significantly with physical function. Several patients who had identifiable psychopathology had undergone multiple operations before the Symes amputation. We hypothesized that this experience—many procedures with a poor outcome followed by an amputation—was likely to cause significant adjustment problems.

What do the results of this study signify in the modern era? First, they set some goals that we must try to attain for patients managed with distraction techniques, comparing their achievements with those of the Symes group. I do not think any of us would argue that some reduction in function after lengthening would still be preferable to amputation. Now, however, we must decide how much function is possible and how much functional loss we are willing to accept.

In addition, I think this study provides some useful warnings for surgeons using the Ilizarov techniques. The boy we studied who was able to play basketball after his bilateral Symes is a case in point. His problem before the amputation was not length, but rather the position and function of his feet. Many of the 17 operations undertaken before amputation had been performed to reposition his feet. At amputation, the talus was coalesced to the calcaneus and articulated very poorly with the tibia. While some of the distortion of his tibiotalar joint may have been caused by earlier surgery, we have seen the same changes in the feet of some patients with fibular hemimelia who were undergoing primary amputation at 9 months of age. While I am

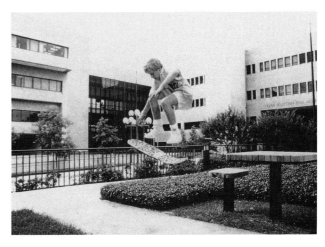

Fig. 1 A boy with a traumatic Symes amputation who is a competitive skateboard athlete.

certain we can restore length and alignment with the Ilizarov methods, I doubt that we can restore ankle function, and I know we cannot produce subtalar joint function.

Another area of concern for those using the new technology involves psychological function. In our study, we observed some psychopathology, which we attributed to repeated hospitalizations, unsightly scars, and stiff, painful feet. Certainly we can now achieve much better results, but the patient still must endure months of the inconvenience of frame wear, a not inconsiderable amount of pain, and some visible scarring. We need to perform significant psychological studies of patients undergoing distraction methods to determine how well they tolerate these interventions.

A third consideration is the question of function following Ilizarov treatment. It is necessary to know if there will be complete restoration of joint range of motion, if the muscles will regain normal function and strength, and if the bone will be strong enough to allow participation in contact sports. We must remember that, as good as the technique is, it has not been shown to have eliminated such problems as disuse atrophy, joint stiffness, and osteopenia of immobilization. As I stated at the outset, to be successful the technique does not have to solve all these problems. Yet, these problems and parameters must be studied and quantitated to allow us to make well-informed decisions.

Knowing what I now know about the Ilizarov technique, I have altered my thinking significantly about early amputation for fibular hemimelia. First, if there is a possibility of eventually being able to reconstruct or salvage a foot, I do not recommend an early amputation. Second, there are still some children for whom I believe early amputation to be the appropriate treatment. I recommend amputation if two or more of the criteria are present: (1) severe shortening in infancy of 35% or more, (2) marked equinovalgus deformity with the heel at the mid-calf level or higher, (3) a deformed talus, fused to the calcaneus and coupled with a very abnormal tibiotalar articular, and (4) a diminutive foot, usually with missing rays.

Before performing an amputation, I always seek the advice of my colleagues who are proficient in the Ilizarov technique, and if they indicate that there is a possibility of successfully keeping the foot, we do so. On the other hand, if the anatomy is so poor that there really is no way to have a functional result, we recommend amputation.

References

1. Herring JA, Barnhill B, Gaffney C: Syme amputation: An evaluation of the physical and psychological function in young patients. *J Bone Joint Surg* 1986;68A:573–578.

CHAPTER 50

Epiphysiodesis for Management of Lower Limb Deformities

Charles E. Johnston II, MD

Matthew J. Bueche, MD

Bryan Williamson, MD

John G. Birch, MD

Epiphysiodesis, which is simple, usually reliable, and has a low surgical morbidity, is a procedure used to achieve angular or limb-length correction of lower extremity deformities. For appropriately selected cases with mild to moderate deformity, epiphysiodesis is the method of choice to correct either angular or limb-length deformity because it is a simple procedure and is well accepted by the patient. This chapter focuses on its use in angular deformity correction. It also deals briefly with its use in the management of limb-length discrepancy, a topic covered in detail elsewhere.[1,2]

Hemiepiphysiodesis

Hemi-arrest of the physis to correct angular deformity in a growing child has been used in one form or another for more than 40 years.[3] Present techniques use percutaneous surgery to produce hemiepiphyseal arrest.[4] The advantages of this approach include correction of angular deformity by subsequent growth of the opposite unarrested physis. Thus, one minor surgical procedure achieves correction and, at the same time, preserves maximum growth potential for the operated bone. Obviously, the timing of the procedure is crucial if over or undercorrection is to be avoided. Errors in this aspect of preoperative evaluation are a major source of failure for this procedure. Two additional causes of failure are inadequate correction of deformity if the opposite unarrested physis is abnormal, as in adolescent Blount disease, and failure by the procedure to achieve arrest of the hemiphysis.

Interest in hemiepiphyseal arrest has been stimulated by the work of Bowen and associates,[5] who reported on use of this procedure primarily for the management of idiopathic genu valgum. By applying trigonometric analysis to a hemiepiphyseal arrest and combining this information with the Green-Anderson chart[6] of growth versus skeletal age, they are able to predict angular deformity correction as a function of remaining

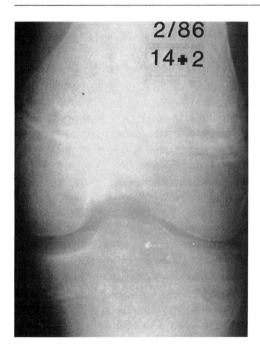
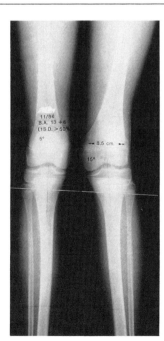
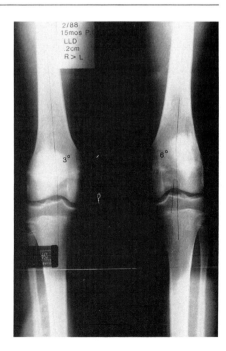

Fig. 1 **Left,** Healed Salter II fracture of the distal femur in a 14-year-old boy. **Center,** Progressive valgus deformity caused by lateral physeal injury. The limb length on the normal side was one standard deviation greater than the 50th percentile at a skeletal age of 13.5 years. **Right,** Correction achieved by hemiarrest of medial distal femur. Correction was achieved by growth of the traumatized but still functioning lateral physis.

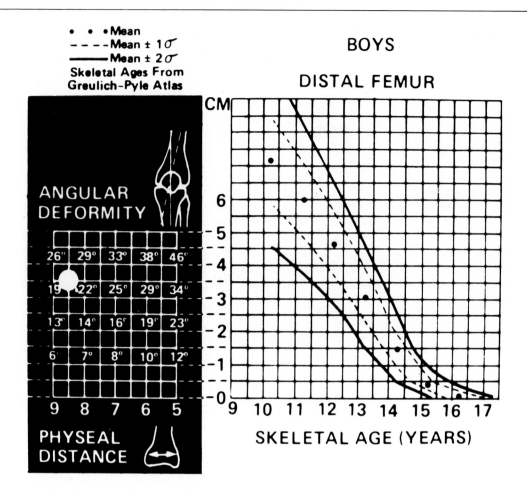

Fig. 2 Predicted correction from the graph of growth versus angular correction was approximately 20 degrees (physeal width = 8.5 cm). (Reproduced with permission from Bowen JR, Leahey JL, Zhang Z-H, et al: Partial epiphysiodesis at the knee to correct angular deformity. *Clin Orthop* 1985;198:184–190.)

growth. The prediction of the amount of correction depends on the bone age and the width of the physis to be arrested. Thus, the technique is limited by the inherent uncertainty in the determination of bone age, which is a subjective evaluation that is based on hand radiographs depicted in the Greulich-Pyle Atlas.[7] Because there is a lack of standardization (i.e., magnification) for radiographs that measure epiphyseal width, this measurement is also subject to inherent error. Nevertheless, Bowen and associates[5] have determined that, in general, a hemiepiphyseal arrest of the distal femur will produce 7 degrees of correction per year of remaining growth, and that 5 degrees per year of remaining growth are available in the proximal tibial physis. These amounts of potential correction are most reliably obtained during the last three years of growth. Additionally, Bowen and associates determined that because undercorrection of angular deformity is the rule rather than the exception, only about 60% of predicted angular correction is usually achieved.[5]

Hemiepiphysiodesis is best used for patients who are nearing skeletal maturity and have an angular deformity caused by documented hemiepiphyseal arrest, as a result of trauma, infection, or developmental causes. Because any of these causes may also subclinically involve the less affected side of the physis, these conditions may not respond reliably to hemiepiphysiodesis (see below). Figures 1 and 2 illustrate the use of hemiepiphysiodesis to correct angular deformity secondary to Salter II fracture of the distal femur.

Because of wide deviations in predicting remaining growth caused by the uncertainties mentioned above, untimed hemiepiphysiodesis is probably more valuable, because with this technique, the deformity is arrested when it is recognized and the correction does not require determinations of bone age or physeal width. The disadvantages of untimed hemiepiphysiodesis are that it requires close observation to avoid overcorrection, and that an age-dependent limb-length discrepancy is a certainty, in some cases requiring possible arrest of growth of the contralateral extremity to avoid a significant discrepancy.

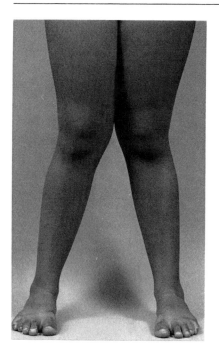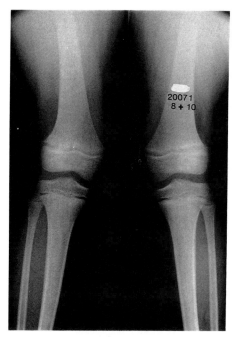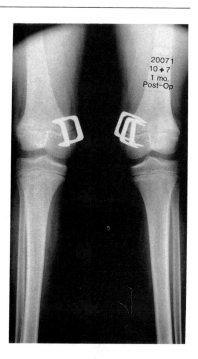

Fig. 3 **Left** and **center,** An eight-year-old female with genu valgum secondary to metaphyseal chondrodysplasia (Schmid type). **Right,** Bilateral medial distal femoral epiphyseal stapling procedures were performed.

Hemiepiphyseal stapling for temporary epiphyseal arrest, introduced by Blount in 1949, has performed admirably in the hands of its inventor.[3,8] Unfortunately, other investigators have reported problems with this technique, including ineffective growth arrest caused by staple extrusion, complete arrest as a result of stapling, and prominence, requiring additional procedures to remove staples.[9-12] Stapling to produce complete physeal arrest is probably contraindicated because of the difficulty in achieving symmetrical simultaneous growth arrest of both medial and lateral physes. Thus, the ability to produce temporary arrest, as reported by Blount, has in fact failed to occur in a significant percentage of cases (Figs. 3 and 4). There is no question that the technique of staple placement is critical to the success of the procedure.[8] The timing of staple removal, and the uncertainty of resumption of growth following staple removal, make this procedure too unpredictable to recommend. Although this technique has been used successfully to treat idiopathic genu valgum,[13] stapling should be considered a method of permanent growth arrest, because the resumption of growth following removal is so uncertain.[10] Staple removal can damage the peripheral physis and perichondrial ring, and it should not be underestimated as a possible cause of subsequent lack of growth.

Technique

Percutaneous epiphysiodesis has enjoyed considerable interest because the minimal surgical exposure produces a very satisfactory cosmetic result. The amount of physis to ablate under fluoroscopic control, and more importantly, how to ensure this ablation, are controversial. Original recommendations by Bowen and associates[5] indicated that a depth of 0.5 cm of the peripheral physis should be removed. Also, in order to achieve the appropriate peripheral bone bridge to produce the hemiepiphysiodesis effect, the physis should be removed anteriorly and posteriorly to include at least 75% of its peripheral extent.

Experimental evaluation of growth-plate ablation by percutaneous technique has shown that it can be difficult to achieve appropriate ablation if the physis is simply curetted (Fig. 5). This is particularly true in the distal femur, where the undulations of the physis make it difficult on fluoroscopy to ascertain how thoroughly the physis has been removed (Fig. 5, *top right*). In order to ensure that enough physis has been ablated, a cavitation technique can be used (Fig. 6, *left*). With this technique, the curette is passed clearly into the metaphyseal and the epiphyseal area, proximal and distal to the physis, creating a large excavation that encompasses the physeal plate (Fig. 6, *center*).

Clinical evaluation of the anatomic damage produced by percutaneous ablation has revealed that, even with cavitation, it is possible to miss the physis almost completely (Figs. 7 and 8, *top left, top right,* and *bottom left*). For this reason, we recommend "mini-incision" epiphysiodesis, which not only provides sufficient exposure for the surgeon to curette the physeal cartilage under direct vision, but also makes it possible to pack me-

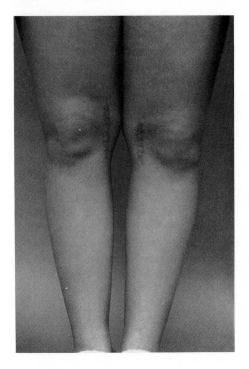
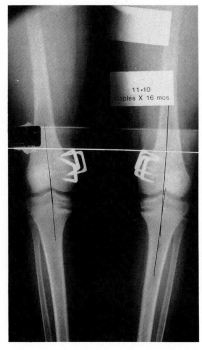
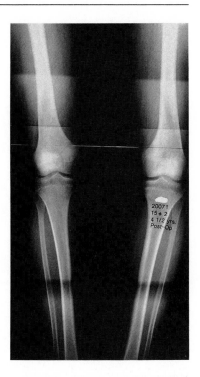

Fig. 4   **Left** and **center,** After 16 months, the deformities were corrected, and staples were removed. **Right,** Progressive varus deformity developed on the left caused by lack of growth resumption following staple removal.

taphyseal bone in the peripheral physeal area to induce peripheral bone bridge formation. With this technique, the physis must be located fluoroscopically before making the skin incision. A 2- to 3-cm incision is then accurately placed, and sharp dissection is carried directly to the physis. The perichondrial layers are excised to allow visualization of the physeal cartilage, including the anterior and posterior extent over a distance of 3 to 4 cm (Fig. 8, *top right*). The perichondrial structures are further elevated by sharp dissection to the extent that the skin incision allows. After blood is removed by suctioning, the physis can be ablated to a depth of 1 cm under direct vision, leaving only the most anterior and posterior peripheral physis intact. Using a small osteotome, bone graft may then be obtained from the metaphysis to produce the peripheral bridge.

In spite of meticulous technique, however, hemiepiphysiodesis may fail to produce angular correction even after successful physeal arrest (Figs. 7 and 8). As mentioned earlier, if the physis on the opposite side of the bone is not normal, correction by its continued growth is uncertain. A recent review of 11 cases of lateral proximal tibial hemiepiphysiodesis for adolescent Blount disease demonstrated complete correction in four, partial correction in two, and no correction in five cases. Four of the five failed cases demonstrated radiographic hemiepiphysiodesis, and no cause for the failure to correct could be identified. The growth potential of the abnormal medial proximal tibial physis

must have been inadequate to produce correction even though the lateral proximal tibial physis had been arrested. There was no correlation between the success of hemiepiphysiodesis and the severity of deformity or the patient's weight. Because of the low morbidity of this procedure compared with the morbidity of a high tibial osteotomy in a massively obese patient, we continue to perform lateral proximal tibial hemiepiphysiodesis in patients with adolescent Blount disease, because a 50% success rate for a procedure of no morbidity compared to the alternative procedure seems worth the risk.

Hemiepiphysiodesis to correct deformity is a simple, safe procedure that has established efficacy for the correction of angular deformity, whether the procedure is untimed or is timed to coincide with an appropriate bone age and physeal width to achieve correction at the end of skeletal growth. Untimed hemiepiphysiodesis has the advantage of correcting the deformity when it is recognized, rather than allowing additional deformity to occur while waiting for the patient's bone age to become more advanced. However, it requires close observation so that the opposite ipsilateral physis can be arrested if more growth remains once correction has been achieved. Obviously, in a young patient, this may cause unacceptable shortening of the affected limb requiring epiphysiodesis of the contralateral extremity to avoid unacceptable limb-length discrepancy. At present, the mini-incision technique is believed to be the

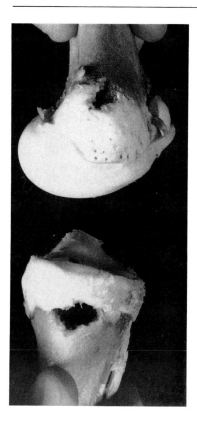
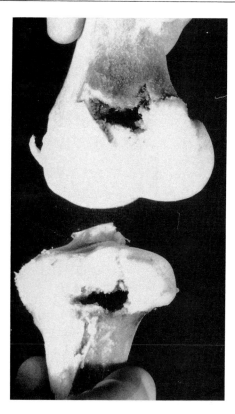
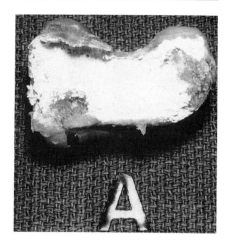
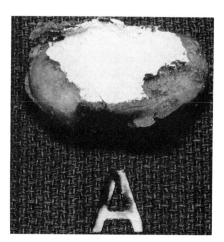

Fig. 5 **Left** and **Center,** Cadaveric knees from a 10-year-old child. The growth plates have been ablated by simple curettage on one side, and by curettage with cavitation on the other. All procedures were carried out under fluoroscopic control through the fenestrations seen here. **Top right,** Resulting amount of physeal cartilage removed by simple curettage, distal femur. ("A" = anterior) **Bottom right,** Physeal cartilage ablation by simple curettage, proximal tibia.

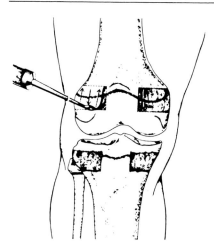
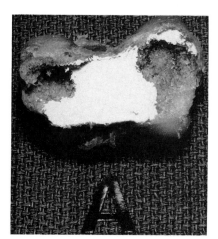
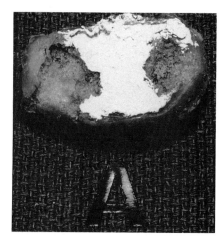

Fig. 6 **Left**, The technique of curettage with cavitation. **Center**, Physeal cartilage ablation by cavitation technique, distal femur. Compare this figure with Figure 5, *top right*. **Right**, Physeal cartilage ablation by cavitation method, proximal tibia. Compare this figure with Figure 5, *bottom right*.

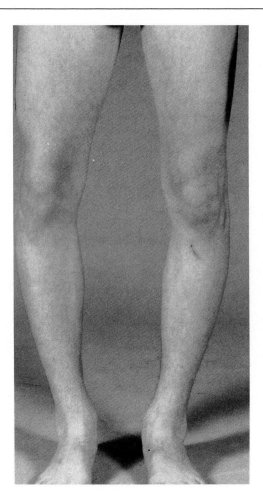 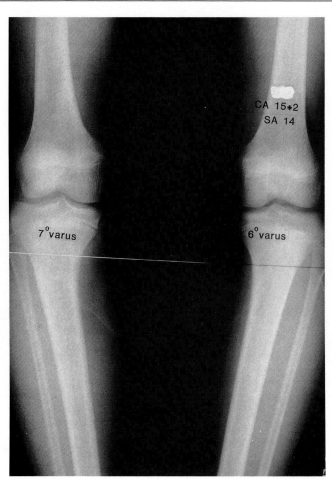

Fig. 7   **Left** and **right**, Bilateral idiopathic tibia vara in a 16-year-old male.

most reliable way to expose and achieve peripheral physeal arrest, although the depth of physeal ablation (0.5 or 1.0 cm) remains controversial. Finally, the surgeon must recognize that abnormality of the physis on the opposite side of the bone may preclude correction of an angular defect in spite of adequate peripheral hemiepiphyseal arrest.

Epiphysiodesis for Limb-Length Discrepancy

This procedure is a standard orthopaedic technique used to manage limb-length discrepancies.[2] It has been well described in the literature since the initial work of Phemister.[14] Presently, the indication for epiphysiodesis to control limb-length discrepancy is a predicted discrepancy at skeletal maturity of between 2 and 5 cm. A difference of less than 2 cm probably requires no treatment. Differences greater than 5 cm, in most cases, would be corrected by lengthening, to avoid excessive shortening.

Timing of the epiphysiodesis is obviously critical, pri-

marily to avoid overcorrection. It is generally recommended that the procedure be performed at a time when slight undercorrection is expected.[2]

The timing depends on the determination of bone age, and either the Moseley or Green-Anderson techniques are used to predict the amount of growth remaining and the probable ultimate discrepancy. The details of these techniques have been reviewed elsewhere and will not be repeated here.[2,10] An important aspect of the Green-Anderson technique to predict how much growth remains in the normal epiphysis is the determination of the standard deviation of the patient's bone length from the mean. This obviously adds an additional source of uncertainty in determining the appropriate timing of the epiphysiodesis. Because overcorrection can be as much as 100% in a patient whose bone length is two standard deviations greater than the mean, the importance of this determination in patients for whom no previous limb-length discrepancy data are available cannot be overemphasized. Finally, the limitations of the Green-Anderson growth data must be recognized. Because the data were based on figures

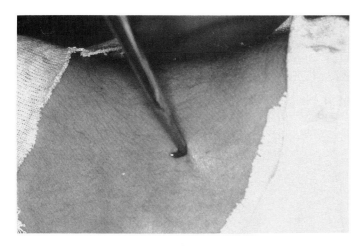
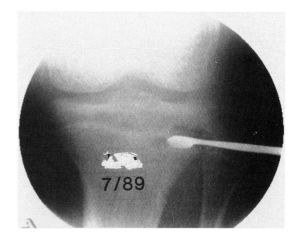

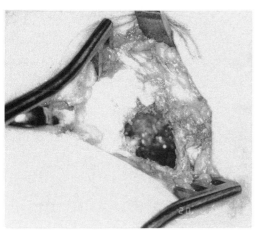
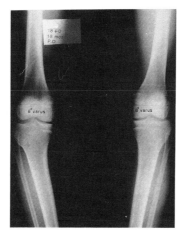
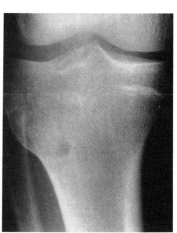

Fig. 8   Top left, The technique of percutaneous lateral proximal tibial epiphysiodesis. The patella is to the right. **Top right**, Fluoroscopic appearance of curettage with cavitation. **Bottom left**, Open exposure of percutaneous procedure. The cavity produced by the curette has missed the physeal plate on the proximal side. Physeal ablation was carried out under direct vision. **Bottom center** and **right**, In spite of open physeal ablation, no correction in the deformity occurred. Radiograph reveals definite evidence of lateral physeal arrest.

using white children in the New England area before 1950, their applicability to children of differing race and body habitus in the 1990s must be cautiously interpreted. No updating of the Green-Anderson data is presently available, and one must keep in mind the increased absolute amounts of growth generally seen in present-day immature patients. The use of the straight-line graph of Moseley eliminates this uncertainty to some extent, because, with appropriate data, the expected discrepancy between the two limbs can be determined arithmetically. Obviously, in patients who are first seen at the end of growth, the straight-line or arithmetical method cannot be used, and the surgeon must use the Green-Anderson data to make the best approximation possible.

The technique of epiphysiodesis for limb-length discrepancy is essentially the same as the technique for hemiepiphysiodesis, except that here the surgeon does not have to limit the ablation to a depth of 0.5 to 1.0 cm. Because the purpose of the procedure is to arrest growth, the surgeon need not spare the ablation. Consequently, the physeal curettage should be carried to a depth of nearly halfway across the physis (radiographic control is useful). If the central ablation is accomplished without excessive damage to the peripheral physis and perichondrial ring, it will not destabilize the epiphyseal-metaphyseal connection sufficiently to warrant formal immobilization after the surgery.

References

1. Green WT, Anderson M: Experiences with epiphyseal arrest in correcting discrepancies in length of the lower extremities in infantile paralysis: A method of predicting the effect. *J Bone Joint Surg* 1947;29A:659–675.
2. Moseley CF: Leg length discrepancy, in Morrissy RT (ed): *Pediatric Orthopaedics*. Philadelphia, JB Lippincott, 1990, pp 767–813.
3. Blount WP, Clarke GR: Control of bone growth by epiphyseal stapling: A preliminary report. *J Bone Joint Surg* 1949;31A:464–478.

4. Canale ST, Russell TA, Holcomb RL: Percutaneous epiphysiodesis: Experimental study and preliminary clinical results. *Pediatr Orthop* 1986;6:150–156.

5. Bowen JR, Leahey JL, Zhang Z-H et al: Partial epiphyseodesis at the knee to correct angular deformity. *Clin Orthop* 1985;198:184–190.

6. Anderson M, Green WT, Messner MB: Growth and predictions of growth in the lower extremities. *J Bone Joint Surg* 1963;45A:1–14.

7. Greulich WW, Pyle SL: *Radiographic Atlas of Skeletal Development of the Hand and Wrist*, ed 2. Stanford, Stanford University Press, 1959.

8. Blount WP: A mature look at epiphyseal stapling. *Clin Orthop* 1971;77:158–163.

9. Brockway A, Craig WA, Cockrell BR Jr: End-study result of sixty-two stapling operations. *J Bone Joint Surg* 1954;36A:1063–1069.

10. Green WT, Anderson M: Skeletal age and the control of bone growth, in American Academy of Orthopaedic Surgeons *Instructional Course Lectures, XVII*. St. Louis, CV Mosby, 1960, pp 199–217.

11. Pilcher MF: Epiphyseal stapling: 35 cases followed to maturity. *J Bone Joint Surg* 1962;44B:82–85.

12. Poirer H: Epiphysial stapling and leg equalisation. *J Bone Joint Surg* 1968;50B:61–69.

13. Howorth B: Knock knees: With special reference to the stapling operation. *Clin Orthop* 1971;77:233–246.

14. Phemister DB: Operative arrestment of longitudinal growth of bones in the treatment of deformities. *J Bone Joint Surg* 1933;15A:1–15.

CHAPTER 51

Surgical Technique of Physeal Bar Resection

John G. Birch, MD

Introduction

Partial physeal arrests or bony bars connecting epiphyseal and metaphyseal bone in the presence of substantial remaining skeletal growth can cause progressive or recurrent angular deformity, progressive joint distortion, and significant limb-length inequality. Surgical options include repeated osteotomies, completion of the epiphysiodesis with lengthening of the involved segment or epiphysiodesis of the opposite extremity, and, more recently, physeal distraction with an external fixator.[1] The concept of surgical resection of these partial physeal growth arrests to minimize or correct their untoward effects was introduced by Langenskiöld.[2] Careful patient selection, preoperative planning, and attention to detail during the surgery are essential to successful bar resection when this mode of treatment is selected.

Classification

Partial arrests are classified anatomically by their relationship to the perimeter of the remaining physis. The two types of partial arrests are peripheral arrests and central arrests.

Peripheral arrests (Fig. 1, *left*) are eccentrically located and involve a portion of the perimeter of the physis. With these lesions, the perichondrium is replaced by a layer of periosteum over the bar itself.

Central arrests are of two types. Type A arrests (Fig. 1, *center*) have a perimeter of healthy physis. These arrests tend to cause "tenting" of the epiphysis with corresponding joint deformity. The principle of surgical resection is to remove the bar without injuring the pe-

rimeter of healthy physis. In type B central arrests (Fig. 1, *right*), the lesions run through the middle of the physis and have healthy physis on either side. This pattern occurs most commonly as a consequence of Salter type III or IV fractures of the medial malleolus.

Partial arrests may also be classified according to etiology (Table 1). Post-traumatic arrests are most common. In my experience, arrests associated with infantile Blount's disease were next most common. Arrests may also occur as sequelae to sepsis or radiation. Occasionally, there is no obvious cause.

Preoperative Evaluation

Considerations

The five major factors to be considered during preoperative evaluation are: (1) the amount of growth remaining; (2) the etiology of the lesion; (3) the location of the lesion; (4) the extent of physeal surface replaced by bar; and (5) the approach, either by cortical window or osteotomy.

Growth Remaining Because bar resection is neither easy nor predictably successful, the surgeon must consider whether or not there is sufficient growth remaining to justify the procedure. In general, I consider bar resection only when more than two years of skeletal growth remain.

Etiology In general, post-traumatic lesions and those associated with infantile Blount's disease have a higher likelihood of successful restoration of growth than lesions associated with more diffuse injury to the physis as a whole, such as after radiation or sepsis.

Physeal Location Central lesions are usually approached from the metaphysis, either by means of an osteotomy or a metaphyseal window. Peripheral lesions are generally approached directly. Knowing exactly where the lesion is within the bone, based on preoperative studies, helps in planning the surgical approach.

Extent The surgeon must determine how much of the surface area of the physis is replaced by bar. In general, lesions that involve more than 25% of the total surface area of the physis are less likely to be successfully removed.[3-5]

Approach The bone involved and the requirement for angular correction will influence whether an osteotomy

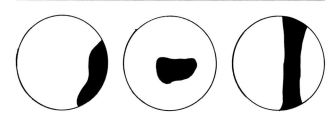

Fig. 1 Anatomic classification of physeal bars. **Left,** Peripheral type lesions. **Center,** Central type A lesion completely within, and surrounded by healthy physis. **Right,** Central type B "through-and-through" lesions with normal physis on either side.

Table 1
Partial physeal arrests by etiology*

Etiology	Number	Resumption of Growth
Trauma	21	5 (3 indeterminate)
Blount's disease	8	6
Radiation	2	0
Enchondromatosis	2	0
Infection	1	1
Unicameral cyst	1	0
S/P Brachial plexus injury	1	— (1 indeterminate)

*12, successful; 20, failed; 4, indeterminate

is part of the procedure. For example, central and posterior peripheral lesions of the distal femur can be exposed via a metaphyseal osteotomy just above the physis (I prefer to approach the metaphysis medially). On the other hand, patients with central lesions, particularly those of the distal tibia or distal radius, will recover from surgery more quickly and easily if the lesion can be removed through a window without osteotomy.

Imaging

The lesion must be well localized by imaging preoperatively to adequately plan the approach, and to aid with orientation during the procedure. Four modalities are used most commonly.

Multiple view plain films Although plain films are usually not sufficient to truly reveal the location or extent of physeal bar, they can sometimes suffice on occasions when the need for surgery, the location, and the etiology of the lesion are well known (such as in infantile Blount's disease), and some circumstance precludes more sophisticated radiologic study.

Hypocycloidal (poly)tomography This technique provides clearer images than can be obtained with routine linear tomography. Anteroposterior and lateral tomograms should be obtained, preferably with narrow (3-mm) cuts. It is important to instruct the radiologist to make these projections perpendicular to the plane of the physis, taking into account any deformity created by the bar. The mapping technique described by Carlson and Wenger[6] can then be used to indicate more graphically the location and extent of the bar.

Computed tomographic scan This modality can provide very nice localization of a bar. Cuts perpendicular to the lesion can be hard to obtain, however, and cuts that enter, leave, and then re-enter the physis can be confusing.

Magnetic resonance imaging Although this modality has tantalizing imaging potential, it, too, may fail to demonstrate the bar as precisely as one would like. T_2-weighted images offer the most visible distinction between physis and the medullary bone of the metaphysis and epiphysis. However, because the bar itself usually has a signal quality similar to that of cortical bone, distinguishing among bar, cortical bone, and physis can be difficult. The physis has a higher signal intensity (and thus appears white) with short T_1 inversion recovery sequences, but the overall image is much less distinct for bone with this technique.

In summary, despite this method's somewhat archaic nature, I currently prefer to use good quality 3-mm anteroposterior and lateral polytomograms to orient myself to the size and location of the physeal bar.

Surgical Technique

For both peripheral and central arrests, the surgical goals are to remove the bone bridging the physis while preserving the remaining healthy physis, to fill the cavity thereby created with some interpositional material that will inhibit reformation of the bridge, and to correct pre-existing bony deformity with osteotomy as necessary.[3–5,7,8] Central lesions are approached from the metaphysis, either through a window created in the cortex or by means of osteotomy. The option selected depends on the surgeon's preference, on which bone is involved, and on whether it is necessary to correct a pre-existing deformity. Peripheral lesions are approached directly, with resection of the overlying periosteum. Osteotomy is usually done for peripheral lesions only when it is necessary to correct a bone deformity.

With either type of lesion, the key is to create an initial cavity within the bar that spans the physis (Fig. 2). The bar itself is located by seeking out the hard, sclerotic bone that is typical of most bars. Once a cavity has been created that spans the healthy physis, the procedure is completed by methodically expanding that cavity at the level of the physis until all the bar is removed and healthy physis lines the cavity throughout its margin. To be able to do this without undue frustration, I find several tools very helpful. Good radiographic and/or fluoroscopic equipment should be readily available in the operating room. Until the initial cavity within the bar spanning the physis has been created, it is very easy for the surgeon to become disoriented. A periodic check with fluoroscopy of the location relative to the physis is most helpful.

Magnification and a brilliant light source will also help make the physis easy to see, especially when abnormal tissue is present. This is often the case in infantile Blount's disease or postseptic arrests, where abnormal cartilage or fibrous tissue may resemble physis to the naked eye.

A small dental or similar mirror can also prove helpful. Particularly, but not exclusively, when a metaphyseal window approach is used for a central type of lesion, it is usually impossible to see the entire perimeter of physis within the cavity unless a small mirror is available that can be inserted into the cavity to allow the surgeon to view it circumferentially. Alternatively, an angled arthroscope can be inserted into the cavity to allow a direct viewing of the physes (Michael Busch, personal communication).

It is a very good idea to insert small metallic markers into the epiphyseal and metaphyseal bone on either side of the remaining physis at the end of the procedure. These markers serve as reference points in recording the extent of growth (Fig. 3). Furthermore, if growth ceases again after an initial resumption, or if angular deformity recurs, these markers will allow the detection of this event radiographically before it is obvious clinically (Fig. 4).

Interpositional Material

Interpositional material is inserted to serve as a spacer to prevent reformation of bony bridges across the physis. Fat (local or harvested from the buttock), cranioplast, and silicone rubber have all been used with success both experimentally and clinically.[3,9-13] The choice of which one to use is a matter of personal preference. Silicone rubber is still considered investigational by the Food and Drug Administration and has not been approved for general use. If you choose to use an inert material (silicone rubber or cranioplast) the principle is to fill the epiphyseal portion of the cavity you have created, and cover the physis, leaving

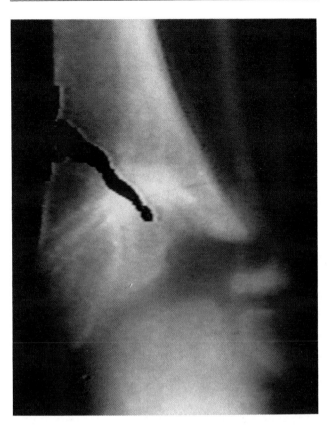

Fig. 2   Technique of bar resection under fluoroscopic control. A cavity is made spanning the physis within the bar. The cavity is expanded peripherally at the level of the physis until all the bar has been removed.

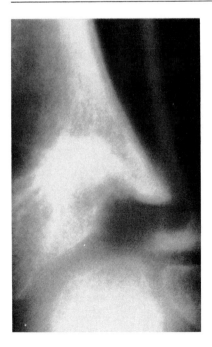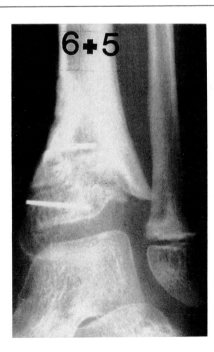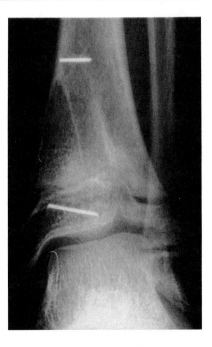

Fig. 3   Central type arrest with restoration of growth. **Left,** Polytomograms of a posttraumatic lesion in the distal tibia. Note typical sclerotic nature of bar and tenting of articular surface **Center,** Immediately after resection via metaphyseal window with fat interposition. Note metaphyseal and epiphyseal metallic markers. **Right,** Three years later, resumption of growth apparent as markers spread apart.

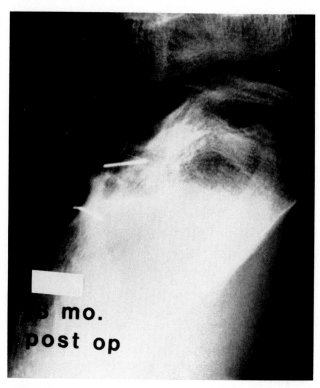

Fig. 4 Anteroposterior radiograph one year after surgery for infantile Blount's disease. Deformity recurring and markers show no change in position, indicating failed resection.

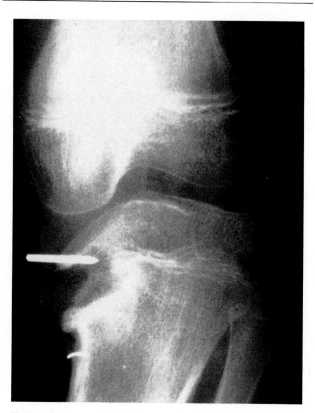

Fig. 5 Anteroposterior radiograph after bar resection for Blount's disease and interposition with cranioplast. Steinmann pins "anchor" inert material to maintain contact with physis.

the material free from the metaphysis. These materials should be pinned to the epiphyseal cavity with a Kirschner-wire or Steinmann pin. This is done so that, with growth, the inert interpositional material will move along with the epiphysis (Fig. 5), and presumably, continue to protect the physis from reformation of the bridge. Because fat tends to stick to the physis, pinning it to the epiphysis is not necessary. Furthermore, Langenskiöld has suggested clinically and experimentally that the fat may actually persist and hypertrophy within the cavity during subsequent growth.[14,15] It is important not to allow the fat to be carried into a metaphyseal cavity. I prefer to fill the surgical cavity completely, covering the fat with soft tissue in the case of peripheral lesions, and sealing it in by replacing the metaphyseal window for central lesions. Alternatively, hemostasis can be achieved with bone wax or other material before the fat graft is inserted.

Results

We reviewed the results of 34 patients with 36 physeal arrests treated by physeal bar resection at Texas Scottish Rite Hospital from 1981 through 1990. The age at the time of surgery averaged 8 years and 9 months (range, 2 years, 4 months, to 15 years).

Follow-up averaged 3 years, 6 months (range, 4 months to 9 years, 1 month). In this review, follow-up for a minimum of 12 months was required before designating a bar resection outcome successful. If follow-up was less than 12 months, the results were classified as indeterminate, unless recurrent bar formation or progressive deformity had occurred, in which case it was classified as failure.

The etiology, frequency, and success of attempted bar resection are compiled in Table 1. In this series, trauma was the most frequent cause of partial arrests, and infantile Blount's disease was the second most frequent. Of 36 physeal bar resections, 12 were successful in restoring growth, 20 failed, and four were indeterminate. Of the 12 successful resections, five have subsequently gone on to physeal closure prior to skeletal maturity.

The location of bar and the number of successful resections is indicated in Table 2. The most common location of physeal bar undergoing resection in this series was the distal femur, with 12 patients. The next most frequent location was the proximal tibia, with ten, which included eight patients who had infantile Blount's disease.

The most common lesion type by location was peripheral, with 23, again including eight patients with

Table 2
Partial physeal arrests by location

Location of Bar	Number	Resumption of Growth
Distal femur	12	3
Proximal tibia	10	6
Distal tibia	9	3
Proximal humerus	2	0
Distal radius	1	0
Distal ulna	1	0
Proximal phalanx	1	0

Table 3
Effect of interpositional material on growth resumption

Interpositional Material	Number	Resumption of Growth
Fat	15	4
Cranioplast	15	8
Silicone rubber	6	0

Blount's disease. Thirteen of the lesions were central. Resumption of growth occurred in eight peripheral lesions, but when the Blount's cases are excluded, the figure is only two of 14. Growth was restored in four central lesions.

Osteotomy either for pre-existing deformity correction, for exposure, or for both was performed in conjunction with resection of 23 lesions. In 13 others, it was not. With the Blount's cases excepted, performance of osteotomy did not influence the likelihood of restoration of growth.

Fat, cranioplast, and silicone rubber were all used in this series as interpositional material. Resumption of growth for the various interpositional material types is shown in Table 3.

Further surgery was performed on 20 of the 34 patients, including six of the 12 patients who had successful physeal bar resections. The majority of these operations involved completion of epiphysiodesis of the involved extremity and contralateral epiphysiodesis. Three patients with Blount's disease underwent final corrective osteotomy.

There were eight patients in this series with peripheral bars of the medial proximal tibia secondary to Langenskiöld stage VI infantile Blount's disease. All of these patients had recurrent varus and internal rotational deformity after at least one previous high tibial osteotomy. The average age at surgery was 8 years, 3 months (range, 6 years, 8 months, to 10 years, 1 month). Growth was restored in six of the eight patients. Growth in these six averaged 13.5 mm (range, 6 to 25 mm) from the proximal tibia. Three of these six patients subsequently ceased growth before reaching skeletal maturity and required a final corrective osteotomy. One had mild recurrent deformity, but did not require corrective osteotomy. Two patients con-

tinue to grow. Follow-up averaged four years (range, one to eight years). Other than one patient with a superficial wound infection that required only local care, there were no complications in this group.

Complications

Complications, which occurred in six of the 34 patients, included three deep wound infections (two with delayed unions), one superficial wound infection, one transient peroneal nerve palsy, and one delayed union. Two of the deep wound infections, one of the delayed unions, and the one nerve palsy occurred after resections of distal femoral lesions. Failure to resume growth or subsequent early closure of the physis was not considered a complication of treatment.

Conclusions

Resection of partial physeal arrest is neither a very easy nor a universally successful procedure. Although some spectacularly good results do occur, in this series, of patients overall followed for longer than one year, only 33% successfully resumed growth. Even then, the growth resumption can abruptly stop, effectively resulting in insignificant improvement. Resection must not be thought of as something to do while doing the osteotomy. Careful preoperative planning and attention to detail during the procedure will help to maximize the opportunity for the resumption of growth. Epiphyseal and metaphyseal markers should be used to help chart growth. The patients should be followed carefully throughout the remainder of growth to deal with early subsequent cessation of growth as necessary and appropriate for the patient.

References

1. de Pablos J: Bone lengthening methods in the treatment of angular deformities of the long bones, in de Pablos J, Canadell J (eds): *Bone Lengthening Current Trends and Controversies*. Pamplona, Spain, Servicio de Publicaciones de la Universidad de Navarra, 1990, pp 331–354.
2. Langenskiöld A: The possibilities of eliminating premature partial closure of an epiphyseal plate caused by trauma or disease. *Acta Orthop Scand* 1967;38:267–279.
3. Langenskiöld A: Surgical treatment of partial closure of the growth plate. *J Pediatr Orthop* 1981;1:3–11.
4. Ogden JA: The evaluation and treatment of partial physeal arrest. *J Bone Joint Surg* 1987;69A:1297–1302.
5. Peterson HA: Partial growth plate arrest and its treatment. *J Pediatr Orthop* 1984;4:246–258.
6. Carlson WO, Wenger DR: A mapping method to prepare for surgical excision of partial physeal arrest. *J Pediatr Orthop* 1984; 4:232–236.
7. Birch JG, Herring JA, Wenger DR: Surgical anatomy of selected physes. *J Pediatr Orthop* 1984;4:224–231.
8. Birch JG, Carduff S: Surgical management of partial physeal

bars. Presented at the 56th Annual Meeting of the American Academy of Orthopaedic Surgeons, Las Vegas, NV, Feb 9–14, 1989.

9. Bright RW: Operative correction of partial epiphyseal plate closure by osseous-bridge resection and silicone-rubber implant: An experimental study in dogs. *J Bone Joint Surg* 1974;56A:655–664.

10. Langenskiöld A, Videman T, Nevalainen T: The fate of fat transplants in operations for partial closure of the growth plate: Clinical examples and an experimental study. *J Bone Joint Surg* 1986;68B:234–238.

11. Lennox DW, Goldner RD, Sussman MD: Cartilage as an inter-position material to prevent transphyseal bone bridge formation: An experimental model. *J Pediatr Orthop* 1983;3:207–210.

12. Osterman K: Operative elimination of partial epiphyseal closure: An experimental study. *Acta Orthop Scand Suppl* 1972;147:7–79.

13. Williamson RV, Staheli LT: Partial physeal growth arrest: Treatment by bridge resection and fat interposition. *J Pediatr Orthop* 1990;10:769–776.

14. Langenskiöld A: Growth plate regeneration, in Uhthoff HD, Wiley JJ (eds): *Behavior of the Growth Plate*. New York, Raven Press, 1988, pp 47–50.

15. Langenskiöld A: Osseous bridging of the growth plate, in Uhthoff HD, Wiley JJ (eds): *Behavior of the Growth Plate*. New York, Raven Press, 1988, pp 259–261.

Orthopaedics in Developing Countries

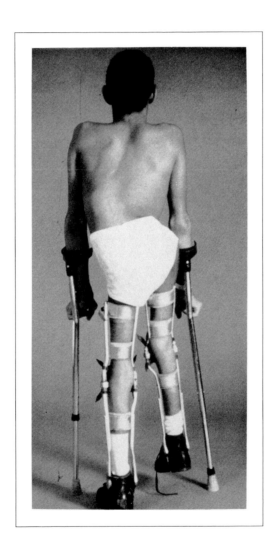

Third World Orthopaedics

Mercer Rang, MB, FRCS

Introduction

The third world presents the orthopaedic surgeon with three problems and three opportunities. The three problems are unfamiliar diseases, suffering people, and minimal resources. The three opportunities are helping those in greatest need, self-education, and the chance to be a pioneer.[1,2]

The Orthopaedic Desert

While thousands of orthopaedic surgeons pursue excellence—a better arthroscope or prosthesis—amid the lavish displays at the Annual Meeting's Exhibit Hall, two thirds of the world goes without orthopaedic care, because they live in an orthopaedic desert. There, the injured and crippled do not have access to an orthopaedic surgeon. Doctors are scarce, and few are available to train in orthopaedics. If the United States had the same ratio of orthopaedic surgeons to patients as exists in Malawi, there would only be 30 orthopaedists for the entire country. For most of the people of the world, an open fracture means an amputation, polio is still common, and osteomyelitis is a fatal or a lifetime disease.

In most of the world, there is a huge deficit of orthopaedic surgeons. The shortfall is 20,000 in Africa alone, and patients go untreated. It has been estimated that for every ten necessary operations, only one gets done.

The problem, of course, is poverty. Expenditure on health care in Canada is $1,600 per person per year. In Malawi, Africa, the figure is $2.00. The cost of one orthopaedic malpractice case in Canada would pay for orthopaedic care for the entire eight million people of Malawi. Because there is so little money for health care, even the most public-spirited doctor cannot survive without outside funding.

The gulf between the rich and the poor nations is widening, not just financially, but also in terms of technology. Thirty years ago the needs of an orthopaedic surgeon were the same in London and Jamaica—an X-ray machine, some hardware, and little more. But now the gulf has widened immensely because the third world has stood still.

Variation exists in the third world countries. Some, like Central Africa, are very poor. Others, like Jamaica, are intermediate. Even some parts of Canada and the U.S. have limited funds.

Traditionally, medical services in the third world, such as they were, were provided by colonial governments, companies, and missions. Now that these countries are independent, medical services are locally supplied, with help from overseas aid programs, service club projects, and volunteers.

The Orthopaedic Imperative

The basis of medicine is helping a fellow person. Here, in Canada and the United States, it is easy to devote too much time to paperwork and to demanding patients who have no need of our services. When there is so much real orthopaedics to be done in the third world, we should be there. Orthopaedic skill should not be wasted.

There is a fundamental contradiction in an ethical system that demands that we treat the terminally ill and the severely handicapped in North America and, at the same time, allows us to ignore a person who may die of an open fracture in the third world.

If orthopaedic planning is to be left to the politicians, these disparities can be regarded as imposed. But if we regard planning as a part of our professional duty we should be pro-active.

Lastly, necessity has been the mother of invention. Some orthopaedic advances, anterior spinal surgery is an example, have come from the third world.

The Orthopaedic Orphan

The difficulties of providing orthopaedic care are great. Why don't these countries do more themselves? They are paying off loans to the rich nations. In a country with surplus people, health care has a low priority. The first priority is security, and a great deal of money is spent on armed forces.

Prevention and primary health care are basic needs[1] and the World Health Organization rightly promotes and funds these activities. Orthopaedics becomes an orphan.

Training programs in orthopaedics are few. There are not enough teachers and not enough candidates. A period of peace is needed, and trained staff must be able to earn a living wage and get paid better for greater skill.

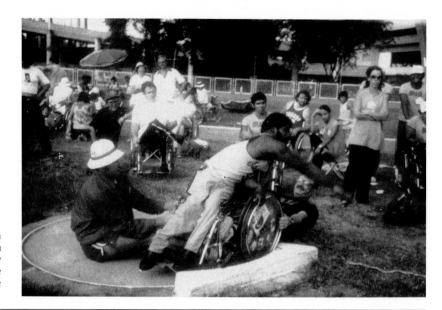

Fig. 1 Sports for the handicapped. Sports can raise the morale of "patients" by turning them into "athletes". The public are shown what they can do and service clubs sponsoring health care have a powerful positive image to encourage fund raising.

Orthopaedic Aid

World Orthopedic Concern is a volunteer world-wide organization founded in 1973 at a meeting organized by Ronald Huckstep and Allan M. McElvie to improve the situation. Orthopedics Overseas, Inc. was started in 1981. The two organizations are affiliated.

Several principles have become clear: (1) The needs are too great to provide purely service assistance. (2) The main thrust must be to teach and set up services that will become self sufficient. (3) Provide help only when invited. (4) Train people in their own country, with their own patients, and with their own resources.

Bringing doctors from the third world to the rich countries often ends up with them not returning home. They learn a lot about osteoarthritis in the elderly—neither the elderly nor osteoarthritis are common in the third world—and about hip replacement, which is unaffordable there. They learn nothing about polio, untreated club feet in a two-year-old child, and neglected trauma. For this reason, sending volunteer teachers overseas to assist in established programs is probably the most useful thing that we can do.[2]

Volunteers arriving on the scene sometimes feel that the situation is asking for a display of behavior that includes ordering people about, banging on the desks of officials, appealing to a sense of shame, and throwing up one's hands. This behavior is no more productive in the third world than it is at home.

Supplies, books, and journals are useful, but complicated devices cannot be serviced and soon break down. Transportation is expensive, and, often, things fail to arrive. Hence, simple, locally produced devices are best. Twinning of hospitals has proven difficult to sustain because the arrangement is too one-sided.

Matching Resources to Needs

Third world orthopaedics is as much a specialty within orthopaedics as hand surgery is. The repertoire of diseases is unfamiliar, most patients are seen only when their disease has progressed to a late stage, and limited facilities require special skill. The technology-dependent, sports-medicine and joint-replacement oriented orthopaedic surgeon will feel at a loss faced with a clinic of 100 patients with advanced examples of unfamiliar diseases, next to no facilities, and only one nurse for the 100 in-patients in 50 beds.

The small budget limits care, and, because of this, the emphasis must be on providing functional care for the whole community, rather than providing Western-standard care for a very few (Fig. 1).

In the very poor countries, orthopaedic paramedics are trained to run a service and perform surgery. They have more interest in orthopaedics than do either the general practitioners or the general surgeons, who are kept busy dealing with life-threatening conditions. The surgical repertoire is limited and repetitive, consisting primarily of closed reduction of fractures, debriding open fractures, draining abscesses, and releases of deformities. Complicated cases are sent to the central hospital.

The advantages of this sort of functional care are shown in the program used in Malawi—a country with a population of eight million that for years had no orthopaedic surgeons. Two courses lasting 18 months each were started five years ago and have put orthopaedic clinical officers in every hospital in the country, a total of about 26 hospitals. Country-wide orthopaedic services could not have been provided in any other way. This solution is quick, inexpensive, and self sustaining.

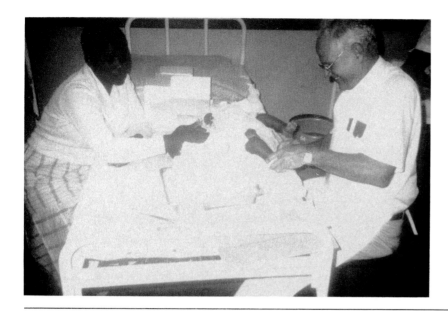

Fig. 2 Volunteers can be helpful with clinics and teaching.

Obviously, the standard of care is not great but, given the facilities that are available, a trained orthopaedic surgeon would find it difficult to do much better.

The surgical repertoire is generally restricted to quick, effective procedures. Poor equipment and a lack of gowns, drapes, and gloves make surgery difficult and, generally, contraindicated. Up to one in five patients are HIV positive. Blood transfusion is difficult. Anesthetic deaths are not rare. Infection rates are high. Most fractures are treated closed. Complex surgery is impossible. The lack of an image intensifier or even a portable X-ray machine makes many procedures, for example, nailing a hip, impossible.

Much organizing is needed. Some kind of regional plan is needed, which means having the support of the neighbourhood doctors and requires setting up outreach clinics and training programs, and arranging for the manufacture of supplies. Recovering patients need rehabilitation and jobs. Service clubs are an important source of help and are able to bridge with the community and set up rehabilitation projects (Fig. 2). The cooperation and help of government is essential.

The doctor needs a lot of ingenuity. The third world doctor has to be an organizer and a scrounger and must have a network of friends to provide help.

References

1. Cobey JC: A guide for short term volunteer medical workers in developing countries. Zimmer and Orthopedics Overseas, Washinton, D.C. 1985.
2. Sandler RH, Jones TC (eds): *Medical Care of Refugees.* New York, Oxford University Press, 1987.

Cultural Differences: North and South

Sir John Golding, OJ, OBE, FRCS, LLD (Hon)

The nations of our planet are rather arbitrarily, if conveniently, considered to belong either to the "North" or "South."

The disparity between these groups, as far as health services are concerned, is immense. The United States, for instance, spends about $2,000 per capita per annum on health, while Mozambique can afford only $7.50. Jamaica, at $60, comes somewhere in between.

We all realize that there is little that we can do personally about such matters. However, it is important to realize that a discrepancy of this order of magnitude, by leading to the destabilization of our world, will be detrimental to our future and must be of concern to us all. I believe that those of us who feel that this is a dangerous situation must try to do what we can to show our concern by making some attempt to redress the balance.

Our own individual contributions may seem small, however, the images that our countries gain abroad are largely derived from the sum total of such small, yet inspiring, personal actions of ordinary people.

I will concentrate on the effects that different cultures have on medical practice and then illustrate this by showing how we have worked to solve some of the orthopaedic problems found in a very poor country.

We can liken culture to the wind, which we cannot see although we readily appreciate the effect it has on the branches of a tree bending before it. Our culture, too, although we are seldom even aware of it, fills and largely determines our lives without intruding into our conscious thoughts. Only when something we do runs counter to prevailing cultural beliefs do we become conscious of unexpected opposition; opposition that seems irrational to us only because we do not understand its origins. Our reaction often implies to our hosts that our behaviour may stem from a lack of respect.

A lack of perspective can make it easy to jump to erroneous conclusions. One thing is certain regarding conclusions that tend to set one group of peoples apart from others. The more experience you gain, the more remarkable you will find it to be that peoples are so alike.

A first world upbringing makes us believe that all of us should be held largely responsible for our futures. We are trained to think of ourselves as "captains of our own ship." If it were not for such beliefs, we would not be here today. What positive steps you finally decide to make will depend largely on whether you come to believe that the time, effort, and money expended will lead to something worthwhile and meaningful. The 35 years that I have spent in the third world have convinced me that it has all been well worthwhile.

There is no doubt that an individual's actions can alter and improve the world others live in. The problem is to gain perspective, to live long enough to see the difference between what was and what is.

It has taken years of effort, but now it can be seen that the pattern of orthopaedic disease has changed from a nineteenth century preponderance of untreated infection, tuberculosis, yaws, and poor fracture treatment, to the present time, in which degenerative conditions and the debilities of old age are our predominant concerns.

Perhaps an even more important change has been the movement away from the unnecessary crippling caused by the lack of appreciation of the importance of surgery of the locomotive system. Surgery was performed by general surgeons, whose training was mainly in the care of abdominal and life-threatening conditions. Often orthopaedic problems were dealt with by even less experienced junior practitioners. This problem has become much less serious than it was, but there is still a long way to go in most third world countries.

I have seen my department change from a few delapidated huts to a modern well-built facility. This has not just happened. These changes have taken place because we have been able to tap the resources of a comparatively poor country by studying the culture, motivation, and beliefs of its population; particularly the decision-making section. During the colonial era, all decisions were made by the colonial government. Now it is the service clubs, business groups, and theologians who provide the thought from which our social decisions originate. Publicity has now supplanted national honours as the motivating force for those who want to be recognized for what they have helped to achieve. It is fortunate that the affluent in our societies want to appear generous, they just need us to convince them that their generosity will not be wasted.

I have to point out that it is characteristic of the sort of society we live in that leadership originates from individuals, the private sector, and what are generally referred to as nongovernment organizations. It has been the lack of this kind of leadership in totalitarian systems that has caused their failure by preventing the responsiveness to individual human needs that is essential for human progress. A healthy, dynamic, and independent volunteer group like ours, which responds to human situations, is characteristic of any healthy democracy. Its absence results in a regimented, controlled, static, and sterile existence for the individual citizen.

For a program to succeed, it must have the outlook of an Einstein rather than that of a Newton. The Newtonian attitude is like a clock—mechanical, rational, centrally directed, and predictable. Its defect is its unresponsiveness to people. Einstein's thinking brings us closer to social and cultural reality in the changing relationships and complexities that are particularly obvious in the third world.

For our overseas orthopaedic programs to succeed, we must want to understand the other man's point of view—his pride, his prejudices, and his thinking, which are vital parts of his cultural heritage.

Let us first consider the effect that independence has had on third world countries. Suddenly, individuals were confronted with the concept of liberty instead of the feeling of inferiority that had prevailed under colonialism. The effect has been to stimulate excessive and, often, rather misdirected activity. Instead of the progress expected to accompany the idea of the "developing world," change has been haphazard, erratic, and often ineffective. It is the sort of situation Edmund Burke once reacted to by saying, "the effect of liberty on individuals has been that they may do as they please. We ought to see what it will please them to do before we risk congratulations."

We have to recognize that the status of successful individuals is very much more important in the third world than it is elsewhere. Surgeons and civil servants, for instance, dress formally and resent visitors who call on them looking like tourists.

Just surviving in a tropical country was almost a miracle in the days before preventive medicine began to play its part. We cannot but respect the way of life and the culture that enabled people to survive in that hostile environment, which so often killed visitors and missionaries not so many years ago. The survival of these people depended on a way of life that fitted their needs extremely well and deserves to be appreciated.

For instance, because paper is destroyed so quickly where the termite abounds, reliance could not be made on the written words. Instead of books, tradition handed down by word of mouth must form the basis of the cultural heritage of such nations.

The senior members of the extended family group, have always been the guardians of life-saving traditions. It is the elderly, therefore, who have the knowledge, experience, and status to assure the group's survival. They are the recognized authorities whose opinions are always sought and who make the decisions. The position of the elderly is therefore one of honour, and it is they, rather than the individuals directly involved, who make decisions. This situation influences the doctor's work. For instance, a child may be brought in with a problem.

After the doctor has explained to the parents and arranged admission for surgery, the child may never be brought back, because the family members did not feel that they knew enough about the doctor.

Therefore, the first thing a program must do is to establish a reputation. This means avoiding anything complex and concentrating on the treatment of problems that can be easily corrected. The volume of problems that present themselves will make it easy to determine priorities and make sure that every moment is used constructively. Cases, in the early days of any program, should be chosen because they are likely to do well, recover quickly, and go home without pain.

Sometimes a surgeon is surprised by being asked to treat an adolescent with an obvious deformity that must have been present from birth. The parents may be unable or unwilling to explain why they have delayed for so long in coming for treatment. Usually this will be because of the prevailing "bride price" system, which is widespread and in many ways eugenic. This sensible arrangement, which is a particular part of the Moslem way of life, allows for more than one wife to be enjoyed by those successful enough to pay for them and to care for them and their children. It is a way of life that promotes the survival of the fittest and helps to prevent much of the abuse that is inherent where poverty makes individuals expendable. Unfortunately, however, because the presence of a deformed brother or sister will lower the bride price, a deformed child may be kept hidden from public gaze until the last girl has been married.

The continuance of a program depends largely on getting on well with one's colleagues. For the majority, great personal effort and cost has had to be borne by the physician's family to enable their son to get into medical school and to graduate. The physician is regarded as the elite of his generation.

A visiting surgeon will be joining a group that has great status in a community where status is as important as income. Any actions that threaten or appear to threaten colleagues will cause a program to fail, because cases that need the visitor's expertise will not be referred. If this happens, the opportunity to train residents and to perpetuate skills will be lost.

It is best to avoid involvement in politics either at a national or a medical level. A doctor who becomes identified with one group will be rejected by the others. What we have to offer is universal, not sectional, and our whole effort should be confined to activities that are clearly for the public good.

The actual way of life influences the advice we should give. For instance, most people squat to defecate, and an arthrodesed hip makes this most difficult. Hip arthrodesis is thus a procedure that should only be advised when there is absolutely no alternative and then performed in more flexion than would ordinarily be considered optimal.

In Moslem communities, the wise and healthy custom of using the left hand only for toilet and activities that carry the risk of infection means that the complete loss of a hand presents severe problems. Every attempt must be made to preserve at least a part of a hand even if it will have little or no real function.

We are in agreement that the purpose of our programs is to educate, to demonstrate by our enthusiasm and determination how difficulties may be overcome, and to show residents; general duty medical officers, who are the back bone of medical services; medical students; and technicians what we have to offer. The most important thing we have to communicate is our caring attitude to all patients, whether rich or poor, a thing that is very obviously lacking in many countries.

The high esteem in which physicians have always been held has depended on their attitude to the weak and needy. An apparent lack of concern for the poor will result in a loss of status that is most undesirable. There is no place for greed in the life of a physician. We all know that those we teach absorb as much from our attitude to patients as from the facts we present to them.

Orthopaedic technicians, if available, can become great allies. They can take responsibility for much routine work, such as applying traction, casts, and club foot treatment. They are particularly useful for the general duty medical officer who works alone.

Often, a visiting surgeon will be so impressed with a resident or student that there is a temptation to help him continue in his training. The visitor may wish to sponsor the younger man in his own department, but this idea must be avoided. After all, one's objective is to improve orthopaedics in a country that desperately needs what we have to offer.

If a man is removed from his home environment at the most formative period in his life, he will usually throw down roots, and if he brings his family with him, they will do so too. If he comes alone he may well marry a nurse who will convince him that, if he returns home, he will never be able to practice the sort of medicine he has been taught to perform. For whatever the reason, of the 14 men I have tried to train in North America, only one has returned to his homeland.

The problems that many patients have in coming for treatment need to be appreciated because they may greatly influence the advice we give. Many of them must travel long distances along bad roads, in a land where transport is in short supply and is very expensive. Having arrived, they may have to take lodgings for some time during their treatment. They may well find it impossible to come back for further treatment after the present course of treatment is ended. For this reason, particularly when treating cases of polio and club feet, if conservative methods do not gain the desired effect rapidly, surgery may well be indicated much earlier than one would advise in one's own practice. If there is only one chance to treat a patient, it is necessary to do all that is possible as quickly as possible.

Late presentation of cases usually occurs because of the difficulties that must be overcome in coming for treatment. Even if a problem is life threatening, once a surgeon has established a reputation for good, effective work, he can safely perform life-threatening procedures, provided he has explained the situation to the patient, often through a trusted interpreter.

When setting up a new program, it is advisable to plan it to be near and closely associated with an academic center, if only because the possibility of influencing the teaching program will be much greater. Also, associating with colleagues with similar interests can make the visit much more enjoyable. It is important to avoid being a burden to one's hosts, who are often very much less affluent than might be expected.

All of us who have been able to mount successful programs have done so by capturing the imagination of the private sector, who are only too glad to assist a pet charity so long as they garner favorable publicity and have confidence in your integrity. If emphasis can be put on the problems of children, the impact will be greater.

There are many ways to make a program attractive to the public so that it can get the sort of support that will sustain it. Sport for the disabled has proved to be the best single means of bringing our patients' problems before the public. Such a program can make it easier to convince employers that a disabled worker is likely to be a better, and certainly a more conscientious, worker than the average. The principal long-term benefit for patients is employment, which allows them to regain the dignity that they lost as the result of their illness or disease.

The final aim must be to develop a complete program that will give the patient a chance to return home and contribute again to his family's needs. Retraining of patients must emphasize activities that can be performed even by severely disabled persons. Farming, the care of livestock, carving, painting, embroidery, and woodwork have all been found suitable and practical.

No program will ever achieve everything we would like for it. Each program will be formed by the interplay of what the men setting up the program have to give and the cultural environment they are working in. What should be common to all programs is the quiet determination of the volunteers and their sense of humour and enthusiasm. These intangible assets set the stage for the sort of program that will continue making a permanent contribution to these societies.

I do not wish to leave the impression that all is "blood, tears, toil and sweat." Most volunteers feel, as I do, that it has all been very much worthwhile. They return home with memories of friendship and beauty that surmount the extraordinary problems that might, at first, have seemed likely to overwhelm them. If nothing else, they will return home realizing how fortunate they are to live in the first world.

The orthopaedic programs we have been running over the last 30 years are the result of a new idea—an idea that formed in the minds of those whose thinking had been permanently altered by their involvement in World War II. This new idea not only became the basis for the development of the Orthopaedic Letters Club Overseas group, which soon developed into Orthopedics Overseas and World Orthopedics Concern; it inspired a whole generation and also resulted in the hospice movement and the Cheshire Homes. As Victor Hugo has reminded us, "there is only one thing stronger than all the armies of the world and that is an idea whose time has come." We should all be proud that our orthopaedic colleagues have led the whole medical world in recognizing and reacting successfully to an idea whose time has certainly come.

Appropriate Surgery and Appliances for Patients With Deformities and Paralysis in Developing Countries

Ronald L. Huckstep, MD, FRCS

Introduction

Poliomyelitis and other paralytic, congenital, and traumatic deformities of the lower limb are common in developing countries. Surgical procedures are often performed by general duty doctors and general surgeons, and surgical facilities can be very limited. Sophisticated procedures are often quite inappropriate for the majority of patients. Millions of paralyzed and deformed patients still require treatment.

Many patients with paralyzed lower limbs require simple, cheap, but effective braces, crutches, wheel chairs, and other appliances to achieve mobility. These devices should be made from locally available materials and should be manufactured by unskilled or partly skilled workers in the developing country itself. Many appliances can be made out of galvanized wire, the iron used for reinforcing concrete, wood, furniture tubing, and bicycle wheels. There is little place for imported expensive braces, wheelchairs, and other supports.

Many patients require simple, mainly subcutaneous, correction of paralytic contractures of the lower limb. The methods I advocate for correcting these deformities are based on a personal series of over 5,000 joint corrections in which over an 85% acceptable long-term result was achieved.

Training of orthopaedic assistants, who are nursing assistants with about one year of practical training in assessment of patients, running of clinics, fitting of supports, simple physiotherapy, muscle charting, and other practical procedures, will also enable the efficient running of clinics for polio and other paralyzed patients. Similarly, locally trained workshop technicians, often paralyzed themselves, can make most of the appliances required, using local materials and with very little formal training.

It is also stressed that there is a great need for visiting orthopaedic surgeons to teach local doctors, orthopaedic assistants, and workshop technicians. Simple appropriate rehabilitation and education is essential after the patients are mobilized, with the aim of making the patients self-supporting.

Correction of Lower-Limb Deformities

The most common deformities in poliomyelitis are a flexed hip and knee and an equinus deformity of the ankle. In the majority of cases a subcutaneous correction of these contractures, combined with an open biceps tenotomy if necessary, will correct these deformities. Fasciotomy of the iliotibial band with a small tenotomy knife seldom requires stitching, except when it is combined with an open biceps tenotomy.

Figure 1 demonstrates the method of correction of hip and knee contractures by a fasciotomy of the iliotibial band. A small tenotomy knife should be inserted behind the tight band and slid down to the femoral shaft just above the knee. The fascia is then cut in an anterior direction keeping lateral to the line of the femur and being careful to avoid the common peroneal nerve, which is located medial to and behind the biceps tendon. This single division will often partially correct a flexed knee as well as hip. An open biceps tenotomy should be performed, in addition, if the knee contracture exceeds 20 degrees to 30 degrees.[1-4]

Other incisions one finger breadth below the anterior superior iliac spine and at points one third and two thirds along the thigh may also be required (Fig. 1). These procedures can usually be performed safely if the anatomy of the neurovascular structures is kept in mind. After surgery, Russell traction, or plaster casting, after one or more manipulations but without putting the knee under tension, will correct most contractures. Contractures greater than 60 degrees can be corrected by a rotation supracondylar osteotomy of the lower femur.[1-4]

Supracondylar Osteotomy for Severe Contractures of the Knee

Figure 2 illustrates a supracondylar osteotomy designed to correct severe knee contractures of up to 110 degrees. The anterior half of the supracondylar area of the femur is resected after osteotomy of the remainder of the femur. The lower femur is then rotated 60 to 110 degrees.

This usually locks the lower femur into a curved resected area of the supracondylar region without requiring any internal fixation or stability other than the backslab. One or two Kirschner wires can be inserted for three to four weeks to give added stability if necessary.

This type of supracondylar osteotomy will shorten the femur, which will also compensate for a posterior soft-tissue contracture. More than 40 patients with severe contractures of more than 60 degrees have been successfully corrected by this method.

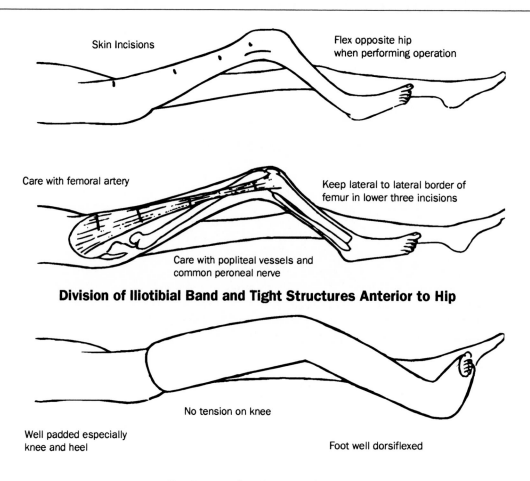

Skin Incisions

Flex opposite hip when performing operation

Care with femoral artery

Keep lateral to lateral border of femur in lower three incisions

Care with popliteal vessels and common peroneal nerve

Division of Iliotibial Band and Tight Structures Anterior to Hip

No tension on knee

Well padded especially knee and heel

Foot well dorsiflexed

Postoperative Plaster Cast

Fig. 1 Subcutaneous fasciotomy for hip and knee contractures.

Ankle Equinus

An equinus ankle without an associated fixed varus deformity is best treated with a simple subcutaneous tenotomy, without tourniquet and with a small tenotomy knife. The patient is supine and the posterior two-thirds of the upper part and medial two-thirds of the lower part of the Achilles tendon are divided. This divides all the fibers, which often rotate through about 90 degrees, as described by White in 1943 (Fig. 3). A full correction can usually then be achieved by dorsi-flexing the foot to allow the tendon to slide. This procedure is followed by six weeks in a plaster cast. Care should be taken not to damage the posterior tibial vessels and nerve. If the tendon does not slide easily, it may be necessary to divide slightly more tendon. In the case of inadvertent complete division of the Achilles tendon, no attempt should be made to repair the tendon, because it will almost always heal without complication. In the case of an associated fixed varus deformity, an open posterior and medial capsulotomy is usually necessary. Most cases, however, achieve an excellent correction by this simple subcutaneous method.[1-3]

The number of patients with lower-limb contractures treated mainly by subcutaneous methods and followed for one to nine years is shown in Table 1. These 3,657 procedures are representative of more than 5,000 lower-limb contractures treated by the author. More than 85% of the 5,000 resulted in an acceptable long-term result.

In the case of a severe equinovarus deformity, a triple arthrodesis may be necessary, requiring extensive resection of the cuboid and cuneiforms and sometimes part of the other hindfoot bones. More sophisticated operations, including tendon transfers, may be required, but these should not be carried out until the backlog of contractures, often numbering many thousands in each developing country, have been corrected by the simple subcutaneous methods described. In addition, correction of contractures in children must take priority over adults. It is essential that a full assessment

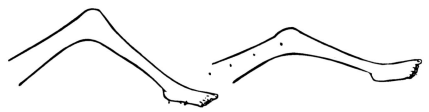

First Stage: Soft-tissue Correction

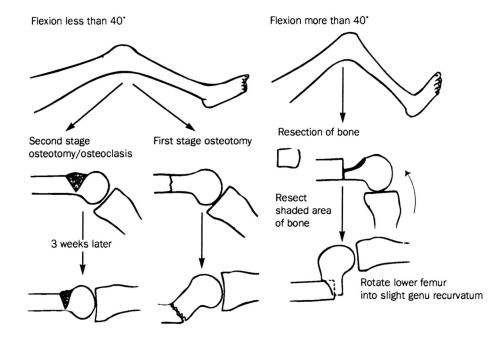

Second Stage: Supracondylar Osteotomy

Fig. 2   Supracondylar osteotomy for difficult flexion contractures of the knee.

of the patient be made before attempting surgery. It is of little use to correct paralyzed lower limbs when weak arms and trunk make it unlikely that the patient will ever walk again.

In the case of a flexed hip and knee and equinus ankle in the spastic patient, from whatever cause, a subcutaneous elongation of the Achilles tendon and bilateral subcutaneous adductor tenotomies will often achieve considerable improvement. A flexed hip and knee will often also improve following this procedure, without the need for any surgical correction on these joints. Postoperatively, the only treatment required is below-knee bracing. In spastic patients, bracing should not extend above the knee.

Treatment of Upper Limb Paralysis and Deformities

In the spastic patient, a flexed elbow, with a pronated forearm and flexed wrist, will often be considerably improved by an open elongation of the biceps tendon alone. In poliomyelitis, a triad of paralysis of the deltoid, triceps, and thenar muscles can occur, although paralysis of the upper limb is often much less severe than that of the lower limb.

In poliomyelitis, a flail shoulder with a useful forearm and hand can frequently be improved by an arthrodesis of the shoulder, provided the patient has sufficient trapezius power. A weak elbow with a useful hand is best treated with a simple detachable splint rather than by sophisticated surgery. Paralysis of opposition is best treated by the relatively simple transfer of the flexor superficialis of the ring finger, provided the rest of the hand justifies the procedure.[1]

Spinal Paralysis

A paralytic scoliosis or kyphoscoliosis is not uncommon. Mild cases require no treatment other than back

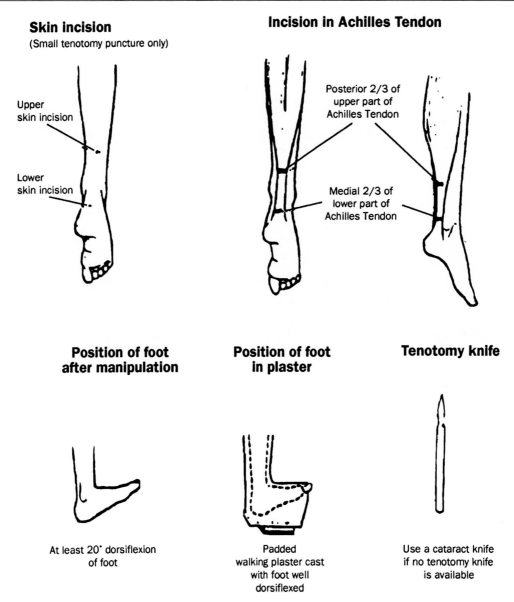

Skin incision
(Small tenotomy puncture only)

Upper skin incision

Lower skin incision

Incision in Achilles Tendon

Posterior 2/3 of upper part of Achilles Tendon

Medial 2/3 of lower part of Achilles Tendon

Position of foot after manipulation

At least 20° dorsiflexion of foot

Position of foot in plaster

Padded walking plaster cast with foot well dorsiflexed

Tenotomy knife

Use a cataract knife if no tenotomy knife is available

Fig. 3   Subcutaneous elongation of the Achilles tendon.

Table 1
Lower-limb contractures—1958 to 1968

Surgical Procedure	No. of Limbs	Acceptable 1 to 9 Year Follow-up
Subcutaneous fasciotomy hip	1,251	89.1% (605 hips)
Fasciotomy	1,253	86.2% (512 knees)
Subcutaneous elongation calcaneus tendon	1,153	87.8% (498 ankles)

In these cases, the patient manages to walk by twisting the spine and pelvis. Arthrodesis of the spine, apart from being a very major procedure in a developing country, will hinder this movement. To do so will make the patient less mobile and can make the patient stop walking altogether. It is much better to give the patient a simple spinal support to wear while sitting and thereby maintain mobility.

Appliances for Paralysis

Braces (Fig. 4) can be made from local materials, (such as galvanized wire, the iron used for reinforcing concrete, and local leather). If possible, they should be

exercises. In severe cases, there is little or no place for arthrodesis of the spine in developing countries, especially if there is severe lower-limb paralysis and the patient is barely able to walk using braces and crutches.

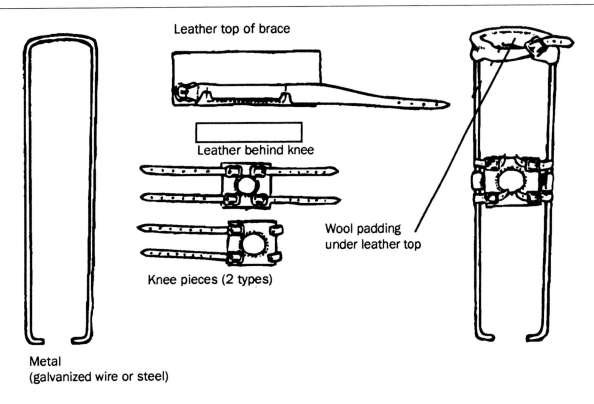

Fig. 4   Manufacture of a simple brace.

worn with a simple wooden clog rather than a boot. The clog (Fig. 5) can be made without heating or welding and by virtually unskilled labor. Braces, made in a range of sizes, can easily be adjusted by bending to compensate for slight varus, valgus, flexion, or genu recurvatum of the knee.[1-7]

The advantage of the clog is that it is less likely to be damaged by water, which makes it much more suitable for patients working in the fields. For patients with paralysis and shortening on one side only, a brace and clog on that side alone, without a clog on the opposite foot, will often be accepted while a boot would not (Figs. 4, 5, and 6).

A simple crutch can easily be made from a piece of split wood or bamboo (Fig. 7). A walking stick can be made from a tree branch or wooden dowel with a handle.

Wheelchairs made from an old frame chair, or furniture tubing, with two bicycle wheels and a bogie wheel at the back, can be made locally (Fig. 8). Full, simple manufacturing drawings are available for this as well as any of the other appliances in this paper.[1,5,7]

Skelecasts

Skelecasts are lightweight devices used for immobilization. Developed in 1966, they have since been used by several thousand patients. They are a new method

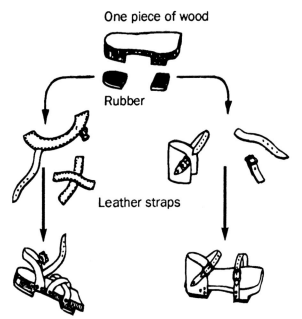

Fig. 5   Manufacture of a clog (carved wood).

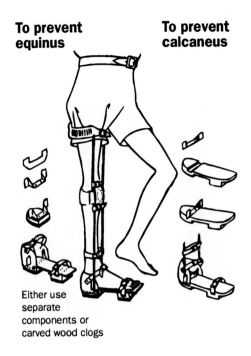

To prevent equinus

To prevent calcaneus

Either use separate components or carved wood clogs

Fig. 6 Manufacture of a backstop for a clog.

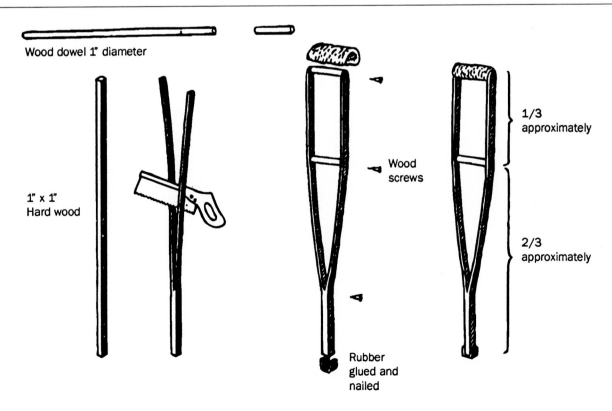

Wood dowel 1" diameter

1" x 1" Hard wood

Wood screws

Rubber glued and nailed

1/3 approximately

2/3 approximately

Fig. 7 Manufacture of a wooden crutch.

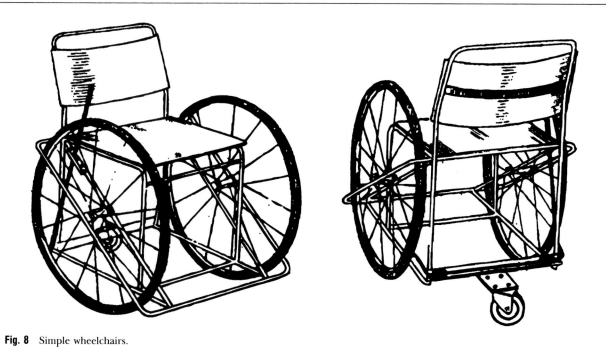

Fig. 8 Simple wheelchairs.

of three- or four-point immobilization of the limbs and trunk and use a variety of waterproof materials as simple strut supports. Skelecasts can supersede plaster of Paris in over 50% of patients requiring immobilization and have many advantages over plaster of Paris. They allow the patient to have a daily shower and to swim. Fractures heal quickly, skelecasts are cooler than circumferential plaster casts, muscles retain their tone, the skin can be observed, and most joints regain their mobility immediately after removal.

Polyester resin thickened with an inert powder is applied onto fiber glass tape or old bandage. The method is cheap, making it ideal for use in developing countries. Thermoplastics are easier to apply but are more expensive. These are dipped into water at approximately 65 to 70 C and are applied directly to the patient over a waterproof lining. Newer plastics can also be applied after dipping into cold water.

Edema caused by trauma can be controlled with a crepe bandage over wool, and the struts can be tightened, loosened, or repositioned easily. Radiographs can be taken without removing the support, if required for the knee and elbow (Fig. 9).

Training

Training of all grades of staff, as already mentioned, is essential. Local surgeons and doctors should be taught how to assess patients and perform simple surgery under supervision, rather than spend time learning sophisticated techniques.

Orthopaedic assistants (nursing assistants without the educational qualifications to become trained nurses) should be taught by apprenticeship a few practical skills, such as taking of orthopaedic histories, muscle charting, simple physiotherapy, fitting of braces, assisting at operations, application of plaster casts, and the follow-up and rehabilitation of patients. One or two of these assistants can be invaluable in each up-country hospital, and more in the main center.[5,6]

The disabled adults themselves can be trained to be orthopaedic technicians and in three to six months can learn how to manufacture such simple appliances as braces, clogs, and crutches. They need little or no education, although basic skills such as wood carving and sewing are useful.

The manufacture of wheelchairs requires more skill, but a local metalworker with a basic knowledge of welding would have this ability. Sophisticated technicians, who can work only with aluminium, and who will refuse to make braces without an expensive knee-bending piece, can be a disaster in a developing country, as most will not lower their standards. One hundred simple, but effective braces may cost the same as a single sophisticated imported support.

The record number of simple braces fitted in a single day under the supervision of the author at an up-country clinic in Uganda was 194 braces for 143 patients with poliomyelitis. In poor countries, most braces can be made for about $1.00 each. By 1971, over 40,000 supports were being made each year, mainly by uneducated disabled laborers. These supports included 500 artificial limbs and 5,000 braces.

Polyester Resin
Polyester resin putty impregnated into
fiberglass tape or bandage

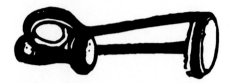

Scaphoid
Patients can bathe and swim
Cast is waterproof and light

Lower Limb
Position of strips are adjustable for ease of dressings

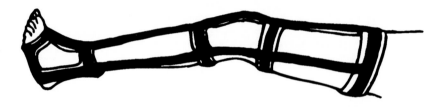

Fig. 9 Skelecasts—a lightweight concept of immobilization. (Reproduced with permission from Huckstep RL: *A Simple Guide to Trauma*, ed 4. London, Churchill Livingstone, 1986, p 155.

Rehabilitation and Education

Rehabilitation and education should be geared to the needs of the individual country. Simple agricultural training, so that patients can grow food, is often important. Other training may include light industry, such as the manufacture of bags and umbrellas. Clerical duties may be appropriate for those with some education. Governments should be encouraged to enroll disabled children into ordinary schools, and mobility with crutches or even a wheelchair can make this possible.[1,3,8,9] In Uganda in 1970 there were 13 rehabilitation centers, where 2,000 patients at a time were learning skills appropriate to their education and needs. Relatives and patients must be shown how to stretch contractures, fit braces, and attend their local dispensary or hospital for repair or changing of supports. Braces can be fitted with new leather and reused many times by different patients.

Voluntary Agencies

Local voluntary agencies, such as Rotary, Apex, Round Table, Lions Club, and Red Cross, will often be of assistance in starting workshops and rehabilitation schemes, as has occurred in Uganda, Malawi, and other developing countries under the supervision of the author. The cooperation and help of governments is also essential.[1,3]

Volunteer orthopaedic surgeons recruited through World Orthopaedic Concern and Orthopaedics Overseas have contributed much to developing countries. All orthopaedic surgeons are encouraged to join one of these organizations. Joining does not commit them in any way, but it does show that they are interested in the aims of these organizations.

Summary

Death before maturity is the usual fate of the untreated crawling crippled child in developing countries. Most children with poliomyelitis, however, when upright and walking with supports, or following surgery, are accepted by the community, educated by parents and relatives, and employable when they reach maturity. It is more economic to prevent 100 polio cases than it is to treat one hopelessly crippled child. It is often quicker to straighten 100 deformed limbs by simple subcutaneous operations, than to treat a single patient by complicated procedures. It costs less for 100 crawling paralyzed children to walk in simple, locally made braces and clogs than for one patient to be mobile in expensive imported appliances and boots. It is essential to educate or rehabilitate patients in addition to making them mobile. The final aim should be a patient returned to his own village or town, accepted and integrated into his own community, and earning his own living among his friends and family.

References

1. Huckstep RL: *Poliomyelitis: A Guide for Developing Countries, Including Appliances and Rehabilitation*, ed 2. Edinburgh, Churchill Livingstone, 1975.

2. Huckstep RL: *Polio in Uganda* [16 mm film & video]. Park Ridge, American Academy of Orthopaedic Surgeons Library.

3. Huckstep RL: The cripple in Africa. *Makerere Med J* 1970;14:9.

4. Huckstep RL: Soft tissue release of hip and thigh, in Crenshaw AW (ed): *Campbells Operative Orthopaedics*, ed 7. St Louis, CV Mosby, 1987, p 2989.

5. Huckstep RL: Simple appliances for developing countries: *Int Rehabil Rev* 1969;XX:5

6. Huckstep RL: Orthopaedic appliances for developing countries. *Trop Doct* 1971;64(2,3):108.

7. Hunt SCM, Huckstep RL: Wheelchairs for developing countries of the world. *J Bone Joint Surg* 1967;49B:595.

8. Huckstep RL: *A Simple Guide to Trauma*, ed 4. Edinburgh, Churchill Livingstone, 1986.

9. Huckstep RL: Orthopaedic problems in the newer world, in *Commonwealth Foundation Paper X*. London, 1970.

Management of Common Third World Orthopaedic Problems: Paralytic Poliomyelitis, Tuberculosis of Bones and Joints, Hansen's Disease (Leprosy), and Chronic Osteomyelitis

Hugh G. Watts, MD

Management of Children With the Residua of Paralytic Poliomyelitis

In spite of the availability of prophylactic vaccination, 250,000 cases of polio were reported to the World Health Organization in 1986 (almost 700 cases each day). Undoubtedly, many more cases go unreported. Approximately ten million people worldwide have some lameness caused by polio. There are many obstacles to vaccine use: (1) Vaccine is thermolabile and needs to be maintained under refrigeration at 4 C (and the highest incidence is in countries where refrigeration is uncommon). (2) Transportation, both roads and vehicles, to take the vaccine to local clinics is usually limited. (3) Techniques of administration often denature the vaccine. For example, chlorox, which is often used to sterilize the spoons used to dispense vaccine, can inactivate the virus. (4) Patient factors, such as malnutrition, frequently reduce seroconversion. (5) Social factors, such as fear of government personnel, lack of education, and the rare child who develops the disease after receiving the vaccine (with the ensuing rumors) can impair vaccination programs, as can political factors, such as the high cost and the lack of glamour of vaccination programs. (6) Lack of awareness by those in developed countries of the extent of polio remaining in the rest of the world has resulted in little help coming from the parts of the world that could best provide it.

An orthopaedic surgeon who has been trained in the developed countries and has seldom, if ever, seen a patient with polio, is often overwhelmed by the multiplicity of problems to be treated. It is particularly important to avoid focusing on a single deformity. First, the surgeon must establish an overall plan, and thorough assessment is the cornerstone of the planning. Check the child's gait (if a walker) both with and without crutches and braces, then the sitting capability, and passive range of motion. Manual testing of the muscles of the extremities and the trunk muscles is basic. This kind of testing is a skill that may require review. The muscle test results should be carefully and individually recorded. A simple worksheet for use in the clinic is a great time saver. A muscle commonly loses one full grade after transfer. To be functionally useful, a grade of at least 4 is necessary, although a grade 3 muscle, when transferred, can be effective in preventing deformity by balancing an opposing muscle.

The most difficult aspects of patient assessment are the social and cultural ones. Patient information, usually gathered through the filtering process of an interpreter, is analyzed by a surgeon whose understanding of local needs, uses, and geography is probably limited. Often these social and cultural factors are the primary ones that can lead to the success or failure of treatment.

The establishment of an overall treatment plan requires priorities. The priorities for polio management are, by and large, sequential: (1) Get the child walking; (2) Correct factors that will create deformity with growth; (3) Correct factors that will obviate or reduce a lifetime dependency on external bracing; (4) Correct upper extremity problems; (5) Treat scoliosis.

Get the Child Walking

First, however, it is essential to determine if the child is likely to ever become a walker. Here, the evaluation of the strength of the upper extremities is paramount. Can the child lift the buttocks off the examining table with the hands placed beside each thigh? Failure to succeed at this simple task bodes ill for a child's ability to help himself walk with crutches (Fig. 1, *left*). If the child has the potential to become a walker, get the child walking in any fashion with the minimal contracture releases necessary to allow use of simple braces. The contracture releases required at this stage are most often the hip flexors and abductors, the fascia lata distally, and the heel cord. Children younger than 3 or 4 years of age often respond to stretching; those a few years older to serial casting; and those older yet will require surgery.

Correction of Hip Flexion and Abduction Contractures Hip flexion contractures can occur in isolation but are more commonly associated with contractures of the tensor and the gluteus medius. Many hip flexion and abduction contractures are relieved by radical release of the iliotibial tract and intramuscular septum at the knee (the Yount procedure). In other cases, proximal release (Ober release) is used. I prefer not to use subcutaneous tenotomies, because the hip abduction contractures require releasing far posteriorly. In younger children, a residual contracture of 20 degrees can usually be corrected with stretching exercises.

Correction of Knee Flexion Contractures There are four ways to correct knee flexion contractures. In the first, serial

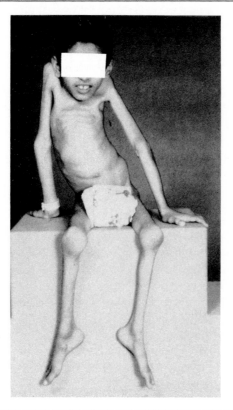

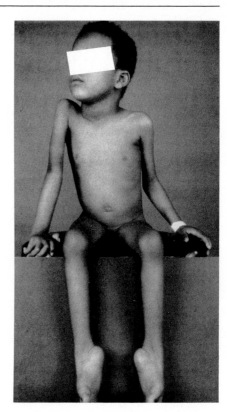

Fig. 1 Left, This boy with polio has obvious weakness of the upper extremities and trunk in addition to his leg weakness. As he presses down on the seat with his hands, his shoulders move proximally, so that he is unable to raise his body off the seat. This boy will not become a walker. Efforts to make him walk will frustrate everyone. **Right**, Note the 90-degree external rotation deformities of the tibias, a common finding. Derotation of the tibias is needed for proper, comfortable brace wearing.

casting, age, degree of contracture, available facilities, and the distance the patient has to travel all influence the treatment. The cast is applied without sedation or anesthesia and is changed at two- or three-week intervals. Approximately 10 degrees of correction can be achieved per cast change. The second mode of correction, surgical release at the knee, can commonly be done laterally. Posterior capsulotomy should usually be avoided or back-knee may become a problem. Number three is surgical release with femoral shortening or followed by skeletal traction. If the contracture is greater than 60 degrees or the neurovascular bundle is very tight, the femur may be shortened or postoperative skeletal traction may be used. It is not necessary to fully correct the contracture by traction. About two to three weeks of traction is ample. Once all but 40 degrees of correction have been achieved, the remainder can be gained by serial casting. When stretching out knee flexion contractures, it is important to avoid hyperextension. The fourth mode of correction, distal femoral extension osteotomy, can be used if the child is near maturity or if the contracture is recurrent. If the child has no active knee extensor, 10 to 15 degrees of hyperextension should be the goal.

Bracing Braces should be kept simple. In deciding whether to brace below the knee or above, it is best to err on the side of more extensive bracing. A child who has never walked may become frustrated without the

instant stability provided by a knee-ankle-foot orthosis. Lack of initial demonstrable success may cause the child and parents to decide against further treatment. For the same reason, a walker may be the best initial choice for an external walking aid. Later, the patient can progress to axillary and then forearm crutches.

The materials used in braces will depend on available facilities. The lightness of plastic has to be balanced against its lack of durability; the relative ease of working steel and leather against its greater weight. Usually a broken metal-and-leather brace can be repaired more readily by local craftsmen than can a fractured plastic brace.

A child who is missing knee extension muscles requires a long-leg brace with a knee lock (or built without a knee joint if the child is young and does not need to sit with a bent knee). If the foot is flail, ankle motion in the brace should be limited to approximately 15 degrees of plantar flexion. If the foot is dropped, use a planter flexion stop at zero. Dorsiflexion spring assists seldom stand even a few months of hard use by an active child, and are unnecessarily expensive. Where the foot and ankle are in balance, a free ankle joint is satisfactory.

If the child cannot balance the trunk over the legs, then a pelvic band and hip hinges can be added. When both hip extensors are paralyzed, a hip lock can be added. As the child improves, it is almost always possible to abandon the pelvic band.

Prevention of Deformity

For a child who is walking confidently, the surgeon should focus on those problems that commonly result in deformity as the child grows.

Foot Foot problems that can lead to deformity include equinus, foot drop, foot valgus, equinovarus, and calcaneus. In most children under the age of 10 years, equinus can be corrected by serial casts (with the foot in inversion to prevent rocker-bottom). In older children it requires a lengthening of the Achilles tendon. It is important to remember that some degree of equinus contracture may beneficially stabilize the knee by forcing the knee into hyperextension on floor contact. If the quadriceps has a strength of 3 or better, the Achilles tendon may safely be lengthened. If the child stabilizes the knee by means of equinus, releasing the Achilles tendon may take away the child's ability to walk without a brace.

After correction of the equinus, foot drop is corrected by tendon transfers to improve dorsiflexion, if suitable muscles are available to prevent the knee from buckling. A drop-foot may be corrected by a brace or by appropriate transfers.

Foot valgus involving an everted heel and valgus forefoot with active peronei and lateral toe extensors is a deforming combination that is seen commonly. A subtalar arthrodesis is effective in stabilizing the heel. The peronei should be transferred to the heel if the knee is likely to give way because of quadriceps weakness, and to the dorsum if the knee is not likely to buckle. Stabilization and transfer should not be delayed too long, because early correction can make a later triple arthrodesis unnecessary. In children younger than 10 years of age, most foot deformities can be corrected by soft-tissue release combined with a subtalar fusion.

As the child approaches maturity, a triple arthrodesis may be needed. In doing a triple arthrodesis for a foot that corrects passively, simple removal of the cartilage surfaces, rather than cutting wedges, will result in much less foot shortening.

Equinovarus in the younger child can be corrected by casts and stabilized by bracing or tibialis posterior transfer. If the deformity returns or correction fails, then a posterior medial release combined with a subtalar fusion may be necessary. It is important to make sure that the resulting fusion is not in varus.

To prevent calcaneus deformity when no muscles are available for transfer, tenodesis of the Achilles tendon to the fibula with the foot in 5 to 10 degrees of plantar flexion will control the heel.

Knee A back-knee deformity in a growing child should be protected by bracing. If there is sufficient quadriceps to maintain stability with the knee in a little flexion, make the brace in 10 to 20 degrees of flexion at the knee. If the recurvatum occurs solely in the tibia, an osteotomy is useful.

Surgery for Comfortable Brace Wearing If the child will always be a brace wearer, aim for comfort in the brace. Because children improve in function with time, enough time should be allowed to determine whether or not the child will always require a brace.

Procedures that will make a brace more comfortable include: (1) release of equinus, (2) stabilization of the subtalar joint so that the medial malleolus does not become abraded by the medial upright of the brace, (3) derotation of an externally rotated tibia, (Fig. 1, right) and (4) correction of calcaneus by an appropriate tendon transfer to prevent a painful heel. Tenodesis of the Achilles tendon to the fibula can be done when a transferable muscle is not available.

The Dangling Leg A child who has a short, flail leg with a normal contralateral leg, normal upper extremities and trunk, may learn to get about remarkably well by using crutches and dangling the affected limb. Often, if such a child is fitted with an appropriate long-leg brace and shoe lift, the child can learn to walk without crutches, thereby freeing up the hands for more useful functions. The change from crutches and a dangling limb to a brace usually requires a period of crutch use along with the brace. Because this combination will appear to the child and the parents as a step backward, clever persuasion on the part of the orthopaedist may be required.

Leg-Length Discrepancies The degree of acceptable leg shortening often depends on the culture. A limb that will always require a brace should be left at least 1 cm short to allow for the thickness of the brace under the sole of the foot for easier swing through. An affected limb may be associated with a dysplastic hip. Leaving the leg short can provide added coverage. Other surgery anticipated for later years should be planned for. For example, a triple arthrodesis or ankle fusion may further shorten a foot, while a bone graft for a subtalar arthrodesis, taken from the proximal tibia, may stimulate growth in the tibia.

The choice of treatment for a leg-length discrepancy is likely to be different in non-Western countries. Shoe lifts are not well tolerated where sandals or bare feet are the custom. Epiphysiodesis might be the obvious treatment for many leg-length discrepancies in the view of the orthopaedic surgeon, but parents may not see the logic of operating on a good limb, even though the procedure may be much simpler than lengthening the short leg.

Leg-length discrepancies in polio do not necessarily increase in a predictable fashion. If lengthening is planned, it is best left until after skeletal maturity is achieved.

Hip Instability Although a great deal has been written about regaining hip joint stability after polio, I have found the need for such surgery to be uncommon. As in the treatment of the unstable hip in myelodysplasia, a dislocated hip may not be a significant impairment to function, but multiple surgical attempts to regain muscle balance leading to hip stiffness can surely be the cause of significant disability. Hip stiffness is much more of a problem in cultures where floor-sitting is an important activity of daily living—the very cultures where polio is rampant.

Decrease Bracing

Once the child is walking with confidence and potential deformities have been cared for, it is time to determine if the child be made brace-free or if the bracing can be decreased. A child with an absent quadriceps can walk brace-free provided there is a hip extensor, an ankle plantar flexor (or block to ankle dorsiflexion), or a combination of both. However, because the presence of a knee-flexion contracture will not allow the knee to support body weight, the first step is to correct the knee-flexion contracture. Contractures cannot be corrected by tendon transfers or by bracing. In a child under the age of 2, contractures can usually be stretched out gradually by physical therapy. Older children respond to serial casting, and teenagers usually require surgery.

In the patient near skeletal maturity, knee extension stability can often be easily obtained by a supracondylar extension osteotomy. This procedure is most effective in a patient who can walk brace-free, but who needs a hand to support the knee.

While a strong hamstring can be transferred anteriorly to act as a knee extensor, transfers of the hamstrings into the patella have not proven to be popular in most societies where polio is still a problem because the patient loses the ability to flex the knee for sitting, squatting-at-toilet, and praying. Commonly, an attempt should be made to improve pushoff by stabilizing the hindfoot and transferring the peroneii and/or the toe flexors posteriorly into the os calcis. In the absence of ankle plantar flexion muscles, sufficient knee stability may be gained by an ankle fusion in slight equinus to discard a knee-ankle-foot orthosis. In a child who is skeletally immature, the same thing can be gained by a tenodesis of the Achilles tendon to the fibula, but this can only work if the subtalar joint is surgically stabilized.

The Upper Extremity

The function of the whole limb must be assessed. Classically, the upper limb is viewed as a mechanism to place the hand where it is needed. In that teaching, a useless hand would lead one away from shoulder surgery. But remember that a child may use the upper extremities to support the body weight with crutches (even with useless hands), or to shift the trunk weight by leaning on the arm rest of a wheelchair. Thus, because shoulder function without hand function can be

well worth striving for (Fig. 2, *left*), I prefer to consider the shoulder first.

Shoulder Theoretically, it is preferable to restore function by tendon transfer rather than by fusion. In practical terms, however, the most frequent solution for a flail shoulder is fusion. With medial scapular muscles, the levator, and the serratus anterior present, a shoulder fusion can be beneficial. In order to gain significant arm elevation after a shoulder fusion, a strong serratus anterior, which rotates the scapula, is the most important factor.

Elbow The function of a normal hand is grossly limited by the absence of elbow flexion. Elbow flexion can be restored by transferring the origin of the wrist flexors or extensors (or both) proximally (Steindler flexor plasty), by transfer of the pectoralis major, or by transfer of the triceps forward to the biceps. A further alternative is to transfer the latissimus dorsi on its neurovascular pedicle.

Care must be taken not to lose an important function with such a transfer. Although moving the triceps forward to act as an elbow flexor is very effective, it can cause a loss of the ability to stabilize the elbow in extension, thereby losing the ability to use crutches. Inability to extend the elbow may also eliminate the ability to reach backward to the starting position for wheelchair propulsion, or the ability to stabilize paper on a desk with one hand while writing with the other. With transfer of the triceps, elevation of the arm will be less functional if the forearm flops into flexion because of an absence of an elbow extensor.

Forearm A pronation contracture causes a functional loss not seen in the west—the child cannot feed himself. In a large part of the world, the main eating utensil is the hand, and the hand must be supinated to get food into the mouth.

With a supination contracture, the child can feed himself, but the absence of pronation means that ordinary hand work is impossible. The balance between a working hand and a feeding hand must be weighed carefully.

Hand The lack of thumb opposition may be dealt with by any of the classic techniques, taking care to correct any abduction contracture of the thumb that may also exist. In crutch walkers, the procedure should be delayed until the patient is able to cooperate. Because there is a real possibility of stretching out the transfer with crutch use, serious consideration should be given to maintaining opposition with a strut graft between the first and second metacarpal rather than with tendon transfers.

Scoliosis

When a curve is noted, baseline anteroposterior and lateral radiographs should be taken with the child sit-

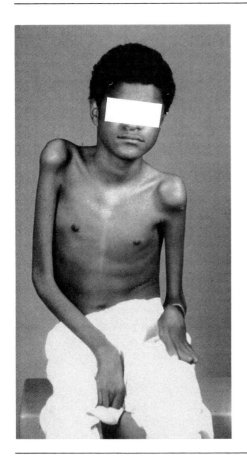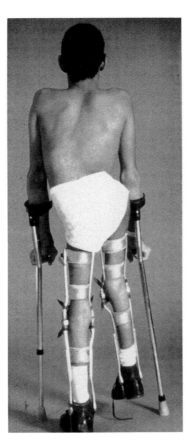

Fig. 2 Left, This boy with polio has unstable shoulder joints and virtually useless hands. Arthrodeses of his shoulder joints made it possible for him to hold crutches under his axillae and allowed him to walk. **Right**, Standing radiographs of this boy's spine will vary from time to time, depending on the amount of pressure he applies to his crutches. In this situation, sitting radiographs are more reproducible.

ting unsupported either by his hands or by an attendant. Standing films can provide valuable information concerning the role played by leg-length discrepancy and pelvic tilt, but the variations in lower extremity brace wear and the degree of spine stretching provided by using crutches to stand makes the standing film less useful for following the progress of a scoliosis (Fig. 2, *right*). A sitting film is more reliably reproducible. Asymmetric hip abduction contractures can cause scoliosis. In such cases, a release of the contracture may be all that is needed to allow the spine to straighten.

Scoliotic spines in children with polio are much more flexible than those seen in idiopathic scoliosis, particularly in younger children. After about the age of 14, the curves tend to become rigid quickly. An increasing curve seen on upright films, which would ordinarily signal the need for surgery, can often be ignored temporarily in younger children. The indication for proceeding to surgery is not when progression is noted, but when stiffening becomes evident in a progressing curve.

Stabilizing the lumbar spine may decrease the patient's ability to walk, whether or not the sacrum is included. Children and parents not warned of this potential difficulty with walking will be justifiably upset if their child stops walking after a spine fusion. Loss of lumbar lordosis following spine surgery can be a major problem if the hip extensors are weak, because there is then no way for the child to lean back and get the mass of the trunk posterior to the hip joints. Every care must be taken to avoid this (Fig. 3).

If the child is a walker and the curve is greater that 30 degrees, is becoming rigid, or is progressing rapidly, then a thoracolumbosacral orthosis should be offered. If the child is only able to sit (rather than to walk) and needs to use his hands to support his trunk, posterior spine fusion should be offered.

In children between 10 years of age and puberty, curves of 30 to 50 degrees should be braced, if possible. Curves greater than 40 degrees that are progressing more than 5 degrees every four months should be fused. The attempt should be made to strike a balance between loss of flexibility caused by waiting too long and the loss of height caused by fusing too early. Clearly, sitters, for whom the final trunk length is less important, can be fused early.

If an older child is seen for the first time who has severe scoliosis and who is also a non-walker, but who could be converted into a walker with appropriate surgery, it is preferable to fuse the spine first, before doing the lower limb releases. If the legs are done first, getting such an older child up and walking may take many

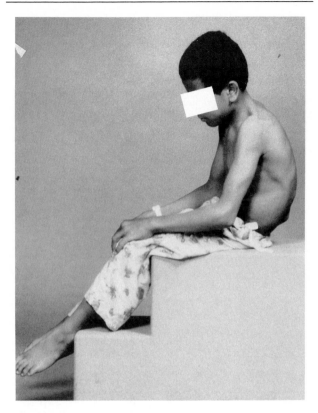

Fig. 3 This boy's spine was fused with lumbar kyphosis. Subsequently, sitting was difficult and walking impossible.

months (during which time the curve is worsening). Then, when the spinal surgery is finally undertaken, the process of learning to walk must be started all over.

Tuberculosis of the Bones and Joints

Tuberculosis has become the world's deadliest infectious disease, killing nearly three million individuals a year. Five percent of patients with tuberculosis have involvement of the bones or joints.

The increasing incidence of HIV infection has made the problem even more serious. In patients who are HIV negative, 5% of tuberculosis is skeletal (with a male to female ratio of 1 to 1). However, in patients who are HIV positive, 60% of tuberculosis is skeletal (with a male to female ratio of 9 to 1).

When tuberculosis involves the bones or joints, the most common site (50%) is in the spine. In the cervical spine the incidence is 5% (this is rare in children); in the thoracic spine it is 25%; and in the lumbar and lumbosacral spine it is 20%. The other common areas are the pelvis, 12%; the hip and femur, 10%; the knee and tibia, 10%; the ribs, 7%; the ankle, shoulder, elbow, and wrist, 2% each; and multiple (3 or more) bones, 3%.

The classic symptoms are pain together with fever and swelling (cold abscess). Radiographs usually show a loss of the normal planes in the soft tissues. Calcification is a late finding. The adjacent bones are frequently osteopenic, and periosteal reaction is usually minimal. In skeletally immature patients, the epiphysis may be enlarged. The joints commonly show areas of erosion, 80% of which is subchondral, 40% of which crosses the physis, and 60% of which crosses the joint. Cysts adjacent to the joints are very common. Joint narrowing is seen in most patients, but only to a slight or moderate degree.

The skin test for tuberculosis can be negative in 10% to 20% of cases, depending on the population and bacillus Calmette-Guerin usage in the country. Because bone or joint involvement is frequently associated with tuberculosis in the lungs (30%) and kidneys, it is prudent to include nonbone samples, such as sputum and urine, whenever taking cultures on these patients. Biopsy for bone and joint tuberculosis is most likely to be productive if a cyst is the site. When doing a biopsy, it is safest to do so under the cover of antituberculous drugs.

Treatment

Treatment of bone and joint tuberculosis is primarily by medicines. Isoniazid, administered at 10 to 20 mg per kg per day (not to exceed 300 mg), and rifampin, administered at 15 to 20 mg per kg per day, are the mainstays. Streptomycin, at 20 mg per kg per day, is added if local progression continues despite treatment or if there is a chronic cavity, because streptomycin demonstrates good penetration into diseased tissues. It is also added to treat such potentially fatal complications as milliary disease or meningitis. The length of drug treatment has been debated, but current recommendations are for the continuation of medication for nine months.

The role of surgery in the management of tuberculosis of the bones and joints is limited. Indications for nonspinal surgery, with the exception of the biopsy, are usually few.

The debate concerning the role of surgery for spinal tuberculosis centers on the issue of cure vs progressive kyphosis. Drugs alone can cure the tuberculosis. The problem is whether there is less disability if late progressive kyphosis can be prevented (Fig. 4).

The probability of late kyphosis depends on the site of the lesion, the age of the patient, and the extent of disease. Kyphosis is more likely to develop if the site of the problem is in the thoracic vertebrae (where there is already kyphosis) than if the site is the lumbar vertebrae (where the spine is already in lordosis). The age of the patient is also important. Because the underlying cartilaginous endplates may be spared, approximately 50% of children will improve their kyphosis. This is especially true in children younger than five years of age. Because destruction of more than two vertebrae portends trouble, a posterior fusion, followed by immobilization, is recommended in such cases.

The role of spinal surgery for tuberculosis also depends a great deal on which country is being considered. Spinal surgery is expensive both in terms of facilities and personnel and requires expertise on the part of the surgeons. Both money and personnel are in short supply in the very countries where tuberculosos is most rampant. There are the countries where patients frequently present late in their disease, compounding the problem. There can also be differences in cultural expectations from medical care—some peoples are less concerned with physical deformity than with cure. Conversely there can be great concern for the lack of marriageability of a daughter who is deformed.

If facilities allow, the absolute indications for spinal surgery are when, despite adequate drug therapy, there is onset of gradual paraplegia, the worsening of paraplegia, the persistence of motor loss after one month, or a severe paraplegia after six months. Uncontrolled spasticity and the onset of any sudden severe paraplegia are also absolute indications. Relative indications are the presence of paraplegia in the elderly (to minimize the related complications of recumbency) and the presence of persisting pain from root pressure or from spasticity.

Hansen's Disease (Leprosy)

Is it called Hansen's disease or leprosy? The term leprosy is well known—perhaps too well so, going back to biblical references. There has always been a dread of contracting the disease, even among professional health personnel. A recent survey in a western country showed that people fear contracting leprosy even more than they fear contracting AIDS. This fear and loathing of leprosy has resulted in a vigorous campaign by patients and their physicians to gain general acceptance for the term Hansen's disease, named for the Norwegian who first discovered the causative bacillus. Their hope is that the name change will lead to less isolation for patients and a greater likelihood that people afflicted with the problem will seek medical care sooner.

It is estimated that there are over 12 million patients in the world with Hansen's disease. Over one fourth of them have disabilities and, of these, half are severely involved.

Although Hansen's disease is a systemic infection, caused by *Mycobacterium leprae*, that has a predilection for skin and nerves, for the treating physician it is easiest to think of it as primarily a disease of the peripheral nerves. The incubation period, usually two to four years, can be from a few months to many years.

The clinical diagnosis of Hansen's disease turns on the finding of thickened peripheral nerves, of skin anesthesia, and of paralysis of muscles in the hands, feet,

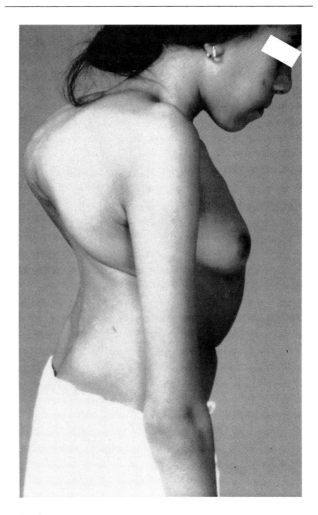

Fig. 4 Moderately severe thoracic kyphosis secondary to spinal tuberculosis in three mid-thoracic vertebrae.

or face. The documentation, by pathology, of the presence of inflammatory granulomas around a nerve or of nerve invasion by *M leprae* confirms the diagnosis.

There are two basic clinical types, and a third, intermediate, type. The lepromatous type is found when the host resistance is low. The organism slowly and insidiously destroys the nerve. In the tuberculoid type, host resistance is high, and nerve destruction appears to be secondary to an intense immune reaction. There may be abscess formation with fusiform or nodular swelling of the nerves. In the intermediate, borderline, type, there are varying degrees of hypersensitivity to the organism. The disease is generalized and many nerve trunks are affected. The deformities caused by nerve damage are the worst.

The nerve lesions can be: (1) purely sensory polyneuritis with the loss of light touch, pain, and temperature, which can be in a "glove-and-stocking" distribution; (2) a mixed sensory polyneuritis plus mononeuritis with paralysis in the peripheral distribution; or (3) purely mononeuritis, which is rare.

The nerves commonly involved are: (1) the ulnar nerve, above the elbow, which results in an intrinsic minus hand with clawing and the loss of pinch; (2) the peroneal nerve, at the fibular head, which causes foot drop; and (3) the posterior tibial nerve, at the medial malleolus, which results in a distal dissolution of the foot bones, associated with ulcers under metatarsal heads, or a proximal dissolution of the tarsal bones.

Treatment

In treating Hansen's disease, drugs are used to control the infection, and protection is provided for the anesthetic parts. Reconstruction is the same as that for the loss of any peripheral nerve function.

Dapsone, rifampin, and clofazimine are usually given for at least six months. Two drugs are usually used because of incidence of resistance, which is as high as 40% in some countries.

The orthopaedic management of hand involvement initially involves the provision of protection for the anesthetic parts. The items and techniques used, such as gloves, vary with local cultural acceptance. Surgery to replace absent power caused by the loss of nerve function is similar to that used to treat other paralyses. Tendon transfers should be splinted after surgery, because the anesthesia of the part makes the strong antagonists likely to disrupt repairs. For the feet, protection of the anesthetic part by proper shoe wear is necessary. Patients must be taught to inspect the soles of their feet. Immobilization, in a cast if needed, can be beneficial for foot ulcers. Surgical options for managing drop foot are the same as for other paralyses. Fusion of the tarsals is useful if disintegration is evident.

Chronic Osteomyelitis

Chronic osteomyelitis, a frequent problem in the third world, stems from poor transportation to health facilities and, often, from poor primary care. The causes of poor primary care can be the use of native medicine for the initial care or the misuse of antibiotics, for example, inadequate doses used for inadequate duration (perhaps because that is all that is available or affordable). All too frequently, the cause is inappropriate surgery resulting from closure of open fractures. Education of third world colleagues has, perhaps, the greatest potential benefit for improving care.

Treatment requires the use of simple and sound orthopaedic principles. Surgical debridement is far more important than antibiotics. Treatment must be aggressive, often involving opening the bone from end-to-end to allow it heal from inside to out. Open wounds can do well under a plaster cast (even while presenting a challenge to the olfactory sensibilities of all concerned), which allows many individuals to be treated as outpatients and avoids inundating the hospital facilities.

Education and History

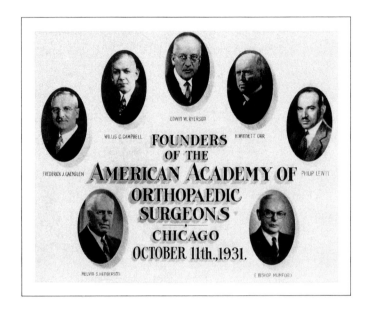

Making Orthopaedic Education Interactive, Problem Oriented, and on Target

James A. Farmer, Jr, EdD

Frederick G. Lippert III, MD

Michael F. Schafer, MD

Introduction

The stereotypic image of an orthopaedic educator lecturing to his residents and medical students falls far short of depicting the many tools, skills, and concepts used in modern orthopaedic education. The orthopaedic educator of today not only teaches but also is involved in planning curricula, evaluating courses, counseling, managing, and administering orthopaedic education in its various forms and settings. In addition to residents and medical students, the learners include patients, the public, attorneys, insurance providers, peer-review organizations, hospital administrators, medical-school deans, and committee members who deal with orthopaedics. In other words, the learners are a wide-ranging group who have varied needs and agendas. Nor is the educational setting limited to the classroom. More often the setting is in the clinical environment. In addition, the courtroom, interviews with the media, or a public forum may be involved. Clearly the format, techniques, and interactions differ, yet the tools, skills, and concepts of orthopaedic education are fundamental to each.

What then do orthopaedic educators need to know and be able to do? They must be able to involve the students and other faculty in the learning process. Interactive techniques facilitate this process. They must be able to structure the learning environment, incorporating the menu of available instructional technology, to suit the needs of learners. Orthopaedic educators must be able to set goals that are on target—goals that are consistent with the national perspective and standards of care. They must be able to evaluate the end product of orthopaedic education, to trouble shoot, and to make necessary modifications for improvement. To the extent that they communicate their intents with precision, they will enjoy more control over their educational environment.

Who should become an orthopaedic educator? Not everyone has the skill or interest to participate in any or all phases of orthopaedic education. One way to develop orthopaedic educators is to encourage and support those who demonstrate an interest. The goal is to assemble a group of orthopaedic educators who will communicate with each other and discuss ideas and problems. To become an orthopaedic educator one needs to be involved in some aspect of the learning process. Some key tools, skills, and concepts that will facilitate the learning process are presented in the following sections.

Modern Trends in Orthopaedic Education

Orthopaedic education begins in medical school, progresses through internship, residency, and/or fellowship, and continues throughout the surgeon's professional life. The traditional approach in medical school, in which the educational process consists of physical diagnosis lectures and clerkships, is being challenged on many fronts. With the increased scientific knowledge base required in all specialties, one skill the students need to learn is informatics, which is the ability to learn to use the tools that allow accessing the information necessary to solve a clinical problem—with or without the assistance of a computer. Decision-making skills, for example the ability to make a differential diagnosis and arrive at an appropriate treatment plan, are also essential. In addition to acquiring these skills and techniques, the student will still be exposed to the physical examination of the musculoskeletal system. Now, however, the core-knowledge base needed may have to be integrated, at least in part, into decision-making courses or incorporated into a multidisciplinary rotation with rheumatology or physical medicine and rehabilitation. The challenge of the 1990s will be to incorporate the core knowledge that must be gained into the overall medical-school curriculum without capitulation of specialized knowledge in musculoskeletal disorders.

The 1980s and 1990s provide a unique challenge to the orthopaedic educator. We are blessed with having the best and the brightest apply to our programs. In addition, the need-to-know information has expanded, and the technology of our field has become increasingly more sophisticated. With changes in the health-care system, the emphasis has switched from large volume inpatient services to smaller inpatient services, same day admissions, and increased outpatient surgery.

To meet these educational challenges, a subcommittee of the American Board of Orthopaedic Surgery, the American Orthopaedic Association, and the Association of Orthopaedic Chairmen has mounted a massive effort to develop a core curriculum. Such a core curriculum would serve as a guide for the program chairmen in identifying what the learners need to know and must be able to do and would help the chairmen in timing the meeting of these educational goals.

The American Academy of Orthopaedic Surgeons has been a valuable resource tool. The *Orthopaedic Knowledge Update* materials and the *Instructional Course Lectures* series provide needed information and give the national perspective. The Summer Institute Program provides valuable educational experience in both cognitive and psychomotor skills. Unfortunately, many program chairmen don't take advantage of this Summer Institute for the teaching of their residents.

The categorical committees of the American Academy of Orthopaedic Surgeons have sponsored many programs that have provided both cognitive and psychomotor instruction. With the development of a candidate membership organization, the cost of attending the courses has become more reasonable for the majority of residents.

However, the mainstay of our teaching is still the responsibility of the residency training program. The basic sciences must be integrated and repeated throughout the residency. In 1988, David Murray[1] compared the role of the orthopaedic surgeon in the operating room with that of a pilot. He defined two terms: safety window and situational awareness. The safety window in flying, which lasts about six minutes, involves takeoff, approach, and landing. More than 80% of airplane accidents occur during these six-minute periods. Focusing simulated training on these critical periods enhances the effectiveness of a pilot's educational program.

A similar safety window situation occurs in the operating room. However, here each surgical procedure consists of a series of "mini windows" that occur through the surgery. Although these experiences cannot be practiced in a simulator, the best surgeons actually prepare in a number of ways, including preoperative review of anatomy, reading about a technique, reviewing video tapes, or practicing with the equipment. A resident must be exposed to this thought process numerous times throughout his training. The attending surgeon can facilitate this experience and make it more meaningful.

Situational awareness, defined as the accurate perception of the factors and conditions that affect the patient and operating room personnel during the procedure, is multifaceted. It can involve the activity of the anesthesiologist and scrub nurse. It may involve the assessment of the equipment. Is the appropriate equipment available and does it work? This concept has been intuitively taught, but it is the attending surgeon's responsibility to instill this awareness in the resident.[2]

The *Orthopaedic In-Training Examination*, taken by all residents in the United States, provides a way of judging the cognitive performance of the residents and also of evaluating the effectiveness of the teaching program. This examination can serve as a powerful learning tool

with multiple spin-offs. It can lead to the formation of discussion groups for the questions or it can lead to the development of a literature search to support the answers.

During the last decade, fellowship programs have proliferated. Unfortunately, it appears that many of these programs are service oriented, instead of being educationally driven. In addition, many of the individuals taking these fellowships point out that they are doing so primarily to improve their own marketability. This situation has been discussed in two candidate-membership forums held in conjunction with the Annual Meeting of the American Academy of Orthopaedic Surgeons. Because of these factors, the Residency Review Committee will inspect the fellowship programs at the time of a residency program review. It is our feeling that this will help to bring the educational and service requirements into line.

In 1988, the American Academy of Orthopaedic Surgeons conducted an educational survey of the membership. The survey demonstrated that the average practicing orthopaedic surgeon spends ten hours or less per week on education. The written word is still the primary vehicle of learning. The survey did identify the need for more in-depth monograph discussion of topics. The Academy has since undertaken publication of a monograph series.

The *Orthopaedic Knowledge Update* materials are widely used to provide need-to-know information quickly. Because each of the *Orthopaedic Knowledge Update* series has been designed to build upon the preceding ones, the Academy has put the past editions, plus a selection of the articles included in reference lists, on a CD-ROM, which is available for purchase by the membership.

The *Self-Assessment Examination*, looked on as an excellent education tool, has had as its primary disadvantage the length of time that elapses between the taking of the examination and the receiving of the answers. The development of computer-assisted examinations will help close the learning loop and should enhance the educational experience.

The use of videotapes of procedures has also increased. The ability to have a procedure demonstrated by an expert has been identified as an important learning tool.

Because of the high expenses associated with multiday meetings, people have expressed a desire for single-day course offerings, preferably held on weekends, which would minimize the amount of time away from a practice and decrease the costs involved. The Academy's Education Committee has taken these factors into account when planning their educational programs.

In summary, the decade of the 1990s will continue a proliferation of knowledge that must be acquired by the orthopaedic surgeon. The use of journals, texts, computers, videotapes, and potentially interactive video will provide the means for home study. Our meetings must be carefully planned to provide the proper mix of cognitive and psychomotor skills. Truly, orthopaedic education is a lifelong experience.

Ways of Making Orthopaedic Education Interactive, Problem Based, and on Target

Innovations in orthopaedic education that do not make it more interactive, problem based, and on target are likely to be counterproductive and problematic. Most professional knowledge, including that concerning orthopaedic surgery, is situated, that is, it is developed over time, reconciled with relevant basic sciences, tested repeatedly in practice, and consensually validated within the profession. Most professional knowledge cannot merely be intuited, derived from logic, or deduced from the basic principles of general knowledge. This section will provide suggestions for making orthopaedic education valid and meaningful (on target) and for handling broad aims and specific objectives in orthopaedic education. It will also describe alternative ways of learning orthopaedics, including the use of guided inquiry and a relatively new technique called cognitive apprenticeship. It will also provide two tools recommended for use in orthopaedic education and will describe their use. These tools are called the cybernetic cycle and the curricular template.

Orthopaedic education is only valid and meaningful to the extent that it: (1) relates to what the learner is doing, needs to be able to do, or wants to be able to do in real life and/or examinations; (2) relates to the structures of knowledge of the learner; and (3) reflects the best of what is known currently about what is to be learned. On-going knowledge acquisition and skill attainment are necessary but are not, by themselves, sufficient to ensure satisfactory performance in orthopaedics. In orthopaedic education, knowledge and skills must be integrated into knowledge in action,[3] which includes, not just the what, but also the how, the when, and the why.[4]

Self-directed learning alone is a relatively unreliable way to acquire situated knowledge. Reception learning, which combines observing, hearing, and reading, is more reliable. Once situated professional knowledge has been attained, however, self-directed learning can be used to allow the learner to develop ways of gaining further knowledge within explicitly acceptable limits established by the profession and society.

Given the knowledge explosion and the immense amount of information that orthopaedic surgeons might need or want to know, there is increasing pressure on orthopaedic educators and learners alike to prioritize what is being taught and what learners seek to learn. It is becoming increasingly important to differentiate between the need to know, ought to know, nice to know, and interesting to know.

Professional and scientific knowledge relevant to orthopaedics moves ahead in a leap-frog manner. What was formerly current and up-to-date at the national level tends to be supplanted by newer information. Often, the supplanted knowledge is not gone but continues to exist at a less-than-current position. Answering the question about what an orthopaedic surgeon really needs to know only on a basis of personal preference, clinical experience, or what is most in fashion locally or regionally does not seem adequate. Of greater importance is what must be known as it is defined from the current national perspective.

So, the broad aim of orthopaedic education is to develop and maintain orthopaedic surgeons who have a currently accepted perspective and who are able to use currently accepted procedures proficiently. Maintenance is as important as development. Acquisition of prerequisite knowledge and attainment of skill alone do not mean that the broad aim has been achieved. Nor do increased learner confidence, positive learner satisfaction, and/or increased competencies per se mean that the broad aim has been achieved.

In oral and written communications about the objectives of orthopaedic education, we have found it important first to provide a significance statement. Such a statement explains why is is important for the learner to attain the knowledge, attitude, or skills specified in the objective. In other words, what will having done so enable the learner to do, and what negative consequences will having done so help the learner avoid? The objective should also specify what the learner is expected to be able to do, under what circumstances, to what level to be considered satisfactory, and according to whom or what.[5]

We have noted the following common errors in oral or written objectives relative to orthopaedic education: (1) stating them as directives, not as objectives (for example, "The residents will apply all casts in accordance with the department's casting manual" is a directive, not an objective.); (2) omitting one or more of the key elements (that is, significance statement, specification of what learners will be able to do, at what level, under what conditions, and to whose satisfaction); (3) developing trivial (nonsignificant) objectives; (4) developing objectives that are not feasible; (5) developing objectives that are too broad in scope; (6) specifying inappropriate content for the objective (for example, specifying knowledge acquisition or skill attainment alone when doing a procedure is intended); (7) specifying content that cannot be measured or observed; (8) focusing on content exposure rather than performance; and, (9) confusing the doing that is a part of the learning method with the doing that is the evidence of having learned what is intended. In the professions, being at a satisfactory level of performance is generally referred to as being "proficient." Proficiency is the ability to do something at least at a minimally satisfactory level (as that is currently defined at the national level), on one's own, while avoiding any difficulties that have been pointed out ahead of time.[6]

Alternative Ways of Learning Orthopaedics

Orthopaedics can be learned through: (1) reception learning (reading, observation, and listening); (2) autonomous (self-directed) learning; (3) guided inquiry; and (4) cognitive apprenticeship. The reader is probably familiar with reception and autonomous learning. The characteristics of guided inquiry and cognitive apprenticeship, which are less widely known, are described briefly below.

Guided Inquiry

This instructional mode[2,7] (process or technique for helping individuals learn) includes the following steps: (1) identifying a problem to be addressed; (2) setting the goal; (3) arraying relevant concepts and, when appropriate, materials; (4) having the learners relate (1) and (3) under guidance, with the instructor providing feedback, until the learners achieve comprehension; (5) evaluating the product and process; and (6) discussion. All of these steps in guided inquiry, except for the fourth one, can be done with or without the help of the learners.

In essence, guided inquiry is an inductive process, because the learners are expected to solve the problem themselves. If the instructor solved the problem for the learners instead of merely providing them with feedback, then the process would be deductive. In other words, it would become a type of reception learning.

Cognitive Apprenticeship

This relatively new form of instruction[8,9] has been found to be a particularly efficient method for teaching clinical orthopaedics.[10]

Cognitive apprenticeship combines and sequences reception learning (particularly seeing and hearing), guided inquiry, and autonomous (self-directed) learning. The six phases in cognitive apprenticeship are: Phase 1: The learner brings to the cognitive apprenticeship experience all past experience and previously acquired knowledge, attitudes, and skills. Phase 2: The procedure to be learned is demonstrated by someone who is already proficient. The demonstrator articulates the thought processes that go along with the procedure, including, if appropriate, any tricks (domain-specific heuristics) that may simplify the procedure. Phase 3: The learner attempts the procedure under scaffolded conditions, also articulating the thought processes that accompany the procedure. The demonstrator from phase 2 coaches and provides remedial instruction as necessary. Phase 4: As the learner demonstrates increased ability to accomplish the procedure unassisted, the amount of scaffolding and coaching is lessened. (This transition is called "fading" in cognitive apprenticeship.) Phase 5: The learner practices alone or with other learners (cooperative learning), doing the procedure in his or her own way within predetermined, acceptable limits. Phase 6: The instructor and the learner finally discuss ways in which what has been learned during this cognitive apprenticeship experience can be applied to other tasks or procedures.

At the heart of cognitive apprenticeship is the demonstration, or modeling, by someone proficient in doing the procedure, who comments on what is being done and why. Any prerequisite or enriching knowledge, attitudes, or skills from the sciences, disciplines, applied fields, or elsewhere taught prior to the modeling of the real thing is kept to a minimum. This is in keeping with the cognitive, holistic, or top-down approach to instruction. Such an approach is intended to let the learner see what a procedure or process looks like, rather than teaching prerequisite knowledge, attitudes, skills, or competencies. It assumes that the learner will know the significance of learning these prerequisites and will eventually be able to apply them.

After watching and listening to the demonstrator, the learner is asked to approximate doing the procedure while verbalizing what is being done and why. Scaffolding and coaching are provided by the instructor. Additional prerequisites are taught as necessary, based on the difficulties evidenced as the learner carried out a scaffolded performance while approximating the procedure.

The individual learner or groups of learners then continue to approximate the procedure, as less guidance and scaffolding are provided as warranted by learner performance. The learner can then practice the procedure in his or her own way (self-directed learning) within predetermined limits.

Recommended Tools

To help make orthopaedic education meaningful, relevant, and valid from the perspective of the learners, the orthopaedic community, and academia, we recommend using the cybernetic cycle and the curricular template.

Cybernetic Cycle

In using the cybernetic cycle, aim is determined first. More specific aims, purposes, goals, and objectives, which are derived from the broad aim, can then be identified.

For example, the broad aim for an orthopaedic residency program may be to graduate residents who are generally proficient in understanding and dealing with musculoskeletal problems. A specific aim may be that each graduate who wishes to do so will have considerable additional knowledge and experience in dealing with at least one specific type of musculoskeletal problem. A specific objective may be that each graduate will be proficient in the use of the arthroscope.

Next, through the use of questionnaires and pretests, or by other means, information is collected about the residents. This information is used to revise the objectives. A particular resident or group of residents, for example, may have special needs or interests that the residency program is able and willing to accommodate. The curriculum can be revised accordingly and instruction provided. On-going evaluation will help all concerned know the nature and extent of progress being made toward achieving the specific aims and objectives of the program within the broad aim. It may also indicate ways of improving the program.

If circumstances change or if evaluative efforts show that the program is not working satisfactorily, the broad aim and specific aims, purposes, goals, and objectives can be revised.

The cybernetic cycle works like a heat-seeking missile (not like a rifle shot) in that it seeks out and corrects for the changing target rather than hoping that the initial aim will hit the valid target. Knowledge, attitudes, skills, and performance change constantly. Learners may look the same but are not.[11]

The faculty of the American Academy of Orthopaedic Surgeons's annual Basic Educator's course uses the cybernetic cycle in an annual up-date process. The cybernetic cycle can also be used in designing, developing, implementing, and evaluating courses, programs, and clinics in which orthopaedics is taught.

Curricular Template

The Curricular Template[11] was developed to help orthopaedic educators design courses or programs. In developing a course or program, several key decisions must be made. The Curricular Template indicates the nature of those key decisions and recommends a sequence for making them. Some decisions involve selecting an appropriate point on a continuum. Other decisions involve selecting an appropriate blend of elements.

The following brief explanation of the decision points that make up the curricular template includes instructions for how each is to be handled.

Driving Factors Identify factors that explain the importance of learning what is to be taught. For example, learning may be essential to providing quality of care or it may be of importance for economic reasons.

Topic—Boundaries of Topic Specify at this point what is to be taught. In specifying the boundaries, define the topic and give examples of what is and is not to be covered in the course or program.

Course Participants Specify the percentage of nonor-

thopaedic specialists, academic orthopaedic surgeons (including orthopaedic residents), and nonacademic orthopaedic surgeons who are expected to be in the course or program. The blend of participants can affect what is taught and how it is taught.

Extent of Participant Involvement Decide the extent to which there is to be high or low participant involvement in the course of program development. Reasons for participant involvement include: (1) to be able to identify and meet student needs; (2) to obtain student perspective on objectives, subject matter content, and learning experiences; (3) to motivate the students, for by incorporating students' suggestions the program becomes their own; (4) to build on the experiences and expertise of the class members; (5) to anticipate and resolve differences about new ideas and procedures you may wish to incorporate into the program; and (6) to build group morale and to provide a favorable climate for learning.

Reasons against participant involvement include: (1) it is more efficient to make a unilateral decision than to attempt to get a group consensus; (2) students have had limited experience with subject matter; (3) planning for the many interests of students can diffuse the learning effort; (4)adult students have a greater resistance to change; and (5) exposure to student-determined procedures may threaten the teacher's authority.

Broad Aim Describe the broad aim of the course or program.

Need to Know or to Do Decide whether the reason it is important to learn what is taught in the course or program is because of its relevance to general orthopaedic practice, to specialized orthopaedic practice, to exams or boards, or to some combination of these.

Pretests Decide whether a written, oral, situational, problem-solving, self-reporting, or other form of pretest is to be used to determine the extent to which the learners already know or are able to do what is to be taught in the course or program.

Specify Objectives Specify the main objectives. As indicated above, we recommend that objectives include a significance statement along with a specification of what the learners will be able to do after the course or program, under what conditions, how good their performance must be to be satisfactory, and who or what is to judge performance.

Curriculum Content Decide to what extent the content in the course or program is to contain theories from the disciplines or sciences, generalizations about orthopaedic surgery, and/or descriptions of or experience in the practice of orthopaedic surgery.

Content and the Uses of Knowledge Decide to what extent what is to be learned in the course or program is to be used tacitly and/or explicitly. A tacit use of knowledge requires one to have a general understanding of what is learned but not a working knowledge of it. An explicit use of knowledge includes the ability to apply that knowledge in the way it is intended to be used.

Clinical Problems Decide to what extent the course or program will teach how to understand and deal with well-defined, moderately well-defined, and/or ill-defined orthopaedic problems. A well-defined problem is one for which there is a diagnosis and treatment of choice. A moderately well-defined problem can be handled by making a differential diagnosis and arriving at an appropriate treatment plan. Problems other than these are ill defined by definition.

Types of Learning Decide what percentages of the course or program will be devoted to autonomous learning, reception learning, guided inquiry, and/or cognitive apprenticeship.

Modalities Select modalities, such as journal club, lecture, or demonstration, to be used in the course or program.

Experience Decide during what percentage of the course or program you intend to have the learners engage in concrete experiences, reflective observation, abstract conceptualization, and/or experimentation.

Instructors Decide what percentage of the instructors are to be basic scientists, orthopaedists, allied health personnel, and/or others.

Tests Decide what percentage of the testing, if any, in the course or program is to be done by formal tests, problem solving, demonstration or performance, oral recall, and/or other means.

Evaluation Decide what percentage of evaluation of the course or program is to be: informal and/or formal; formative (to improve the course or program) and/or summative (to decide whether or not to repeat it, and if so, at what level); and internal (evaluated by the instructors and learners) and/or external (evaluated by outside experts).

The Curricular Template can be used to help make courses and programs in orthopaedic education on target. Increasing participant involvement can make the course more interactive (responsive to the learners' needs) as can the use of cooperative learning.[12] Relating what is taught to solving well-defined, moderately well-defined, and/or ill-defined orthopaedic problems, as well as teaching how to deal with such problems proficiently through the use of cognitive apprenticeship, can help make the course or program more problem based.

References

1. Murray DG: Aircraft management, OR management, and the surgical safety window. *Bull Am Coll Surg* 1988;73(7):13–15.
2. Ausubel DP, Novak JD, Hanesian H: *Educational Psychology-A Cognitive View*, ed 2. New York, Holt, Rinehart & Winston, 1978.
3. Ruesch J: *Knowledge in Action*. New York, Jason Aronson, 1975.
4. West CK, Farmer JA, Wolff PM: *Instructional Design: Implications from Cognitive Science*. Englewood Cliffs, Prentice Hall, 1991.
5. Mager RF: *Preparing Objectives for Instructions*, ed 2. Belmont, CA, Fearon, 1975.
6. Lippert FG III, Farmer JA: *Psychomotor Skills in Orthopaedic Surgery*. Baltimore, Williams & Wilkins, 1984.
7. Gagne RM: *The Conditions of Learning*, ed 2. New York, Holt, Rinehart & Winston, 1970.
8. Brown JS, Collins A, Duguid P: Situated cognition and the culture of learning. *Educational Researcher* 1989;18A:32–43.
9. Collins A, Brown JS, Newman SE: Cognitive apprenticeship: Teaching the craft of reading, writing, and mathematics in Resnick LB (ed): *Cognition and Instruction: Issues and Agendas*. Hillsdale, Lawrence Erlbaum Associates, in press.
10. Johnson AL, Farmer JA: Teaching veterinary surgery in the operating room. *JVME* 1989;16A:11–14.
11. Lippert FG, Farmer JA, Schafer MF: *Handbook for Orthopedic Educators*, ed 12. Park Ridge, American Academy of Orthopaedic Surgeons Committee on Graduate Education, 1990.
12. Johnson DW, Johnson RT: *Learning Together and Alone: Cooperation, Competition, and Individualization*. Englewood Cliffs, NJ, Prentice Hall, 1987.

What We Have Learned From the Wars

Leonard F. Peltier, MD, PhD

Introduction

We should begin any discussion of what we have learned from the wars by reviewing how these lessons have been taught. Before the late 1700s, wars were fought by small professional armies whose medical services were for the most part primitive or nonexistent. While kings, princes, great nobles, and generals included surgeons in the entourage that accompanied them to the wars, the rank and file had no organized medical services. Such surgeons as there were learned their trade by experience or by serving an apprenticeship. Ambroise Paré gives an anecdotal account of his experiences in such a system.[1] It was not until large armies conscripted from the general population became the rule that organized military medical services came into being. Surgeons to provide these services came from the general population also. The differences between civilian and military practice were and remain substantial, and, because of this, all military medical services have developed strong educational components to teach those skills that, although of small value in civilian practice, are vital to the military.

One of the greatest of the military medical educators was Dominique Jean Larrey, surgeon to the revolutionary armies of France and to Napoleon.[2] Between campaigns, during winter encampment, and at every opportunity, he held instructional courses for the young medical officers in which he, among other things, outlined the principles of debridement and wound care. Over the long period of these wars, physicians from almost every country in Europe served under Napoleon's aegis, which made the impact of Larrey's program very important. Larrey, like Paré, has left a good account of his experiences during this turbulent period.[3]

At the outset of the American revolution, civilian physicians were poorly prepared for their role as military medical officers. To help educate them for military service, John Jones, a surgeon in New York, wrote a surgical textbook entitled, "Plain Concise Remarks on the Treatment of Wounds and Fractures to Which is added, a Short Appendix on Camp and Military Hospitals; principally designed for the use of young military surgeons in North America."[4] This little volume has the distinction of being the first book on surgery written in this country, and its appendix is the first American work on public health and hygiene.[5] It is the progenitor of all subsequent surgical manuals written for our

armed forces. First published in 1775, it summarized the best surgical opinion of the day in a simple and useful way.

The American Civil War produced a flurry of books directed to the newly mobilized medical officers in the Union and Confederate armies.[6-9] One of the most enduring is that of Silas Weir Mitchell, George Morehouse, and William W. Keen,[10] which contains a clear description of causalgia. This work was made possible by the policy of directing the injured to special hospitals where large numbers of patients with similar injuries could be concentrated and studied. After the war, a massive report was published, which described the medical and surgical care rendered to the soldiers.[11] This exhaustive compilation was patterned after the report made by the British War Office after the Crimean War.[12] Similar reports were published after World Wars I and II.[13,14] Publications such as these provide a mine of information about the types of problems encountered in military service in war time and provide good follow-up studies of the end results of treatment.

During times of peace, mobilization, and war, the military services continually train their personnel by means of directives and instructional courses. The establishment of the Uniformed Services University of Health Sciences has resulted in the formation of a nidus of military medical educators whose task is to provide instructional services for the armed forces. The Society of Military Surgeons promotes programs where new developments of importance in military surgery are presented.

Shock

The syndrome of "shock" was studied intensively during World War I, but no clear explanation of the phenomena was forthcoming. The experiments of Bayliss and Cannon,[15] who concluded that shock was caused by the absorption of some toxic depressant substance from the area of injury, were given the most credibility. The concept that shock resulted from the loss of blood and fluid into the local sites of injury was discounted. The work of Alfred Blalock,[16] carried out at Vanderbilt during the 1930s, put the toxic theory of shock to rest and clearly demonstrated that shock caused by trauma results from the sequestration of large amounts of blood and fluid in the area of the wound. At the onset of World War II, it was believed that shock could be effectively treated by volume expansion with plasma, plasma substitutes, and fluids alone. The report of the Board for the Study of the Severely Wounded in the North African-Mediterranean,[17] often called "the Beecher Report" after its author Henry K. Beecher, a professor of anesthesiology at Harvard, concluded that transfusion of whole blood was superior to the use of plasma and fluids alone. The studies of the United States Army's Surgical Research Team of Korea, headed by Curtis P. Artz, demonstrated again the value of giving large amounts of whole blood throughout the period of resuscitation and treatment of the seriously injured.[18] These studies have had an enormous influence on civilian practice.

Blood Transfusion

Although the value of transfusion of whole blood from human donors into patients in "collapse" as a result of hemorrhage was known before 1900, it was not until introduction of sodium citrate, as an anticoagulant, and the discovery of the four major blood types, that the clinical use of blood transfusions in medical practice became feasible.[19,20] The experience with the use of blood transfusion for the severely wounded in World War I was not extensive, but it did demonstrate to physicians and the public that such a technique was practical. It was not until the Spanish Civil War (1936–1939) that a system for supplying front-line installations with fresh bank blood was developed on a large scale. While not the originator, one of the major proponents and publicists for the system developed by the Republic Army Medical Corps was the Canadian surgeon Norman Bethune (1890–1939), who later earned the veneration of the Chinese and is the only westerner buried in the Chinese pantheon.[21] This system is well described by Trueta.[22] World War II programs in the military services profited by this experience. Late in the war transfusion services became very extensive, especially in the Pacific Theater.[23] There is no question that the development of civilian blood banks and large numbers of willing donors are the direct result of the programs organized by the armed forces in World War II.

Therapeutic Use of Oxygen

Although Roswell Park[24] had urged that oxygen be used to treat fat embolism as early as 1884, its use in hospitals was very limited because of the lack of proper apparatus to deliver the gas.[24] During World War I there was great concern regarding the management of victims of poison gas and carbon monoxide. John S. Haldane,[25,26] a British physician and physiologist, who had developed a method of analyzing respiratory gases

as early as 1892, introduced into hospital use a metered system by which oxygen could be delivered to patients through a mask. In his article, Haldane warned of the risk of the prolonged administration of pure oxygen. The establishment of the United States Air Force School of Aerospace Medicine in January 1918 provided for the continued study of the effects of high altitude flying and the development of methods of administering oxygen and other gases.[27] The use of the Boothby-Lovelace-Bulbulian (BLB) mask, developed at the Mayo Clinic, became commonplace in hospitals and in aviation prior to World War II.[28,29]

Treatment of Fractures

One of the most important developments in the treatment of fractures to emerge from World War I was so subtle and simple that it frequently has been overlooked. That is the use of the Thomas splint. This splint, devised by Hugh Owen Thomas in 1875 for the treatment of tuberculosis of the knee, was also used by him to treat fractures of the femur. It was introduced into the British army medical service on the western front by Robert Jones, Thomas's nephew, in 1915. Early in World War I, the mortality from shock and sepsis in cases of open fracture of the femur in the British forces was an appalling 80%! Then the Thomas splint was introduced into the front lines, and by 1917 this mortality had been reduced to less than 16%.[30] This traction splint limited local blood loss into the extremity by tightening the fascial envelope and by using local pressure to restrict the bleeding. After World War I, the use of the Thomas splint in civilian emergency services gradually became standard. It was widely used by military services in World War II, the Korean War, and the Vietnam War. It has been superseded by the improvements incorporated in the Hare splint, a traction splint designed by a San Diego police officer, Glenn Hare, in 1967.[31]

The large numbers of open fractures seen during wartime have provided an opportunity to study and evaluate many methods of wound care. The principles of debridement enunciated by Pierre Joseph Desault at the Hotel Dieu in Paris in 1790 were tested and taught to medical officers all over Europe during the Revolutionary and Napoleonic Wars by Larrey, one of his students.[32] Like many other basic principles, debridement was neglected and had to be rediscovered again during World War I. By the end of this war, there was a clear understanding of what the procedure of debridement was all about.

"In performing debridement an anatomic dissection should be done. The skin and subcutaneous tissues should be incised over the wound track and the tissues exposed by sharp dissection, down to the tissue which is evidently devitalized. Devitalization is indicated by hemorrhagic infiltration of the muscle, and by failure to contract and bleed when pinched with tissue forceps or cut. Muscle, the seat of gas gangrene, has a peculiar waxy appearance and is rigid. It looks somewhat like muscle which has been boiled a short while. Muscle which is the seat of such changes should be entirely removed.''[33]

This surgical procedure forms the basis for the treatment of all sorts of wounds and must be a part of the repertoire of all surgeons, military or civilian.

Bitter experience has taught that war wounds and dirty open fractures in civilian practice cannot be primarily closed safely. Local care must be directed toward preparing the wound for delayed primary closure or secondary closure. Two diametrically opposed methods of wound care were developed in World War I.

The first, the continuous irrigation of the wound with a dilute solution of a buffered hypochlorite (Dakin's solution), was initiated by the surgeon Alexis Carrel and Henry D. Dakin, a biochemist.[34] Their irrigation device consisted of a rather complex system of small perforated rubber tubes used to distribute the solution throughout the depths of the wound. The wounds were dressed daily and cultures were taken. When the bacterial count dropped to a low level, the wound was ready for secondary closure. This method was labor intensive and posed real problems for the immobilization of associated fractures. It made the transfer of patients from hospital to hospital very difficult and required long periods of hospitalization. It was used to some extent in civilian practice but was slowly abandoned because of these problems. This system was the early prototype of all of the drip and drip-suck systems that have been used since that time, employing the original Dakin's solution or solutions of antibiotics.

The second, the closed plaster method, was developed by H. Winnett Orr[35,36] on the basis of his experience with the treatment of open fractures at a base hospital in France. After thorough debridement, the wound was packed with a sterile vasoline gauze pack, and the fractured extremity was enveloped in a plaster dressing. These wounds were left undisturbed for weeks at a time and often were allowed to granulate in from below so that secondary closure could be quite simple. The smell was the major inconvenience of this method and Dr. Orr was once quoted as saying: ''When the nurses can't stand the smell any more, send the patient home, but don't change the plaster.'' Orr carried his experience into civilian life and used his method with great success to treat acute and chronic hematogenous osteomyelitis.

In 1934, Jose Trueta revived the closed plaster method for treating open fractures. The onset of the Spanish Civil War gave him an opportunity to test his method, which was quite similar to that of Orr's except that dry gauze was substituted for the vasoline gauze pack.[22] The Orr-Trueta method for the closed plaster

treatment of open fractures had a very broad application in the treatment of the wounded in World War II. It was not labor intensive. It did not interfere with the transfer of patients. It was simple enough that when there were mass casualties they could be treated literally on an assembly line.[37] As experience accumulated, it was learned that delayed primary closure or secondary closure could be done early, which shortened the healing period significantly. This technique remains a valuable one in civilian practice, particularly when sophisticated facilities are not available and when there are mass casualties.

It should be remembered that the use of plaster of Paris dressings in the treatment of fractures was developed by two military surgeons, Antonius Mathijsen and Nikolai Ivanovitch Pirogov, and employed extensively by the latter during the Crimean War.[38] Its use for the treatment of fractures became widespread in civilian hospitals and led to the development of the ambulatory management of fractures of the lower extremities. In France, Pierre Delbet's plaster of Paris splint for the treatment of ankle and tibial fractures was widely used during World War I. Lorenz Bohler in Vienna elevated the use of plaster of Paris to a fine art, and his closed methods of fracture treatment dominated this area of therapeutics until well after World War II. In the United States, the use of plaster of Paris in the ambulatory treatment of fractures was championed in the military by Ernst Dehne and in civilian practice by Augusto Sarmiento.[39,40] Such methods were proven to be safe, were easy to apply to both closed and open fractures, and were economical, both in cost of materials and in personnel.

Little has been learned from wars regarding the use of external skeletal fixation or the internal fixation of fractures, except that these methods have a very limited role in the management of military casualties. These techniques require optimum operating facilities, an extensive armamentarium, and especially skilled personnel. Complications that can result from a failure of the methods are costly in terms of life and limb. For these reasons, in mass casualty situations reliance should be placed upon the simplest and safest effective methods of treatment.

Vascular Injuries

In 1902, Alexis Carrel[41] developed the suture method of blood vessel anastomosis, for which he received the Nobel Prize. The technique was widely used in the laboratory for years before it was applied clinically on a large scale. At the end of World War II, Michael E. DeBakey and Fiorindo A. Simeone[42] published an analysis of 2,471 cases of vascular injury and reviewed the experience with such injuries in previous wars. The reported incidence of such injuries was small, perhaps because of underreporting. It is surprising to note that in only 81 of their 2,471 cases was the performance of an arterial suture recorded. The amputation rate following ligation of the arteries was 48.9%. In the very few cases in which vein grafts or tube anastomoses were attempted, the amputation rate was even higher. In the 81 cases in which suture repair was attempted, the amputation rate was 35.8%.

In the short period between the end of World War II and the Korean War, a revolution occurred in vascular surgery. Frank C. Spencer, the current President of the American College of Surgeons, and his colleague Ray V. Grewe, demonstrated as young medical officers in Korea that methods of vascular repair could be applied to war casualties. They reported the results in the management of 97 arterial injuries in 85 patients.[43] They were able to repair 89 of the injuries, and ligated the artery in only eight. Their overall amputation rate was 22%. In a review of the results of arterial repair in the Korean War, Carl W. Hughes reported that in 304 patients with arterial injuries, 269 were repaired with an amputation rate of 13%, while in the 35 patients treated by ligation the amputation rate was 51.4%.[44] The results of the treatment of such injuries in the Vietnam War were even better. The amputation rate had dropped to 13.5%.[45] What is most interesting about the report by Norman M. Rich and his colleagues[45] is that these results were obtained, not by a small special team of surgeons, but by more than 400! You can be sure that these young surgeons returned to their homes with experience and skills that have benefited their civilian patients. The long-term follow-up studies pursued by Norman M. Rich in the Vietnam Vascular Registry have helped to clarify the role of venous ligation carried out concomitantly with arterial ligation.[46] The value of this procedure has been debated for decades. It appears from these studies that sparing the vein or venous reconstruction is preferable to ligation.

Conclusion

In times of war, the United States has always depended on the mobilization of a largely civilian military force for its security. The medical portion of this force also, for the most part, comes from and returns to civilian practice. As special skills are brought into the service, so too, do special experiences return. One of the hardest qualities to estimate is the quality of leadership forged in the stress of service. While no one has made a study of the orthopaedists who served in World War II, Korea, and Vietnam, we know a good deal about the fate of those orthopaedic surgeons who served in the American Expeditionary Force in France in World War I. Fourteen of them became presidents of the American Orthopaedic Association, six were presidents of the American Academy of Orthopaedic Surgeons,

and 28 became distinguished professors of orthopaedic surgery.[47]

References

1. Paré A: *The Apologie and Treatise of Ambroise Pare, Containing the Voyages Made Into Divers Places, With Many of His Writings Upon Surgery.* Edited and with an introduction by Geoffrey Keynes. Chicago, University of Chicago Press, 1952.
2. Richardson RG: *Larrey DJ: Surgeon to Napoleon's Imperial Guard.* London, John Murray Ltd, 1974.
3. Larrey DJ: *Memoires de Chirurgie Militaire et Campagnes.* Paris, J Smith, 1812–1817.
4. Peltier LF: Jones J: An extraordinary American. *Surgery* 1966; 59:631–635.
5. Jones J: *Plain, Concise, Practical Remarks on the Treatment of Wounds and Fractures; to which is added an appendix, on camp and military hospitals.* Philadelphia, R Bell, 1776.
6. Gross SD: *A Manual of Military Surgery.* Philadelphia, JB Lippincott, 1861.
7. Hamilton FH: *A Practical Treatise on Military Surgery.* New York, Bailliere Brothers, 1861.
8. Chisholm JJ: *A Manual of Military Surgery.* Richmond, West & Johnston, 1861.
9. Tripler CS, Blackman G: *Hand-book for the Military Surgeon.* Cincinnati, R Clarke & Co, 1861.
10. Mitchell SW, Morehouse G, Keen WW: *Gunshot Wounds: And Other Injuries of Nerves.* Philadelphia, JB Lippincott, 1864.
11. United States, Surgeon-General's Office: *The Medical and Surgical History of the War of the Rebellion, (1861–65).* Washington, DC, U.S. Government Printing Office, 1870–1888, vols 1–6.
12. Great Britain, War Office, Medical Services: *Medical and Surgical History of the British Army Which Served in Turkey and the Crimea During the War Against Russia, in the Years 1854–6.* London, Harrison & Sons, 1858, vols 1–2.
13. United States, Surgeon-General's Office: *The Medical Department of the United States Army in the World War.* Washington, DC, U.S. Government Printing Office, 1921–29, vols 1–17.
14. United States, Army Medical Service: *The Medical Department of the United States Army in World War II.* Washington, D.C., Office of the Surgeon General, Department of the Army, 1952.
15. Bayliss WM, Cannon WB: Sections IV, V, and VI, in Medical Research Committee: *Report VIII: Traumatic Toxaemia as a Factor in Shock, Special Report Series No. 26.* London, HM Stationery Office, 1919.
16. Blalock A: *Principles of Surgical Care, Shock and Other Problems.* St. Louis, CV Mosby, 1940.
17. United States Army, Mediterranean Theater of Operations, the Board for the Study of the Severely Wounded: *The Physiologic Effects of Wounds.* Washington, DC, Office of the Surgeon General, Dept. of the Army, 1952.
18. Prentice TC, Olney JM Jr, Artz CP, et al: Studies of blood volume and transfusion therapy in the Korean battle casualty. *Surg Gynecol Obstetr* 1954;99:542–554.
19. Lewisohn R: Blood transfusion: 50 years ago and today. *Surg Gynecol Obstetr* 1955;101:362–368.
20. Landsteiner K: Zur Kenntnis der antifermentativen, lytischen und agglutinierenden Wirkungen des Blutserums und der Lymphe. *Zentralbl Bakteriol* 1900;28:357–362.
21. Allan T, Gordon S: *The Scalpel, the Sword: The Story of Dr. Norman Bethune.* Boston, Little, Brown, 1952.
22. Trueta J: *The Principles and Practice of War Surgery, With Reference to the Biological Method of the Treatment of War Wounds and Fractures.* St. Louis, CV Mosby, 1943.
23. Kendrick DB: *Blood Program in World War II.* Washington, DC, Office of the Surgeon General, Dept. of the Army, 1964.

24. Park R: On fat embolism, in *Selected Papers, Surgical and Scientific From the Writings of Roswell Park.* Buffalo, privately printed, 1914, pp 54–65.

25. Haldane JS: A new form of apparatus for measuring the respiratory exchange of animals. *J Physiol* 1892;13:419–430.

26. Haldane JS: The therapeutic administration of oxygen. *Br Med J* 1917;1:181–183.

27. Peyton G: *Fifty Years of Aerospace Medicine.* Brooks Air Force Base, TX, US Air Force School of Aerospace Medicine, 1968.

28. Lovelace WR Jr: Oxygen for therapy and aviation: An apparatus for the administration of oxygen or oxygen and helium by inhalation. *Proc Mayo Clin* 1938;13:646–654.

29. Bulbulian AH: Design and construction of the masks for oxygen inhalation apparatus. *Proc Mayo Clin* 1938;13:654–656.

30. Sinclair M: *The Thomas Splint and Its Modifications in the Treatment of Fractures.* London, Oxford University Press, 1927.

31. Weber D: S.D. Officer Makes New Type of Splint. *The San Diego Union*, Wednesday morning, Nov 8, 1967.

32. Reichert FL: The historical development of the procedure termed débridement. *Bull John Hopkins Hosp* 1928;42:93–104.

33. Lewis DD: Débridement. *JAMA* 1919;73:377–383.

34. Carrel A, Dehelly D: *The Treatment of Infected Wounds.* New York, Paul B Hoeber, 1917.

35. Orr HW: *Osteomyelitis and Compound Fractures and Other Infected Wounds.* St. Louis, CV Mosby, 1929.

36. Orr HW: *Wounds and Fractures: A Clinical Guide to Civil and Military Practice.* Springfield, IL, Charles C Thomas, 1941.

37. Yudin SS: The treatment of war fractures of the femur. *Surg Gynecol Obstetr* 1944;78:1–8.

38. Peltier LF: *Fractures: A History and Iconography of Their Treatment.* San Francisco, Norman Publishing, 1990.

39. Dehne E, Metz CW, Deffer PA, et al: Nonoperative treatment of the fractured tibia by immediate weight bearing. *J Trauma* 1961; 1:514–535.

40. Sarmiento A, Latta LL: *Closed Functional Treatment of Fractures.* Berlin, Springer-Verlag, 1981.

41. Carrel A: La technique opératoire des anastomoses vasculaires et la transplantation des viscères. *Lyon Med* 1902;98:859–864.

42. DeBakey ME, Simeone FA: Battle injuries of the arteries in World Ward II: An analysis of 2,471 cases. *Ann Surg* 1946;123:534–579.

43. Spencer FC, Grewe RV: The management of arterial injuries in battle casualties. *Ann Surg* 1955;141:304–313.

44. Hughes CW: Arterial repair during the Korean War. *Ann Surg* 1958;147:555–561.

45. Rich NM, Baugh JH, Hughes CW: Acute arterial injuries in Vietnam: 1,000 cases. *J Trauma* 1970;10:359–369.

46. Rich NM: Principles and indications for primary venous repair. *Surgery* 1982;91:492–496.

47. Peltier LF: The Division of Orthopaedic Surgery in the A.E.F.: a.k.a. The Goldthwait Unit. *Clin Orthop* 1985;200:45–49.

The History of the American Academy of Orthopaedic Surgeons

Edward D. Henderson, MD

We are indebted to Charles V. Heck, MD, the Academy's first Director, for a detailed history of the organization. His book, entitled *Fifty Years of Progress*, was published by the Academy in 1983 on the fiftieth anniversary of the first meeting of the Academy and during the presidency of David G. Murray. The book reflects Dr. Heck's intense interest in the organization and its ramifications and in the interrelationships of its various departments and committees.

The Beginnings

The American Orthopaedic Association is a venerable organization, founded in 1887 by 14 orthopaedic surgeons. By the turn of the century, it was well established and prestigious. It was and remains an organization whose membership is limited and where membership is by invitation only. During the early part of this century, the Central States Orthopaedic Society (later Clinical Orthopaedic Society) was formed under the leadership of John Porter of Chicago and, under the leadership of Albert Freiberg of Cincinnati, the Orthopaedic Section of the American Medical Association was formed. During those years the American Orthopaedic Association grew, but its membership was limited to 100. Despite the fact that members were allowed to invite guests to the annual meetings, there was a considerable amount of dissatisfaction among those not invited to become members. Another problem, which became more serious as the years went on, was that the president of the American Orthopaedic Association was expected to pay the expenses of the annual banquet from his own pocket. At the meeting held in April of 1931 only 60 members were present, but there were 165 guests. This total of 225 surgeons attending the meeting brought the problems of the American Orthopaedic Association to a head, and a committee was formed to decide what to do about the number of guests attending the meetings.

At the same time, some members of the American Orthopaedic Association were concerned about those who had not been invited to join, and there was a growing feeling that a national organization open to all qualified and ethical orthopaedic surgeons was needed. The first meeting of a committee appointed by the American Orthopaedic Association to consider this matter was held at the Lake Shore Athletic Club in Chicago in 1931 at the time of a meeting of the Clinical Orthopaedic Society. The committee formed a new organization, named it the American Academy of Orthopaedic Surgeons, and elected Edwin Ryerson of Chicago to be the first president and Willis C. Campbell of Memphis to be the first secretary. Dr. Campbell probably deserves credit for the rapid development of the Academy, because it was he who wrote letters to all the known orthopaedic surgeons in the country inviting them to join. He was aided by a group of midwestern surgeons (Fig. 1), who included Melvin S. Henderson of Rochester, Minnesota, E. Bishop Mumford of Indianapolis, Edwin Ryerson and Philip Lewin of Chicago, Frederick J. Gaenslen of Milwaukee, and H. Winnett Orr of Lincoln, Nebraska. They were joined by Philip D. Wilson, then of Boston and later of New York City, and by John C. Wilson of Los Angeles.

Edwin Ryerson was an excellent surgeon and a vigorous proponent of organized medicine. He originated the triple arthrodesis procedure and popularized that name. He worked at St. Luke's Hospital in Chicago. Willis Campbell was elected president at the first meeting of the Academy in 1933. The other officers elected at that meeting were: Philip D. Wilson, vice-president: Philip Lewin, secretary; and Bishop Mumford, treasurer. It is of interest that, at the same time, the American Orthopaedic Association appointed another committee to study the formation of standards and curricula for orthopaedic residency training programs. This action resulted in the formation of the American Board of Orthopaedic Surgery, which issued its first certificates in 1934. Dr. Campbell had singlehandedly built up the Campbell Clinic Foundation in Memphis, Tennessee, the largest orthopaedic practice in that part of the country. Campbell was an excellent speaker, who knew how to impress the local practitioners in nearby Tennessee and northern Mississippi when he gave talks about orthopaedic subjects at the meetings of local medical societies. He hired a medical student, Hugh Smith, to drive him in his car on his frequent trips into the countryside. As partial payment, Hugh Smith was given a room in the Campbell building to live in. Later, when Smith had finished his residency, Dr. Campbell turned to him again for considerable help in writing his famous textbook, *Campbell's Operative Orthopaedics*.

In addition to the standardized examinations for certification of orthopaedic surgeons, the American Board of Orthopaedic Surgery was instrumental in the efforts to standardize the educational programs in all ortho-

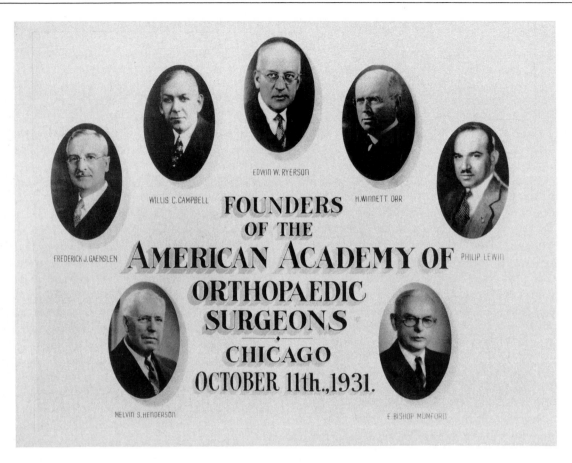

WILLIS C. CAMPBELL

EDWIN W. RYERSON

H. WINNETT ORR

FREDERICK J. GAENSLEN

PHILIP LEWIN

FOUNDERS OF THE AMERICAN ACADEMY OF ORTHOPAEDIC SURGEONS CHICAGO OCTOBER 11th., 1931.

MELVIN S. HENDERSON

E. BISHOP MUMFORD

Fig. 1 Founders of the American Academy of Orthopaedic Surgeons.

paedic residency programs, a concern that led to the establishment of the Residency Review Committee.

The Early Years

The first meeting of the American Academy of Orthopaedic Surgeons was held in Chicago on January 11, 1933. At that meeting a constitution and by-laws were adopted as two separate documents. The definition of orthopaedic surgery adopted on that date was "Orthopaedic Surgery shall be defined as that branch of surgery especially concerned with the preservation and restoration of the skeletal system, its articulations and associated structures." In the intervening years, that definition has been revised, expanded, and restated many times. Those of you who have been asked as an expert witness to define orthopaedic surgery in a courtroom know that it now reads, "Orthopaedic Surgery is the medical specialty that includes the investigation, preservation and restoration of the form and function of the extremities, spine and associated structures by medical, surgical and physical means." When you are on the witness stand, this statement is about as easy to remember as the Gettysburg Address.

The next controversy in orthopaedics had to do with the spelling of the word. There are those who think that the diphthong "ae" should be scrapped and replaced with "e." There are also those who think the term "orthopaedic surgeon" should be replaced by "orthopedist." Because orthopedists do much more than surgery, some people feel that surgeon should not be part of the title. The fact remains that after all the arguments, the official title remains American Academy of Orthopaedic Surgeons. It would be a waste of time to review the arguments and the motions proposed at Academy meetings and elsewhere. Suffice it to say that there are at this time departments of orthopedics, orthopaedic surgery, orthopedic surgery, etc., on this continent. There are also departments of orthopedics and orthopedic sections of departments of surgery. The question of whether orthopedics should be a division of departments of surgery or should be a free-standing department of orthopedics is still a major point of discussion. It is also important to make the distinction between the Academy and the American Board of Orthopaedic Surgery, which is an entirely separate organization.

The officers were aided in running the Academy by an Executive Committee. Organized in 1934, once the

Bylaws had been approved, the Executive Committee originally consisted of the four officers and five others. A president-elect was added in 1935, and in 1938 a Librarian-Historian was added. Then, in 1947, two junior guests were added. The president's term has always been for one year with one exception. In 1945, during World War II, there was no annual meeting, so Bishop Mumford served as president for two years.

In 1972 the Executive Committee was designated the Board of Directors. It was at that time that the idea of a president, first vice-president, and second vice-president was adopted. A second vice-president, elected annually, serves six years, moving up automatically to first vice-president and president and then serving for three years on the Board of Directors as a past president. The other officers of the Board—the secretary and the treasurer—are elected for three-year terms. The office of librarian-historian has been eliminated. There are now three members at large. The chairman, chairman-elect, and secretary of the Board of Councilors and the chairman and chairman-elect of the Council of Musculoskeletal Specialty Societies are also on the Board.

The Board of Councilors

Also in 1972, the Board of Councilors was organized to replace the Regional Committees, which had been appointed to assist the Membership Committee in screening applicants for fellowship in the Academy. The original idea was that because these committee members lived in close proximity to the applicants, they would be good sources of information about such matters as the candidates' practice patterns and ethics, and could advise the Membership Committee. The membership at large, which was approaching 10,000, expressed concern about their lack of direct access to the Board of Directors and officers of the Academy. Although the Regional Committees had been established to advise the Board of Directors, they had no direct representation on the Board. Walter Hoyt of Akron, Ohio, was the First Vice-President at that time, and he deserves credit for leading the efforts to change the situation by developing the Board of Councilors. Phillip D. Wilson, Jr., was the president, and the two worked together to accomplish this important task. As a result the Regional Committees were abandoned and the organization called the Board of Councilors was established. Each state was to have at least one member on the Board of Councilors, and, for every 150 members in addition to the original 150, the state would be entitled to another member. The Board, which was to meet at least one a year, would elect its own officers. Members were to be elected by the state organization for a three-year term and could be re-elected once, extending the term to a total of six years. The three

officers—the chairman, chairman-elect, and secretary—serve on the Board of Directors of the Academy.

Eugene Nordby, of Madison, Wisconsin, was the first Chairman. A fortunate choice, he proved to be witty and personable. He and his successors, Herbert Stark of Los Angeles and Jerome Cotler of Philadelphia, were leaders in the best sense of the word in that they brought the grassroots messages to the Board of Directors firmly and effectively, but without causing any major upheaval. Although at first some members of the Board of Directors were concerned that the Board of Councilor members might be disruptive and would not understand the deliberations and actions of the Board, this concern has given way to a healthy regard for the advice of the Councilor members, who now play a much bigger role in Academy affairs than had been originally anticipated.

The Role of Education

In the early years, the Academy was so involved with the evolution of its educational efforts that it had little time or energy left to consider the socioeconomic forces that were relentlessly changing the environment in which orthopaedic surgeons practice. Shortly after the formation of the Academy, the principle was established that the educational and other functions were to be accomplished by volunteer contributions of fellows of the Academy and that all functions would be initiated, overseen, and managed by committees. The index of *Fifty Years of Progress* lists 94 committees. In addition there are four ad hoc committees, four advisory committees, and four joint committees with other organizations. These committees have been remarkably effective and useful. Some of them have had a profound effect on the activities of the Academy and have contributed in a significant way to the betterment of orthopaedics.

The Academy Office

The complexity of providing support for the activities of the Academy, its committees, and the Annual Meeting and other educational activities required the Academy to establish a permanent office. Called the Central Office, it was originally established by past president Dr. J.E.M. Thompson in his home city of Lincoln, Nebraska, in 1947. A generous grant of $5,000 from the Academy and a considerable amount from his own pocket enabled Thompson to set up the office.

Once the office had been established, data on members was accumulated and files were established. The following year, however, the decision was made to move the Central Office to Chicago, where it was supervised by Dr. John Norcross. This office was located at 122

South Michigan Avenue. The major purposes of the office at that time were to support the secretary, to assist in planning and implementing the Annual Meeting, and to keep files containing information on all orthopaedic surgeons in the established orthopaedic organizations and in the training programs. At that time the offices of the American Board of Orthopaedic Surgery were housed at the same address. In 1954 the Orthopaedic Research and Education Foundation moved into the offices. This trend has continued, and now the Academy office also houses most of the orthopaedic specialty societies. On April 1, 1955, the Central Office moved to 116 South Michigan Avenue. Next it moved to 29 East Madison Street and then, in 1968, it moved to 430 North Michigan Avenue. The move to 444 North Michigan took place in 1978. When Dr. Heck took over as executive director, he tried to get orthopaedic surgeons to call the office the Academy Office rather than the Central Office. Although the Academy was only one of the organizations using the space, he wanted it to be identified as the Academy. It took years for him to get many old timers to break the habit of calling it the Central Office.

The move to the Academy's own office building in Park Ridge, Illinois, in 1985, was made necessary by a number of factors. The Academy membership was growing by nearly 500 members per year, the space in downtown Chicago was increasingly expensive to rent, and, because of the increasing activity of the Academy, the staff was growing and the demands for space were becoming much greater than before. Also, the other orthopaedic specialty societies had grown and now needed more space than was available at the Michigan Avenue location. As the Academy continues to grow, it remains to be seen how long the present building will be able to meet its demands.

The Executives

The Academy office was run by orthopaedic surgeons until 1955, when John K. Hart was hired as executive secretary. He served as executive secretary until 1974. When he left the Academy, that position was ended. Dr. Heck, who had been employed as medical director in 1968, became the chief executive officer. That title caused some confusion among the public, so it was changed to director in 1970 and to executive director in 1972.

The top leadership of the Academy Office was increased by the addition of Thomas C. Nelson as assistant executive director in 1971. He has an MPA and proved to be a very effective executive and a great help to Dr. Heck. Unfortunately, he left the Academy to start his own medical society administrative business in 1978. Dr. Fred Featherstone, an internist by training, joined the staff as deputy executive director in 1978

and has also been exceedingly valuable, particularly in the field of education. When Charlie Heck retired, the Academy was able to entice Tom Nelson to return as executive director, the position he still holds.

Throughout the history of the Academy, the secretary has been a pivotal figure. In the early days of the Executive Committee, the secretary frequently held office for several years. In a real way, the Secretary was the glue that held the Academy together and made the Annual Meeting and other functions go.

The secretaries, who for 50 years carried this enormous burden cheerfully and well, must be mentioned by name. They are: E. Bishop Mumford, 1932–38; Carl E. Badgely, 1938–41; Rex L. Dively, 1941–43; Myron O. Henry, 1944–47; Harold B. Boyd, 1948–52; John R. Norcross, 1953–57; Clinton L. Compere, 1958–62; Charles V. Heck, 1963–66; John J. Hinchey, 1967–69; William F. Donaldson, 1970–73; Mason Hohl, 1974–76; E. Burke Evans, 1977–78; Herbert H. Stark, 1979–82; Reginald R. Cooper 1983–85; William H. Salott, 1986–88; Robert N. Hensinger, 1989–90; and Robert E. Eilert, 1990–92.

Some of these secretaries deserve special acknowledgement because of their personalities and accomplishments. Harold Boyd followed James Spencer Speed as chief at the Campbell Clinic. Most of the alumni of that program consider him the best teacher of all time. He was a kindly, intellectual man, who was a stickler for details. As an example, he would admonish a young resident "to rub the back of the cast, the front will take care of itself."

Clinton Compere of Chicago might be said to have grown up with the Academy. He lived and worked in Chicago and became chief at Northwestern. His older brother, Edward, was also active in organized orthopaedics, but it was Clint who dedicated himself to the Academy and, in addition to being secretary, also served as Treasurer and, later, President.

John Hinchey is a statesman and demonstrated this as secretary and president. He joined Walter Stuck in San Antonio on completion of his residency, and the combination of his ability and his willingness to champion good young orthopaedists in Texas has taken him to the top in his state and in the Texas university system.

Early in his career, William Donaldson showed the energy and ability as a surgeon and administrator that have carried him through the secretaryship and presidency of the Academy. He currently holds the medical directorship of the Children's Hospital of Pittsburgh. He has also been very effective as the Chairman of the Orthopaedic Advisory Board of the Shriners Hospitals for Crippled Children.

The Annual Meeting

The early meetings of the Academy were held in such cities as New York, Cleveland, and Baltimore. In the late 1940s and during the 1950s, the meetings were held in the Palmer House Hotel in Chicago. Because they were held in midwinter, fellows from milder climates complained. Air transportation, too, was frequently uncertain. Finally, the Palmer House became too small for all the functions of the Annual Meeting. At present, the Academy rotates its meeting among those warm-weather cities in the United States, including San Francisco, New Orleans, Atlanta, Dallas, Las Vegas, Anaheim, Orlando, and Washington, D.C., that have convention facilities large enough to handle a meeting with up to 25,000 registrants.

Because of the complexity of the Annual Meeting, numerous individuals and committees share the load in planning and implementing them. The Annual Meeting Committee oversees the work of the Program Committee, the Instructional Course Lectures Committee, the Local Arrangements Committee, the Exhibits Committee, and the Spouse Committee. These member committees in turn are helped greatly by staff members of the Academy, who carry out the complex job of getting the Annual Meeting together and running the meeting once it has been developed.

The Annual Meeting is only one of the educational functions of the Academy, but it is the largest, the most important, and the most costly of the Academy's functions. Its costs are partially defrayed by fees from visitors, and its major source of revenue is the rental of space in the Technical Exhibit Hall to such exhibitors as instrument and pharmaceutical houses. In the early days of the Academy, the programs consisted solely of papers, mostly on clinical matters. Papers submitted by the authors were judged and were selected or rejected by the Program Committee. From the beginning, the meeting was open to all physicians interested in the program and was also open to the press. The number of nonfellows increased rapidly, and the decision was soon made to charge a fee for those attendees who were not fellows of the Academy. Philip D. Wilson, Sr., was the president when the first formal contacts with the press were made by Carl L. Levinson of New York City. Dr. Levinson abstracted all the papers and relayed them to the press at the meeting in 1935 in New York City. The interest in public education and public recording of the Academy meeting then waned until 1942, when a standing committee was formed to handle relations with the press.

For the first few years the arrangements for the Annual Meeting were handled by a paid contractor in the city where the meeting was held. This practice continued until the Academy office was staffed well enough to make arrangements for itself. The contractor arrangements were not always satisfactory, and in 1942 it was decided to develop an arrangements committee within the Academy. The scope of the Academy Annual Meeting changed rather quickly. The technical exhibits, which became a part of the meeting in 1935, have

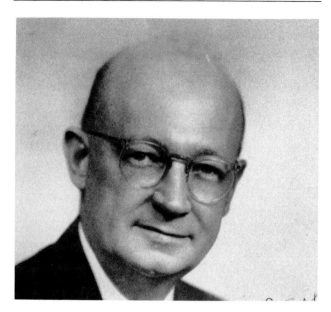

Fig. 2 J. Albert Key

grown increasingly important, both in terms of information delivered and in financial support.

In the 1930s and 1940s the quality of scientific exhibits was good, but, due to their elaborate design and construction, they were quite expensive and few in number. Later, the trend was to have more, less costly exhibits. Also, poster exhibits became popular, and these are now strongly encouraged by the Academy.

The instructional courses, in-depth presentations of particular subjects, were incorporated into the program of the Annual Meeting in 1943, and they have proved to be very popular. These courses have been published in the *Instructional Course Lectures* volumes. For a time, there were instructional course dinners that featured lively presentations of difficult or unusual cases by such masters of repartee as J. Albert Key and H. Relton McCarroll, who could keep a crowd enthralled for hours by their quick wit.

J. Albert Key (Fig. 2), of St. Louis, was one of the most cordial of men and had a great many friends, but he was outraged by fools. He sat in the front row during Academy meetings. If the presenter was unable to back up his conclusions with facts or if his work was poorly done, Key would rise to his feet and point out to the speaker the weaknesses of his arguments. It was a great way to ensure quality in the papers, and there were those who attended the Academy meeting just to hear what J. Albert Key had to say.

H. Relton McCarroll (Fig. 3), also from St. Louis, was another force to be reckoned with. A superb speaker, McCarroll memorized and thoroughly rehearsed each talk before he gave it, even after he had given hundreds of talks. He was so good that he served as master of ceremonies for the instructional course

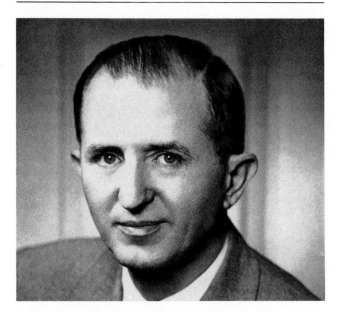

Fig. 3 H. Relton McCarroll

orthopaedics, trauma surgery, and later, anatomic areas, such as surgery of the hand, foot, knee, hip, spine, shoulder, and elbow, began to attract orthopaedic surgeons as areas of primary interest. This tendency to fragment the field was resisted strongly by the Academy, and several of the presidential and first vice-president addresses have dealt with this subject. The result of this concern was an elaborate system of courses that were developed and presented in various locations throughout the country. The usual format was for the course to be given under the sponsorship of one of the "categorical" committees. The committee identified a course chairman, who, with Academy staff help, would prepare an agenda, recruit the faculty, and make arrangements for the time and place for the course to be given. Lately, with the rules of the Accreditation Council for Continuing Medical Education in force, this mechanism has become more structured and more directed toward the perceived and actual needs of the course registrants. The courses have routinely been three days in length, although recently one-day courses also have been offered.

As a part of the Academy's concern for the educational needs of the fellows, the utility of hands-on courses to teach surgeons specific surgical techniques was debated in the committees and by the Board of Directors. This concern led to an effort to supplement the educational functions of the Annual Meeting, through what was called the Summer Institute. Broader in scope than the other courses, the Summer Institute also includes courses in which psychomotor skills and specific techniques are taught.

The Academy has not confined itself to the education of orthopaedic surgeons. The Committee on Injuries, interested in improving the training of emergency medical technicians (chiefly ambulance drivers and personnel), began to present courses in 1964. The first of these was held in September 1964 in New York City. In 1968 there were eight courses given for EMT-Paramedics. The success of these courses and the obvious need for a good education for these emergency medical technicians led the Academy to develop a textbook on the subject, *Emergency Care and Transportation of the Sick and Injured*, first published in 1971. Charles Rockwood of San Antonio was the editor of the first edition. Walter Hoyt was instrumental in bringing it to fruition. In addition to this manual or textbook, specific courses with training manuals were developed. The manual, courses, and tests have been adopted by many states as the educational standards to be used for certification of emergency medical personnel. This effort has not only been an outstanding educational success, but it has also contributed significantly to the financial well-being of the Academy. It has allowed the Academy to advance aggressively into many other areas of education and public affairs.

dinner. A series of difficult or unusual cases was flashed on the screen and McCarroll made the solving of the problem more interesting than a Sherlock Holmes story. Later he was a member of the Residency Review Committee and chaired a subcommittee designed to reconstruct the patchwork organization of orthopaedic residencies that existed at that time.

From 1943 to 1961, Edwards Brothers, Inc., published the *Instructional Course Lectures* in a bound volume. From 1962 to 1969, they appeared in the *Journal of Bone and Joint Surgery*. From 1970 through 1986, they were published by the C. V. Mosby Co. Since 1987, the Academy has published the *Instructional Course Lectures*. Dr. J.E.M. Thompson was the father of the instructional courses. He was honored for this accomplishment at the Annual Meeting in 1962, and he died several months later.

Another feature added to the Annual Meeting was the showing of movies, which usually described specific surgical procedures. With the advance of technology, these were replaced by slide programs and, more recently, by video presentations. The Academy has for years been interested in making this type of presentation part of the armamentarium of undergraduate and postgraduate orthopaedic programs, but with little success. Most orthopaedic residency programs have a video library, but surveys indicate that many residents fail to take full advantage of this useful tool.

Other Continuing Medical Education

Shortly after the end of World War II, orthopaedics began to be specialized, and areas such as pediatric

Controversies

No history of any organization can be interesting enough to be worth recounting without revealing some of the major controversies that have arisen in the course of 57 years. The course of the Academy has not always been a smooth one, although most of the storms appear to have been weathered with little damage.

A good place to start is in the area of educational standards and certification. The American Board of Orthopaedic Surgery was founded in 1934 and is not related in any way to the Academy, except that Academy fellows must be Board certified to be eligible for fellowship. The Board proposed recertification in 1974. This resolution of the Board did not sit well with the Academy's Board of Directors or with the Board of Councilors. The Academy is on record as opposing any recertification based upon an examination alone. There have been several attempts by the Board of Directors of the Academy and the American Board of Orthopaedic Surgery to negotiate these differences of opinion and to develop methods of recertification that will be fair and nonthreatening to practicing orthopaedic surgeons. The Board has developed alternative methods for recertification that will allow fellows to choose the method of their achieving recertification.

In a related field, the Academy learned in 1958 that the American Board of Orthopaedic Surgery was negotiating with the American College of Surgeons for that organization to become sponsor of the Residency Review Committee along with the Board and the American Medical Association. William Green of Boston represented the Academy in the discussions, and, initially, the Academy did not object to this change. A year later, however, the Academy decided that it would like to be a sponsor of the Residency Review Committee and agreed to a quadripartite sponsorship of the Residency Review Committee. This was not accomplished, and, in 1972, the American College of Surgeons objected to the rules of the Orthopaedic Residency Review Committee because it accepts osteopathic physicians into orthopaedic residency programs. This objection led the orthopaedic community to object to the inclusion of American College of Surgeons as a sponsor, because the orthopaedic community would not change the rules to exclude osteopaths. In 1973, the Academy became the third sponsor of the Residency Review Committee in Orthopaedics, and American College of Surgeons was not accepted as a sponsor.

A major controversy arose in 1969 over the report of an ad hoc Committee on a National Health Program for Orthopaedics. This report was a sincere attempt by a group of 140 prominent orthopaedic surgeons from all over the country, with help from workers at the National Institutes of Health, the U.S. Public Health Service, and the University of Missouri, to develop plans for the future of orthopaedics in this country.

Charles Herndon of Cleveland, president of the Academy at the time, strongly supported this effort. Because it included suggestions for regionalization of services and education, national certification, and some other features that were taken by some to favor a national health system, it created a storm of protests. Entitled *A National Health Program for Orthopaedics: A Preliminary Report*, it was withdrawn from the Academy agenda and can now be found only in some personal libraries such as mine at home.

Although not a major controversy, the increasing specialization in orthopaedics has caused the Board of Directors to face the possibility that specialty societies might break away from the Academy's Annual Meetings and go their own way. In addition to the problems with the Annual Meeting, there has been the controversy about specialty certification by the certifying Boards. The response of the Academy has been to offer space and administrative staff support at the Academy's office building in Park Ridge for any specialty society that wishes to use these services. Also, at its Annual Meeting, the Academy has designated the Sunday in the middle of the meeting as Specialty Day, during which each specialty society has a formal scientific program. In addition to these measures, the Academy has added two of the elected officers of the Council of Musculoskeletal Specialty Societies to the Board of Directors of the Academy.

Finally, there has been some continuing controversy in the Academy about an appropriate level of activity in the socio-economic or health policy arena. Some of our fellows have argued for a higher profile in Washington, D.C.; others have argued against it. And, given the not-for-profit tax status of the Academy as an educational organization, the Academy's activities in this arena are limited in scope by the Internal Revenue Code. However, in 1979, the Academy hired Nick Cavarocchi to open an office in Washington to maintain contact with the Congress and the Administration. Also, the Board of Councilors meets each year in Washington, and at that time the Councilors have a briefing session and an opportunity to visit their own congressmen and senators. Academy officers have for the past 20 years appeared and testified at various congressional hearings. This kind of activity has been effective in establishing in 1986 an Institute of Arthritis and Musculoskeletal and Skin Diseases in the National Institutes of Health. Formerly, musculoskeletal research and funding had been housed in the National Institute of Arthritis, Digestive Diseases and Kidney Diseases.

Membership

The Academy was formed with the idea that all qualified and ethical orthopaedic surgeons are eligible to be members. In determining how to identify those who are qualified and ethical, the main criterion has been that the applicant must be certified by the American Board of Orthopaedic Surgery, once that Board was established in 1934. Canadian surgeons were welcomed, but they, too, must be certified by the American Board of Orthopaedic Surgery. There was an argument over whether the Royal College of Surgeons of Canada criteria are equivalent to the American Board certification.

Early in the history of the Academy it was important to recruit new members and to let the orthopaedic community know that the Academy existed. Soon, however, this kind of solicitation was no longer necessary. A Membership Committee was established to examine the credentials of those applying for fellowship. This committee was later assisted by the regional committees, which reported to the Membership Committee. The regional committees assumed duties other than membership screening, and when the Constitution and Bylaws were drastically revised in 1968, the Board of Councilors was formed and the regional committees became the Regional Admission Committees. The actions of the Admission Committee were challenged in court in the 1970s, and this has led to entirely different admission procedures, chiefly by eliminating the confidential nature of the information upon which decisions are based. Recent changes bring "candidate membership" to surgeons before they have taken the Board examinations, and efforts have been made to involve the entire orthopaedic community in Academy affairs.

Another important issue regarding attendance at the Annual Meetings has been the status of our Latin American colleagues. For several years a great effort was made to invite contingents of the Society of Latin American Orthopaedics and Traumatology to the Academy's Annual Meetings. Buses were hired and an elaborate program of pre- and post-meeting visits to various United States and Canadian orthopaedic centers were arranged. To my knowledge, there still has not been a satisfactory resolution of the relationship between the Academy and the Latin American orthopaedic community.

Acknowledgments

I would like to acknowledge the debt that I have to Charlie Heck who was my dear friend for many years, since we took our Boards together in Chicago in 1953. His book on the history of the Academy has been a primary source of information. I also want to thank Dr. George W. Brindley of Temple, Texas, who supplied me with an informal history of orthopaedics written by my friend Bob Murray. This history is accompanied by a bibliography which has been most useful. I would also like to thank Rocco Calandruccio for his support and suggestions and his offers to supply me with photographs. Finally, I cannot express adequately my admiration for the staff of the Academy, headed by Tom Nelson, for their willingness to help in this project.

References

1. Heck CV: *Fifty Year of Progress.* Chicago, American Academy of Orthopaedic Surgeons, 1983.
2. Wickstrom JK: *History of the American Board of Orthopaedic Surgery, 1934–1984.* Chicago, American Board of Orthopaedic Surgery, 1986.
3. Chatterton CC: Early orthopaedic surgery in Minnesota. *Minn Med* 1953;36:360–363.
4. Cleveland M, Winant EM: Orthopaedic Surgeons of the 19th Century in New York City, in Thomson JEM (ed): American Academy of Orthopaedic Surgeons *Instructional Course Lectures, IV.* Ann Arbor, JW Edwards, 1948, pp 228–239.
5. Freiberg JA: Reflections on orthopaedic surgery. *J Bone Joint Surg* 1962;44A:1699–1702.
6. Harris RI, Gallie WE, McLachlin A, et al: Fifty years of Orthopaedic Surgery in Canada. *J Bone Joint Surg* 1950;32B:587–600.
7. Lewin P: John Ridlon (Historical dinner symposium), in Thomson JEM (ed): American Academy of Orthopaedic Surgeons *Instructional Course Lectures, IV.* Ann Arbor, JW Edwards, 1948, p 244.
8. Mayer LJ: Reflections on some interesting personalities in orthopaedic surgery during the first quarter of the century. *J Bone Joint Surg* 1955;37A:374–383.
9. Orr HW: History and biography of orthopaedic surgery, in Pease CN (ed): American Academy of Orthopaedic Surgeons *Instructional Course Lectures, IX.* Ann Arbor, JW Edwards, 1952, pp 423–447.
10. Brown T: *The American Orthopaedic Association: A Centennial History.* Park Ridge, American Orthopaedic Association, 1987.
11. Coventry MB: The American Orthopaedic Association and the written word. *J Bone Joint Surg* 1977;59A:1116–1123.

Computers

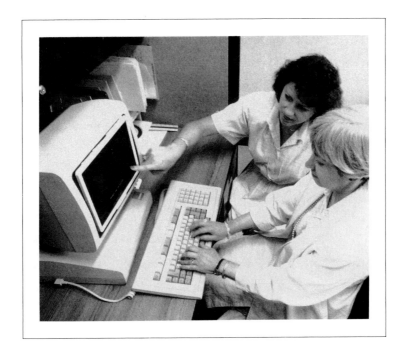

Assessing Your Office

Robert H. Haralson, MD

The question used to be, "How big should my practice be before I consider a computer?" Now the question is, "How big a computer should I consider for my practice?" Not long ago, a computer system was not cost-effective unless a practice was a certain size (normally three or four physicians). Because the price of computers has dropped dramatically and the advantages of computerized practice management systems are so great, now even the small office will probably benefit from computerizing business aspects. If you have a small office, you simply buy a smaller computer.

Before deciding to purchase a computer, a physician should assess the office to see what size computer is needed. The first step is to assure that the office is run efficiently. Sound accounting principles should be in use, and office personnel should be dedicated to improving whatever system is in place. A computer will not correct a sloppily run office. If coding is inaccurate, if booking of charges is not timely, and if insurance forms are not completed accurately, the computer will only compound those problems and the office will run even less efficiently. If there is any question about the efficiency of the office, the services of a practice management consultant may prove worthwhile. In addition, most offices should implement a strategic plan. Without anticipating the future needs and goals of an office, decisions can be made that will be regretted in the future.

The price of the computer system is an important factor. It is difficult to say how much should be spent on a computer system, but, in general, unless the cost is totally unreasonable, the computer will pay for itself within the first year or two. Computerization will not reduce the number of employees needed. At best, it will save hiring additional employees in the future. But the cost of the computer cannot be offset by immediately reducing your office staff. Savings will come through more efficient posting of charges, billing, and completing of insurance forms.

Look out for "lowballing" by computer vendors. Because computer systems are fairly expensive, there is a tendency on behalf of vendors to quote a price that is low enough, but that does not provide all the needed hardware. The purchaser then must purchase additional equipment to make the system run properly. Be aware of this and make sure the cost calculations include the ultimate system. Once the office staff becomes accustomed to the computer, each person will want a separate screen. In addition, it is unusual to be able to

get by with one printer. Most systems require at least one dot matrix printer and one letter quality printer (probably a laser printer). Plan to spend enough money to purchase a system that will function well for both current and future needs.

Using a Request for Proposal

It is standard in the computer industry as well as other industries to complete a request for proposal (RFP). This is a document that tells the vendor what sort of computer system is wanted. The proposal then explains what sorts of computer systems the vendor has available. RFPs are available through many vendors. After carefully completing the customer's portion of the RFP, select approximately ten vendors and ask each of them to complete the RFP. When they are returned, it is normally possible to thin out the list of potential vendors to three or four, using the data on the RFP. The remaining three or four vendors are then asked to demonstrate their product personally. This is much more efficient and much less confusing than trying to assess ten systems personally. Following are some concerns that should be addressed before completing the customer's portion of the RFP.

The number of physicians in the practice is important, and obviously, it is necessary to consider any plans to add physicians in the near future. The number of employees, now and in the future, must also be indicated. In addition, some effort must be made to decide which personnel will be working with a computer terminal. This may include some of the physicians. Data input by physicians is not particularly common at this time but will become common in the future when data input is by scanner, optical character recognition, or voice interpretation.

The RFP should also indicate how many patients are seen presently and how that figure will probably change in the future. The frequency of patient visits is another important piece of information. If a physician sees patients for only half a day, but sees the same number of patients as other physicians see in a full day, then this fact may affect whether data input is done "on line" or "batch."

The number of statements sent out each month should be assessed. Statements are not necessary for all active patients. Some of them may have been previously billed or have some sort of financial arrangement that does not require monthly billings.

The number of offices or treatment locations (such as the emergency room, hospital, operating theater, etc.) is important. Obviously, office expansion requires advance planning.

What Do You Wish the Computer to Accomplish?

While assessing the office and negotiating with vendors, it is also necessary to decide what the computer is to do. There are several functions that might be available but that can be omitted from a system. Furthermore, any system will be better at some functions than at others. Although objectives can change as more is learned about the capabilities of computers, early assessment is best.

One way of deciding how to use the computer most efficiently is by comparing the strengths and weaknesses of humans and computers. Human strengths include the ability to do high level integrated tasks well, identify goals, perceive relationships, deal with exceptions, establish priorities, and complete inferential tasks. Computers are very fast, have perfect memories, and handle repetitive tasks efficiently.

Humans have weaknesses. They tire of repetitive tasks, they have imperfect memories, and they perform some tasks relatively slowly. A human, placed in a room with no distractions and asked to copy figures from one page to another, will have a 3% error rate. Computers can accomplish such a task with essentially no errors.

The main weakness of the computer is that it is stupid. It cannot think for itself, doing only exactly what it is told to do by a human. Therefore, any system that does not relieve your staff of repetitive tasks like copying names and addresses from the file, does not give value for the money spent. If, however, the system expects the computer to think, it will fail.

Billing and Accounts Receivable

Computers should be able to handle a variety of billing situations. Several patients in an office may be under treatment for different conditions at the same time. For instance, a patient may have injuries secondary to a car wreck that are covered by one insurance, another condition that is covered by Medicare or Medicaid, a third condition that is covered by worker's compensation, and a fourth condition for which the fees are reduced. Printing of bills should take no more than three hours. A complicated "month end" that takes the computer out of service for several hours must be avoided.

Electronic Billing

Electronic billing, or "paperless claims," is an extremely important function. Many insurance companies allow transmission of billing data to their computer over telephone lines. This is extremely efficient, saves mailing costs, and allows confirmation of properly completed insurance data within 24 hours. Obviously, this shortens reimbursement turnaround time.

The computer can provide sorting by zip code, which makes it possible to obtain bulk rates from the postal service. The computer can also allow multiple billing dates, so that a certain percentage of the bills are sent out each week rather than all of them at the end of the month. This can even out cash flow and ease tension at the front desk the day after the bills go out.

The computer should be able to handle multiple fee schedules, because Medicare, Medicaid, worker's compensation, and private insurance may all have different fee schedules. The computer should also be able to handle multiple carrier combinations.

Medical Records

The processing of medical records on the computer has several advantages. More will be mentioned on this subject later, but computerized records allow you to assess outcomes in your own practice. In the near future, insurance companies will require the data included in computerized medical records. In addition, the patient and referring physician letters generated by such a system can be a tremendous marketing tool.

Appointment Scheduling

Appointment scheduling modules are commonly available but not frequently used. One should understand the difference in appointment scheduling versus appointment logging. Logging merely means using the computer as a substitute for the manual appointment log. Scheduling is a more sophisticated procedure. The appointment scheduling module should be able to look up "the next available appointment," "the next available Thursday afternoon," "the next open 30-minute appointment," or "when Mrs. Jones' next appointment is." One common problem in both a manual system and computerized logging system is that when patients call in to check on their next appointment time, if the appointment clerk is very busy, and cannot locate that appointment quickly, there is a tendency just to book another appointment. This makes for double booking and no-shows. You should discuss with the vendor the number of physician or office computer installations that use the appointment scheduling, because if the appointment scheduling is inefficient and time-consuming, then it will not be used.

The appointment clerk must understand that even though it takes a few more minutes to book an appointment on the computer than it does to write it down on an appointment book, appointment scheduling on a computer saves time "down the line." For instance, a computerized appointment schedule can generate the next day's patient list with names, addresses, and phone numbers, a task that must be done by hand on a manual system.

Word Processing

Word processing is now common, extremely efficient, and time-saving. It should be an essential part of the computerized office management system. There are two ways to address word processing. The first is to have an integrated system that works within the practice management system. The second way is to have word processing done on a stand-alone personal computer (PC). Either way is satisfactory. Because word processing is memory intensive and can slow the computer, many vendors have elected to implement word processing on a stand-alone PC.

Accounts Payable

Most vendors have in their packages a module for accounts payable. This module can be part of an integrated system or done on a stand-alone PC. Either way is acceptable.

Payroll

Another item frequently offered is a payroll module. Again, this module can be integrated or it can be stand-alone, using a PC and an off-the-shelf software package. An advantage to having payroll on your computer is that tax accounting is frequently included, which saves time at the end of the year.

Management Reports

Management reports are another useful by-product of computerized financial data. Vendors have elected to produce reports one of three ways. In the first way, preprogrammed reports, the software is programmed to produce certain reports, which are obtained by asking the computer to produce them. In the second way, the software includes a report generator, which can allow the user to design reports other than those that have been preprogrammed. In the third way, an off-the-shelf package, such as Lotus 1 2 3, Excel, or another spreadsheet, is used. The software should allow the computer to download the data into the spreadsheet, saving the operator from retyping the data.

Each of the three types of reports has advantages and disadvantages. The preprogrammed report is easiest to use but does not allow customization of reports. The off-the-shelf approach allows unlimited customization but requires the user to be familiar with the spreadsheet. The report generator is a middle-of-the-road approach that allows some customization but does not require the user to know so much about spreadsheets.

Of the reports available, the most important is the aged accounts receivable. This listing includes all patients who owe money, and tells how much they owe, which accounts are 30 days, 60 days, and 90 days old, when the last payment was, and the amount of the last payment. Practice management consultants believe this is the most important document available, and it is rarely produced in a manual system.

Another important report lists production by physician, office, treatment location, or activity. This report makes it possible to assess how much each of these areas is producing.

Another interesting report is production by referring doctor. This report, which tells who is referring patients and how much income the referrals provide, lets the office know if one physician is referring only nonpaying patients.

Another report lists production by carrier or company. It is also possible to report patients by zip code, which shows the geographical area from which patients are coming. A decision to open an office in another location may be based on such a report.

Another important report is insurance claims sent but not paid. In a manual system, many of the insurance claims submitted have been improperly completed. The insurance company returns these unpaid. In many offices, a surprising number of these claims are not resubmitted. This report alone will frequently pay for the computer.

I strongly believe that computerization of the medical office is efficient, cost-effective, and will be essential in the not-too-distant future. Before computerizing, it is important first to make a complete assessment of the medical office and practice and to assure that the office is being run efficiently. Intensive negotiations with potential vendors will also be necessary. It is essential to visit a practice (in the absence of the vendor) that has an up-and-running system like the one being considered. Expect to spend significant time discussing the system with employees who use it (not the doctors). These people will say how much they like the system and can point out its advantages and disadvantages.

CHAPTER 60

Why Computerize?

Charles B. Darling

Overview

Computers have become an integral part of everyday life, from the microchips in microwave ovens to the data processing behemoths that help run the world's financial markets. Small wonder, then, that many orthopaedic surgeons have introduced computer systems into their practices.

Unfortunately, some computer systems are purchased for the wrong reason, leading to disappointment, frustration, and financial loss. Computer systems purchased for the right reasons are far more likely to live up to the physician's expectations. This chapter will discuss four bad reasons and four good reasons to computerize a practice.

Bad Reasons

Bad Reason #1: "Get organized."

The first bad reason stems from a dangerous misconception about computer systems: that having one somehow magically increases organization in a practice. The reasoning seems to be that pencil and paper, forms, and filing cabinets somehow defy the employees' natural inclination for neatness, and that a computer system will somehow remove this supposed barrier to orderliness.

It is said that "it is a poor workman who blames the tools," yet isn't that what is happening here? It is not reasonable to believe that a lack of organization will be reversed by substituting an electronic tool for a centuries-old manual method. An appropriate level of method and organization can be achieved with well-planned policies and procedures. Computerization is not a prerequisite to an organized office.

A computer system reinforces and magnifies the present level of organization. If a person is disorganized, the computer will make things more disorganized—when something is lost in a computer, for example, it stays lost! Because of this, a new computer system often provides the necessary incentive to revise policies and procedures, thereby encouraging organization, but the computer alone cannot organize the office.

Bad Reason #2: "Get efficient."

Efficiency and organization are certainly closely related but are not synonymous. It is possible to be organized without being efficient. Once again, a computer cannot make a person efficient. Efficiency comes from working policies and procedures and from the way in which resources are used.

A computer system certainly offers many new opportunities to improve efficiency, but it does not create efficiency. If anything, it creates inefficiency by adding another step—entering data into the computer—to many processes. To counter this inefficiency, many current policies and procedures will have to be redesigned. The computer simply provides the incentive and the tools for greater efficiency.

Bad Reason #3: "Get well-managed."

Management is an art, and good management is a blessing. Once again, a computer system can assist in better management of the office. As it records the minutiae of an office practice, a computer can become indispensable.

Bad Reason #4: "Get in step."

The belief that every practice must have a computer is another poor reason to install a computer system. Each practice is different, and not every practice needs a computer system. Like any other major decision, the purchase of a computer system must be weighed carefully, considering such relevant factors as the current and projected size and resources of the practice, the background and goals of the physician(s), and the strengths and weaknesses of the employees.

Good Reasons

Good Reason #1: Achieving automation by changing work practices

One fundamentally good reason to computerize the office is to improve work practices. If used wisely, the computer allows for new procedures that can greatly improve the quality of work and can increase the volume of work completed without increasing costs.

The most obvious way in which a computer can improve the quality of the staff's work is during data entry time. A good computer system reduces the opportunity for data entry errors in many ways, by: (1) Reducing the amount of typing by looking up names and descriptions in master tables; (2) Eliminating typing by using nonkeyboard data entry devices such as bar code wands and optical scanners; (3) Validating important codes against master tables; (4) Making sure the data fall within prescribed parameters or follow important rules of the practice; and (5) Checking for mathematical errors.

As a "backstop" to all of these steps, a computer system should also provide the opportunity to review the day's work. This final check for errors is vital to ensure 100% accuracy of data entered. The system's menu usually includes a "journal" or "edit list" that will print out recently entered transactions for review.

Automation also helps protect against the negative effects of increased workload when the practice grows. An increase in patient load normally magnifies any problems with organization, efficiency, or quality. What was a minor annoyance when the practice was small can, if left uncorrected, become a debilitating problem when the practice grows. Automation helps keep the quality of work constant, thereby eliminating many of the small problems that would normally loom larger as the practice grows.

Although automation is the obvious reason to computerize, it is the least important asset of the computer. If you purchase a computer only for its automation capabilities, you will have overlooked the more important and highly leveraged advantages it can offer. The good reasons that follow will explain this point further.

Good Reason #2: Achieving information by applying data

Information comes from assembling and analyzing data. Automation is helpful and necessary, but it is information generated that starts to provide serious dividends on your investment.

Medical research is one important example of how you can use a computer to turn data into information. An inexpensive computer will allow you to use your own practice's data for outcome studies, retrospective studies, trend analysis, and a wide range of other types of investigations.

The computer's ability to assimilate information has a profound effect on imaging in the medical field. Whether you look at the storage, presentation, or analysis of images, adding a computer introduces an important new modality for dealing with the information in the images. This revolution, which is currently in its early stages, merits close attention. As more and more "artificial intelligence" techniques come online, the availability and practicality of computer-assisted imaging will soar.

Many physicians are concerned about identifying and reaching potential patients. Automation won't help you there, but information will. Using the computer to study the health-care needs of your area or to analyze the changing patterns within your own practice can have a profound impact on the services you offer and who you offer them to.

Automation is only the foundation for the ultimate benefits of computerization. Interpretation of information is the first step you can take beyond automation toward realizing the full usefulness of a computer.

Good Reason #3: Achieving communication by moving information

Computer technology has undoubtedly increased the speed at which we live our lives. Using the computer to move information rapidly and efficiently can help you be active and effective in the medical field. There are many ways in which this capability can be of use.

(1) Availability of information at the press of a key improves communication between patients and staff.

(2) Information that moves at the press of a key improves communication between staff and insurers, practice, and hospital.

(3) Electronic mail can greatly enhance communication within the organization.

(4) Computers can be used as effective delivery vehicles for education: computer-based training for staff, computerized continuing medical education for doctors, and health-care information for patients.

(5) Access to computerized libraries of information across the country can have a profound effect on the practice of medicine.

Information builds on and leverages your investment in automation. By the same token, using your computer for communication is the necessary next step beyond interpreting information.

Good Reason #4: Achieving satisfaction by reducing drudgery

Probably the most profound and important result of a good computer system is its ability to free us, to some very small extent, from the menial tasks that eat up our valuable time. Assuming that we then wisely invest the time we've saved, the "satisfaction factor" of a computer may well be the biggest benefit of all.

By reducing drudgery, the computer gives everyone in the practice more time to interact with the patients. By providing better information and communication capabilities, the computer enables each member of the staff to do a better job of filling the patients' needs. For many people, these benefits contribute to an increased sense of accomplishment and self-worth.

This seemingly abstract benefit of computers can translate into a very concrete bonus. Given a shrinking and less-educated labor pool and the soaring costs of education, including on-the-job training, there is a clear incentive to attract and retain the best and the brightest employees. Because a computer system contributes to job satisfaction, it also can make it easier to build a top-notch team.

Summary

Computers can be a great benefit or an insufferable burden to your practice. The first step in the right direction is to realize what a computer can and cannot do for your practice.

A computer cannot organize a disorganized practice,

make an inefficient practice efficient, or make a poorly managed practice run smoothly.

A computer can redesign everyday tasks through automation; assemble and analyze data to produce information; deliver information quickly and easily to improve communication; and attract the best and the brightest employees by increasing job satisfaction.

If there is one item on this list that will help your practice, then you are probably ready to start looking into computers. If you keep all of these last four items in mind, you will maximize the benefit to be gained from your investment in computer technology.

CHAPTER 61

Making It Work

Robert H. Haralson, MD

Once the decision is made to purchase a computerized practice management system, several issues must be addressed before its arrival. How these issues are handled will depend on the particular system purchased.

Dedication

It is essential that at least one physician in the office be dedicated to making the system work. There is a learning curve when implementing any system, and unless a physician in the office is determined to make this venture successful, the office staff and other physicians will become frustrated with the system, and it will fail.

It is equally important that the office be organized and efficient. The computer will not organize a disorganized office. If the billing and insurance functions are not run efficiently, the computer will only magnify mistakes. If necessary, a professional practice management consultant can be engaged to develop a strategic plan.

Personnel

Someone in the office must be in charge of the computer. Although this would seem to go without saying, there have been several offices in which no one was in charge of the computer, and the system floundered. Generally, the office manager is in charge; however, this is not necessarily the case.

Faced with the task of acquiring computer skills, it is likely that some office personnel will leave. Although most of the younger generation are quite computer literate, many of the older generation are not. Many older office employees become frustrated with the complexities of a computer system and the rigid detail that the computer requires. These can be senior, valued employees. In one case, the office manager could not cope with the computer, and the insurance clerk discovered that she knew more about the computer than the office manager did. In this unacceptable situation, the office manager chose to leave.

It is important to designate tasks for each employee. Five important financial functions are posting charges, posting payments, opening the mail, preparing deposits, and making deposits. These five functions should be separated so that, if possible, each is performed by a different employee. If one employee performs several functions, and if the physicians do not understand the computer very well, there is considerable risk of fraud. Separating the functions cannot prevent fraud, but it certainly makes it much more difficult and requires employees to be in collusion.

Physical Considerations

Before purchasing a computer, it is necessary to decide where it will be stationed in the office. Computers no longer need double floored, air-conditioned rooms, but some space considerations are important. Even today's smaller computers generate heat and noise. Special air handling equipment may not be necessary, but computers cannot be placed in a small room with no air circulation. In addition, because the heat of the computer is dissipated by an electric fan, some amount of background noise is present. Although at first the noise may not seem particularly obtrusive, a full day of listening to it can become irritating.

Aesthetic considerations are also important. Even though computers are smaller and very attractive when viewed from the front, the wiring required to attach these computers to multiple screens and printers sometimes can be unsightly when viewed from the side. A good solution is to place the computer in a large room and screen it off with 6-foot decorative screens. This hides the computer and muffles the noise, while allowing plenty of air circulation.

Another physical consideration is the placement of computer terminals. Placement is determined to some degree by first deciding which employees will use them. Once these decisions are made, the office can be wired before the computer system arrives. It will be necessary to point out to the electrician where peripherals (terminals and printers) will be located. If there is doubt, remember that it is much less expensive to put in too many wires at first than it is to rewire later if decisions are changed.

The type of storage mechanism used by your particular system may become an issue. Some storage systems require larger hard disk drives and take up more space than others. Each office should have ten megabytes of storage per physician for each year that the records are kept on line. Many systems purge data every two to three years, which reduces the need for massive storage requirements, but others do not. Therefore, the need

511

for increased hard disk drives (and extra space) should be assessed at the outset.

The type of back-up used by your particular system is also an important space consideration. Some systems use an extra hard disk, which requires more space. Other systems have a tape drive, which is more time-consuming to use but obviates the need for extra space.

Training

Once the computer arrives, employees must be trained to use the system. The two options available are either to have the vendor come to the office and train personnel during office hours, or to have personnel travel to the vendor's shop for training. The first option seems to be less expensive because you do not have to pay employees' travel and housing costs. However, when employees are trained during busy and often hectic office hours the training is much less efficient than if the employees can go off site and have some time set aside to learn the system.

Entering Initial Data

Once the computer is operational, the first task is to enter the initial data. Here the choice must be made whether to enter only active accounts or to include old and closed accounts. If only active accounts are entered, the data for former patients can be entered when and if they schedule a return appointment.

Most vendors will give you the option of either allowing your personnel to enter the initial data or entering the initial data themselves for a fee. Although it may seem worthwhile to pay the vendor to enter the initial data, it is less expensive to have the employees do it, and doing so provides them with useful learning experience.

Service Contracts

Service contracts are extremely important. One of the most consistent things about computers is that they break down. Unfortunately, two separate service contracts are needed. Assuming you have purchased your system from a value-added reseller or an original equipment manufacturer, it will be necessary to have a service contract for the hardware through a local field service and a software service contract from your vendor. Some vendors will instruct you to report hardware service calls directly to the field service. They then will accept all software service calls. Because the user can rarely determine the nature of a problem, the vendor should be required to handle all service calls. The vendor must then decide whether the problem is with the software or the hardware. If it is a hardware problem, the vendor then contacts the hardware field service and arranges repair. The hardware contract should guarantee repair of your system within two working days.

The software service contract is generally required by the vendor. Most of the time, the vendor will be able to repair software problems through a telephone modem without coming to the office. The vendor often has diagnostics that may not be available at the office. Although it may seem unusual for vendors to indicate that they rarely have to come back to your office for software repairs, it is a common practice. Service contracts generally cost from 1% to 2% of the original cost of the entire system for each of the two service contracts. This means that a $50,000 system will require service contracts costing $1,000 to $2,000 per month.

Transition

Entering data can be done one of two ways, on-line or batch. On-line data entry is done during the day as the patients come in and leave. In batch entering, the data are allowed to accumulate and are then entered at the end of the day or on the next day. Either system is acceptable. Many vendors believe that the on-line feature is important and tout their systems because they have this capability. However, in a busy office, on-line entering of data sometimes causes a backlog at the front desk. For this reason, some offices prefer to enter data in the batch mode.

Once the system is running, the decision must be made whether or not to parallel. Paralleling means that the manual system or previous computer system is run along with the new system. Paralleling is usually continued for about three months. At the end of each month, the two systems are reconciled, which makes it possible to determine if mistakes are being made with the new system.

It is also quite acceptable not to parallel. Often, discrepancies exist between the old system and the new. Once employees have gone through the painful process of reconciling the records and determining where mistakes have been made, they usually find that the errors are in the manual system.

What If the System Does Not Work?

Sometimes, because of one of several factors, the system just does not work. If the system selected has already been installed in a number of offices, this is usually not the case. A second reason for failure is that some offices just are not the kind of office that can use a computer system. Every contract should have a clause stipulating that if the system is not functioning properly after six months for any reason (including the fact that the purchaser doesn't like it or the office staff cannot learn to use it), the system can be returned with full refund of your money. If the vendor will not write such a contract, another vendor must be found who will. If the system is not running satisfactorily after three months, the return process should be initiated, because it will probably take at least three months to complete.

Conclusion

Finally, once the decision is made to computerize, an all-out effort should be directed to making the system work, because it will make the office run much more efficiently and will help to attract young and vigorous employees. Properly done, the entire experience will be financially and intellectually rewarding.

CHAPTER 62

Choosing a Computer System

Charles B. Darling

Overview

Nothing can make choosing a computer for a medical practice easy—it is inherently difficult and risky. This chapter provides basic guidelines to understanding the range of people, programs, and equipment involved when considering purchase of a computer for a medical office.

Who Can Help

Consultants

There are two main sources of help for the physician in search of an office management system. The first and perhaps more obvious of these is consultants. If you are considering a consulting firm, you are probably considering one of the following:

Practice management consultants Before selecting practice management consultants to help with your search for a computer, make certain that they are experts on automation and information. If they don't have a full-time specialist in this area, they may not add enough value to your search to justify their fees.

Accounting firms Major accounting firms usually have close ties to the computer world, but once again be sure that they have the depth and experience, not only in computers but also in medical office management, to justify the investment in their services. For the amount of money these firms charge, it is important to get someone with a solid track record in both computers and medical office management.

Computer consulting firms While it is reasonable to expect computer consultants to be very clever with computers, do they really understand the needs of a medical office? Beware of the generalist in this area! You need someone who has in-depth knowledge of medical office management in addition to having computer expertise.

Two very important caveats apply when dealing with any consultant. First, because many consultants are really just salespeople in disguise, it is important to assess their independence. Check their references to see if they recommend different solutions for different situations. If not, they may just come up with the same recommendation that their last three clients paid them for.

Second, beware of the well-intentioned friend, brother-in-law, or other acquaintance who offers to help. Judge such people by the same stiff tests previously suggested for the other consultants. If they aren't bona fide independent computer and medical office management experts, then you can't afford them, no matter how low their fees are.

Staff

The second source of help in selecting an office management system is your own staff. They are the ones who will have to use the system, and they will be much more likely to have a positive approach to a new system if they have been involved in its selection.

Also, involving the staff can have benefits beyond laying the groundwork for their acceptance of the system. Your staff are the experts on how your medical office is run, and they are best qualified to evaluate whether a particular feature in a particular package will be a benefit or a hindrance. Also, any experience they may have had in another medical practice lends further perspective to the search. If their prior experience includes working on a medical office management system, their help can be very valuable.

Choosing Help

No matter where you turn for help, make sure that it is of the highest caliber. Because mediocre help in selecting an office management system can bring dire consequences, it is important to look for the following characteristics in anyone who offers advice:

Understanding of your practice Do they understand in detail what makes your practice unique, or are they just giving you warmed-over general advice? And of course, are they experts in medical office management?

Understanding of medical office management software Many aspects make this highly specialized part of the software industry unique. Is your advisor very knowledgeable about this special part of the industry?

Understanding of the computer industry How computers and software get sold, installed, and serviced can be a mystery to the novice. You need someone who understands the distribution channels in the computer industry, their revenue streams, profit margins, and pressure points, so that the right hardware and software are purchased, and are purchased from the right source.

Understanding of computer technology Making a wise investment in computer technology requires not only knowing the current state of the art, but also understanding where it is going. Your advisor must be in a position to evaluate your choices from the broad perspective of technology trends as well as from the more specific one of system features.

What Software Should I Buy?

Most medical offices should consider four different types of software: a medical office management system, a word processing package, a database package, and a spreadsheet package. While not every practice will need or use all four types of software, the practice that is getting the most out of their investment will.

Medical Office Management Applications

Volumes could be written about selecting the right medical office management system and still not cover the subject in enough detail. But the volumes would all boil down to three simple words: "Know your practice!" Not just how it works, but why it works that way, and what would happen if you changed it. Every medical office management system will require you to make some compromises in the way you currently do things. Without a ready grasp of the implications of every little compromise a given package requires, it is impossible to evaluate its value to your practice.

A good tool to use when analyzing your practice is the sample Request for Proposal, which is available from the Academy office. This document asks several questions that constitute a good starting point in understanding your practice, continues with a list of features for potential vendors to score themselves on, and includes a worksheet for tabulating replies.

Word Processing

Given the importance of communications today, a good word processor is essential. For relatively straightforward needs, such as letters and short reports, one of the simpler models on the market will suffice. For long reports, articles, or books, a full-featured word processor is better. For in-house creation of newsletters or marketing materials, a desktop publishing package is invaluable.

In selecting packaged tools, such as a word processor or desktop publisher, keep in mind that choosing one of the more popular brands can significantly reduce the expense of training, both initially and over the years. Popular brands usually have a variety of training options, from self-study books and training diskettes to videotapes and classes at the local high school or college. Also, with one of the popular choices, there is a better chance that the next person hired will already know how to run the package.

Database

If you need to handle data that is beyond the scope of what your office management application can handle, then you will need a database management package. There is a lot to know about choosing the right database package, but the major deciding factor is ease of use versus depth and sophistication. Analyze carefully the type of data to be stored and the types of questions that will be asked, and then buy a little more capability in a database package than is really needed.

Another important dimension in selecting a database package is its multimedia capabilities. Some databases can now store free-form text, graphics, still video, sound, and even moving video, capabilities that make possible major new applications for databases.

Spreadsheet

For heavy-duty number-crunching, a spreadsheet is excellent. Unless very strenuous analysis is required, any of the popular ones will do a fine job.

Choosing Your Software

In choosing any software, consider several important factors:

Fit Does the software fit your needs? It is foolish to buy a complicated package when you have a simple need, and it is frustrating and damaging to buy too simple a package when you have a sophisticated need. Assess your needs carefully before shopping around.

Credibility No-name software may seem to be a bargain, but if an application is important enough to computerize, it is probably worth the few extra dollars it costs to get software from a well-known company. Look for a manufacturer that has been in the business for a number of years, has a strong market share and happy customers, updates the software regularly, and can provide help when necessary.

Flexibility Because needs can change over time, look for software that has the flexibility to change. Don't buy a lot of unnecessary features, but do look for software that provides choices in the areas that really matter.

Portability As your practice and the computer hardware field grow and change, it is likely that the time will come when you will need to move to another family of computers. Choosing software that is compatible with many different families of computers can save a lot of money on software licenses, retraining, reprogramming, and reentry of data. The computer field shows no sign of slowing its rate of change, so this kind of flexibility can be a significant advantage in the future.

What Hardware Should I Buy?

Many people spend too much time evaluating computer hardware. It is the choice of software, particularly the medical office management system, that is critical. The wrong software package can cause major disruptions in running the office, resulting in lost income and unnecessary expense. The wrong choice of hardware, on the other hand, is rarely more than an inconvenience. There are so many good choices of hardware that just a little thought and planning should get you the equipment you need.

There are at least four families of computers from which to choose, and each family is divided into numerous subfamilies, configurations, and manufacturers. The size of the practice, expected growth rate, and budget will help you choose from one of the following categories:

Single-User Personal Computer

The smallest reasonable computer for a medical office is a single-personal computer (PC) running a single-user operating system like DOS, OS/2, or the Macintosh operating system. While only one person at a time can use this system, it is probably adequate for a very small practice. If any growth is foreseen, it is essential to plan which of the multi-user computers (described below) is best to grow into, and to take this into account in purchasing a single-user computer. With careful planning, little or nothing will be lost in moving from single-user to multi-user.

Network of PCs

This multi-user configuration makes a lot of sense for an office that already has a handful (or more) of single-user PCs and wants to tie them together so they can share such resources as printers, programs, and data files. In addition to the PCs you already own, you will probably have to buy a powerful PC to be the "server" or traffic cop that manages the other PCs in their use of the shared resources. In addition, you will have to buy a network operating system to run on the server, and enough cable to connect the PCs together.

A network of PCs is a very strong solution in an environment where a lot of people use their computers as personal productivity tools, for activities such as running spreadsheets, word processors, desktop publishers, and graphics packages. Applications such as medical office and database management can also run on networks, but if these types of applications are the majority of the work you'll be doing, you should also seriously consider multi-user PCs and minicomputers.

Multi-user PC

Today's more powerful PCs are successfully encroaching on what once was minicomputer-only territory (just as 20 years ago the minicomputer began encroaching on the mainframe's territory). A properly configured PC running a multi-user operating system such as Unix can support a number of terminals. For medical office management and database applications,

this can be a very sound and economical approach. The more personal productivity applications you run, however, the more you should consider networks or a hybrid system.

Minicomputer

If you need more than 10 or 20 users on your computer system, you probably should consider a minicomputer. The low-end minicomputers, particularly those based on the reduced instruction set computer (RISC) processors, compete effectively with the high-end multi-user PCs. Avoid proprietary operating systems in the minicomputer world if possible; stick to a Unix derivative, which virtually every manufacturer offers.

Hybrid Systems

If your needs are so diverse that none of the previously mentioned categories provides the whole solution you are looking for, then you should investigate a hybrid system. With the powerful networking and communication software available today, there are very few limitations to the types of computer hardware that can work productively together.

Choosing Hardware

No matter what family (or families) of hardware is chosen, it should have the following characteristics:

Position in Computer Industry

The computer industry is brutally competitive. By buying from a clear winner, it is possible to avoid having to find a new vendor when it is time to expand.

Penetration Into Office Management Marketplace

Look for a hardware vendor that is widely used in medical offices. All the people in the vendor's organization, from the salespeople to the service people, are more likely to be attuned to your special needs if they are used to dealing with medical offices on a daily basis.

Maintenance Options

There are many ways to obtain and pay for routine maintenance and emergency repairs. Be sure that the plans your vendor offers make sense and will work well in your situation.

Conformance to Industry Standards

The clear direction in the computer industry is toward "open systems" and away from proprietary approaches. Select a vendor with a strong track record in building systems that exploit agreed-upon industry-wide standards, such as SCSI, SQL X-Windows, Unix, and PostScript, for example.

Who Should I Buy From?

Finding the right computer system is only half the battle. Finding the right company to buy it from is equally important. The dynamics of medical office management dictate a continued involvement with the vendor long after the initial sale for a variety of reasons. Changes in laws could necessitate changes to your software. Your growing practice may require additional hardware or software. New employees may need training, or your staff may need help with a computer problem.

There are many ways to acquire computer hardware and software. Some of these are far more appropriate than others for buying a medical office management system.

Mail order

The computer segment of the mail order industry is no better or worse than the mail order industry as a whole. There are truly outstanding companies that will make you a customer for life, and there are others you can hope never to deal with. But even the best of them is not in the business of providing the total solution that you should be looking for in a complete office management system.

Consultants

Taking advice from consultants who also sell what they recommend is questionable. Buying equipment from such persons is equally questionable.

Computer Store

The local computer store may be a reasonable place to begin to learn about computers, or to purchase a piece of equipment or a popular software package, but computer stores rarely have the focus and track record you are looking for. Because theirs is a particularly high turnover segment of the computer industry, the buyer must be cautious.

Hardware Manufacturers

Hardware manufacturers are the household names that everyone thinks of when considering computers. Because these manufacturers do not normally take the lead in selling the type of total solution you are looking for, they usually call in a value-added reseller to see that you get what you need.

Original Equipment Manufacturers and Value-Added Resellers

These value-added resellers are the solutions-oriented specialists that you need. The good ones are very tightly focused—they should only do medical office management systems—and are also very committed because all of their revenue comes from the one market segment they have chosen. A good value-added reseller will have the depth and expertise required to get you and your staff adjusted to a new computer system.

However, value-added resellers have a notoriously high turnover. Because it is very easy for them to underestimate the amount of capital, hard work, and time required to build a stable business, many of them fail in their early years. The buyer should look long and hard at their track record and current position in the marketplace before picking one.

Choosing Your Vendor

Invest as much energy in evaluating a prospective vendor's ability to create and keep a satisfied customer as you do in evaluating what they want to sell you. Be sure that you cover the following points, to avoid going off course.

Longevity Newcomers in any field, but especially in computers, have a higher risk of failure. Be certain that your vendor has a substantial track record doing exactly what they will be doing for you. And talk to the references they give you—all of them—at length.

Stability Even the oldest businesses can make a false step that can imperil their future, especially in the fast-changing, competitive computer field. Be sure that you are comfortable with their current financial position.

Expertise Nothing is worse than being told how to run your practice by a group of computer experts. Your vendor's support and training staff must all be former medical office managers and the like. Don't settle for a group of computer people who think they know a lot about medical offices!

Focus Prefer the specialist over the generalist. Market penetration is an important factor in any business's success, and this is especially true in the value-added resale business. Trying to be all things to all people, or even many things to many people, almost guarantees failure in the computer systems world.

Commitment A single-minded dedication to their chosen area should grow out of a vendor's focus, and you will benefit from this dedication. Medical office management and computers are both changing rapidly, and it is your vendor's responsibility to keep you up to date on the important changes in both fields. Be sure that they have the focus and commitment to do so.

Availability Value-added resellers have a history of trying to grow too rapidly. Be sure that the vendor you are considering will be available when needed. Can they adequately serve a multi-location practice? Do they have enough people to service a client of your size? Are they proficient on all the different hardware configurations your practice will be using? If they have difficulty covering you in any of these areas, they are introducing risk into the equation.

Summary

If you can set aside the intense marketing and the appealing gadgetry that surround computer systems, you will still be left with a complex and challenging set of choices. Investigate the hardware and software carefully, certainly, but pay especially close attention to the quality of the people involved, from the consultants to the vendors. Be as skeptical and cautious as any good customer, and make your decisions as though the future of your practice depended on it.

Database Technology for Medical Records

Charles B. Darling

Overview

Although computers have achieved good results in medical office management, they have made relatively little impact in organizing medical records for the orthopaedic practice, which is puzzling because computers usually organize records well.

This chapter suggests appropriate goals for a computerized medical records system and examines barriers that might stand in the way of achieving them. It also reviews the various database technologies available for computerizing medical records and compares in detail the ways in which the two most popular technologies handle common medical record queries. The chapter concludes with some advice on choosing a database technology and suggests future developments to watch for.

Appropriate Goals of Computerized Medical Records

Unfortunately, the most obvious goals of computerizing a practice's medical records are also the least appropriate. At present, it is not economically feasible to store a patient's entire medical record in the computer, to replace rooms full of charts with a single large computer disk, and to place a terminal at every desk and in every examining room. Yet this is what most people envision when thinking of "computerized medical records." Fortunately, computerization of medical records has several valuable (although less glamorous) benefits.

Self-Quality Assurance

The most important benefit of computerized medical records is improved quality of the records. Computerizing medical records normally involves arranging the data. This structuring can contribute greatly to the completeness and consistency of a practice's medical records. But structure does not require a computer— a good set of manual forms, conscientiously applied, will bring the same benefit. However, the computer can add another level of quality assurance.

For example, if a certain blank on a form must be filled out, or the blank must contain a number between 0 and 90, or if Blank A is greater than 0 then Blank B must be between 1 and 10, then the computer will not process a form that fails to meet these standards. The computer can impose a level of completeness and con-sistency that even the most disciplined practice would have difficulty matching.

Data Analysis

Every practice has the potential to generate a wealth of valuable medical data. It is impossible to put that data to good use if it is not stored in a computer.

Because a computerized medical records system arranges the data collected and can assure high quality of data, it makes meaningful data analysis possible. Using the variety of data analysis tools available with even the simplest of office computers, a practice can organize and summarize information to search for interesting and suggestive patterns.

Data Sharing

Only when data is well-structured and of good quality does it become truly valuable, because at this point it becomes possible to use the computer's ability to communicate with other computers to share data with other practices. Your practice may need a bigger data set to find meaningful patterns, or other practices may need more specialized data. In either case, computerized medical records can help achieve the goal of studies based on data collected across many practices.

Paper Truncation

Anything that allows a practice to run more efficiently and economically is a worthwhile goal, and the introduction to this section was not intended to imply otherwise. However, it is important to understand that the very obvious goal of cutting down on paper record-keeping is also the least practical and most costly goal to attain.

A computerized medical records system can easily increase the amount of paper a practice uses. If major changes in office policies and procedures are not designed and enforced, the computer can end by printing beautiful pages of well-structured data captured during each office visit, which are then added to the patient's chart along with handwritten notes and forms from which the computerized medical record was transcribed.

If paper truncation is an important goal, then having terminals on every desk and in every examination room, and entering medical data directly into the computer, with no intermediary worksheets, are serious considerations. You should also plan on an absolutely foolproof backup and security system for your valuable data. Because of costs, training time, and difficulty in changing employees' deeply ingrained habits, most practices will find the paper truncation potential of computerized medical records less than compelling.

Barriers to Computerized Medical Records

Lack of Standards

The greatest barrier to widespread use of the computer as a medical records tool is the lack of consensus on what goes into a medical record. Each practice must decide which aspects to computerize, which hardware and software technologies to use, and how best to introduce a computerized medical record system into the workflow of an established practice. Solving these problems is difficult and expensive. As long as each practice essentially starts from scratch to deal with these issues, computerized medical records will continue to be widely ignored.

The good news is that these economic barriers will fall rapidly once doctors show signs of seriously working toward a consensus. Given the highly competitive nature of the computer software industry, its love of broad standards (with room for competition), and the vast potential that medical records-keeping represents, you can expect to see software companies leaping on the bandwagon as soon as a serious effort is made within the medical community to create a bandwagon. But until the medical community makes a real effort to define what goes into medical records, the economic barriers will remain insurmountable.

Data Entry

Another major barrier to the wide acceptance of computerized medical records is the logistics of data entry. Traditionally, a second step is created in which the written records are transcribed in some form into the computer. The expense, inconvenience, and inaccuracy of this approach have contributed to the lack of interest in computerized medical records.

Many promising one-step approaches and new technologies are being used. Unfortunately, none of them to date has been good enough to sweep all the competition aside and present an easy and obvious answer, an industry standard for all to embrace.

Data Retrieval

Once data have been entered into a computer, the fun begins—or does it? While computers have an unsurpassed potential for analyzing and synthesizing large amounts of data, provoking a computer to do so is still largely beyond the skills of the average person. As long as it requires a "rocket scientist" mentality to extract meaningful data from a computer, computerized medical records will continue to be the exception rather than the rule.

The science of database management has been moving forward slowly but steadily for the past 25 years, and the industry is close to agreeing on a standard approach to database management. With standardization of this vital area, more and more energy will be devoted to adding "user-friendly front ends" to the standard back end. In the foreseeable future, a person won't have to be a "rocket scientist" to get information from a database.

Common Business Practices

Medical practices do not exist in a vacuum. Rather, they are a key element in the complex web of products and services that makes up the health-care industry and the economy as a whole. A major change, such as computerization of medical records, cannot be contemplated without considering how this change will affect the practice in its dealing with the "outside world."

While more and more information moves electronically every day, the majority of electronic information is financial in nature and is highly structured. Nonfinancial information of a much less structured nature, such as a medical record, is still largely recorded on paper. This aspect of the economy will change slowly over time. As long as records from dealings with insurers, lawyers, hospitals, and other doctors must remain mostly paper-based, computerized medical records will be irrelevant to your dealings with the "outside world."

Choosing a Database

Once some reasonable goals for a computerized medical records system have been set, the next problem is selecting a database. First, you must understand what you are looking at. There are several types of database management systems available, and each has its own strengths and weaknesses. The basics of each system must be understood before looking at any one package in detail.

Next, it is necessary to examine carefully just what the database is to do. By understanding the dynamics of the data that will be input and retrieved from the database, you can better match needs to the capabilities of a given package.

Flat File Databases

Flat file databases are the simplest and least expensive databases on the market, but they are also the most limited. Flat file technology, which dates back at least to the 1960s, is simply an outgrowth of the way records were handed in the days before disks, when information was stored on 80-column punchcards.

A flat file is no more complex conceptually than a set of punchcards or a telephone book. Data, stored as a long list, can be sorted into different orders (physically

Outline 1
How many back operations in 1990?

dBASE	SQL

USE Oper
COUNT TO Answer FOR OperCode = 'BACK'
         .AND. OperDate >= CTOD('01/01/90')
         .AND. OperDate <= CTOD('12/31/90')
? Answer
	SELECT COUNT(*)
	FROM Oper
	WHERE OperCode = 'BACK'
	AND OperDate BETWEEN '01-Jan-90' AND '31-Dec-90'

or logically), and a single record can be located very quickly.

A drawback of this simplicity is lack of sophistication. A flat file system will not handle repetitive information easily ("List each patient and the medications currently prescribed") nor will it allow linking of files based on common data elements. While there may be some medical record applications that are so straightforward that a flat file database would be sufficient, these simple applications are clearly the exception, not the rule.

The Relational Database Paradigm

By far the most common type of database is the relational database. Relational database theory was originated in the late 1960s by Dr. E. F. Codd at IBM. A mathematician, Codd combined set theory and the predicate calculus to create a theory of database management that proved complete and correct.

The key to relational databases is their ability to link together separate files, which Codd called tables, based on a common data element. For example, you could have a table of patient names and numbers in your relational database, and another table where each record is a patient number and the name of a medication that patient takes. A relational database will allow you to "join" the two tables by their common data element (patient number) in order to see a list of all the medications for each patient. The ease with which a relational database can assemble information about a patient and the medications taken is a major advance over flat file technology.

dBASE-style Relational Databases

Currently, there are two major families of relational database products in the marketplace. The better-known family of the two includes such products as dBASE, Paradox, and R:Base. This family evolved on personal computers from the flat file world without the benefit of Codd's conceptual foundation. Each product is based on its own proprietary language (although dBASE has suffered some legal setbacks in that regard lately), and they do not attempt to truly implement Codd's theory of relational databases. As a result, as the complexity of the question increases, additional effort is required from the user to extract data from the database.

Structured Query Language-Style Relational Databases

The older (and less well known) of the two families of relational databases originated from Codd's work and is based on the widely accepted Structured Query Language (SQL). This family includes products such as ORACLE, Ingres, Informix, and Sybase. These products, which implement Codd's theories, provide better support for complex data structures and complex queries than do the dBASE family of relational databases. The level of skill required of the user in posing more difficult questions to more complex data structures rises slowly, at a low linear rate.

Comparing dBASE and SQL

The difference in the way the two types of relational databases respond to increasing complexity can be seen by comparing the dBASE language to SQL in each of three situations. Outline 1 answers a simple query from a single table: "How many back operations did I perform in 1990?" Both dBASE and SQL scan the Oper file looking for the word "BACK" in the field called OperCode and for a date in 1990 in the field called OperDate.

In Outline 2 the code for a two-table query reads: "How many back operations did I perform on male patients in 1990?" Assuming that a patient's sex is stored in the Patient (Pat) master file, the Pat file must be "joined" with the Oper file to find the answer. While the dBASE solution seems a little more complex than the SQL solution, the two are still essentially comparable.

Outlines 3 and 4 present a more complex query: "List the male patients who had back operations and also took propoxyphene." In this query the computer is not just counting—it is retrieving a list of names from the Patient master table. But to pick a given name, the computer must first read all the related records for that patient in the Oper file, as well as all the related records for that patient in the Rx file.

In this example, SQL is the clear winner. dBASE requires a long list of convoluted commands that only a programmer can fully understand. SQL accomplishes the same task by finding the list of names of males who had back operations, finding the list of males taking propoxyphene, and selecting only the common names ("INTERSECT") in the two sets.

Outline 2
How many back operations on male patients in 1990?

dBASE	SQL
SELECT A	SELECT COUNT(*)
USE PAT INDEX PatID	FROM Oper, Pat
SELECT B	WHERE Oper.PatID = Pat.PatID
USE Oper	AND OperCode = 'BACK'
SET RELATION TO PatID INTO Pat	AND OperDate BETWEEN '01/01/90' AND '12/31/90'
COUNT TO Answer FOR OperCode = 'BACK'	AND Sex = 'M'
.AND. OperDate >= CTOD('01/01/90')	
.AND. OperDate <= CTOD('12/31/90')	
.AND. Pat->Sex = 'M'	
? Answer	

How to Choose a Database

Understanding the relative merits of various database technologies is only part of the challenge in choosing a database. In the next step, it is necessary to consider some very important questions about the data to be stored and the ways in which it will be used.

How complex is the data set? Designing a proper data structure for medical records is a vital first step, and one in which professional guidance is warranted. The most important things to consider at this stage are the number of different files or tables needed to capture the data, the number of one-to-many relationships these tables contain, and the degree of interrelatedness among the tables.

At one extreme, you may find you can do a good job with one or two tables, no one-to-many relationships, and no interrelatedness. In that case, a flat file database should work well. The next level would be a two-table database with a simple one-to-many relationship. As previously discussed, the dBASE-style databases can handle this challenge perfectly well. Finally, for multiple tables with much interrelationship, a SQL-based database should be seriously considered.

How complex is the data analysis? As shown in Outlines 1 through 4, the type of questions asked of a database have a lot to do with the type of database used. For simple questions like the first two (Outlines 1 and 2) a computer may be unnecessary, or a medical office management package may suffice. In my opinion, the third question (Outlines 3 and 4) marks the lower boundary of the type of data analysis that would justify building a medical records system at all.

In any case, the first question can be handled by any type of database software. The second requires at least a relational package, and the third seems to work much better in a SQL-based relational database. If you think carefully about how you want to use the data stored, then you should see which database best fits your needs.

How well planned is the data analysis? If most of the data analysis will be planned ahead of time and produced on a regular schedule, then the nature of the database's user interface is not of major importance in selecting a database. The worst that can happen is that a consultant will have to write some reports for you to run again and again. If, on the other hand, you never know what kind of questions you will need to ask the database, then choosing a database with a powerful, easy-to-use interface is very important.

Who will do the data analysis? If a lot of data analysis is to be done, it is advisable to have a staff member devote the time and effort to learn thoroughly the database package selected. In that case, the ease of the user interface is not a critical issue—it is better to spend a little more time to learn the database than to spend a lot of hours using it.

If, on the other hand, the database will not be used daily, it is best to select one that is easy to learn and hard to forget. An intermittent pattern of usage does not lead to the proprietary feelings that would inspire one employee to become the "database person," so having several people (perhaps including yourself) who are fairly proficient at using the database will work best.

Future Developments

Several trends in the computer industry can have a significant impact on computerized medical records over the next several years. This paper concludes with a list of technologies to watch for.

More Flexible Data Entry Tools

Everyone seems to agree that the keyboard is not the way to capture data for medical records. However, no one can agree on what is correct. The following list covers some interesting contenders and points out the strengths and weaknesses of each:

Mouse Excellent pointing device, good for checking off boxes and picking items from a list. Awkward when you have to switch between mouse and keyboard, alternately typing words and pointing.

Touch screen Same strengths and weaknesses as the

Outline 3
List the male patients who had back operations and also took propoxyphene.

dBASE*

```
SELECT A
USE Pat
SELECT B
USE Oper INDEX OpPatID
SELECT C
USE Rx INDEX RxPatID
SELECT A
DO WHILE .NOT. EOF() .AND. .NOT. BOF()
    IF Sex = 'M'
       BackOper = .F.
       Propox   = .F.
       SELECT B
       SEEK Pat->PatID
       DO WHILE PatID = Pat->PatID .AND. .NOT. EOF()
          IF OperCode = 'BACK'
             BackOper = .T.
          ENDIF
          SKIP
       ENDDO
       IF BackOper
          SELECT C
          SEEK Pat->PatID
          DO WHILE PatID = Pat->ID .AND. .NOT. EOF()
             IF MedCode = 'PROPOX'
                Propox = .T.
             ENDIF
             SKIP
          ENDDO
          SELECT A
          IF BackOper .AND. Propox
             ? PatID, PatName
          ENDIF
       ENDIF
       SKIP
ENDO
USE
SELECT B
USE
SELECT C
USE
```

*NOTE: This example must be written as a program, then executed using the DO command. Unlike the preceding examples, this one CANNOT be entered interactively.

Outline 4
List the male patients who had back operations and also took propoxyphene.

SQL

```
SELECT Pat.PatID, PatName
FROM Oper, Pat
WHERE Oper.PatID = Pat.PatID
AND    OperCode = 'BACK'
AND    Sex = 'M'
       INTERSECT
SELECT Pat.PatID, PatName
FROM Rx, Pat
WHERE Rx.PatID = Pat.PatID
AND    MedCode = 'PROPOX'
AND    Sex = 'M'
```

mouse, with the added drawbacks of being less precise and more physically taxing. Wonderful solution for a casual encounter between a computer and a computerphobe, however.

Pen Pen-based computers are a very new technology that is maturing rapidly. These may be an excellent keyboard alternative if the writing-recognition software really works.

Voice Years of unfulfilled promise have tarnished this technology's reputation somewhat. Don't count it out yet, however. The rewards of making it work are huge, which keeps the research going.

Bar code Mature, effective technology, but the logistics in a practice are less than ideal. Still requires a keyboard for entering words.

Mark sense Same strengths and weaknesses as bar code.

Optical character recognition A reasonably effective technology, but not very useful for most medical records applications.

Digitizing scanners A vital tool for storing images in computerized medical records. The technology is maturing rapidly, and the usefulness of digitized images in many applications should continue to drive it forward for years to come.

More Usable Data Retrieval Tools

The computer software industry continues to make great strides in making the computer easier to use. A number of different trends are converging to make the future look very bright for computerized medical records in this area.

There is a strong industry-wide trend toward graphical user interfaces (GUIs). The Apple Macintosh was the first popular computer to sport a GUI, and its GUI is what caught everyone's attention. Now, most of the rest of the world is hastening along the same path, greatly enhancing the computer's accessibility and ease of use in the process.

Another important trend in the software industry is the movement toward "nonprocedural" or "fourth generation" languages (4GLs), which do not require traditional, step-by-step instructions (programs) that tell them how to do their job. Instead, they can figure out an answer based on a very structured and precise description of what you want. You can see this qualitative difference (as well as the associated quantitative difference) by reading through Outlines 3 and 4 carefully. The dBASE language is a 3GL that tells the computer how to get the answer; SQL is a 4GL that describes what we want to know and leaves it to the computer to figure out how to get it. The 4GLs are yet another trend that will make data retrieval and analysis simpler in the future.

There is one other major trend that enhances and reinforces the others. The database sector of the software industry is rapidly turning structured query language (SQL) into an entrenched standard. Because everyone agrees that SQL is the best way to store data, software developers must turn their attention and resources elsewhere to create the vital competitive advantage that keeps them going. Currently, much of that energy is going into building better user interfaces. This trend should lead to improvements in GUIs and 4GLs for years to come.

Intelligent Systems That Mimic Human Thought Processes

The last category of future developments worth watching is a very broad one. There is substantial progress on many fronts, both commercially and in the research labs, in the drive to make computers better able to mimic human mental processes. Four areas in particular will have a significant impact on computerized medical records.

Rule-based programs were the first to demonstrate that computers are not just number crunchers—they can use symbolic logic to solve problems that other systems could not. The tools for building rule-based systems (also called knowledge-based or expert systems) have evolved rapidly recently, and their newfound ability to integrate with standard data processing programs to create intelligent systems assures that they will start appearing everywhere. Look for intelligent systems that will allow even a new employee to perform certain tasks quickly and easily.

Pattern-based programs pick up where rule-based programs leave off. If a rule-based program can be thought of as left-brain because of its orderly, logical nature, then a pattern-based program is clearly right-brain. As the name implies, these programs are best used for spotting trends and predicting outcomes. Pattern-based tools are rapidly catching up with rule-based tools, and an intelligent system should be able to use either or both.

Hypermedia programs are able to present textual or multimedia information flexibly. Hypermedia tools have the potential of being the linking mechanism for an intelligent computerized medical records system. By establishing connections between diverse pieces of data on different kinds of media (textual data on disk, audio on CD-ROM, video on laser disks, for example), a hypermedia system would allow the user to move rapidly and intuitively from a patient's test results to an appropriate reference in an on-line physician's desk reference, to a related reference in an on-line journal, to a video image of the procedure under consideration, to a summary of other patients' records that follow the same pattern as this patient's. With the new CD-ROM players and hypermedia tools, this is not as farfetched as it sounds.

Fuzzy logic tools are changing the way users look at their data. One problem with a good deal of medical records data is its excessive granularity. The facts that the patient is 74″ tall, weighs 175 pounds, and has a 180-degree range of motion are important details for the chart, but the data's real significance is obscured by its focus on detail. Fuzzy logic is a mathematically sound approach that lets us see who this patient really is: a tall, thin person with a normal range of motion. Summarizing and comparing "fuzzy" data (tall, thin, normal, and so on), which is often much more meaningful than comparing precise data, is one more way in which computers are beginning to learn to think.

Summary

Paper truncation may be the first goal that comes to mind when people think of computerized medical records, but this is probably the least realistic goal at present. Structuring a medical records system to improve record quality and to open the door to data analysis are two more realistic goals.

Of the many significant barriers to computerized medical records, the most serious is the lack of agreement in the medical community regarding what should go into a medical record. Even small steps in that area should bring major improvements in available medical records software.

Choosing a database for medical records requires familiarity with database principles and a detailed understanding of data needs. The safe choice is an SQL-based relational database, but a smaller system will suffice if present and future medical records challenges are small enough.

The rate of change in the computer world is increasing all the time. Emerging and maturing technologies that can have a significant impact on medical records software include data entry tools such as the mouse, pen, and voice; better data retrieval tools such as GUIs and 4GLs; and software tools that use rules, pattern-matching, hypermedia links, and fuzzy logic to create systems that seem to think like humans.

While computerized medical records systems are not yet comparable with medical office management systems, they should be someday. In the meantime, smart physicians will begin exploring possibilities on their own in order to reap some benefits at an early stage and to be better prepared when the tide finally turns.

Computerized Medical Records

Robert H. Haralson, MD

The advancement of office medical recordkeeping is at a turning point. Early office records were short notes that were jotted down by the physician or by assistants while patients were being treated. These notes were often illegible and contained scant data at best. The development of dictation and transcription technology improved the task of medical recordkeeping significantly. The physician could take the time to include more complete data in dictated records. In addition, the typed record was much easier to read, and the advent of the word processor made it easy to correct mistakes. These anecdotal or "text-oriented" records have been the standard in one form or another since physicians began keeping records. In the past they have served physicians well. Physicians could mark the typed record with notes or flags that served to remind them of some unique or unusual aspect of a patient's case.

On the other hand, the text-oriented record frequently lacks detailed information. Unless the physician follows closely some form of written questionnaire or template, exact details of the patient's care can be omitted. The need to continually assess the appropriateness, quality, and cost of medical care in the office setting requires the collection of large amounts of detailed and accurate data. A text record containing this level of detail takes too long both to dictate and to transcribe. One solution is to use data-oriented records that are in a computer rather than on paper. In the computer, data elements can be stored as characters (numbers or letters) rather than as words. For instance, instead of dictating that a patient "has a $3+$ right knee effusion," the character "3" can be stored in a field that represents the answer to a question on the questionnaire about the presence and volume of an effusion in the patient's right knee. Entering this one character obviously takes much less time than it takes to type in the entire text phrase. This shortcut allows collection and storage of a great deal more detailed information than can be included in the text record.

Computerized records have several other advantages. As mentioned, more complete and accurate medical records will be available if the need arises to defend one's action, either to insurance companies, to other third-party payors, or to the courts. The increase in the amount of information available and the ease of retrieving it from the computer make it possible for the physician in private practice to review patient data and assess outcomes. Assessment of outcomes in the private practice setting, rarely done at present, should be more

common, because it is the only way to know if a physician's results are as good as those of other physicians.

There is an increased need for this sort of system in the medical office. Computerized medical records have been developed to some degree in many hospitals, especially in hospitals associated with teaching programs. Unfortunately, patients who are cared for in a teaching setting are in the minority. In most private practices, follow-up of hospitalized patients is carried out in private offices, and the hospital has no way of tracking the outcomes of these patients unless the patient is rehospitalized for complications. Accurate outcome assessment of most patients will require that a data-oriented medical record be developed for the office environment.

Third-party payors and even certain industries now frequently require that any hospital that participates in the company's managed health care plan must have in place a computerized quality assurance and utilization review system. This system allows the third-party payor and/or industry to assess outcomes of patient care and the cost of patient care in the individual hospitals. Because most health care will be under some form of managed health plan in the near future and because industry and third party payors will want the same data on outpatients, implementation of computerized medical recordkeeping in the office setting will become a necessity.

Lastly, the computerized medical record can serve as a valuable means of educating both physician and patient. The private practitioner who can carry out meaningful outcomes research is able to accumulate proof of the efficacy of the methods and techniques used and can use that information to answer questions and to allay the concerns of prospective patients.

Versions of Computerized Medical Records

There are three basic versions of computerized medical records. The first is the generic record, available as a part of a practice management package. The second is an off-the-shelf database management package, and the third is a turnkey system. There are advantages and disadvantages to each version.

The first version, the generic system, is available as a part of some computerized practice management packages. One of its big advantages is that this system is integrated with the billing package. In addition, it is extremely versatile. Because these packages were not developed for any particular specialty, the medical record must be quite versatile to allow different specialties to adapt the system to a particular purpose. The main disadvantage of this type of system is the fact that because the medical record was not developed for a specific specialty, each physician must spend significant time customizing the record to fit a particular specialty and practice. To do so requires some knowledge of computers and of the particular software package.

The second version is one that could be developed from an off-the-shelf database management package, such as dBASE, R:Base, ORACLE, or Ingress. A system developed in this manner would also be extremely versatile, because the developer has free rein in developing the package. The big disadvantage, of course, is that this package also requires significant knowledge of database management techniques.

The third version is the turnkey system. A few of these systems are available today, and they have the distinct advantage of being ready for use. The big disadvantages are that they are not integrated with a billing system and are not nearly as versatile as the other two versions. The medical record that comes with the system is the only one that can be used. Although the developers have written into the software ways that the user can customize the medical record to some degree, this system is not as versatile as the other two systems.

Each of these systems has advantages for different types of practices. The generic system has advantages for a private office that also needs a billing system. The off-the-shelf package is a good choice for a physician who is already on a billing system, wants a very versatile medical record, and doesn't mind the learning curve required to become expert in database management. (The alternative to developing database management skills is to hire someone with these skills, but this can be fairly expensive.) The turnkey system is probably best for a physician who is already on a billing system, who does not wish to learn database management techniques, and who does not mind the restrictions involved in using a medical records system developed by someone else.

Types of Computerized Medical Records

There are five types of computerized medical records, which differ in the way the computer stores the data. The first is a text record, the standard anecdotal record in which the computer is merely used to store the full text. This use of the computer is rather inefficient, because the computer must store massive amounts of data, and it is very difficult to search the full text. Therefore, this form of computerized medical record has few advantages.

The second type is a text record with user-defined fields. Here, the computer stores the full text, but the user can define certain fields (such as diagnosis or procedure) that will be stored in separate tables in a database. For instance, if the diagnosis field is chosen, the stenographer would mark that field with a special character, such as question marks or brackets. This character notifies the computer to store this field in a specific table. A list can then be developed of all patients who have a particular diagnosis. Some rather innovative ways to gather data have been developed, but the product of a search is still a list of patients. Manual abstraction of other data from the record is required in order to do research.

The third type is an attached database with user-defined fields. This is the first of the data-oriented records or parameterized records. In this type of record, the computer does not store text but merely stores characters that represent fields. The example used earlier was to indicate that if a patient has a 3+ effusion of the right knee, one simply enters in the right knee effusion field the character "3" and the computer stores that character. Now the computer has stored one character that would represent an entire sentence in a text record. This significantly reduces the amount of data that a computer must store and search if one wishes to do research. With word-processing techniques, the computer can be instructed to use this data to reproduce a full text record.

The fourth type is an attached database with user-defined fields and text fields. Computerized medical records must include some text fields, because it is impossible to ask all the questions that are necessary to uniquely identify each patient. There must be an area in the record that allows the physician to include the anecdotes that supplement the finite data elements. Though techniques have been developed to make searching of text somewhat easier, enough problems remain to make searching difficult and not completely satisfactory.

The fifth type of computerized medical record is somewhat futuristic. This is the attached database with user-defined fields and searchable text fields. As artificial intelligence techniques become more sophisticated, physicians will eventually be able to search these text fields.

The Perfect Medical Record

In investigating or developing a computerized medical records system, a list of features emerge that would make up the "perfect" medical record. Most importantly, the record should be easier to use than a text record would be. Unfortunately, up to this point, if the learning curve is included, this feature has not been accomplished. It takes a fair amount of training for the physician and stenographer to implement computerized medical records. Frustrations associated with the learning curve frequently cause the project to be abandoned. If one persists, however, and makes it through the learning curve, the advantages of the computerized medical record will surface.

Medical records should be parameterized with text fields. As mentioned in the previous section, a text field is believed to be an essential feature of a computerized medical record. The record must be printed in an understandable text form. If the computer merely prints out what is stored (characters), then attorneys and other third parties will be unable to interpret the record. For this reason, the computer must be able to produce a text record.

The computer should not print empty fields. If the physician elects not to answer a question, the computer should skip that question and not print it with a blank space where the answer should be.

The computerized medical record should be time-oriented. That is, the data element should be attached to a particular date. This provides the computer with a means of separating events and attaching them to a particular diagnosis or procedure.

It is essential for the package to allow a user to customize the medical record and add or subtract fields. It is impossible to develop a medical record that includes all the questions asked by different practitioners based on their particular specialty or practice.

The computer should produce a tickler file. This serves to remind the physician that certain events are due. For instance, if a patient is taking an anti-inflammatory drug, it might be time for a laboratory check.

Another interesting feature is that the computer can generate follow-up letters to patients. In addition, some systems can produce prescriptions if drugs are prescribed.

If the computer defaults to normal data, only abnormal data must be entered, which can significantly decrease the amount of data that must be input. Another helpful feature is to have the computer default to the last visit, so that at a follow-up visit, only the data that have changed must be entered.

Work Forms and Logistics

A study of computerized medical records leads to the conclusion that there is no way around the use of forms. These forms are templates or questionnaires that are followed by the patient and by the physician or an assistant. Forms are required because so much must be collected and it is essential to collect the data in exactly the same order each time. It is impossible and unnecessary for anyone to memorize all the pieces of data to be collected and the order in which they must be collected. At present, most systems use dictation, followed by manual input of the data by a stenographer. As voice recognition technology and scanner technology become more sophisticated, it will soon be possible to bypass the stenographer. Eliminating this step will significantly increase efficiency, decrease the number of errors, and reduce the overall cost.

In developing forms, there are three options. The first is to develop a form with every question that might ever need to be answered. This would require a form several hundred pages in length. The second option, to develop a separate form for every question, is obviously just as ludicrous. The third, and reasonable, option is somewhere in between, that is, to develop forms that are divided by diseases, procedures, conditions, or anatomic areas. Orthopaedics is conveniently divided into six anatomic areas: spine, shoulder-elbow, hand, hip, knee, and foot-ankle. Unfortunately, in the spine area, the cervical and lumbar spine are completely different, and scoliosis is different from either of these. A child's hip and an adult hip are completely different, and so are children's feet and adult feet. One also must decide how to handle, for instance, a fractured femur (is it a hip or is it a knee). Each system handles these problems differently but the end result is a finite number of forms. The exact number has not been defined, but should be in the range of 20 to 25.

Forms

Each patient will need to complete a variety of forms during treatment and follow-up. A general history and physical is also done. Therefore, specific forms must be used for the history and physical. Each should have some sort of evaluation system, such as the Harris hip scale or the Iowa knee scale. Otherwise, outcomes cannot be compared. It is hoped that these evaluation systems will be standardized in the future, but at this point, several exist and only one can be chosen for a particular situation. Radiograph and laboratory forms are also needed. When the patient returns for follow-up, an interim history and interim physical are necessary. This can be a brief note and in some systems is handled quite well by text fields. Eventually, however, a form that details a complete follow-up history and physical is required. At this point, a repeat of the evaluation system is used to allow comparison with the original evaluation. An operative note that details the specific surgical procedure is important. Again, this should not be a text record but should be data-oriented (parameterized). A surgical follow-up history and physical may be different from a nonsurgical follow-up history and physical, and, as a result, additional forms may be necessary. In addition, a form detailing any complications will be needed.

Although a computerized medical record does eliminate some paperwork, its primary advantage is that it enables the office to collect and store increased amounts of data, and the data collected are more detailed and accurate than those found in a text record.

The advantages of accumulating complete and accurate data are becoming more and more obvious, and in the near future, computerized medical recordkeeping will probably be a necessity.

Index